AF249143

NEW ADVANCES IN THE BASIC AND CLINICAL GASTROENTEROLOGY

Edited by **Tomasz Brzozowski**

New Advances in the Basic and Clinical Gastroenterology
Edited by Tomasz Brzozowski

Published by InTech
Janeza Trdine 9, 51000 Rijeka, Croatia

Publishing Process Manager Vana Persen

Technical Editor Teodora Smiljanic

Cover Designer InTech Design Team

Additional hard copies can be obtained from orders@intechopen.com

New Advances in the Basic and Clinical Gastroenterology, Edited by Tomasz Brzozowski
p. cm.
ISBN 978-953-51-0521-3

Meet the editor

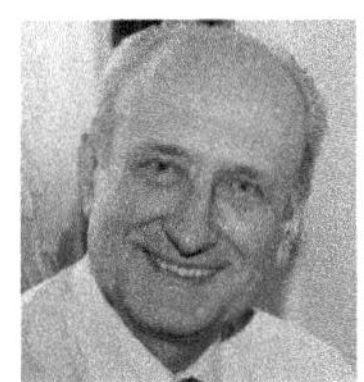 Professor Dr Thomas Brzozowski works as a professor of human physiology and holds the position of Chairman of the Department of Physiology and is v-Dean of Medical Faculty at Jagiellonian University Medical College, Cracow, Poland. His major area of interest is physiology and pathophysiology of gastrointestinal (GI) tract with the major focus addressed to the mechanism of GI mucosal defense, protection and ulcer healing. He was a postdoctoral NIH fellow at University of California and Gastroenterology VA Medical Center, Irvine and Long Beach, CA, USA and at Gastroenterology Clinics at Erlangen-Nuremberg and Munster in Germany. He published 290 original articles in most prestigious scientific journals and 7 book chapters in the field related to pathophysiology of GI tract, gastroprotection, ulcer healing, drug therapy of peptic ulcer, hormonal regulation of the gut and inflammatory bowel disease.

Contents

Preface

The purpose of writing this book was to overview recent hot topics in gastroenterology with a focus directed towards information derived from the bench and used at the patient's bedside. To address these issues, scientists who are working on a daily basis in the field of experimental gastroenterology and clinical investigators, with their chapter proposal's being *peer-reviewed*, all have integrated their attempts to summarize the recent advances in the pathophysiology and therapy of upper and lower gastrointestinal tract disorders. Such an integrative approach in basic and clinical gastroenterology seems to be essential for the pathomechanism, proper diagnosis and management of patients who suffer from gastrointestinal disorders. The potential reader will not only find in this book the recent advances in the physiology and pathomechanism of GI tract disorders, but also the treatment options based on pharmacological and surgical intervention and the recent advances in the biological therapy with probiotics and prebiotics, which nowadays is a rapidly growing area of interest. For instance, *Betta and Vitaliti* described in their review, the direct and indirect effects of probiotics in the functional interactions between bacteria, gut epithelium, gut mucosal immune system and systemic immune system. The direct effect of probiotics in the lumen include the competition with pathogens for nutrients, production of antimicrobial substances and in particular organic acids competitive inhibition on the receptor sites, change in the composition of mucin hydrolysis of toxins, receptor hydrolysis, and nitric oxide (NO). The indirect effect of probiotics largely depends on the site of interaction between the probiotic and the effectors of the immune response. *Thantasha et al.*, presented the number of specific properties or criteria a microbial strain has to fulfill in order for it to be regarded as a probiotic. These criteria are classified into its safety profile, performance within the GI tract and technological aspects of its development. The criteria are further dependent on the specific purpose of the strain and on the location for the expression of the specific property. With regards to safety, the probiotic strain must be of human origin, isolated from the gastrointestinal tract (GIT) of healthy individuals. The strain itself, its fermentation products or its cell components after its death, should be non-pathogenic, non-toxic, non-allergic, non-mutagenic or non-carcinogenic even when given to immunocompromised individuals. The detailed criteria for the probiotic is underlined with respect to their performance, acid-tolerance and survival in the human gastric juices and bile. Probiotic bacteria must be able to survive in sufficient numbers and adhere to the intestinal mucosal surface in order to survive within the gastrointestinal tract.

The historical background of probiotics can be traced back to when the first definition of probiotic bacteria was given by Russian scientist Elie Metchnikoff who stated that probiotics are considered to exert a beneficial effect on the host. This was confirmed later on by an official statement by FAO/WHO. In their reviews, two group of investigators *Matur et al.* and *Boaventura et al.,* presented the impact of probiotics on the physiology of the GIT and the underlying mechanism of action of this microflora and the benefits derived with the use of probiotics in human and animal nutrition. Until now there is a growing list of probiotic bacteria involved in the regulation of gastrointestinal tract. Among them *Lactobacillus* and *Bifidobacterium* species were most frequently cited and have been implicated in many human GIT disorders and have become commercially promoted to improve the health of the host. The mode of action of probiotics involves a mutual interaction with intestinal cells and other microflora present in the gut. In these two chapters, the influence of probiotics on digestion, absorption and barrier function, secretory functions and the postnatal maturation of intestinal mucosa are described. Probiotics may exert a multidirectional effects affecting the gene expression in intestinal cells. A number of positive effects of probiotics have been indicated, particularly their beneficial effect in the pathologic conditions including antibiotic-associated traveler's diarrhea, irritable bowel syndrome (IBS), lactose intolerance, dental caries, gastroduodenal ulcers due to *Helicobacter pylori,* hepatic encephalopathy, intestinal motility disorders and neonatal necrotizing enterocolitis. Authors evaluated a variety of probiotics functions for the control of morphological characteristics and the proliferation capacity of crypt and villous epithelium as well as their effects on enteric nervous system. Since the microorganisms located within the digestive tract during the postnatal period have been shown to decrease villi length and increased crypt depth in many species, one of the aims was to overview the effects of probiotics on villous and crept depth. Indeed, the evidence from literature indicated that the villous height was increased in piglets inoculated with probiotics, *Lactobacillus fermentum* or *Pediococcus acidilactici* and some *Bifidobacterium* species but it was not the case for another probiotics such as *Saccharomyces boulardii.* Major inconsistency still exist as to whether probiotics could affect the crypt depth because some studies have reported that crypt depth decreased in mice supplemented with moderate and high doses of probiotic, however there were reports to the contrary as some failed to confirm those findings. All this information was important for the determination of the villous height /crypt depth ratio that may indicate the proper development of intestinal epithelia regulated by probiotics. Authors also deliberate on the villous surface area parameter that may contribute to the enhancement of the intestinal absorptive area which seems to be positively regulated by probiotics in a majority of the available evidence. From the perspective of the functionality of the GIT, particularly that which is affected by probiotics the most important being cell proliferation, migration and turnover regulated by apoptosis. Probiotics can increase number of cells in intestinal mucosa and affect the migration of cells in crypt to the tip of the villous. The GIT motility constituents such as migrating motor complex in the stomach and the one way peristaltic movements in small intestine are significantly influenced by the bacterial colonization. Moreover, the decrease of intestinal motility may cause a small intestinal bacterial overgrowth (SIBO). Therefore the use of *Lactobacillus* or *Bifidobacterium*, which caused an enhancement in intestinal contractility could be of interest in the modification of several functions of the upper GIT including gastric emptying, probiotics-induced normalization of motor disorders associated with IBS causing gastrointestinal dysfunction.

Rudil and Isaksen presented a comprehensive overview on the methods of detection, cultivation of the bacteria and pathogens and molecular techniques of laboratory bacterial detection including quantitative PCR. The authors explored the current focus on the human gut microbiota screenings that are based on explorative deep sequencing and by probes targeting the gene encoding 16S ribosomal RNA. The conserved regions provide information for classification of the higher taxa, while the variable regions can be used for differentiation between closely related species. *Mortavasian et al.,* have provided an update on the mechanism of delivery of probiotics by food products, which has recently been considered as a physiological way to transport beneficial compounds such probiotic bacteria to the organism of the host. Because of that, this mechanism of probiotics delivery is also termed 'functional foods'. The authors define the viability of probiotic bacteria in food, which depends mostly upon the number of viable and active cells per g or mL of probiotic food products, at the moment of consumption. This is essentially a measure of the transport efficiency discussed in this chapter. It has been documented that the consumption of probiotic bacteria using food products, mainly probiotic dairy products, could be beneficial to the health of the host. The probiotic bacteria must be viable to affect the health, but the non-viable bacteria could also affect the immunological status of the host. It is believed that the arrival of probiotic bacteria with food to different parts of intestine can increase probiotic bacteria adherence and the rate of colonization. Food products may contain many forms of probiotic bacteria, including culture concentrate that is added to a food (dried or deep-freeze form), the fermented or non-fermented food products, and dietary supplements in the form of drug products-powder, capsules or tablet. It is estimated that probiotic foods comprise between 60 and 70% of the total functional food market. Among food products probiotic bacteria is distributed in a variety of products including fermented milks, ice cream, various types of cheese, baby-food milk powder, frozen dairy desserts, whey-based beverages, sour cream, butter milk, normal and flavored milk, and concentrated milk. Currently, yogurt is the major probiotic which is sold to consumers. *Mortavasian et al.* attempted to characterize the probiotic microorganisms used in food products exploring the most common, bifidobacteria and lactic acid bacteria. *Lactobacillus* and *Bifidobacterium* are the probiotic organisms which are the normal constituents of the human intestinal microbiota. Some other strains considered by the authors of being equally beneficial are *Lactococcus*, *Enterococcus*, *Saccharomyces* and *Propionibacterium*. The predominant organisms in the intestinal tract of breast-fed babies, *L. acidophilus* is so far the most widely used probiotic. The dominant overall flora in human intestines in bifidobacteria, *B. longum*. The information provided by the Authors are very useful in understanding the process of probiotic adaptation with regards to the fermentation conditions, in milk and other food substrates. Among the factors influencing the viability of probiotic microorganisms in food products, the most important are: pH, titrable acidity, molecular oxygen, redox potential, hydrogen peroxide, bacteriocins and short chain fatty acids.

Azzaroli et al. dedicated their chapter to the most prescribed medications worldwide, namely non steroidal anti-inflammatory drugs (NSAIDs). These drugs are prescribed for pain management in musculoskeletal or osteoarticolar pathologies because of their analgesic and anti-inflammatory properties, however, major side effect associated with NSAIDs include gastrointestinal bleedings from both the upper and lower gastrointestinal tract. The authors provided evidence regarding NSAIDs mechanism of action and NSAIDs management including low-dose aspirin therapy. The discovery of safe NSAIDs with reduced upper GI toxicity such as selective COX-2 inhibitors is also presented in this chapter. *Vanaskova et al.*, described the functional disorders of the GIT, focusing on swallowing dysfunctions in human beings. It is well known that these disorders are not only difficult to verify and quantify but also difficult to treat. There are a great deal of problems associated with functional disorders related to psychosomatic, morphological and mechanical alterations as the real causative background for these diseases. The authors decided to describe in detail the relationship between the clinical disability of locomotor system and functional dysphagia. They provided detailed anatomic and functional characteristics of the esophagus including the extrinsic and intrinsic innervations. Moreover, they had concentrated on the reflex part of swallowing involving both the afferent and efferent pathways. The afferent signals apparent during the swallowing reflex are directed from sensitive fibers of the trigeminal nerve, *n. glossopharyngeus* and *n. vagus*. The major nerve constituents of the efferent pathway are nerves in the hypoglossal motor fibers, *n. trigeminus, n. facialis, n. glossopharyngeus* and the *n. vagus*. Subsequent physiology phases of swallowing are listed by *Vanaskova et al.* in proper order and the role of autonomic and enteric system is emphasized. Finally they explore the physiology of the lower esophageal sphincter (LES) and its neurohumoral control. Among the swallowing disorders, dysphagia is the most prevalent and dangerous due to the fact it can lead to tumor formation. The classification of swallowing disorders into obstructive and non-obstructive including e.g. lower motor neuron dysfunction, autoimmune disease and achalasia were discussed in this chapter. The authors also referred to motility disorders in diabetic neuropathy, alcoholism, psychiatric illness and scleroderma – an autoimmune disease that causes weakening of the tissues of the esophagus.

Charisis et al. dedicated their review to the various textures which entails substantial information regarding the structural arrangement of surfaces and their relationship to the surrounding environment. Texture is an innate property of virtually all surfaces;

the grain of the wood, the weave of a fabric, the pattern of crops in a field, rugae on the mucous membrane of the stomach, the mucosa of colon and small intestine. This structural information and image color property has been proven essential for the purpose of medical image analysis and interpretation, perhaps the eroded ulcerous region or a protruded cancerous tissue is visually distinguished, mainly, by its alternated texture. *Akimov and Bezuglov* described existing models for the evaluation of protein digestibility with a major focus on the evaluation of enzymes involved in protein digestion in stomach and intestine. Moreover, a special emphasis is placed on the characterization of the intestinal wall peptidases (surface as well as intracellular) with description of their specificities and their role in overall protein digestion.

Thrombosis in the gut is a serious disorder which may have fatal consequences. *Jomha and Schmidt* presented the most common cause of arterial mesenteric ischemia, which is embolization to the SMA. The Authors evaluated the mechanism of arterial emboli, intracardiac mural thrombus and specific circulatory disorders such as mural thrombus in proximal aneurysms within the thoracic or proximal abdominal aorta. Since SMA arises at the lesser acute angle from the abdominal aorta compared with other mesenteric vessels, it appears to be the most common final destination for mesenteric emboli. Arterial thrombosis constitutes the next most common cause of AMI and occurs in 20% to 35% of cases. The authors provided the tools for the diagnostic evaluation in the form of Duplex ultrasonography and color Doppler, scanning used to assess the flow velocities and resistance index. Another method is Computed tomography (CT) and Magnetic resonance angiography (MRA), which provides an accurate, noninvasive imaging modality for diagnosing mesenteric ischemia and mesenteric occlusive disease.

It is well known that the GIT regulates the absorption of microelements, which are essential for the maintenance of body homeostasis and a failure in natural nutrient absorption in the intestine, resulting in anemic diseases. One of the major functions of intestine is the control of the mechanism of iron uptake and iron loss. In the chapter by *Freiberg et al.*, the pathomechanism of microcytic anemia and the major causes of this blood disorder are described. The physiology of red blood cells (RBC), hemoglobin and gas exchange at the level of tissues and lungs as well as pathology of various anemia's based on the gender and race of the patient are presented. This blood disease is usually attributed to iron deficiency resulting mainly from the dysfunction of iron absorption in the intestine leading to anemia. The reader is informed that apart from nutritional deficiency, the greatest cause of iron deficiency worldwide and in the United States, is a slow or "silent" gastrointestinal bleed. Based on the basic and clinical criteria that categorizes anemia's there are three important pathological processes: decreased or ineffective erythropoiesis, increased hemolysis, and blood loss. Evidence based medicine indicates that especially in poor countries, infestation by hookworm (mostly Necator americanus and Ancylostoma duodenale) is the leading cause of gastrointestinal blood loss causing the iron deficiency and iron deficiency anemia. The authors consistently classified the anemia from a pathological point of view into: 1) iron deficiency anemia, 2) thalassemia trait, 3) lead poisoning, 4) chronic disease, 5) sideroblastic anemia. Since iron deficiency anemia is almost always due to chronic blood loss, they also made the distinction between acute and chronic blood loss that can occur externally by any route or internally into any anatomical space, including intracranial, intrathoracic, retroperitoneal and abdominal spaces. The paper is logically divided into sections concerning epidemiology of iron deficiency in children affecting large population worldwide, health conditions of population suffering from iron deficiency and clinical cases of the genetic disorders affecting the uptake of iron and the formation of hemoglobin.

Turki and Kallel dedicated their work to malabsorption, which could be defined as a state arising from abnormalities in the absorption of food nutrients across the GIT. Depending on the abnormality, impairment can be of single or multiple nutrients leading to malnutrition and a variety of anemia's. General symptoms may include loss of appetite (anorexia), weight loss, fatigue, shortness of breath, dehydration, low blood pressure, and swelling (edema). The authors describe the nutritional disorders that may cause anemia such as lack of iron, foliate and vitamin B_{12}, bleeding tendency such as lack of vitamin K, or bone disease due to deficiency of vitamin D. Gastrointestinal symptoms include flatulence, stomach distention, discomfort, diarrhea, steatorrhea (excessive fat in stool) and frequent bowel movements. Intestinal malabsorption may result in mucosal damage (enteropathy), congenital or acquired reduction in absorptive surface, defects of specific hydrolysis, defects of ion transport, impaired enterohepatic circulation or pancreatic insufficiency. Their major focus was directed towards fat malabsorption caused by severe pancreatic insufficiency. These authors provide the drawbacks of therapeutic use of currently available lipase preparations, as a new oral enzyme substitution that will be helpful in the treatment of intestinal fat malabsorption caused by exocrine pancreatic insufficiency.

Kota et al. attempted in their chapter to describe the development of traditional remedies as a alternative to mainstream pharmaceuticals. In recent years, a number of research papers have been published on herbal medicines to provide experimental evidence for their traditional claims. Authors provide the experimental (animal and human studies) evidence for the plants that have been traditionally used to treat most notable gastrointestinal diseases, namely, peptic ulcer, diarrhea and inflammatory bowel syndrome. Besides the medical usefulness, some of this knowledge on herbal medicine is updated constantly and transferred from one generation to another generations.

It is know that inflammatory bowel disease (IBD) consists of ulcerative colitis (UC) and Crohn's disease (CD) but the role of lymphoma genesis in the pathogenesis of IBD has not been thoroughly investigated. *Prasada et al.* have focused on several lower GIT disorders attributed to UC, the non-Hodgkin's lymphoma (NHL) known as hepatosplenic T-cell lymphoma (HSTCL) and CD and the potential treatment modalities linked to commonly used drugs for the management of IBD, namely thiopurines and tumor necrosis factor (TNF) antagonists. IBD is a global disease affecting a number of Western population and the highest prevalence in developed countries. Interestingly, several reports before revealed that the chronic inflammation seen in IBD itself may be the cause of lymphoma and also the drugs possessing immunosuppressive effects used in the treatment of IBD were suspected to confer this risk. Other diseases that might be associated with a risk of lymphoma are rheumatoid arthritis (RA), primary Sjogren's syndrome, systemic lupus erythematosus (SLE) and Hashimoto's thyroiditis. These authors focused on pathogenesis and etiology of IBD discussing the bacterial aspect and enteric microflora including potential microbial triggers, which have been studied in the past such as the enteroadherent *Escherichia coli* and *Mycobacterium paratuberculosis.* There is no doubt that the particular combination of susceptible genes and environmental triggers which greatly vary between individuals with IBD and can lead to different patterns and severity of disease. The pharmacological treatment mainly with anti-inflammatory and immunomodulatory drugs has been indicated to majority of IBD patients. This include corticosteroids, 5-aminosalicylates, azathioprine, mercaptopurine, methotrexate and cyclosporine A, which have been the most commonly used medications. Since recently the biological therapy with infliximab and adalimumab were recommended, the advantages and disadvantages of the treatment with these agents is emphasized. Later part of this review is dedicated to the cancer risk associated with IBD and the classification of lymphomas. An increased risk of certain non-colorectal malignancies has been shown amongst IBD patients. There is also literature disputing the malignancies associated with thiopurines therapy, which needs a final clarification. In the last part of the review by *Prasada et al.*, a broad spectrum of lymphomas appearing in the form of a variety of neoplasm's due to proliferation of lymphoid cells is discussed. The terminology difference between *leukemia* and *lymphoma* is clearly presented for the readers. Furthermore, the historical background for the classification of various type of lymphoma based on the morphological and functional features of the neoplastic cells is presented. The authors describe in details non-Hodgkin's Lymphoma and the pathogenic factors associated with its formation, such as infectious agents, immunosuppressive therapy, autoimmune conditions and the genetic susceptibility. Finally, they point out the recent global factors, mainly the chemical carcinogen exposure of human beings and problems of diet and obesity are implicated in NHL.

Lee et al., have focused their review on medications recommended to treat cancer currently, such as paclitaxel, which at present seems to be an effective anticancer drug belonging to the taxane family. This drug has been successfully used in the treatment of a wide variety of cancers including breast and ovarian cancers. The current formulation of this drug could induce adverse patient reactions such as hypersensitivity, the nonlinear pharmacokinetic behavior and paclitaxel-induced precipitation during infusion procedure. This group of investigators have been looking for more effective and convenient ways to administer paclitaxel with less formulation-related toxicities than the parent drug. For this purpose, paclitaxel and its analogs have been prepared in many different ways for various intravenous administration.

The chapter by *Gancarcikova et al.*, was designed to evaluate the effects of age and various diets including natural feeding, artificial feeding and gnotobiotic conditions on the development of microflora, and the production of short-chain fatty acids (SCFAs). Moreover, authors studied the postnatal morphological development and disaccharidase enzymes activity in the small intestine in piglets reared under the sow, piglets fed on milk replacement, as well as in gnotobiotic piglets. Important information on the mechanism of stress in the early postnatal period and just after weaning affecting gut development, the microbial colonization of the digestive tract and the absorption capacity. The changes in colostrums, that contains a high levels of several hormones and growth promoting peptides like insulin, epidermal growth factor (EGF), insulin-like growth factor-I and II (IGF-I and II), transforming growth factor-β (TGF- β), glucagon-like peptide-2 (GLP-2) and leptin are discussed. These factors were proved to play an important role in the postnatal development of the digestive tract in newborn animals. On the other hand, the morphologic changes combined with certain types of enterobacteria, can be responsible for post-weaning *diarrhea*. It has recently been recognized that probiotics such as *Lactobacillus, Bifidobacterium, Bacillus, Enterococcus* and *Streptococcus* may be effective in preventing various forms of diarrheic diseases of dietetic and bacterial origin. In the experimental part of the chapter, the authors collected sections of jejunum, ileum and caecum and processed them for microbial counting and short-chain fatty acids (SCFAs) determinations. These experiments were carried out in the contents from jejunum, ileum and colon of gnotobiotic and conventionally bred piglets. Furthermore, the association between the digestive enzyme activity in relation to pH and other constituents of the intestinal contents in various breeds of pigs were studied and suggested that the gnotobiotic animals are a very useful model in studying the physiology of the digestive tract, based on established microbial population affecting the postnatal intestinal development. The authors gave insight into the mechanism of the beneficial effects of probiotic microorganisms that may interact with colostrums, milk containing growth factors, hormones and other bio-active compounds to maintain the proper growth and development of GIT.

Sophia and Bashir described what mostly occurs in adolescent or young adults and is classified as a rare disorder, termed superior mesenteric artery syndrome (SMAS). This syndrome was first described by the Von Rokitansky in 1842 and since then about 400 cases has been reported in literature. In their overview, Sophia and Bashir have underlined the epidemiology of this disorder, and have reported it to be around 0.013-0.3 %. The Authors refer to the high rate of morbidity caused by this syndrome and the difficulty in diagnosing it, and convincingly warned clinicians to be aware of this disorder.

Marte Antonio et al. presented a case report on the mucosa associated lymphoid tissue (MALT) lymphoma involving the appendix in a 6-year-old girl, a rather rare disease in the children in young age. The complications appearing after MALT lymphomas includes approximately 40% of adult developing non-Hodgkin lymphomas (NHL), with the disease being more prevalent in females than males. The primary diagnosis was appendicitis and the patient underwent laparoscopic appendectomy using the three-trocar technique. The authors recommend simple appendectomy as a first line treatment that also endoscopic surveillance seems to be essential for control of a low grade MALToma that can progress into IBD.

The review by *Burmeister et al.* was dedicated to the pathogenesis and therapy of chronic pancreatitis (CP), which has been defined as a continuing inflammatory disease of the pancreas. This disease is characterized by irreversible morphological changes, often associated with pain and loss of exocrine and endocrine function, which may be clinically relevant. The mechanism of pancreatitis involves multiple factors including excessive generation of reactive oxygen-derived metabolites (ROM), tissue hypoxia and acidosis. The development of pancreatitis includes tissue inflammatory infiltration, accompanied by impaired transmission of pain sensation *via* neural ascending pathway and the development of pancreatic ductal and tissue fluid hypertension. Pancreatic disorders are the most difficult diseases to treat, and there is a lot of concerns regarding how to manage the pancreatitis patients from the first symptoms to hospital admission and proper handling those patients either symptomatically or surgically. Pain together with pancreatic insufficiency may have a significant deleterious effect on a patient's quality of life as well as their ability to work and contribute to society, often leading to a loss of their' social support network. *Burmeister et al.* proposed surgery of the pancreatic head containing altered neural fibrotic tissue and diseased ducts as an option to bring relief of pain, due to a resection of inflamed pancreatic tissue and the prevention of the glycoprotein plug formation that may calcify leading to pancreatic ductal hypertension. They also critically analyzed their own surgical attempts and data on pancreatic surgery in humans that exists so far in the literature, and paid major attention to the risk of post-operative pancreatic functional insufficiency and in some cases the surgically related morbidity and mortality for the patient. Furthermore, *Burmeister et al.* described the pathophysiology of pain in CP, and discussed the rationale and indications for surgical intervention and detailed the procedures currently available.

Uchiyama-Tanaka have addressed his review of colonic hydrotherapy with a major focus on colonic irrigations. These procedures are performed using an instrument in combination with abdominal massage, but without drugs or mechanical pressure. The Author explored the events associated with colonic irrigation, for instance, a lymphocyte transmigration from gut-associated lymphoid tissue (GALT) into the circulation, which may improve the functions of both the colon and immune system. Colonic irrigation was developed approximately 40 years ago with no serious complications associated with its use being reported. The author made a substantial contribution to the field of colonic irrigation and shares with readers his experience with this method, which is employed in subjects with no history of malignant or inflammatory disease. The impact of this method, which uses a large amount of water, on the function of intestinal microbiota and serum electrolytes remains, however, unknown.

Nguyen have overviewed the pancreato-biliary cancers that may arise from cancer of the pancreas, bile duct and major ampullae. These tumors uniformly carry a poor prognosis due to its late presentation. Despites many medical advances in imaging diagnosis, chemo-radio-therapy, surgical technique and post-operative care over the last 2 decades, the overall survival of patients with pancreato-biliary neoplasm has not improved significantly. Surgical resection is only possible in less than 20% of patients. The Author's discussed in his review the current techniques and approaches to the diagnosis and management of pancreato-biliary neoplasm. The aim of the chapter by *Jablonska and Lampe* was to present different types of biliary reconstructions used in the surgical treatment of iatrogenic bile duct injuries (IBDI). IBDI remain a critical issue in gastrointestinal surgery due to the fact its a frequent cause of laparoscopic cholecystectomy, which is one of the most commonest surgical procedure in gastroenterology. The early and proper diagnoses of IBDI is very important for surgeons and gastroenterologists, because unrecognized IBDI can lead to serious complications such as biliary cirrhosis, hepatic failure and in some cases to death. The authors refer to the non-invasive, percutaneous radiological and endoscopic techniques as a recommended options for the initial treatment of IBDI. When endoscopic treatment is not effective, surgical management is considered. The major goal of surgical treatment is to reconstruct the proper bile flow to the alimentary tract.

Parkash et al. explored in their review, the most common liver diseases, namely, acute liver failure (ALF) and the chronic liver disease (cirrhosis), however, these authors also considered herein the extra hepatic manifestations of liver disease such as hepatic encephalopathy (HE). This latter occurs in 50-70% of patients with chronic liver disease indicating decompensated chronic liver disease. Among symptoms of HE, the most important are alterations in psychomotor functions, personality changes, cognitive impairment and disturbed sleep patterns. Authors provide the recent standings on classification of HE into 3 types: A, B and C, respectively. Type A is associated with acute liver failure; type B observed mainly in patients with porto-systemic bypass and no intrinsic hepatocellular disease; and type C is linked with cirrhosis or portal-hypertension or porto-systemic shunts, respectively. The proposed mechanism of pathophysiology for HE includes the generation of ammonia, inflammatory cytokines, benzodiazepine among them manganese like substances, which impair neuronal function. The ammonia hypothesis includes dietary nitrogenous components producing ammonia, bacterial metabolism of these nitrogenous products in the colon and in small intestine from glutamine by glutaminase enzyme. Ammonia can activate peripheral type benzodiazepine receptor (Trasnslocator proteins) giving rise to neurosteroids and the GABA/benzodiazepine receptor complex theory. Other mechanisms include the contribution to HE of the microelements such as zinc and manganese as well as oxidative and the nitrosative stress effects *via* a mechanism involving their effect on translocator proteins. Overall, other possible mechanisms of HE have been also carefully analyzed and explained.

Hernandez et al. have focused their review on common adverse drug reactions of the GIT, mainly hemorrhages and peptic ulcer disease. These Authors propose proper clinical problem recognition and management of the most common drugs affecting the gastrointestinal tract. Moreover, they attempted to identify epidemiology, the true incidence in hospitalized and non-hospitalized patients and the main concerns about their causes and the treatment modalities. The problem is of great clinical interest because less common and, usually less severe disorders such as liver disease and pancreatitis can be induced by adverse drug reactions.

In the overview by *Rakus-Andersso*, the subject of Computational Intelligence development in recent years is described. Computational Intelligence has been divided into five main regions, namely, neural networks, evolutionary algorithms, swarm intelligence, immunological systems and fuzzy systems. The author's attention has been attracted by the possibilities of medical applications provided by immunological computation algorithms. Immunological computation systems are based on immune reactions of living organisms in order to defend the bodies from pathological substances. Especially, the mechanisms of T-cell reactions to detect strangers, have been converted into artificial numerical algorithms. In this chapter, another hybrid between the NS algorithm and the chosen solutions coming from fuzzy systems is proposed. This hybrid constitutes their own model of adapting the NS algorithm to the operation decisions "operate" contra "do not operate" in gastric cancer surgery.

In summary, we hope that this book with divergent thematic gastroenterology chapters will be beneficial to all those who share our interest in basic and clinical medicine, translational medicine and health care as well as it serving to trigger the attention of medical students, and potential patients to understanding the recent advancements in the field of gastroenterological disorders of human beings, and the therapeutic options offered by conventional and interventional medicine.

Tomasz Brzozowski
Professor of Medicine, Chairman, Department of Physiology,
Jagiellonian University Medical College, Cracow
Poland

Section 1

Emerging Impact of Probiotics in Gastroenterology

Intestinal Microbial Flora – Effect of Probiotics in Newborns

Pasqua Betta* and Giovanna Vitaliti
U.O UTIN, Department of Pediatrics,
University of Catania
Italy

1. Introduction

The surface of the human gut has a surplus area of 200-250 m² in order to contain, between intraepithelial lymphocytes and lamina propria, Peyer's patches and lymphoid follicles, the lymphoid tissue, while hosts a flora of about 800 different bacteria species with over 7000 strains. The 99% are obligate anaerobes and varies species were then classified using traditional anaerobic culture techniques. More than 50% of the dominant gut microbiota (corresponding to 10 ^{8}-10 ^{11} per gram of faeces) cannot be identified using traditional colture ,but molecular approaches, based on the use of 165 ribosomal DNA molecular (Mai & Morris, 2004). Most of these bacteria colonizes the large intestine (in a range of 10-^{12} bacteria/g). The bacterial count of the small intestine (duodedum and jejunum) is considerably lower (approximately 10$^{4-7}$ bacteria/ml) than Streptococcus Lactobacillus, Enterobacteriaceae corresponding to the transient microbiota.

The main bacterial species represented in the human large intestine (colon) are distributed with densities higher than 10 $^{9-11}$ per gram of contents, and these high densities can be explained by the slow transit and low redox potential . In this intestinal tract we can mostly find bifidobacteria and bacteroides ,bifidobacterium clostridium. The fecal microbiota contains 10 ^{9} -10 ^{11} CFU per gram, and microorganism in about 40% of their weight. The dominant microbiota is represented by strict anaerobes , while the sub-dominant microbiota by facultative anaerobes. In addition to the resident microbiota (dominant and sub dominant), the faeces contain the transient microbiota, that is extremely variable, including Enterobacteriacee (Citrobacter, Klebsiella, Proteus) and Enterobacter (Pseudomonas) and yeast (Candida) CFU per gram (Table 1) (Zoetendal et al, 2004).

2. Intestinal microbiota in newborn

The normal human microflora is a complex ecosystem that somehow depends on enteric nutrients for establishing colonization. At birth ,the digestive tract is sterile. This balance of the intestinal microflora is similar to that of adult from about two years of age (Hammerman et al, 2004).

---

* Corresponding Author

Mouth	200 species	
Stomach,duodenum	pH 2,5-3,5 destructive to most of bacteria 10^1-10^3 unit /ml Lactobacillus,Streptococcus,	
Jejunum,ileum	10^4-10^6 unit /ml bifidobacteria and bacteroides ,bifidobacterium clostridium	Aerobes
Colon	300-400 several species 10^{10}-10^{11} unit /ml Enterobacteriacee (Citrobacter, Klebsiella,Proteus)o(Pseudomonas) Candida.	Anaerobes

Table 1. Composition and topographical features of intestinal microbiota

Diet and environmental conditions can influence this ecosystem. At birth intestinal colonization derives from microorganism of the vaginal mucoses of the mother and faecal microflora . The microbial imprinting depends on the mode and location of delivery. Literature data shows that infants born in a hospital environment, by caesarean section, have a high component of anaerobic microbial flora (Clostridia) and high post of Gram-negative enterobacteria. Those born prematurely by vaginal delivery and breast-feed have a rather rich in Lactobacilli and Bifidobacteria microflora. (Grönlund et al, 1999; Hall et al, 1990)

Diet can influence the microbiota, while breast-feeding promotes an intestine microbiota in which Bifidobacteria predominate, while coliform, enterococci and bacteroides predominate in formula bottle-fed baby.

Escherichia coli and Streptococcus are included among the first bacteria to colonize the digestive tract. After them, strict anaerobes (Bacteroides, Bifidobacteri ,Clostridium) establish during the first week of life, when the diet plays a fundamental role. (Mackie et al, 1999). The pattern of bacterial colonization in the premature neonatal gut is different from the one of healthy, full term infant gut. Aberrant pre-term infants admitted to NICU, born by caesarean section, are more often separated from their mother and kept in an aseptic intensive care setting, treated with broad-spectrum antibiotics. This is the reason why they show a highly modified bacterial flora, consisting of less than 20 species of bacteria, with a predominance of Staphylococcus (aureus and coagulase negative) among aerobic micro-organisms, and Enterobacteriaceae (Klebsiella), among enterococci and anaerobic Clostridia (Dai et al, 1999; Gothefor, 1989).

It is believed that microbial diversity is an important factor in determining the stability of the ecosystem and that the fecal loss of diversity predisposes the preterm gastrointestinal colonization of antibiotic-resistant bacteria and fungi colonization with a consequent potential risk of infection, thus contributing to the development of necrotizing enterocolitis (NEC) (Fanaro et al, 2003; Sakata et al, 1985)

2.1 Structure and function of intestinal microbial flora

The intestinal microbial flora has numerous functions, even if the most of them has not yet been identified. Among these functions, we can report its anatomical –functional role, its protective function, in particular the "barrier effect", referring to the physiological capacity of the endogenous bacterial microflora to inhibit colonization of the intestine by pathogenic microorganism. It is already known that the intestinal microbial flora influences food digestion ,absorption and fermentation, the immune system response, peristalsis, production of vitamins such as B-vitamins, influencing moreover the turnover of intestinal epithelial cells. In addition the metabolism of gut microflora influences hormonal secretion.

Bacterial colonization of human gut by environmental microbes begins immediately after birth; the composition of intestinal microbiota, relatively simple in infants, becomes more complex with increasing in age, with a high degree of variability among human individuals. It is believed that microbial diversity is an important factor in determining the stability of the ecosystem and that fecal loss of diversity predisposes the preterm gastrointestinal colonization of antibiotic-resistant bacteria and fungi with the consequent potential risk of infection (Cummings & Macfarlane, 1991; Montalto et al, 2009; Neish, 2002).

2.2 Gut microflora and immunity

The mucosal membrane of the intestines, with an area of approximately 200 m^2, is constantly challenged by the enormous amount of antigens from food, from the intestinal microbial flora and from inhaled particles that also reach the intestines. It is not surprising therefore that approximately the eighty per cent of the immune system is found in the area of the intestinal tract and it is particularly prevalent in the small intestine. The intestinal immune system is referred as GALT (gut-associated-lymphoid tissue). It consists of Peyer's patches, which are units of lymphoid cells, single lymphocytes scattered in the lamina propria and intraepithelial lymphocytes spread in the intestinal epithelia.

The immune system of infants is not fully developed. The structures of the mucosal immune system are fully developed in utero by 28 weeks gestation, but in the absence of intrauterine infections, activation does not occur until after birth. Maturation of the mucosal immune system and establishment of protective immunity is usually fully developed in the first years of life. In addition the exposure to pathogenic and commensal bacteria, the major modifier of the development patterns in the neonatal period, depends on infant feeding practices. (Brandtzaeg, 2001; Gleeson et al, 2004)

Bacterial colonisation of the intestine is important for the development of the immune system. The intestine has an important function in working as a barrier.This barrier is maintained by tight-junctions between the epithelial cells, by production of IgA antibodies and by influencing the normal microbial flora. It is extremely important that only harmless substances are absorbed while the harmful substances are secreted via the faeces.

Studies show that individuals allergic to cow´s milk have defective IgA production and an increased permeability of the intestinal mucosa. This results in an increased absorption of macromolecules by the intestinal mucosa. The increased permeability is most probably caused by local inflammations due to immunological reactions against the allergen. This damages the intestinal mucosa

2.3 Modification of the intestinal flora micro-ecosystem

During the past century our lifestyle has dramatically changed regarding hygienic measures, diet, standards of living and usage of medical drugs. Today our diet largely includes industrially produced sterilized food and the use of different kinds of preservatives. This has led to a decreased intake of bacteria, particularly lactic acid producing bacteria .

The widespread use of antibiotics in healthcare and agriculture, antibacterial substance is also something new for human kind. We have in so many ways sterilized our environment, which is detrimental to the microbial (Cummings & Macfarlane G.T., 1997; Vanderhoof & Young, 1998).

3. What are probiotics?

The term 'probiotic' was proposed in 1965 to denote an organism or substance that contributes to the intestinal microbial balance. The definition of probiotics has subsequently evolved to emphasise a beneficial effect to health over effects on microbiota composition, underscoring the requirement of rigorously proven clinical efficacy. Most probiotic bacterial strains were originally isolated from the intestinal microbiota of healthy humans and the probiotics most thoroughly investigated thus far belong to the genera lactobacilli and bifidobacteria (Caramia G., 2004).

Probiotics have several effects, including modulating the gut microbiota, promoting mucosal barrier functions, inhibiting mucosal pathogen adherence and interacting with the innate and adaptive immune systems of the host, which may promote resistance against pathogens. The intestinal microbiota constitutes an important aspect of the mucosal barrier the function of which is to restrict mucosal colonisation by pathogens, to prevent pathogens from penetrating the mucosa and to initiate and regulate immune responses

3.1 Proved beneficial effects on the host

Prerequisites for probiotics' efficacy are human origin, resistance transit gastric capacity to colonize survival in and adhesion, competitive exclusion of pathogens or harmful antigens to specific areas of the gastrointestinal tract, vitality, verifiable and stability conservation, production substances with antimicrobial action, exclusion of resistance transferable antibiotic. No pathogenicity and / or toxicity has ever been demonstrated on the host.

3.2 Effect of probiotics

Among their effects, the most important are: competition to the more valid nutrients and enteric epithelial anchorage sites; reduction of intestinal pH values for high production of lactic acid from lactose and acetic acid from carbohydrates, which selects the growth of lactobacilli; production of bacteriocins, peptides with bactericidal activity towards related bacteria species; metabolism of certain nutrients in the volatile fatty acids; activation of mucosal immunity, with increased synthesis of secretory IgA, and phagocytosis; stimulation of production of various cytokines

3.3 Mechanism of action of probiotics

The functional interactions between bacteria, gut epithelium, gut mucosal immune system and systemic immune system are the basis of the mechanisms of direct and indirect effects of probiotics. The direct effect of probiotics in the lumen are: competition with pathogens for nutrients, production of antimicrobial substances and in particular organic acids competitive inhibition on the receptor sites, change in the composition of mucins hydrolysis of toxins, receptorial hydrolisis, and nitric oxide (NO), while the indirect effect largely depends on the site of interaction between the probiotic and the effectors of the immune response, topographically located in the intestinal tract.

There is evidence, in vitro and in vivo, on effects of different probiotics on specific mechanisms of the immune response. The starting point is the interaction between probiotic and the host intestinal mucosa, but it seems clear that not all probiotics have the same initial contact (immune cells, enterocytes, etc.).

There are several literature data that have demonstrated the interaction between probiotics and the immune system, in particular it has been demonstrated their capacity to stimulate the production of intestinal mucines, their trophic effect on intestinal epithelium, the re-establishment of the intestinal mucosa integrity, the stimulation of the IgA-mediated immune response against viral pathogens. All these effects have been demonstrated in experimental studies and in some clinical studies, even if it is not still clear the main mechanism of action and it is conceivable that different mechanisms of action contribute to the efficacy of probiotics, with a different role in different clinical situations (Vanderhoof & Young, 1998).

3.4 Safety

The oral consumption of viable bacteria in infancy naturally raises safety concerns. Products containing probiotics are widely available in many countries and, despite the growing use of such products in recent years, no increase in Lactobacillus bacteraemia has been detected. Nevertheless, the average yearly incidence of Lactobacillus bacteraemia in Finland between the years 1995 and 2000 was 0.3 cases/100,000 inhabitants. Importantly, 11 out of the 48 isolated strains were identical to Lactobacillus GG, the most commonly used probiotic strain. Lactobacillus bacteraemia is considered to be of clinical significance; immune-suppression, prior prolonged hospitalisation and surgical interventions have been identified as predisposing factors. Nonetheless, clinical trials with products containing both lactobacilli and bifidobacteria have demonstrated the safety of these probiotics in infants and children, and in a recent study, the use of L. casei was found to be safe also in critically ill children

In a trial assessing the safety of long-term consumption of infant formula containing B. lactis and S. thermophilus, the supplemented formulas were demonstrated to be safe and well tolerated. No serious adverse effects have been reported in the trials involving premature neonates, but it should be noted that the studies were not primarily designed to assess their safety (Hammerman et al, 2006)

4. Probiotics and gastrointestinal disorders

The presence of Bifidobacteria in artificial milk can contribute to the induction of a significant increase of Bifidobacteria in the intestinal tract, promotes the development of a protective microflora, similar to that one of the breast- fed newborn, contributes to the modulation of immune-defenses, giving them a major efficiency (Langhendries et al, 1995; Fukushima et al, 1998).

In early 2002, the United States Food and Drug administration accepted a "generally regarded as safe (GRAS) the use of *Bifidobacterium lactis* and *Streptococcus thermophilus* in formula milk for healthy infants aged 4 months or more" (Hammerman et al, 2006).

The clinical efficacy of probiotics in the prevention and treatment of infectious disease in infancy has most comprehensively been documented in diarrhoeal disease. *Lactobacillus* GG or *Lactobacillus reuteri* (ATCC 55730) supplementation has been demonstrated to be effective in the prevention of acute infantile diarrhoea in different settings. *Lactobacillus* GG has also been reported to significantly reduce the duration of acute diarrhoea and the duration of rotavirus shedding after rotavirus infection. Bifidobacteria have also shown promising potential in preventing both nosocomial spread of gastroenteritis and diarrhoea in infants in residential care settings. Meta-analyses of double-blind, placebo-controlled clinical trials have concluded that probiotics, particularly *Lactobacillus* GG, are effective in treatment of acute infectious diarrhoea in infants and children. Probiotics appear also to have some protective effect against antibiotic-associated diarrhoea and acute diarrhoea in children, but the heterogeneity of the available studies precludes drawing firm conclusions (Vanderhoof, 2000).

5. Probitics and atopic disease

Probiotics acts on atopic diseases modulating initial colonisation, intralumenal degradation of allergens, promoting intestinal barrier function, enhancing immune maturation with induction of IgA production, induction of regulatory T cells. In infancy, food allergy and atopic eczema are the most common atopic disorders. Even though atopic disease often becomes manifest during the course of the first year of life, it is well established that the immune pathology leading to clinical disease has its origins in early life, possibly already in the immune environment prevailing *in utero*. Indeed, infantile food allergy could be considered a manifestation of a primary failure to establish tolerance to dietary antigens rather than loss of tolerance characteristic of allergies in later life. Therefore, measures aimed at reducing the risk of atopic diseases should be started in the perinatal period. Thus far, the rationale of most studies assessing means of primary prevention of atopic diseases has been to reduce exposure to the allergens known to most often be associated with sensitisation and provocation of symptoms in allergic individuals, but the success of such measures has been relatively poor. Consequently, probiotics have been investigated as a novel approach with a number of potential effects which might beneficially affect the host immune physiology to a non-atopic mode.

The immune pathology of atopic diseases is characterised by T helper (Th)2-driven inflammatory responsiveness against ubiquitous environmental or dietary allergens. The factors leading to inappropriate Th2 responsiveness, and thus atopic disease, in early immune development remain poorly understood. Th2-type responsiveness is counter-regulated both by Th1 responses, which are usually directed against infectious agents and immunosuppressive, and by tolerogenic regulatory T cell responses. Prescott and colleagues demonstrated that infants with high hereditary risk who subsequently developed atopic disease are characterised by an impaired capacity (compared with healthy infants) to produce both Th1 and Th2 cytokines in the neonatal period. During the first year of life, an increase in Th2 responsiveness is seen in infants developing atopic disease, whereas a reverse development takes place in healthy infants.

5.1 Use of probiotics for prevention of atopic diseases

As previously mentioned, the sequence of bacterial intestinal colonization of neonates and young infants is important in the development of the immune response. Recognition by the immune system of self and nonself, as well as the type of inflammatory responses generated later in life, are likely affected by the infant's diet and acquisition of the commensal intestinal bacterial population superimposed on genetic predisposition.

During pregnancy, the cytokine inflammatory-response profile of the fetus is diverted away from cell-mediated immunity (T-helper 1 [Th1] type) toward humoral immunity (Th2 type). Hence, the Th2 type typically is the general immune response in early infancy. The risk of allergic disease could well be the result of a lack or delay in the eventual shift of the predominant Th2 type of response to more of a balance between Th1- and Th2-type responses (Neaville, 2003).

Administration of probiotic bacteria during a time period in which a natural population of lacticacid– producing indigenous intestinal bacteria is developing could theoretically influence immune development toward more balance of Th1 and Th2 inflammatory responses (Majamaa & Isolauri, 1997). The intestinal bacterial flora of atopic children has been demonstrated to differ from that of nonatopic children. Specifically, atopic children have more Clostridium organisms and fewer Bifidobacterium organisms than do nonatopic study subjects (Björkstén et al, 1999; Klliomaki et al, 2001), which has served as the rationale for the administration of probiotics to infants at risk of atopic diseases, particularly for those who are formula fed.

In a double-blinded RCT, LGG or a placebo was given initially to 159 women during the final 4 weeks of pregnancy. If the infant was at high risk of atopic disease (atopic eczema, allergic rhinitis, or asthma), the treatment was continued for 6 months after birth in both the lactating woman and her infant (Kalliomäki et al, 2003). A total of 132 mother-infant pairs were randomly assigned to receive either placebo or LGG and treated for 6 months while breastfeeding. The primary study end point was chronic recurrent atopic eczema in the infant. Atopic eczema was diagnosed in 46 of 132 (35%) of these study children by 2 years of age. The frequency of atopic eczema in the LGG-treated group was 15 of 64 (23%) versus 31 of 68 (46%) in the placebo group (RR: 0.51 [95% CI: 0.32– 0.84]; P = .01). The number of mother-infant pairs required to be treated with LGG to prevent 1 case of chronic recurrent atopic eczema was 4.5. By 4 years of age, eczema occurred in 26% of the infants in the group treated with LGG, compared with 46% in the placebo group (RR: 0.57 [95% CI: 0.33– 0.97]; P =.01). However, only 67% of the original study group was analyzed at the 4-year follow-up. These results support a preventive effect for giving a probiotic to mothers late in pregnancy and to both mothers and infants during the first 6 months of lactation for the prevention of atopic eczema in infants who are at risk of atopic disease.

Conversely, Taylor et al (2007) found that probiotic supplementation did not reduce the risk of atopic dermatitis in children at high risk with the report of some increased risk of subsequent allergen sensitization. As concluded in a review by Prescott and Björkstén (2007) and in a 2007 Cochrane review (Osborn & Sinn, 2007) despite the encouraging results of some studies, there is insufficient evidence to warrant the routine supplementation of probiotics to either pregnant women or infants to prevent allergic diseases in childhood. Explanations for varied study results include host factors such as genetic susceptibility, environmental factors such as geographic region and diet, and study variables including probiotic strains and doses used (Prescott & Björkstén, 2007; Penders, 2007).

5.2 Use of probiotics in the treatment of atopic diseases

In an RCT, 53 Australian infants with moderate-to-severe atopic dermatitis were given either Lactobacillus fermentum or placebo for 8 weeks. At final assessment at 16 weeks, significantly more children who received the probiotic had improved extent and severity of atopic dermatitis as measured by the Severity of Scoring of Atopic Dermatitis (SCORAD) index over time compared with those who received placebo (P = .01) (Weston et al, 2005; Viljanen et al, 2005). These results are encouraging, but as summarized in a 2008 Cochrane review (Boyle et al, 2008), probiotics have not yet been proven to be effective in the treatment of eczema.

6. Probiotics and premature infants

Prematurity compromises the anatomical and functional development of all organs, in inverse proportion to the gestational age. Some peculiarities of the preterm are the high incidence of respiratory diseases, the multi-systemic immaturity, even if nutrition constitutes one of the major actual problem to afford.

The preterm infant lacks of the sucking reflex, has a restricted gastric and intestinal capacity, insufficient absorption of the main food, that contribute to both quantitative and qualitative nutritional deficiencies.

The lack of an adequate nutrition decreases the synthesis of surfactant and anti-oxidant molecules, thus causing a delayed lung maturation and both cellular and humoral immune response, responsible for an increase of the catabolism, promoting the use of endogenous proteins. Therefore, the goal of the nutrition of the ELBW infant is the manteinance of his post-natal growth, similarly of what happens in utero, preventing the protein catabolism (through the use of endogenous proteins: lean body mass), avoid the weight loss during the first 2 weeks after birth, assuring a high energetic rate since his first day of life, thus reducing the percentage of preterms with a weight less than 10° percentile at discharge.

Nowadays the first approach to ELBW preterms is the parenteral nutrition since their first day of life (with the prompt introduction of glucose as it is the main source of energy and it reduces the catabolism of endogenous proteins since the first 2 hours after birth, and the introduction of lipids since the first 24 hours after birth). It is also important the introduction of low quantities of milk (minimal enteral feeding) via oral or nasal-gastric way in order to promote the feeding tolerance and the increase of enteral production of cholecystokinin that stimulates the bile function, protecting the liver from hepatic steatosis due to parenteral nutrition.

It is important that these procedures are managed in a gradual way in order to avoid the tiredness of the infant and the aspiration of milk with regurgites. For this reason it is conceivable using a fortified maternal formula for premature infants, with a daily increase of the feeding, paying attention to abdominal distension, vomit, gastric stagnation, apneas, and diarrhea.

It is conceivable to stop the parenteral nutrition when the energetic rate reach a quote of 80cal/Kg/die and the daily increase of milk must not be more than 10ml/Kg/die, and sometimes it is necessary the continuous or discontinuous enteral feeding, via nasal-gastric tube, in order to suspend the parenteral nutrition.

The passage from enteral nutrition to nursing depends on the acquisition of sucking, deglutition, epiglottis and larynx closure ability and on the nasal passage, as well as the esophageal motility and a synchronized process is usually absent before 34 weeks of gestation. The sucking ability is usually reached when the infant has a weight over 1500 gr even if sometimes it is necessary to proceed with the tactile stimulation of the infant tongue (Tsang et al, 2005).

Enzymatic digestive functions in preterm more than 28 weeks of gestation are mature enough to allow the adequate digestion and absorption of proteins and carbohydrates. Lipids are well adsorbed and unsaturated fatty acids and lipids in maternal milk are better adsorbed than the components of the formula milk.

The weight gain in infants with a birth weight less than 2000 gr should be adequate when the mother shows a protein intake of 2.25-2.75/Kg/die, because they should provide a good intake of essential aminoacids, in particular tryptophan and threonine, that are important for the cerebral development.

The maternal milk, through specific immunologic factors, can potentiate the defensive mechanisms of preterms, contributing to ameliorate the immune defense against infectious agents. Recent studies highlighted that the maternal milk not only promote a passive protection, but can directly modify the immunologic development of the infant.

The maternal milk contains immunologic and non-immunologic factors, and immune-modulant factors, such as the bifidogenic factor, that promotes the development of the *Lactobacillus Bifidus,* that by competition promotes the decrease of the intestinal pH and inhibits the growth of *Escherichia Coli*. The maternal milk must be fortified, while the formula for preterm infants do not contain the bifidogenic factor (Heiman & Schanler, 2007).

It is also well established that the composition of the intestinal microbiota is aberrant and its establishment delays in neonates who require intensive care, with an increased risk of developing NEC. As discussed above, probiotics have been shown to enhance the intestinal barrier, inhibit the growth and adherence of pathogenic bacteria and to improve altered gut micro-ecology In preterm infants, administration of the probiotic *Lactobacillus* GG has been shown to affect colonisation patterns. Data from experimental animal models suggest that bifidobacteria reduce the risk of NEC in rats. Consequently, it could be hypothesised that probiotics might have potential in reducing the risk of NEC in premature infants.

The supplementation of probiotics since the first day of life represents a valid help in influencing the growth of a favourable intestinal ecosystem, decreasing the quote of Clostridium, Bacillus and Bacteroides Fragilis and increasing the rate of bifidobacteria, also improving the intestinal barrier with a way of action similar to that of the maternal milk, protecting the gut from bacteria and fungal colonization, avoiding the development of NEC.

7. Probiotics and necrotizing enterocolitis

Necrotizing enterocolitis (NEC) is a serious anoxic and ischemic disease particularly affecting premature newborns, affecting almost the ileo-colic area, with bacteria proliferation, production of gas inside gastric walls (cystic pneumatosis), associated with edema and inflammation. Its incidence rate is 1-3 cases for 1000 newborns, with a mortality rate ranging between 10-50%. The prematurity is the most important risk factor, as well as the low birth weight (< 1500 gr). This risk increases after the colonization or the infection of pathogens such as Clostridium, Escherichia, Klebsiella, Salmonella, Shigella, Campylobacter, Pseudomonas, Streptococcus, Enterococcus, Staphylococcus aureus and coagulase negative Staphylococcus. Other factors that can increase its incidence are the intestinal immaturity, the decrease of the intestinal motility, the increase of permeability to macromolecules and the excessive volume of milk. Certainly breast feeding represents a protective factor, as it is shown by the decreased incidence of NEC in breast-fed infants. Moreover literature data supporting the benefits of probiotics are increasing in the last decades.

The role of intestinal micro-organisms has been largely described, even if it is still not clear. Advances in molecular biology and intestinal microbiology allow a better characterization of the intestinal microbiota in children affected by NEC. Nowadays, literature data describe different methods of characterization of the microbic genotype and of identification of its genes, expression of the specific proteins and production of metabolites. The application of these techniques on bioptic samples of infected and non-infected subjects could better the comprehension of the persistence of NEC in premature newborns. Deshpande et al. (2007) published a meta analysis that confirms the benefit of probiotic supplements in reducing death and disease in preterm newborns.

The mechanism of action of probiotics in the protection of NEC seem to be the increased production of anti-inflammatory cytokines, blockage of the passage of bacteria and their products through the mucose, competitive action with some pathogen groups, modification of the response of the host towards microbial products, improving the enteral nutrition, decreasing the duration of the parenteral nutrition, responsible for late sepsis.

Different studies highlight that the supplementation of probiotics reduces the risk of NEC. In the most recent literature, the study of Bin-Nun et al. (2005) showed a lower frequency of serious diseases in newborns with a low birth weight when in their feeding was added a probiotic mixture. Desphande's meta analysis, published in Lancet in 2007, showed the same results. As a matter of fact the first studies on probiotics in premature children were leaded in order to reduce the incidence of NEC in this group of children.

8. Probiotics and infections

The most valid indication of the probiotic remains the decrease of intestinal infections. In fact, the literature shows that the probiotic can reduce the severity and number of episodes of diarrhea.

Weizman & Alsheikh made a double-blind placebo-controlled study using a formula supplemented with L. reuteri or B. bifidium for 12 weeks. In the group of infants in therapy with probiotics, less gastrointestinal infectious episodes have been detected, fewer episodes of fever compared to placebo, with consequent reduce of antibiotic therapy. The fetus and the newborn are particularly vulnerable to the injuries caused by infectious agents or immunological mechanisms related to the immaturity of the immune system. The improvement of perinatal care has led to increased survival of high-risk infant (ELBW, respiratory distress, surgery), neonatal research priorities on the prevention and treatment of sepsis in NEC and bronchopulmonary dysplasia (CLD) (Weizman & Alsheikh, 2006).

In view of the role of mediators of inflammation in CLD and in sepsis is therefore important to modulate the immune response in these young patients. Some studies have shown that probiotics can alter the intestinal microflora and reduce the growth of pathogenic microorganisms in the intestines of preterm infants, decreasing the incidence of necrotizing enterocolitis and sepsis. Moreover, a study performed in rats with immune deficiency has shown that the administration of LGG reduced the risk of colonization and sepsis by Candida.

One of our retrospective study, performed in 2002 at the University of Catania TIN, showed that supplementation from birth for at least 4-6 weeks of a symbiotic (lactogermine plus 3.5 x109 ucf / day) decreased the incidence and intensity of gastrointestinal colonization of Candida, and subsequently its related infections in a group of preterm infants. Another randomized study on 80 preterm infants has confirmed that the administration of LGG (at a dose of 6 billion cfu / day) from the first day of life for a period of six weeks reduced the fungal enteric colonization with no side effects (Romeo et al, 2011).

Newborns submitted to greater surgical interventions (esophageal atresia, hernia diaframmatica, intestinal malformations) have an increased risk of bacterial and/or mycotic infections due to the use of drains, central venous catheter, NPT, persistent nose-gastric probe that can be the cause of serious sepsis and pneumonias.

In a recent study that we presented at ESPHGAN, we demonstrated that surgical infants admitted to our NICU and supplemented with probiotics have a reduced risk of bacterial and *Candida* infections and an improved clinical outcome (Figure 1) (Betta et al, 2007)

In another recently published study on preterm infants, the use of probiotics appeared to be effective in the prevention of both bacterial and mycotic infections, in the attenuation of gastrointestinal symptoms and in a more rapid weaning from total parenteral nutrition with a reduction in the central venous catheter time and the number of days in hospital. These results were evident both in a group of preterm newborns and in a group of surgical newborn treated with a supplementation of probiotics (Figure 2).

9. Probiotics and respiratory tract infections (RTI)

Two studies have examined the effect in adults of a combined multi-strain probiotic and multivitamin/mineral supplement containing L. gasseri, B. longum and B. bifidum on the incidence, duration and severity of common cold infections and aspects of immune function (de Vrese et al, 2006; Winkler et al, 2005). Both studies found a reduction in severity and duration, as well as enhanced expression of immune cells, while only Winkler et al. (2005) found a reduction in incidence. The major difference between studies is dose — the same probiotic strains were used for both, as well as the same assessment methods for the illness — suggesting that although the dose used by de Vrese et al. (2006) (5 9 107 CFU) was enough to attenuate symptoms and duration, a higher dose such as that used by Winkler et al. (2005) (5 9 108 CFU per day) was needed for prevention of infections. The lower dose may promote a systemic immune response sufficient to reduce severity and duration but not incidence, while the higher dose may stimulate systemic immunity via the mechanism of

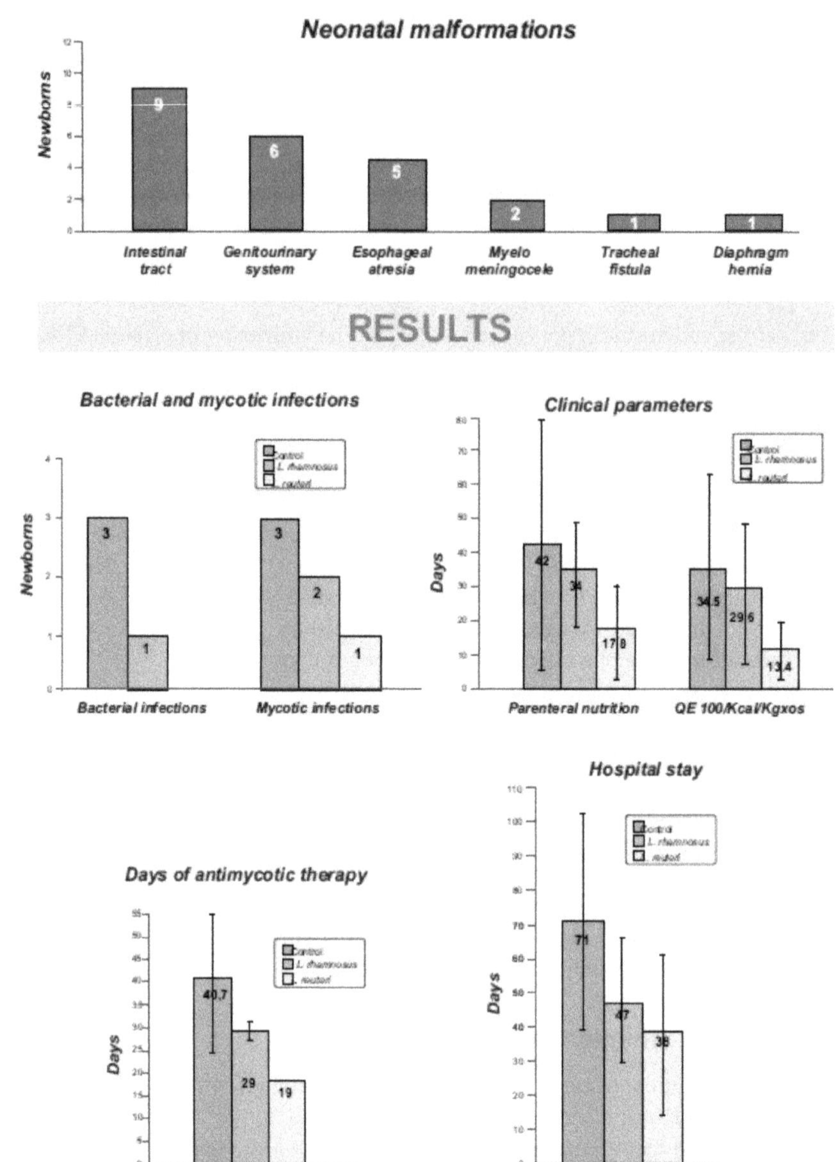

Fig. 1. The direct introduction of probiotics, that positively influences the intestinal microbial population, determining a reduction of more pathogenic species in the bowel reservoir, can improve enteral nutrition reducing time of dependence on intravenous nutrition and might contribute to a better outcome in high risk newborns.

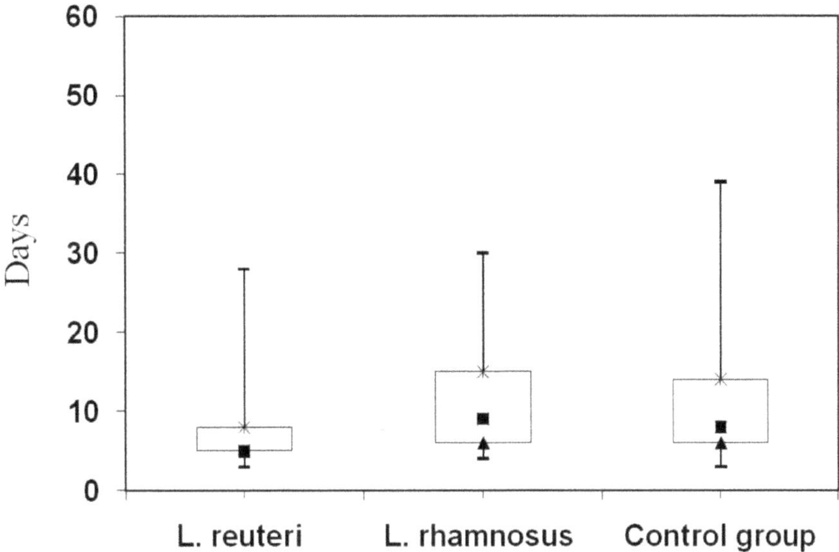

Fig. 2.

distribution of T and B lymphocytes, primed in the gut, which proliferate to the mucosal-associated lymphoid tissue (MALT), where the B cells differentiate into immunoglobulin-producing cells after specific antigenic exposure, leading to an inhibition of colonisation by pathogenic strains.

Olivares et al. (2006) also found an immunostimulatory effect in subjects given a multistrain probiotic containing L. gasseri and L. corniformis, compared with a standard yoghurt containing S. thermophilus and L. bulgaricus, although this study provides no evidence for the efficacy of a greater number of strains, since two non-comparable treatments were used.

Gluck and Gebbers (2003) investigated colonisation by nasal pathogens and showed a 19% reduction in the group given probiotics (L. rhamnosus GG, Bifidobacterium lactis, L. acidophilus, S. thermophilus) compared to no reduction with placebo. Despite this reduction in colonisation, no data are given as to whether subjects became unwell during the study period, making conclusions as to actual health benefits difficult to draw. In a similar study, Hatakka et al. (2007) found no effect of a probiotic mixture on incidence and duration of otitis and upper respiratory infections on children aged 6 months to 10 years; a lower dose than that used by Gluck and Gebbers (2003) may explain the disparity between results. It may also be that ingested probiotics have less effect on the aural mucosa compared to that on the nasal mucosa, or that the effects are strain-specific.

In a 7-month study with over 1,000 subjects, Lin et al. (2009) examined the protective effect of two single probiotics (L. casei and L. rhamnosus, given individually) and one multi-strain mixture containing the 2 lactobacilli and 10 other organisms. Reduced physician visits, as well as decreased incidence of bacterial, and viral respiratory disease were seen in all groups compared with placebo, but there was no significant difference in effectiveness between the preparations even though the multi-strain probiotic was given at a tenfold higher dose than the individual strains. However, in the case of prevention of gastro-intestinal tract infections, the probiotic mixture was significantly more effective than the single strains. This may be due to the exceptionally high dose given in the multi-strain treatment, resulting in larger numbers of probiotic bacteria competing with pathogens for binding sites and or nutrients in the gut.

Another point of interest in this study is that despite large differences in dose, the two single strains did not have statistically different effects, suggesting strain-specificity in dose and effect for individual species. These data support the theory that supplementation with certain multi-strain probiotics can reduce severity, duration, and possibly incidence of RTIs, and in the case of Lin et al. (2009) that a multi-strain probiotic may be more effective than a single-strain. There is some evidence for immunostimulation, even in cases where illness still occurs. Further consistency could be added to this evidence with the establishment, by testing varied concentrations of probiotic bacteria, of an optimum dose that prevents pathogenic colonisation of the mucosa as well as the incidence and severity of illness. Testing this dose with and without vitamin and mineral supplementation may reveal a synergy between both types of supplement.

Further work should be done to determine the relative efficacy of single- and multi-strain probiotics in this area.

10. Conclusion

The direct introduction of probiotics, can positively influence the intestinal microbial population, include a reduction in the bowel reservoir of more pathogenic species, improve enteral nutrition, and reduce dependence on intravenous nutrition, favour an increased gut mucosal barrier to bacteria and bacterial products, and up regulation in protective immunity.

It is important to establish what probiotic it should be used, the right dosage, the right time of use, and furthermore controlled studies should answer to these questions, in order to describe specific indications on the type of probiotic that must be used in a specific situation, thus better clarifying the structure of the probiotic and its characteristics, selecting the right probiotic for each kind of disease.

It is important to underline that the use of probiotics is safe even at high dosages, without any side effect in preterm infants. After birth the rapid development of the intestinal microflora regulates all the different gastro-intestinal and immunologic functions that are included in the so called mutualism bacteria- host organism. This kind of relationship starts from birth and regulate different aspects of the immune system of the newborn.

Recent epidemiologic data support the hypothesis that in the last 20 years some immunologic modification can find a cause in the modification of the intestinal microflora.

Different therapeutic actions could be potentially able to alter the normal relationship between the intestinal microbiota and the host organism. The international medical community has to be aware of the increasing importance that initial colonising intestinal microflora could have on the health and well-being of the host later in life. It is of great importance to know that the initial bacterial colonisation of the neonate appears to play a crucial role in inducing immunity in the immature human being, and that a suboptimal process could have definite consequences. The optimal early interface between the microbes and the intestinal mucosa of the host may have been somewhat disturbed by modern perinatal care. It is fundamental to try to decrease these possible negative influences and to discover in the near future the possible means to help manipulate positively the gut microbiotia of infants (Rautava, 2007).

11. References

Betta, P.; Sciacca, P.; Trovato, L. et al. (2007) Probiotics in the prevention of Bacterial and Candida infections in newborns submitted to greater surgical interventions and admitted in NICU. Retrospective Group Controlled Study. ESPGHAN, Barcelona, May 9-12, 2007

Bin-Nun, A.; Bromiker, R.; Wilschanski, M. et al. (2005) Oral probiotics prevent necrotizing enterocolitis in very low birth weight neonates. J Pediatr, 147(2):192-6.

Björkstén, B.; Naaber, P.; Sepp, E. & Mikelsaar, M. (1999) The intestinal microflora in allergic Estonian and Swedish 2-year-old children. Clin Exp Allergy, 29(3):342–346

Boyle, R.J.; Bath-Hextall, F.J.; Leonardi-Bee, J. et al (2008). Probiotics for treating eczema. Cochrane Database Syst Rev, (4):CD006135

Brandtzaeg, P. (2001) Nature and function of gastrointestinal antigen-presenting cells. Allergy,56 Suppl 67:16-20.

Cummings, J.H. & Macfarlane, G.T. (1991) The control and consequences of bacterial fermentation in the human colon. J Appl Bacteriol, 70:443-59.

Cummings, J.H. & Macfarlane, G.T. (1997) Colonic microflora: nutrition and health. Nutrition, 13:476-8.

Dai, D. & Walker, W.A. (1999). Protective nutrients and bacterial colonization in the immature human gut. Adv Pediatr,46:353-82

Deshpande, G.; Rao, S. & Patole, S. (2007) Probiotics for prevention of necrotising entercolitis in preterm neonates with very low birthweight: a systematic reiew of randomised controlled trials, Lancet, 369:1614-20

de Vrese, M.; Winkler, P.; Rautenberg, P. et al, (2006) Probiotic bacteria reduced duration and severity but not the incidence of common cold episodes in a double blind, randomized,controlled trial. Vaccine, 24(44–46):6670–6674

Fanaro, S.; Chierici, R.; Guerrini P. & Vigi, V. (2003) Intestinal microflora in early infancy :composition and development Acta Paediatr Suppl, 91:48-55.

Fukushima, Y.; Kawata, Y.; Hara, H.; Terada, A. & Mitsuoka, T. (1998) . Effect of a probiotic formula on intestinal immunoglobulin A production in healthy children, 42:39-44.

Caramia, C. (2004) Probiotics: from Metchnikoff to the current preventive and therapeutic possibilities. Pediatr Med Chir, 26:19-33.

Gleeson, M.; Pyne, D.B. & Callister R. (2004) The missing links in exercise effects on mucosal immunity. Exerc Immunol Rev, 10:107-28.

Gluck, U. & Gebbers, J.O. (2003) Ingested probiotics reduce nasal colonization with pathogenic bacteria (Staphylococcus aureus, Streptococcus pneumoniae, and beta-hemolytic streptococci). Am J Clin Nutr, 77(2):517–520

Gothefors, L. (1989) Effects of diet on intestinal flora. Acta Paediatr Scand Suppl, 351:118-21.

Grönlund, M.M.; Lehtonen, O.P.; Eerola, E. & Kero, P. (1999) Fecal microflora in healthy infants born by different methods of delivery: permanent changes in intestinal flora after cesarean delivery. J Pediatr Gastroenterol Nutr, 28:19-25

Hall, M.A.; Cole, C.B., Smith, S.L.; Fuller, R. & Rolles, C.J. (1990) Factors influencingthe presence of faecal Lactobacilli in early infancy. Arch Dis Child, 65:185-8.

Hammerman, C.; Bin-Nun, A. & Kaplan, M. (2004) Germ warfare: probiotics in defence of premature gut. Clin Perinat,31: 489-500.

Hammerman, C.; Bin-Nun, A. & Kaplan, M. (2006). Safety of probiotics: comparison of two popular strains. , 11;333:1006-8.

Heiman, H. & Schanler, R.J. (2007) Enteral nutrition for premature infants: the role of human milk. Semin Fetal Neonatal, 12:26-34.

Hatakka, K.; Blomgren, K.; Pohjavuori, S. et al. (2007). Treatment of acute otitis media with probiotics in otitis-prone children-a doubleblind, placebo-controlled randomised study. Clin Nutr, 26(3):314–321

Kalliomäki, M.; Kirjavainen, P.; Eerola, E. et al. (2001) Distinct patterns of neonatal gut microflora in infants in whom atopy was and was not developing. J Allergy Clin Immunol, 107(1):129 –134

Kalliomäki, M. ; Salminen, S. ; Poussa, T. et al (2003) Probiotics and prevention of atopic disease: 4-year follow-up of a randomised placebo-controlled trial. Lancet, 361(9372):1869 –1871

Karvonen, A.; Casas, I. & Vesikari, T (2001). Safety and possible antidiarrhoeal effect of the probiotic Lactobacillus reuteri after oral administration to neonates, Clin Nutr ,20;63:abstract 216.

Langhendries, J.P.; Detry, J.; Van Hees, J. et al (1995) Effect of a fermented infant formula containing viable bifidobacteria on the fecal flora composition and pH of healthy full-term infants. J Pediatr Gastroenterol Nutr, 21:177-81.

Lin, J.S.; Chiu, Y.H.; Lin, N.T. et al. (2009) Different effects of probiotic species/strains on infections in preschool children: A double-blind, randomized, controlled study. Vaccine, 27(7):1073–1079

Mackie, R.I.; Sghir, A. & Gaskins, H.R. (1999) Developmental microbial ecology of the neonatal gastrointestinal tract. Am J Clin Nutr, 69:1035S-1045S.

Mai ,V.; & Morris, J.G. (2004). Colonic bacterial flora: changing understandings in the molecular age, J Nutr, 134:459-64

Majamaa, H. & Isolauri, E. (1997) Probiotics: a novel approach in the management of food allergy. J Allergy Clin Immunol, 99(2): 179 –185

Manzoni, P.; Pedicino, R.; Stolfi, I.; Decembrino, L.; Castagnola, E.; Pugni, L.; Corbo, M. & the Neonatal Fungal Infections Task Force of the Italian Neonatology Society. (2004). Criteri per una corretta Diagnosi delle Infezioni Fungine Sistemiche Neonatali in TIN: i suggerimenti della Task Force per le Infezioni Fungine Neonatali del G.S.I.N, Pediatr Med Chir, 26:89-95.

Montalto, M.; D'Onofrio, F.; Gallo, A.; Cazzato, A. & Gasbarrini G. (2009) Intestinal microbiota and its functions. Digestive and Liver Disease Supplements 3: 30–34

Neaville, W.A.; Tisler, C.; Bhattacharya, A. et al. (2003) Developmental cytokine response profiles and the clinical and immunologic expression of atopy during the first year of life. J Allergy Clin Immunol, 112(4): 740 –746

Neish, A.S. (2002) The gut microflora and intestinal epithelial cells: a continuing dialogue. Microbes Infect, 4: 309-17

Olivares, M.; Diaz-Ropero, M.P.; Gomez, N. et al (2006) The consumption of two new probiotic strains, Lactobacillus gasseri CECT 5714 and Lactobacillus coryniformis CECT 5711, boosts the immune system of healthy humans. Int Microbiol 9(1):47–52

Oliveri, S.; Trovato, L.; Betta, P.; Romeo, M.G. & Nicoletti, G. (2008). Experience with the Platelia Candida ELISA for the diagnosis of invasive candidosis in neonatal patients, Clinical Microbiology and Infection,14:377-397.

Osborn, D.A. & Sinn, J.K. (2007) Probiotics in infants for prevention of allergic disease and food hypersensitivity. Cochrane Database Syst Rev, (4):CD006475

Pappas, P.G.; Rex, J.H.; Sobel, J.D.; Filler, S.D.; Dismukes, W.E.; Walsh, T.J. & Edwards, J.E. (2004). Guidelines for treatment of Candidiasis, Clin Infectious Disease,38:161-89

Penders, J.; Stobberingh, E.E.; van den Brandt, P.A. et al. (2007) The role of the intestinal microbiota in the development of atopic disorders. Allergy, 62(11):1223–1236

Prescott, S.L. & Björkstén, B. (2007) Probiotics for the prevention or treatment of allergic diseases. J Allergy Clin Immunol, 120(2): 255–262

Ramesh, A.; Nidhi, S.; Rama, C.; Ashok, D.; Vinod, K.P.; Ira, G.H. & Pinaki, P. (2003). Effect of oral Lactobacillus GG on Entyeric Microflora in Low Birth-Weight in Neonates. JPGN, 36:397-402.

Rautava, S. (2007) Potential uses of probiotics in the neonate. Semin Fetal Neonatal Med, 12(1):45-53.

Romeo, M.G.; Romeo, D.M.; Trovato, L. et al. (2011) Role of probiotics in the prevention of the enteric colonization by Candida in preterm newborns: incidence of late-onset sepsis and neurological outcome. J Perinatol, 31(1):63-9.

Sakata, H.; Yoshioka, H. & Fujita, K. (1985) Development of the intestinal flora in very low birth weight infants compared to normal full-term newborns. Eur J Pediatr,144:186-90.

Taylor, A.L.; Dunstan, J.A. & Prescott SL. (2007) Probiotic supplementation for the first 6 months of life fails to reduce the risk of atopic dermatitis and increases the risk of allergen sensitization in high-risk children: a randomized controlled trial. J Allergy Clin Immunol, 119(1): 184 –191

Tsang, R.C.; Uauy, R.; Koletzko, B. & Zlotkin, S.H. Nutrition of the Preterm infant. Scientific Basis and Pratical Guidelines. Cincinnati, Digital Educational Publishing 2005.

Vanderhoof, J.A. & Young, R.J. (1998) Use of probiotics in childhood gastrointestinal disorders Journal of pediatrics, 27:323-332

Vanderhoof, J.A. (2000) Probiotics and intestinal inflammatory disorders in infant and children. Journal of Pediatric Gastroenterology and Nutrition, 30:534-38

Viljanen, M.; Savilahti, E.; Haahtela, T. et al. (2005) Probiotics in the treatment of atopic eczema/dermatitis syndrome in infants: a double-blind placebo-controlled trial. Allergy, 60(4):494 –500

Weizman, Z. & Alsheikh, A. (2006) Safety and tolerance of a probiotic formula in early infancy comparing two probiotic agents: a pilot study. J Am Coll Nutr, 25(5):415-9.

Weston, S.; Halbert, A.; Richmond, P. et al (2005) Effects of probiotics on atopic dermatitis: a randomised controlled trial. Arch Dis Child. 90(9):892– 897

Winkler, P.; de Vrese, M.; Laue, C. et al. (2005) Effect of a dietary supplement containing probiotic bacteria plus vitamins and minerals on common cold infections and cellular immune parameters. Int J Clin Pharmacol Ther, 43(7):318–326

Zoetendal, E.G.; Collier, C.T.; Koike, S.; Mackie, R.I. & Gaskins, H.R. (2004) Molecular ecological analysis of the gastrointestinal microbiota: a review. J Nutr, 134:465-72.

2

Probiotics – What They Are, Their Benefits and Challenges

M.S. Thantsha, C.I. Mamvura and J. Booyens
University of Pretoria
South Africa

1. Introduction

This chapter reviews literature on probiotics. Probiotics are defined and different microbial cultures used as probiotics will be considered. It further discusses delivery vehicles for probiotic cultures, with their advantages and disadvantages. Since the presence of viable probiotic cultures in products is vital to their functionality, different methods used for their detection in products will be examined. The beneficial health effects of probiotics, the methods that are currently used in an attempt to overcome some of the challenges faced will also be discussed. Different strategies for protection of probiotic cultures and challenges for the probiotic industry are highlighted. In addition to these, alternative strategies increasing numbers of beneficial microorganisms through administration of prebiotics and synbiotics are briefly mentioned.

2. What are probiotics?

The definition of probiotics has been modified with increasing knowledge in the field of how they function. The term is derived from the Greek language meaning 'for life'. In the past there have been many attempts to define the term 'probiotic', one of the first being described by Lilly & Stillwell in 1965. They defined probiotics as "substances secreted by one microorganism, which stimulates the growth of another". The focus of this definition was to distinguish them from and make it clear that they are the opposite of antibiotics. Subsequently, in 1974, Parker defined them as "organisms and substances which contribute to intestinal microbial balance" (Schrezenmier & de Vrese, 2001). In 1989, Fuller tried to improve on Parker's definition by proposing the following definition: "live microbial feed supplement, which beneficially affect the host (animal or human) by improving its intestinal microbial balance" (Salminen et al., 1999; Vilsojevic & Shah, 2008). Then, Havenaar & Huis In't Veld (1992) defined probiotics acceptably as 'a viable mono- or mixed culture of microorganisms which applied to animal or man, beneficially affects the host by improving the properties of the indigenous microflora'. Schrezenmeir & de Vrese (2001) defined the term probiotic as "a preparation of or a product containing viable, defined microorganisms in sufficient numbers, which alter the microflora by implantation or colonization, in a compartment of the host and by that, exert beneficial effects on host health". Among these descriptions and definitions, there were many others, until the Food and Agriculture Organization of the United Nations-World Health Organization (FAO-WHO) officially defined probiotics as: "live microorganisms that when administered in adequate amounts confer a significant health benefit on the host" (FAO, 2001). This definition was later endorsed by the International Scientific Association for Probiotics and Prebiotics (ISAPP) and is currently the most accepted definition of probiotics by scientists worldwide (Reid, 2006).

Probiotic food cultures have become popular due to appreciation of their contribution to good health (Desmond et al., 2002). In probiotic therapy, these beneficial microorganisms are ingested and thereby introduced to the intestinal microflora intentionally. This results in high numbers of beneficial bacteria to participate in competition for nutrients with and starving off harmful bacteria (Mombelli & Gismondo, 2000). The probiotics take part in a number of positive health promoting activities in human physiology (Chen & Yao, 2002).

The beneficial effects of the ingested probiotic bacteria are provided by those organisms that adhere to the intestinal epithelium (Salminen et al., 1998). The presence and adherence of probiotics to the mucous membrane of the intestines build up a strong natural biological barrier for many pathogenic bacteria (Chen & Yao, 2002). Adhesion is therefore regarded as the first step to colonization. Adhesion to the epithelium can be specific, involving adhesion of bacteria and receptor molecules on the epithelial cells, or non-specific, based on physicochemical factors.

2.1 Desirable properties for a probiotic strain

A microbial strain has to fulfil a number of specific properties or criteria for it to be regarded as a probiotic. These criteria are classified into safety, performance and technological aspects (Gibson & Fuller, 2000). The criteria are further dependent on specific purpose of the strain and on the location for the expression of the specific property. With regards to safety, the probiotic strain must be of human origin, isolated from the gastrointestinal tract (GIT) of healthy individuals. They should possess GRAS (generally regarded as safe) status, be non-pathogenic, and without previous association with diseases such as infective endocarditis or gastrointestinal disorders. Probiotic strains must not deconjugate bile salts and they should carry no antibiotic resistance genes that can be transferred to pathogens (Collins et al., 1998; Saarela et al., 2000). The strain must not induce an immune reaction in the host, i.e. the host must be immuno-tolerant to the probiotic (Havenaar & Huis int'Veld, 1992). The strain itself, its fermentation products or its cell components after its death, should be non-pathogenic, non-toxic, non-allergic, non-mutagenic or non-carcinogenic even in immunocompromised individuals (Collins et al., 1998; Havenaar & Huis int'Veld, 1992). It must have antimutagenic and anticarcinogenic properties and not promote inflammation in individuals (Collins et al., 1998). A probiotic strain should possess a desirable antibiogram profile. It must also be genetically stable with no plasmid transfer mechanism (Havenaar & Huis int'Veld, 1992; Ziemer & Gibson, 1998).

With respect to their performance, potential probiotic strains should be acid-tolerant and therefore survive human gastric juice and bile. They must be able to survive in sufficient numbers and adhere to the intestinal mucosal surface in order to endure the GIT. They should have antagonistic activity against pathogens such as *Salmonella* species, *Clostridium difficile* and *Listeria monocytogenes* that adhere to mucosal surfaces. Lastly, probiotic strains should also stimulate an immune response, thereby positively influencing the host (Biavati et al., 2000; Kolida et al., 2006; Mattila-Sandholm et al., 2002; Saarela et al., 2000;). The probiotic should survive the environmental conditions in their target site of action and proliferate in this location (Havenaar & Huis int'Veld, 1992). That is, they should be able to adhere to and colonise the epithelial cell lining to establish themselves in the colon (Guarner & Schaafsma, 1998; Parracho et al., 2007). The ability to adhere to the epithelium secures the strain from being easily flushed out by peristaltic movements (Gupta & Garg, 2009). Technologically, a good probiotic strain should be easily, inexpensively reproducible (Charteris et al., 1998; Havenaar & Huis int'Veld, 1992). It must be able to withstand stress during processing and storage, with process and product application robustness (Charteris et al., 1998). The organism should be able to survive, in particular, the harsh environmental conditions of the stomach and small intestine (e.g. gastric and bile acids, digestive enzymes) (Dunne et al., 2001; Parracho et al., 2007).

In addition, technological aspects must be taken into account before selecting a probiotic strain. Strains should be capable of being prepared on a large scale and should be able to multiply rapidly, with good viability and stability in the product during storage. The strains must not produce off flavours or textures once incorporated into foods. They should be metabolically active within the GIT and biologically active against their identified target. Probiotic strains must be resistant to phages and have good sensory properties (Collins et al., 1998; Kolida et al., 2006; Lacroix & Yildirim, 2007; Mattila-Sandholm et al., 2002; Saarela et al., 2000;). Therefore probiotic containing foods and products need to be of good quality and must have high enough numbers of viable probiotic cells to ensure that consumers get the optimal benefits from the product (Alakomi et al., 2005). Probiotic strains have to be good vehicles for specific target delivery of peptides and recombinant proteins within the human GIT (Dunne et al., 2001; Parracho et al., 2007).

2.2 Common probiotic microorganisms

A number of microorganisms are currently used as probiotics. However, the most commonly used are bacteria belonging to the genera *Lactobacillus*, the first and largest group of microorganisms to be regarded as probiotics (Mombelli & Gismondo, 2000; Wolfson, 1999) and *Bifidobacterium*. These bacteria are indigenous to the human GIT (Bielecka et al., 2002; Tannock, 2001). They are known to have no harmful effects, which is in contrast to other gut bacteria (Kimoto-Nira et al., 2007). Species of Lactobacilli include *L. acidophilus, L. rhamnosus, L. casei, L. delbrueckii* ssp. *bulgaricus, L. johnsonii , L. reuteri, L. brevis, L. cellobiosus, L. curvatus, L. fermentum, L. gasseri* and *L. plantarum* (Krasaekoopt et al., 2003; Meurman & Stamatova, 2007). The most recognized bifidobacteria species used are *Bifidobacterium breve, B. animalis* subsp *lactis* formerly *B. lactis* (Masco et al., 2004) and *B. longum* biotypes *infantis* and *longum* (Masco et al., 2005).

Probiotics now include other lactic acid bacteria (LAB) from genera such as *Streptococcus, Lactococcus, Enterococcus, Leuconostoc, Propionibacterium,* and *Pediococcus* (Krasaekoopt et al., 2003; O'Sullivan et al., 1992; Power et al., 2008; Vandenplas et al., 2007; Vinderola & Reinheimer, 2003). Some countries are, however, concerned about the possible transfer of antibiotic resistance genes by some members of the *Enterococcus* (Lund & Edlund, 2001). Other non-related microbes used include bacteria such as non-pathogenic *E. coli* Nissle 1917 and *Clostridium butyricum* (Harish & Varghese, 2006), yeasts (*Saccharomyces cereviciae, Saccharomyces boulardii*), filamentous fungi (*Aspergillus oryzae*), and some spore forming bacilli (Fuller, 2003; Mombelli & Gismondo, 2000; Wolfson, 1999).

2.3 Probiotic products

Probiotics can be consumed either as food components or as non-food preparations (Stanton et al., 1998). Foods containing probiotics are referred to by others as functional foods. This refers to foods with nutrient or non-nutrient components that affect targeted function(s) in the body resulting in a positive health effect (Bellisle et al., 1998). Thus, functional foods have a physiological or psychological effect beyond basic nutritional value (Clydesdale, 1997). Several probiotic LAB strains are available to consumers in both traditional fermented foods and in supplemented form (Kourkoutas et al., 2005). The majority of probiotics are incorporated into dairy products such as milk powders, yoghurt, soft-, semi-hard and hard cheeses and ice cream (Desmond et al., 2005; Dinakar & Mistry, 1994; Stanton et al., 2001; Stanton et al., 2005). These products offer a suitable environment for probiotic viability and growth (Özer et al., 2009; Ross et al., 2002). There is an increase in use of other foods as vehicles for probiotics. This is partly due to allergenicity of some consumers to milk products. Non-dairy products such as malt-based beverages and fruit juices (Champagne & Raymond, 2008; Rozada-Sanchez et al., 2007; Sheehan et al., 2007), meat sausages (Ruiz-Moyano et al., 2008), capsules, and freeze-dried preparations (Berni-Carnani et al., 2007) are among these alternatives. Growing vegetarian alternatives have also led to soy-based probiotic foods (Farmworth et al., 2007). Recently, Aragon-Alegro et al. (2007) added probiotic chocolate mousse to the list of alternatives.

2.4 Beneficial effects of probiotics

The benefits attributed to probiotics can either be nutritional or therapeutic (Prasad et al., 1998). Benefits associated are, however, strain specific (Saarela et al., 2000).

2.4.1 Nutritional benefits

Microbial action in the gut, specifically by beneficial cultures, has been shown to enhance the bioavailability, quantity and digestibility of certain nutrients (Parvez et al., 2006). Ingestion of probiotics is associated with improved production of riboflavin, niacin, thiamine, vitamin B_6, vitamin B_{12} and folic acid (Gorbach, 1997; Hargrove & Alford, 1978). Probiotics play a role in increasing bioavailability of calcium, iron, manganese, copper, phosphorous (Alm, 1982; McDonough et al., 1983) and increase the digestibility of protein and fat in yoghurt (Fernandes et al., 1987). Enzymatic hydrolysis of protein and fat leads to an increase in free amino acids and short chain fatty acids (SCFAs). Organic acids such as acetate and lactate produced during fermentation by LAB lower the pH of intestinal contents thereby creating undesirable conditions for harmful bacteria (Mack et al., 1999; Parvez et al., 2006).

2.4.2 Therapeutic benefits

Patients prefer medicine with little or no side effects for treatment of their ailments. Probiotics provide such an alternative, being living, non-pathogenic organisms, which are extremely safe as indicated by their GRAS status. Probiotic bacteria are claimed to alleviate and prevent conditions such as lactose intolerance, allergies, diarrheal diseases, lowering of serum cholesterol, reduction of the risk associated with mutagenicity and carcinogenicity and inhibition of pathogens, as well as stimulation of the immune system (Collins & Gibson,

1999; Shah, 2007). Positive effects of probiotics are not confined to the gut only, but can extend to other parts of the body. For instance, probiotics are known to have anti-inflammatory benefit when administered parenterally (Shiel et al., 2004).

Lactose malabsorption (also referred to as lactose intolerance or lactose indigestion) is the inability to hydrolyze lactose (Adams & Moss, 2000; Salminen et al., 1998a). It is caused by a deficiency of the enzyme β-D-galactosidase (lactase) (Buller & Grand, 1990). The undigested lactose passes to the colon where it is attacked by resident lactose fermenters (Adams & Moss, 2000). Colonic lactose fermentation results in high levels of glucose in blood and hydrogen gas in breath (Buller & Grand, 1990; Mombelli & Gismondo, 2000; Scrimshaw & Murray, 1988; Shah, 1993; Vesa et al., 2000). Probiotics strains and the traditional yoghurt cultures, *Lactobacillus delbrueckii* spp. *bulgaricus* and *Streptococcus thermophilus* produce β-D-galactosidase thereby improving tolerance to lactose (Adams & Moss, 2000; Fooks et al., 1999, Shah, 2000c)

Constipation, a disorder of motor activity of the large bowel characterized by bowel movements that are less frequent than normal (Salminen et al., 1998b), pain during defecation, abnormal swelling and incomplete emptying of colon contents (Salminen et al., 1998a), can also be relieved by probiotic use. *Lactobacillus reuteri, Lactobacillus rhamnosus* and *Propionibacterium freudenreichii* are probiotic strains shown to improve the condition (Ouwenhand et al., 2002).

Incidences of antibiotic associated diarrhoea caused by *Clostridium difficile* (Fuller, 2003; Tuohy et al., 2003; Vasiljevic & Shah, 2008) and rotavirus diarrhoea (Salminen et al., 1998a) can also reduced by administration of probiotics. Strains associated with reduction of diarrhoea include *Bifidobacterium* spp, *B. animalis* Bb12 (Fuller, 2003, Guandalini et al., 2000), *L. rhamnosus* GG, *L. acidophilus, L. bulgaricus* (Fuller, 2003; Goldin, 1998; Gorbach, 2000; Sazawal et al., 2006) and *Saccharomyces boulardii* (Kotowska et al., 2005, Sazawal et al., 2006). The effect of probiotics against diarrhoea is the most researched and substantiated claim, with documented clinical applications (BergogneBérézin, 2000; Cremonini et al., 2002; Marteau et al., 2001, McNaught & MacFie, 2001; Reid et al., 2003; Sullivan & Nord 2005).

Inflammatory bowel disease (IBD) and irritable bowel syndrome (IBS) are other intestinal disorders that can be treated with varying degrees of success using probiotics. IBD is a collection of disorders including ulcerative colitis, Crohn's disease and pouchitis, characterized by chronic or recurrent inflammation, ulceration and abnormal narrowing of the GIT resulting in abdominal pain, diarrhoea and gastrointestinal bleeding (Hanauer, 2006; Marteau et al., 2001). IBS is typically characterized by abdominal pain, excessive flatus, variable bowel habit and bloating (Madden & Hunter, 2002). Several studies have been conducted to investigate the efficacy of probiotics in treatment of IBD (Guandalini, 2002; Ma et al., 2004; Zhang et al., 2005). The tested strains against IBD include among others VSL#3 probiotic (Gionchetti et al., 2000), *Bifidobacterium longum* (Furrie et al., 2005) and *Lactobacillus rhamnosus* GG (Gupta et al., 2000). Combination of *Lactobacillus acidophilus and Bifidobacterium infantis* (Hoyos, 1999) and of *Bifidobacterium bifidus, Bifidobacterium infantis* and *Streptococcus thermophilus* were shown to reduce incidences of ulcerative colitis (Bin-Nun et al., 2005). Several studies reported the success of bifidobacteria for the alleviation of IBS (O'Mahony et al., 2005; Brenner et al., 2009; Jankovic et al., 2010). Alfredo (2004) demonstrated the efficacy of *Lactobacillus plantarum* LP01 and *Bifidobaccterium breve* BR0 as short-term therapy for IBS. Although some of the results obtained were very encouraging, there is need for larger, randomized, double-blinded, placebo-controlled clinical trials to substantiate these claims.

Hereditary allergic conditions of increasing importance in developing countries such as eczema, asthma, atopic dermatitis and rhinitis can be treated with probiotics (Holgate, 1999; Kalliomaki et al., 2003; Salminen et al., 1998a). Tested probiotics with antiallergenic properties include *Bifidobacterium lactis* Bb-12 (Isolauri et al., 2000) and *Lactobacillus* GG (Isolauri et al., 2000; Kalliomaki et al., 2001; Kalliomaki et al., 2003; Lee et al., 2008; Mirkin, 2002; Vanderhoof & Young, 2003). However, contradictory studies report on the poor efficiency of probiotics in allergy alleviation (Helin et al., 2002; Vliagoftis et al., 2008) and highlight the need for more convincing and conclusive research in allergy treatment.

Probiotics have the ability to lower levels of cholesterol in serum, contributing to the prevention of cardiovascular disease (Fooks et al., 1999; Proviva, 2002). This ability has been shown for *Lactobacillus johnsonii* and *L. reuterii* using animal models (Mombelli & Gismondo, 2000). They also reduce the risk of cancer (Sanders, 1999) due to their activity against certain tumors (Chen & Yao, 2002). Several studies indicated that probiotics in a diet reduces the risk of cancer (Sanders, 1999). Anticarcinogenic effects of *Bifidobacterium bifidum* and *Lactobacillus acidophilus* were shown using clinical trials in humans (Fooks, 1999).

2.5 Mechanism of action of probiotics

Probiotic bacteria beneficially affect the individual by improving the properties of the indigenous microflora and its microintestinal balance (Betoret et al., 2003; Frost & Sullivan, 2000; Matilla-Sandholm et al., 2002; Saarela et al., 2000). They compete with disease causing bacteria for villi attachment sites and nutrients (Chen & Yao, 2002). Probiotic bacterial cultures encourage growth of beneficial microorganisms and crowd out potentially harmful bacteria thereby reinforcing the body's natural defence mechanisms (Saarela et al., 2000). They provide specific health benefits by modifying gut microflora, strengthening gut mucosal barrier, e.g. adherence of probiotics to the intestinal mucosa thereby preventing pathogen adherence, pathogen inactivation, modification of dietary proteins by intestinal microflora, modification of bacterial enzyme activity, and influence on gut mucosal permeability, and regulation of the immune system (Betoret et al., 2003; Krasaekoopt et al., 2003; Salminen et al., 1998).

The probiotic effect is accredited to their production of metabolic by-products such as acid, hydrogen peroxide, bacteriocins, e.g. lactocidin, and acidophilin that manifest antibiotic properties and inhibit the growth of a wide spectrum of pathogens and/or potential pathogens such as *Escherichia coli*, *Klebsiella*, *Enterobacter*, *Pseudomonas*, *Salmonella*, *Serratia* and *Bacteroides* (Chen & Yao, 2002; Krasaekoopt et al., 2003). Lactic acid bacteria inhibit growth of pathogenic microorganisms by producing short chain fatty acids such as acetic, propionic, butyric as well as lactic and formic acids which reduces intestinal pH. Lactic acid produced by bifidobacteria in substantial amounts has antimicrobial activity against yeasts, moulds and bacteria (Adams & Moss, 2000; Percival, 1997). These species are also active in reducing the faecal activity of enzymes implicated in the production of genotoxic metabolites such as β-glucoronidase and glycolic acid hydroxylase (Collins & Hall, 1984; Mombelli & Gismondo,

2000). Probiotic organisms produce enzymes that help in digestion of proteins, fats and lactose (Frost & Sullivan, 2000). They also produce β-galactosidase, an enzyme that aid lactose intolerant individuals with breaking down or digestion of lactose (Krasaekoopt et al., 2003).

Production of short chain fatty acids in the colon during fermentation by colonic microflora is the main process that prevents colorectal cancer (Holzapfel & Schillinger, 2002). Probiotic strains also reduce levels of some colonic enzymes such as glucoronidase, β-glucoronidase nitroreductase, azoreductase (Adams & Moss, 2000; Chen & Yao, 2002; Fooks et al., 1999; Gorbach, 2000) and glycoholic acid hydrolase. These enzymes convert procarcinogens to carcinogens such as nitrosamine or secondary bile acids (Chen & Yao, 2002). Low levels of these enzymes therefore decrease chances of cancer development in the colon (Gorbach, 2000; Kasper, 1998).

2.6 Methods for quantification of probiotic cultures

The methods used for detection of viable probiotic cells include conventional plate counts (culture dependent) and molecular techniques (culture-independent). The culture dependent method has been criticized for underestimation of counts due to bacteria forming chains and/or clumping and unsuitability (inappropriateness) of media for growing of viable but non-culturable cells (Auty et al., 2001; Lahtinen et al., 2006; Veal et al., 2000). Isolation media used may be insufficiently selective, affecting the reproducibility of results (Roy, 2001). These limitations of plate counting techniques prompted the use of molecular techniques and other alternative methods (Vitali et al., 2003). New methods include molecular based techniques such as quantitative real-time polymerase chain reaction (PCR), fluorescent *in situ* hybridization (FISH) (Boulos et al., 1999; Veal et al., 2000), confocal scanning laser microscopy (CSLM) (Auty et al., 2001; Gardiner et al., 2000; Palencia et al., 2008), flow cytometry (Alakomi et al., 2005) and microplate scale fluorochrome staining assay (Filoche et al., 2007; Mättö et al., 2006).

Flow cytometry is a rapid and sensitive technique that measures physiological characteristics such as membrane integrity, enzyme activity, respiration, membrane potential and intracellular pH (Bunthof et al., 2001) of each cell individually (Bunthoff & Abee, 2002). Microplate scale fluorochrome staining assay is appropriate for assessing viability of fresh, freeze-dried and stressed cells. It can detect changes in the condition of probiotic cells earlier than can be done with conventional cultivation methods (Filoche et al., 2007; Mättö et al., 2006).

The fluorescence based molecular techniques are used in conjunction with viability staining techniques. A number of commercial techniques are available. LIVE/DEAD® *Bac*Light™ and BD Cell viability assay kit (BD Biosciences, Oxford, UK) are some examples. LIVE/DEAD® *Bac*Light consists of two nucleic acid stains SYTO® 9 and propidium iodide (PI). Green-fluorescent SYTO9 (excitation and emission maxima, 480 and 500 nm, respectively) penetrates both viable and nonviable cells. Red-fluorescent PI (excitation and emission maxima, 490 and 635 nm, respectively) penetrates cells with damaged cell membranes (Auty et al., 2001). The BD Cell viability assay kit (BD Biosciences, Oxford, UK) contains the stains, thiazole orange and propidium iodide (Doherty et al., 2009). Cells stained using these kits can also be assessed using microscopes, which will also distinguish between 'live' (e.g. green-stained) from 'dead' (e.g. red-stained) cells (Berney et al., 2007).

All the above mentioned methods have their own disadvantages. For example, the viability kits and real time PCR are based on bacterial DNA which is not only present in live cells but can also be retained by dead cells in significant amounts. Both PCR and FISH are not independent as they require determination of a standard curve which is determined most of the times using standard plate counts. PCR requires expensive reagents which cannot be afforded by everyone in the industry. Detection limits for PCR and FISH are relatively high, being about 10^4 cells/ml and 10^6 cells/ ml, respectively. FISH is based on detection of 16s rRNA whose presence is not a direct proof of metabolic activity but rather an indication of potential viability (Biggerstaff, 2006). Real-time PCR and FISH have a limitation whereby counts of bacteria decreased but PCR and FISH results remained higher over the experimental period. This is due to detection of high levels of rRNA and DNA in dead cells. The intensity of rRNA in dead cells may still be strong enough for visually counting (detection) though it is expected to decrease upon cell death. Thus, the RNA content of the cell detected by fluorescent probes cannot be regarded as reliable indicator of cellular viability (Vives-Rego et al., 2000). Also, real time PCR detects both viable and non-viable bacteria, thus does not provide information on the condition of the cells and results in an overestimation of metabolically active cells (Kramer et al., 2009; Masco et al., 2007).

The appropriateness of PCR for quantification of viable cells can be improved by staining the samples with DNA binding dyes prior to DNA extraction and amplification. Treatment with DNA-binding dyes and subsequent PCR analysis uses membrane integrity as the criterion in determining viability of cells. Live cells are able to exclude DNA-binding dyes such as ethidium monoazide (EMA) and propidium monoazide (PMA), while dead cells or those whose membrane integrity has been compromised are able to pick-up these stains (Kramer et al., 2009). These dyes form covalent bonds with DNA upon exposure to visible bright light and thus inhibit subsequent PCR amplification. Only DNA from live cells with intact membranes is selectively amplified (Nocker et al., 2009).

Despite some of its drawbacks, the plate count method is traditionally used to assess cell viability in probiotic preparations (Alakomi et al., 2005). Though plate counting is arduous and time consuming, no method has yet been found that completely replaces it. Therefore it is still being routinely used in assessing viability of probiotic cultures in various foods, often in conjunction with culture-independent methods (Lopez-Rubio et al., 2009; Masco et al., 2005; Temmerman et al., 2003b).

2.7 Probiotic challenges

Commercially, viable probiotic strains are incorporated into fermented food products or are supplied as freeze-dried supplements or pharmaceutical preparations (Holzapfel & Schillinger, 2002). The basic requirement for probiotics is that products should contain sufficient numbers of microorganisms up to the expiry date (Fasoli et al., 2003). Thus, probiotics must contain specific strains and maintain certain numbers of live cells for them to produce health benefits in the host (Mattila-Sandholm et al., 2002). Different countries have decided on the minimum number of viable cells required in the probiotic product for it to be beneficial. In Australia, a minimum viable count of 10^6 organisms per gram should be available in fermented milk products at the end of the shelf life (Wahlqvist, 2002). However, according to Krasaekoopt et al. (2003), there are no specifications as to how many probiotics should be available in Australian fermented products. The same minimum count (10^6

organisms per gram) was approved by countries of MERCOSUR which includes Argentina, Paraguay, Brazil and Uruguay (Krasaekoopt et al., 2003). In products containing multiple probiotic organisms, at least a million of each of them per gram should be present to produce required beneficial effects (Wahlqvist, 2002). In Japan, a minimum of 10^7 viable cells per millilitre of fresh dairy product is required. The South African legislation states that functional foods containing probiotic bacteria must deliver 1×10^8 bacterial cells per day. A daily intake of 10^9 to 10^{10} cfu viable cells is considered the minimum dose shown to have positive effects on host health (Fasoli et al., 2003). This could be achieved by consuming 100 g of a product containing between 10^6 and 10^7 viable cells g^{-1} daily (Boylston et al., 2004).

Low viability of probiotic cultures in yoghurt has been reported (Kailasapathy & Rybka, 1997; Lourens-Hattingh & Viljoen, 2001; Shah, 2000).

Retention of viability of the probiotic bacteria presents a major marketing and technological challenge for application of probiotic cultures in functional foods (Desmond et al., 2002; Mattila-Sandholm et al., 2002). Many active cultures die during manufacturing, storage or transport of the finished product (Siuta-Cruce & Goulet, 2001) and also during the passage to the intestine (Sakai et al., 1987; Siuta-Cruce & Goulet, 2001; Park et al., 2002). Thus, the majority die even before the consumer receives any of the health benefits (Siuta-Cruce & Goulet, 2001). A serious problem of shelf instability had been encountered with dried cultures. Refrigerated products also have short lives due to negative effects of low temperature and formation of crystals on bacterial cells. The numbers of viable bacteria continually decrease with time during refrigerated storage (Porubcan et al., 1975). Market surveys have revealed much lower counts in the products even before the expiry date (Talwalkar et al., 2001). Shelf life for probiotics is thus unpredictable; hence, the industry has had difficulty backing up label claims (Siuta-Cruce & Goulet, 2001). Excesses of 50 to 200 % cells have been incorporated into products in an attempt to make-up for cells that die during storage. For example, in tablets containing dry cells, where the tablets are labelled as containing a certain minimum count of active cells per tablet, to be safe, the manufacturer must incorporate an excess of cells at the time the tablets are manufactured, thereby assuring that the labelling will remain accurate while the product is in stock by the retailers. This practice increases the cost and makes the use instructions inaccurate (Porubcan et al., 1975).

Probiotics, after surviving food processing, are upon consumption then exposed to conditions prevailing in the stomach and small intestine before they reach their site which is the colon (Siuta-Cruce & Goulet, 2001; Hansen et al., 2002; Lian et al., 2002). The microbes may die during their transit through the upper intestinal tract to the colon and therefore they may not be able to colonize the colon (Talwakar et al., 2001). They must therefore survive gastric acidity and bile salts which they encounter during their passage through the GIT (Hansen et al., 2002; Lian et al., 2002; Sakai et al., 1987; Siuta-Cruce & Goulet, 2001;). Their survival in the GI T depends on the strain and species-specific resistance to low pH (pH values ranging from 1.3 to 3.0) in gastric juice and to bile salts found in the small intestine (Hansen et al., 2002; Lian et al., 2002).

Probiotic bacteria can only perform when they find adequate environmental conditions and when they are protected against stresses (e.g extreme temperatures, high pressure, shear forces) they encounter during their production at the industry level or in the GIT (gastric acids and bile salts) (Siuta-Cruce & Goulet, 2001). Factors affecting viability during storage such as temperature, moisture, light and air should also be taken into consideration (Percival, 1997; Mattila-Sandholm et al., 2002). Oxygen toxicity is another major problem in the survival of probiotic bacteria in dairy foods. High levels of oxygen in the product are detrimental to the viability of these anaerobic bacteria (Talwakar et al., 2001).

Manufacturers of probiotics are facing the challenge that they should produce probiotic cultures that can survive for long periods, and are resistant to acidity in the upper intestinal tract so that they can reach the colon in high numbers to colonize the epithelium. Probiotic cultures should therefore be produced in a way that will protect these sensitive bacteria from unfavourable interactions with detrimental factors (Siuta-Cruce & Goulet, 2001).

In view of the health benefits associated with probiotics, it is not surprising that there is increasing interest in their viability. Probiotics do not have a long shelf life in their active form. Refrigeration is required in most cases to maintain shelf life as high temperatures can destroy probiotic cultures (Saxelin et al., 1999). However, most probiotics still have a short shelf-life even under low temperature storage (Lee & Salminen, 1995). There is low recovery of viable bacteria in products claiming to contain probiotic bacteria (Hamilton-Miller et al., 1999; Temmerman et al., 2003a).

The preservation of these probiotic microorganisms presents a challenge because they are affected by exposure to temperature, oxygen and light (Bell, 2001; Chen et al., 2006). Survival of most bifidobacteria in most dairy products is poor due to low pH and/or exposure to oxygen (Gomes & Malcata, 1999). Naturally many LAB may excrete exo-polysaccharides to protect themselves from harsh conditions but this is usually not enough to give them full protection (Shah, 2002).

2.8 Methods for improving probiotic viability

In view of the health benefits associated with probiotics, it is not surprising that there is an increasing interest in their viability. The common practice is storage at refrigerated temperatures to prolong their shelf life (Saxelin et al., 1999). Nevertheless, most of them still have a short shelf-life (Lee & Salminen, 1995). There is low recovery of viable bacteria in products claiming to contain probiotic bacteria (Hamilton-Miller et al., 1999; Temmerman et al., 2003a).

Viability of probiotics is reduced as a result of their exposure to high temperature, oxygen, low pH and light (Bell, 2001; Chen et al., 2006; Gomes & Malcata, 1999). Naturally many LAB may excrete exo-polysaccharides (EPS) to protect themselves from harsh conditions. However, protection afforded by these EPS is not sufficient (Shah, 2002). As a result, researchers are continuously searching for ways to improve survival of probiotic cultures during processing, storage and GIT transit. Different approaches are used in an attempt to preserve viability of probiotic cultures. These include among others, pre-exposure of probiotic cultures to sub-lethal stresses (Desmond et al., 2002) and incorporation of micro-nutrients such as peptides and amino acids (Shah, 2000). The disadvantage of pre-exposure to sublethal stresses is that it may result in significant decreases in cellular activity, cell yield and process volumetric productivity (Doleyres & Lacroix, 2005). Other alternative methods for improving probiotic viability are genetic modification (Sheehan et al., 2006; Sheehan et al., 2007; Sleator & Hill, 2007), immobilization (Doleyres et al., 2004), two-step fermentations, use of oxygen-impermeable containers and microencapsulation (Özer et al., 2009). Of these techniques, microencapsulation is relatively new and has been investigated by various researchers.

Microencapsulation is a process by which solids, liquids or gases are packaged into miniature, sealed microcapsules that can release their contents at controlled rates under influences of specified conditions (Anal et al., 2006; Anal & Singh, 2007). It stabilizes the probiotics, increases their survival during processing and storage, controls the oxidative reaction, ensures sustained or controlled release at a specific target site (both temporal and time-controlled release) and improves shelf life (Anal & Singh, 2007; Dembczynski & Jankowski, 2002). The encapsulated probiotics are released from the microparticles as a result of many factors such as changes in pH and/or temperature (Gibbs et al., 1999; Vasishtha, 2003). These changes may cause microcapsule walls to swell and rupture or dissolve (Franjione & Vasishtha, 1995; Brannon-Peppas, 1997).

Microparticles reduce loss of probiotic cell viability by blocking reactive components such as atmospheric moisture, oxygen (Kim et al., 1988; Krasaekoopt et al., 2003; Reid, 2002; Siuta-Cruise & Goulet, 2001; Vasishtha, 2003), high temperature, pressure, bacteriophage attack and cryoeffects (Krasaekoopt et al., 2003). Studies have indicated that probiotic cultures enclosed within solid fat microcapsules retain both their activity and vitality (Krasaekoopt et al., 2003).

Methods of microencapsulation used in pharmaceutical and food industries are classified as either physical or chemical. Physical methods include pan coating, air-suspension coating, centrifugal extrusion, vibrational nozzle and spray drying (Anal & Singh, 2007), spray coating, annular jet, spinning disk, spray cooling, spray drying and spray chilling (Versic, 1988), extrusion coating, fluidized bed coating, liposome entrapment, coarcervation, inclusion complexation, centrifugal extrusion and rotational suspension separation (Vasishtha, 2003). Chemical methods include interfacial polymerization, *in-situ* polymerization, matrix polymerization(Vidhyalakshmi et al., 2009) and extrusion. Extrusion and emulsion techniques are the mostly commonly used methods (Krasaekoopt et al., 2003).

There is a diversity of materials used for encapsulation of probiotics. These include among others, alginate (Chandramouli et al., 2004; Dembczynski & Jankowski, 2002; Hansen et al., 2002; Krasaekoopt et al., 2003; Sultana et al., 2000), κ-carrageenan, locust bean gum, cellulose acetate phthalate, chitosan, gelatin (Krasaekoopt et al., 2003), cellulose (Chan & Zhang, 2002), pectin, whey protein (Guerin et al., 2003) and rennet (Heidibach et al., 2009). These materials are used either as supporting materials or gelling agents by different investigators.

Although generally there are positive effects of microencapsulation, this method is not without disadvantages. Some types of the resulting microparticles may shrink and lose mechanical strength due to their sensitivity to acids (Sun & Griffiths, 2000), may present problems for large scale production, others require use of potassium ions that should not be taken in large amounts in diet, (Sun & Griffiths, 2000), some of the polysaccharides used are prohibited in specific foods in other countries (Picot & Lacroix, 2004). Additionally and possibly the key disadvantage, is that the mentioned microencapsulation methods use water and other organic solvents whose use is less favoured due to their high costs and concerns about their negative environmental impacts (Sihvonen et al., 1999).

Progress towards elimination of use of organic solvents has been made with development of microencapsulation technique using supercritical technology (Moolman et al., 2006). This microencapsulation technique is based on the formation of an interpolymer complex between poly (vinyl pyrrolidone) (PVP) and poly (vinyl acetate-co-crotonic acid) (pVA-CA) in supercritical carbon dioxide ($scCO_2$). A supercritical substance is neither a gas nor a liquid but possesses properties of both, making it unique (Moshashaee et al., 2000). Since supercritical fluids have a wide spectrum of solvent characteristics, they can be used as solvents in different techniques (Frederiksen et al., 1997). Microparticles produced using this method have suitable morphological characteristics, encapsulation efficiency and affords encapsulated probiotic cultures protection in simulated gastrointestinal fluids (Mamvura et al., 2011; Thantsha et al., 2009).

2.9 Concerns about probiotics

Although there are numerous advantages and health benefits associated with probiotics or probiotic food products, there are risks associated with probiotic therapy. These risks are mainly concerned with respect to safety in vulnerable target groups such as immunocompromised individuals (pregnant women, babies and the elderly) or critically ill or hospitalized patients (Boyle et al., 2006; Jankovic et al., 2010).

Probiotic cultures are resistant to some antibiotics. There is concern about the possible transfer of antimicrobial resistance from probiotic strains to pathogenic bacteria in the gut. For example, many *Lactobacillus* strains are naturally resistant to vancomycin, which poses a potential threat of transfer of this resistance to other pathogenic bacteria such as *Staphylococcus aureus*. However, these vancomycin-resistant genes in lactobacilli are chromozomal and not readily transferred to other species.

Another important area of concern is the risk of sepsis. There have been several reports of cases of *Lactobacillus* sepsis and other bacterial sepsis due to the intake of probiotic supplements (Boyle et al., 2006). One case included a 67 year-old man who was taking probiotic capsules daily for mitral regurgitation and developed *Lactobacillus rhamnosus* endocarditis after a dental procedure (Borriello et al., 2003; Mackay et al., 1999). In another case, a 4-month old infant with antibiotic-associated diarrhoea, who was given *Lactobacillus rhamnosus* after cardiac surgery, developed *Lactobacillus* endocarditis 3 weeks after *Lactobacillus rhamnosus* treatment (Boyle et al., 2006; Kunz et al., 2004). However, there have been no reports to date on the occurrence of *Bifidobacterium* sepsis. All cases of bacterial sepsis from the use of probiotics (*Lactobacillus* spp.) have occurred in immunocompromised individuals or patients who have a chronic disease or debilitation. No cases have been reported in healthy individuals (Boyle et al., 2006). There have also been several cases of fungemia associated with *Saccharomyces boulardii*. However, investigation of these cases revealed that the infection was due to contamination of inserted catheters. It is therefore now recommended that *Saccharomyces boulardii* probiotics be prepared in powdered form under stringent hygienic conditions to prevent contamination (Borriello et al., 2003; Salminen et al., 1998). There is a small risk of adverse metabolic effects from manipulation of the microbiota with the use of probiotics, although probiotic studies to date have not shown significant adverse effects on growth or nutrition (Boyle et al., 2006). A review of safety assessments of probiotics was recently published (Sanders et al., 2010).

3. Prebiotics

Prebiotics are non-digestible food ingredients that beneficially affect the host by selectively stimulating the growth and/or activity of one or a limited number of colonic bacteria and thereby improve host health (Femia et al., 2002; Gibson & Roberfroid, 1995; Roberfroid, 1998; Theuer et al., 1998; Tuohy et al., 2003; Young, 1998). Gibson et al. (2004) redefined them as 'a selectively fermented ingredient that allows specific changes; both in the composition and/or activity in the gastrointestinal microflora that confers benefits to host well-being and health'. The refined definition takes into account both the microbial changes and the nutritional and physiological benefits attributed to prebiotics. Just like probiotics, they modulate the composition of the natural ecosystem though probiotics does so through introduction of exogenous bacteria into the colon (Bouhnik et al., 2004). Prebiotics pass through the upper GIT unfermented and are only utilized in the colon and are therefore called 'colonic food' (Roberfroid, 2000). Non-digestibility can be demonstrated *in vitro* by subjecting the carbohydrates to pancreatic and small intestinal enzymes. It can be shown *in vivo* on human subjects with an ileostomy (i.e people who have had their large intestine removed and have a stoma at the end of the ileum) (van Loo et al., 1999). Compounds that are not digested and absorbed by the host but are preferentially fermented by *Bifidobacterium* species in the colon are called 'bifidogenic' factors (Shah, 2007). Prebiotics are not readily digested by pathogenic bacteria (Annika et al., 2002; Farmer, 2002; Femia et al., 2002). They favour or promote growth of potentially health-promoting bacteria such as lactobacilli and bifidobacteria, thereby allowing them to be predominant (Bouhnik et al., 2004; Flamm et al., 2001; Gibson et al., 1999; Roberfroid, 1998; Wang, 2009). This subsequently leads to predominant numbers of the stimulated endogenous bacteria in faeces as well (Femia et al., 2002; Losada & Olleros, 2002). Scientific studies in Japan indicated that consumption of prebiotics increases the populations of bifidobacteria and other beneficial microorganisms even in the absence of probiotics in diet. The selective stimulation of growth of bifidobacteria by prebiotics is characterized by a substantial decrease in numbers of potentially pathogenic bacteria (Losada & Olleros, 2002).

The following criteria are used for selection of a carbohydrate as a prebiotic: It must not be absorbed in the stomach or small intestine; It must be selectively fermented by the beneficial gut microflora; It should also stimulate the growth and/or activity of beneficial bacteria; Its fermentation should induce the beneficial luminal or systemic effects within the host; It must be resistant to gastric acidity and mammalian enzyme hydrolysis (Kolida, et al., 2002; Manning and Gibson, 2004).

Classes of non-digestible oligosaccharides (NDOs) commercially available are cyclodextrins, fructooligosaccharides (FOS), gentiooligosaccharides, glycosylsucrose and isomaltulose (also known as palatinose). Other classes include lactulose, lactosucrose and maltooligosaccharides (Sako et al., 1999). NDOs such as inulin, fructooligosaccharide, lactulose and dietary fibre are common prebiotics (Davis & Milner, 2009). There are conflicting views on the prebiotic classification of resistant starch. Some researchers classify it as a prebiotic (Douglas & Sanders, 2008) while others (Shah, 2004) differ, arguing that resistant starch is not digested by some beneficial bacteria, and therefore cannot be classified as a prebiotic. Inulin and FOS are the only NDOs that have been sufficiently studied to give adequate data to analyze their functional properties (Roberfroid, 2000). Galacto-oligosaccharides (GOS), gluco-oligosaccharides, lactulose, isomalto-oligosaccharides, raffinose, transgalacto-oligosaccharides, xylo-oligosaccharides, soya bean oligosaccharides and oat β-glucans are considered as prebiotic candidates (Lomax & Calder, 2009). Other NGOs such as lactulose (Crittenden & Playne, 1996) and xylobiose (Vazquez et al., 2000) are also included in the prebiotic category. All the prebiotic candidates except maltooligosaccharides, glycosylsucrose and cyclodextrins are reported as being bifidogenic (Ziemer & Gibson, 1998).

Prebiotics are found naturally in a number of materials. Honey, fruits and vegetables such as artichoke, asparagus, banana, barley, chicory, garlic, leeks, oats, onion, rye, soybeans, tomatoes and wheat are sources of non-digestible oligosaccharides, especially inulin (Davis & Milner, 2009; Femia et al., 2002; Losada & Olleros, 2002; Manning & Gibson, 2004; Mussatto & Mancilha, 2007; Sangeetha et al., 2005). They are also present in burdock, Chinese chives, garlic, graminae (fodder grass), pine, even bacteria and yeasts (Bengmark et al., 2001; Ziemer & Gibson, 1998). Honey and bamboo shoots are natural sources of isomaltulose (Lina et al., 2002). Raffinose and stachyose can be found in soyabeans and other leguminous seeds and pulses (Voragen, 1998). Milk is a good source of glycoproteins and oligosaccharides (lacto-N-tetraose and lacto-N-neotetraose), including those believed to be prebiotic (Alander et al., 2001; Newburg, 2000; Petschow & Talbott, 1991). Human milk contains more galactooligosaccharides than cow's milk. Oligosaccharides can be found in levels as high as (12g/l), making them the third bulkiest constituent of human milk (Newburg et al., 2004). Taking foods containing prebiotic oligosaccharides is not enough for modulation of gut flora as they are present in only small concentrations in these foods. Instead, prebiotics are extracted from these foods and transferred into more commonly ingested foodstuffs like biscuits and other carbohydrate based materials (Taylor et al., 1999).

These natural compounds can also be produced commercially through enzyme hydrolysis and extraction processes (Losada & Olleros, 2002; Mussatto & Mancilha, 2007; Sako et al., 1999). The enzymes employed include β-D-fructofuranosidase or fructosyltransferase, which joins the fructose molecules by means of transfructosylation mechanisms (Losada & Olleros, 2002). These mechanisms are employed for production of oligosaccharides with the exception of raffinose, soybean oligosaccharides and lactulose (Mussatto & Mancilha, 2007; Sako et al., 1999). Raffinose and soybean oligosaccharides are extracted directly from plant materials using solvents such as water, aqueous methanol or ethanol (Johansen et al., 1996; Mussatto & Mancilha, 2007). Lactulose is produced by enzymatic action of β-galactosidases (E.C 3.2.1.23) on lactose. The glucose moiety is converted to a fructose residue by alkali isomerization and the process results in a lactulose disaccharide (Villamiel et al., 2002). Inulin can also be extracted from chicory (*Cichorium intybus*) and then partially hydrolyzed to short-chain fructans (oligofructose) using inulase (E.C 3.2.1.7) or to long chain fructans by applying an industrial separation technique (Roberfroid, 2000). Additionally, inulin type fructans can be manufactured through transfer of fructosyl residue to and between sucrose molecules using fungal fructosyl transferases (E.C 2.4.1.9) (Cummings & Roberfroid, 1997). FOSs are manufactured from sucrose using the trans-fructosylation activity of β-fructofuranosidase (E.C 3.2.1.26). Alternatively, FOS can are produced by controlled enzymatic hydrolysis of inulin (Crittenden & Playne, 1996; Frost & Sullivan, 2000). Lactose is also used in the industrial production of GOS through the transgalactosylation activity of β-galactosidases (Sako et al., 1999). The production of FOS and GOS requires high concentrations of the starting material for efficient transglycosylation (Park & Almeida, 1991). GOS are synthesized from lactose syrup using the enzyme β-galactosidase (Frost & Sullivan, 2000; Gibson, 2004). They are neither hydrolyzed nor absorbed in the human intestine and act as a substrate for bifidobacteria (Frost & Sullivan, 2000). Soy oligosaccharides are extracted directly from soybean whey. Their bifidogenecity has been confirmed in humans (Frost & Sullivan, 2000).

3.1 Beneficial effects of prebiotics

In the last decade there have been numerous investigations on the health-promoting effects of prebiotics. Bifidogenic oligosaccharides increase the level of nutrient supplementation and enhance nutrient solubility (Farmer, 2002). Some of these effects include better mineral absorption, alleviation of constipation and irritable bowel syndrome, protection against colon cancer, enhancement of the immune system, anticarcinogenic effects and lowering of cholesterol (Davis & Milner, 2009; Manning & Gibson, 2004; Tuohy et al., 2003; Venter, 2007). Supplementation of diet with oligofructose and inulin-type oligosaccharides significantly lowers serum triglycerols and phospholipids. This hypotriacylyglycerolaemic effect could be caused by a decrease in the concentration of plasma very low-density lipoproteins (VLDL) (Delzenne et al., 1993; Fordaliso et al., 1995). Prebiotics acidifies colonic contents by increasing the concentration of short-chain carboxylic acids. They also aid in colonic absorption of minerals, particularly Mg^{2+} and Ca^{2+}. Mineral absorption is promoted through establishment of an osmotic effect whereby entry of water into the colon increases dissolution of minerals (Roberfroid, 2000).

Ingestion of prebiotics is also associated with relief of constipation due to faecal bulking and possible effects on intestinal motility, aiming at daily defecation. They suppress diarrhoea when it is associated with intestinal infections. They also reduce the risk of osteoporosis when improved bioavailability of calcium due to use of inulin-type fructans is followed by significant increase in bone density and bone mineral content. Prebiotics reduce the risk of obesity and possibly type-2 diabetes (van Loo et al., 1999).

Most of the studies on prebiotic effects on bone development have been done on animal models, particularly rats (Scholz-Ahrens, 2007). *In vivo* studies carried out on humans showed that inulin and oligofructose increase the absorption of calcium but not iron, zinc or magnesium (Coudray et al., 1997). More research needs to be done to substantiate these claims, including that of bowel cancer prevention (Ziemer & Gibson, 1996). Studies that have been carried out on animal models so far have shown promise, though human studies are required (Reddy et al., 1997; Rowland et al., 1998). It is vital for studies conducted *in vitro* on prebiotic effects to be carried out *in vivo* in well-designed and reproducible experiments.

Prebiotics, unlike probiotics, are not living organisms, and therefore they do not have survival problems both in the products and the gut (Frost & Sullivan, 2000). Prebiotics have an advantage over probiotics in that they are not affected by factors such as oxygen and heat in industrial applications. This attribute led to increased interest in their health issues (Kolita et al., 2002). Some commercially available prebiotic supplements are water-soluble. Solubility in water allows their possible incorporation in any type of food and also renders them undetectable once dissolved (Douglas & Sanders, 2008).

However their excess levels can cause symptoms such as flatulence, bloating and diarrhoea. This may be caused by a change in osmotic potential or due to excessive fermentation.

Undesirable effects occur when very high doses are ingested. This is advantageous as it allows a relatively broad "therapeutic window", i.e. the dose above the minimal effective level (Holzapfel & Schillinger, 2002). However, FOSs are slightly laxative and produce flatulence when taken in high doses (Losada & Olleros, 2002).

4. Synbiotics

Synbiotics are preparations containing a mixture of a probiotic and a prebiotic, or a combination of probiotics and prebiotics (Davis & Milner, 2009; Holzapfel & Schillinger, 2002; Touhy et al., 2003). These preparations aim to improve the viability of the proven probiotic *in vivo* as well as stimulate the indigenous gut microflora. They provide both the beneficial microbial culture and a specific substrate that can be readily available for fermentation by this culture (Gallaher & Khil, 1999). The presence of the readily fermentable substrate could enhance the survival of the probiotic. The prebiotic ingredient could also offer protection of probiotic against gastric acidity and proteolysis, probably through steric hindrance and coating of the probiotic.

Synbiotic supplements available include combinations of bifidobacteria and FOS, *Lactobacillus* GG and inulin and a combination of bifidobacteria lactobacilli with either FOS or inulin. Fermented milks contain both live beneficial bacteria and fermentation products that may positively stimulate the intestinal microflora also fall within this category. Crittenden et al. (2006) encapsulated a *B. infantis*-FOS synbiotic within a film-forming protein-carbohydrate-oil emulsion to improve its survival and viability during non-refrigerated storage and GIT transit. Gallaher et al. (1996) observed a comparable synbiotic effect with oligofructose and bifidobacteria. Lactobacilli/lacitol, and bifidobacteria/GOS combinations have also been tried as synbiotics in addition to bifidobacteria/FOS (Mountzouris et al., 2002). A well-known benefit of synbiotics is that they increase the persistence of the probiotic in the GIT (Tuohy et al., 2003). The use of synbiotics has not been extensively explored, though studies indicated positive results with regard to maintenance of gut microflora (Shimizu et al., 2009). Their possible use for prevention of allergic diseases is just an example of the studies that still needs to be covered (Johannsen & Prescott, 2009).

5. Conclusion

Probiotics are beneficial microorganism with a host of benefits for the consumer though some of these benefits still have to be confirmed using clinical trials. There is however still a problem of maintenance of viability of these cultures both in storage and in the gastrointestinal tract. The search for methods that can protect and retain viability of probiotic cultures is still on going. There are also concerns about the negative effects of probiotics on sensitive consumers but there is insufficient evidence to support the raised concerns. Prebiotics and synbiotics are alternative mechanisms for increasing the levels of beneficial microorganisms in the gut.

6. References

Adams, M.R. & Moss, M.O., 2000. Food Microbiology. Second Edition, The Royal Society of Biochemistry, Cambridge, UK, pp. 318-323.

Alakomi, H-L, Matto, J, Virkajarvi, I & Saarela, M 2005, 'Application of a microplate scale fluorochrome staining assay for the assessment of viability of probiotic preparations', Journal of Microbiological Methods 62, 25-35.

Alander M., Mättö J., Kneifel W., Johansson M., Kögler B., Crittenden R., Mattila-Sandholm T. & Saarela M. 2001. Effect of galactooligosaccharide supplementation on human faecal microflora and on survival and persistence of *Bifidobacterium lactis* Bb-12 in the gastrointestinal tract. International Dairy Journal 11, 817-825.

Alfredo S. 2004. Probiotics in the treatment of irritable bowel syndrome. Journal of Clinical Gastroenterology 38, S104-S106.

Alm L. 1982. Effect of fermentation on lactose, glucose and galactose content in milk and suitability of fermented milk products for lactose-deficient individuals. Journal of Dairy Science 65, 346-352.

Al-Saleh, A.A., 2003. Growth, bile tolerance and enzyme profiles of various species of Bifidobacteria. Internet:
http://ift.confex.com/ift/2000/techprogram/paper_2983.htm.

Anal A.K. & Singh H. 2007. Recent advances in microencapsulation of probiotics for industrial and applications and targeted delivery. Trends in Food Science & Technology 18, 240-251.

Anal A.K., Stevens W.F., & Remuñán-López C. 2006. Ionotropic cross-linked chitosan microspheres for controlled release of ampicillin. International Journal of Pharmaceutics 312, 166-173.

Annika, M., Tarja, S. & Outi, V., 2002. Combination of probiotics. World Patent no. WO02060276.

Auty M.A.E., Gardiner G.E., McBrearty S.J., O'Sullivan O.E., Mulvihill D.M., Collins J.K., Fitzgerald G.F., Stanton C., Ross R.P. 2001. Direct in situ viability assessment of bacteria in probiotic dairy products using viability staining in conjunction with confocal scanning laser microscopy. Applied and Environmental Microbiology 67, 420-425

Bell L.N. 2001. Stability testing of nutraceuticals and functional foods. In R.E.C Wildman (Ed.), Handbook of nutraceuticals and functional foods. New York: CRC Press, 501-516

Bengmark, S., García de Lorenzo, A. & Culebras, J.M., 2001. Use of pro-, pre-and synbiotics in the ICU: Future options. Nutrición Hospitalaria. 6, 239-256.

BergogneBérézin, E., 2000. Treatment and prevention of antibiotic associated diarrhea. International Journal of Antimicrobial Agents 16, 521-526.

Betoret, N., Puente, L., Díaz, M.J., Pagán, M.J., García, M.J., Gras, M.L., Martínez-Monzó, J. & Fito, P., 2003. Development of probiotic-enriched dried fruits by vacuum impregnation. Journal of Food Engineering 56, 273-277.

Biavati, B, Vescoco, M, Torriani, S & Bottazzi, V 2000, 'Bifidobacteria: history, ecology, physiology and applications', Annals of Microbiology 50, 117-131.

Bielecka M., Biedrzycka E., Majkowska A. 2002. Selection of probiotics and probiotics for synbiotics and confirmation of their in vivo effectiveness. Food Research International 35, 125-131.

Biggerstaff, J. P., Puil, M. L., WEidow, B. L., Prataer, J., Glass, K., Radosevich, M. & White, D.C. 2006. New methodology for viability testing in environmental samples. Molecular and Cellular probes 20, 141-146.

Bin-Nun A., Bromiker R., Wilschanski M., Kaplan M., Rudensky B., Caplan M., 2005. Oral probiotics prevent necrotising enterocolitis in very low birth weight neonates. Journal of Paediatrics 147, 192-196.

Borriello, S.P., Hammes, W.P., Holzapfel, W, Marteau, P, Schrezenmeir, J, Vaara, M & Valtonen, V 2003, 'Safety of probiotics that contain lactobacilli or bifidobacteria', Clinical Infectious Diseases 36, 775-780.

Bouhnik, Y., Vahedi, K., Achour, L., Attar, A., Salfati, J., Pochart, P., Marteau, P., Flourié, B., Bornet, F. & Rambaub, J-C., 1999. Short chain oligosaccharides administration dose dependently increases bifidobacteria in healthy humans. Journal of Nutrition 129, 113-116.

Boulos, L., Prévost, M., Barbeau, B., Coallir, J., & Desjardins R. 1999. LIVE/DEAD® BacLight ™: application of a new rapid staining method for direct enumeration of viable and total bacteria in drinking water. Journal of Microbiological methods 37, 77-86.

Boyle, R.J, Robins-Browne, R.M & Tang, M.L.K 2006, Probiotic use in clinical practice: what are the risks?, American Journal of Clinical Nutrition 83, 1256-1264.

Boylston, T.D., Vinderola, C.G., Ghoddusi, H.B. & Reinheimer, J.A., 2004. Incorporation of bifidobacteria into cheeses: challenges and rewards. International Dairy Journal 14, 375-387.

Bunthof, C.J., Bloemen, K, Breeuwer, P, Rombouts, F.M & Abee, T 2001, 'Flow Cytometric Assessment of Viability of Lactic Acid Bacteria', *Applied and Environmental Microbiology*, vol. 67, no. 5, pp. 2326-2335.

Brannon-Peppas, L. 1997. Polymers in controlled drug delivery. Biomaterials 11, 1-14.

Brenner D.M., Moeller M.J., Chey W.D., Schoenfeld S. 2009. The utility of probiotics in the treatment of irritable bowel syndrome: A systemic review. American journal of Gastroenterology 104, 1033-1049.

Bryers, J.J. 1990. Biofilms in Biotechnology. In: Characklis, W.G., Marshall, K.C. (Eds.), Biofilms, Wiley and Sons, New York, pp. 733-734.

Buller H.A. & Grand R.J. 1990. Lactose intolerance. Annual Reviews in Medicine 41, 141-148.

Champagne C.P and Raymond Y. 2008. Viability of Lactobacillus Rhamnosus R0011 in an apple-based fruit juice under simulated storage at the consumer level. Journal of Food Science 73, M221-M226.

Chan E.S. and Zhang Z. 2002. Encapsulation of probiotic *Lactobacillus acidophilus* by direct compression. Food and Bioproducts Processing 80, 78-82.

Chandramouli V., Kailasapathy K., Peiris P., Jones M., 2004. An improved method of microencapsulation and its evaluation to protect *Lactobacillus* spp. in simulated gastric conditions. Journal of Microbiological Methods, 56, 27-36.

Charalampopoulos, D., Wang, R., Pandiella, S.S. & Webb, C., 2002. Application of cereals and cereal components in functional foods: a review. International Journal of Food Microbiology 79, 131-141.

Charteris W.P., Kelly P.M., Morelli L. & Collins J.K. 1998. Development and application of an in vitro methodology to determine the transit tolerance of potentially probiotic

Lactobacillus and Bifidobacterium species in the upper human gastrointestinal tract. Journal of Applied Microbiology 84, 759-768.

Chen, B.H. & Yao, Y.Q., 2002. Beneficial microbe composition, new protective material for the microbes, method to prepare the same and uses thereof. US Patent 6368591.

Collins, E.B. & Hall, B.J., 1984. Growth of Bifidobacteria in milk and preparation of *Bifidobacterium infantis* for a dietary adjunct. Journal of Dairy Science 67, 1376-1380.

Collins M.D. & Gibson G.R. 1999. Probiotics, prebiotics, and synbiotics: approaches for modulating the microbial ecology of the gut. American Journal of Clinical Nutrition 69, 1052S-1057S.

Collins J.K, Thornton G and Sullivan G.O. 1998. Selection of probiotic strains for human applications. International Dairy Journal 8, 487-490.

Coudray C., Bellanger J., Catiglia-Delavaud C, Remesy C., Vermorel M. & Rayssignuier Y. 1997. Effect of soluble and partly soluble dietary fibre supplementation on absorption and balance of calcium, magnesium, iron, and zinc in healthy young men. European Journal of Clinical Nutrition 51, 375-380

Cremonini, F., Di Caro, S., Santarelli, L., Gabrielli, M., Candelli, M., Nista, E.C., Lupascu, A., Gasbarrini, G. & Gasbarrini, A., 2002. Probiotics in antibiotic-associated diarrhea. Digestive and Liver Disease 21, S78-S80.

Crittenden R.G & Playne M.J. 1996. Production, properties and applications of food grade oligosaccharides. Trends in Food Science & Technology 7, 353-361.

Cummings J.H & Roberfroid M.B. 1997. A new look at dietary carbohydrate: chemistry, physiology and health. European Journal of Clinical Nutrition 51, 417-442.

Dairy Council of California, 2003. Probiotics: Friendly Bacteria with a Host of Benefits. Internet: http://www.dairycounsilofca.org/media/medi_topi_probio.htm. Access date: 14/04/2003

Davis, D.C & Milner, J.A 2009, 'Gastrointestinal microflora, food components and colon cancer prevention', Journal of Nutritional Biochemistry 20, 743-752.

Delzenne N.M., Kok N., Fiordaliso M.F, Deboyser D.M., Goethals F.M., Roberfroid M.B. 1993. Dietary fructooligosaccharides modify lipid metabolism. American Journal of Clinical Nutrition 57, S820.

Dembczynski R. & Jankowski T. 2002. Growth characteristics and acidifying activity of *Lactobacillus rhamnosus* in alginate/starch liquid-core capsules. Enzyme and Microbial Technology 31, 111-115.

Demirbaş, A., 2001. Supercritical fluid extraction and chemicals from biomass with supercritical fluids. Energy Conversion and Management. 42, 279-294.

Desmond, C., Stanton, C., Fitzgerald, G.F., Collins, K. & Ross, R.P., 2002. Environmental adaptation of probiotic lactobacilli towards improvement of performance during spray drying. International Dairy Journal 12, 183-190.

Dinakar P. and Mistry V.V. 1994. Growth and viability of *Bifidobacterium bifidum* in cheddar cheese. Journal of Dairy Science 77, 2854-2864.

Doherty S.B., Gee V.L., Ross R.P., Stanton C., Fitzgerald G.F., Brodkorb A. 2010. Efficacy of whey protein gel networks as potential viability-enhancing scaffolds for cell immobilisation of Lactobacillus rhamnosus GG. Journal of Microbiological Methods 80, 231-241.

Doleyres Y., Fliss I., and Lacroix C. 2004. Increased stress tolerance of *Bifidobacterium longum* and *Lactococcus lactis* produced during continuous mixed-strain immobilized-cell fermentation. Journal of Applied Microbiology 97, 527-539.

Doleyres Y. & Lacroix C. 2005. Technologies with free and immobilised cells for probiotic bifidobacteria production and protection. International Dairy Journal 15, 973-988.

Douglas L.C. and Sanders M.E. 2008. Probiotics and prebiotics in dietetics practice. Journal of the American dietetic association 108, 510-521.

Dunne C., O'Mahony L., Murphy L., Thornton G., Morrissey D., O'Halloran S.Feeney M., Flynn S., Fitzgerald G., Daly C., Kiely B., O'Sullivan G.C., ShanahanF. & Collins J.K. 2001. *In vitro* selection criteria for probiotic bacteria of human origin: correlation with *in vivo* findings. American Journal of Clinical Nutrition 73, 386S-392S.

Food and Agriculture Organization of the United Nations (FAO). 2001. Health and Nutritional Properties of Probiotics in Food including Powder Milk with Live Lactic Acid Bacteria,
http://www.who.int/foodsafety/publications/fs_management/en/probiotics.pdf

Farmer, S., 2002. Probiotic, lactic acid-producing bacteria and uses thereof. US Patent no. 6461607.

Fasoli, S., Marzotto, M., Rizzotti, L., Rossi, F., Dellaglio, F. & Torriani, S., 2003. Bacterial composition of commercial probiotic products as evaluated by PCR-DGGE analysis. International Journal of Food Microbiology 82, 59-70.

Femia, A.P., Luceri, C., Dolara, P., Giannini, A., Biggerei, A., Salvadori, M., Clune, Y., Collins, K.J., Paglierani, M. & Caderni, G., 2002. Antitumorigenic activity of the prebiotic inulin enriched with oligofructose in combination with the probiotics *Lactobacillus rhamnosus* and *Bifidobacteriun lactis* on azoxymethane-induced colon carcinogenesis in rats. Carcinogenesis 23, 1953-1960.

Fernandes C.F., Shahani K.M., Amer M.A. 1987. Therapeutic role of dietary lactobacilli and lactobacillic fermented dairy products. FEMS Microbiology Reviews 46, 343-356

Filoche S.K., Angker L., Coleman M.J., Sissons C.H., 2007. A fluorescence assay to determine the viable biomass of microcosm dental plaque biofilms. Journal of Microbiological Methods, 69, 3, 489-496.

Finch, C. A., 1993. Industrial Microencapsulation:Polymers for microcapsule walls. In: Karsa, D. R., Stephenson, R. A. (Eds), Encapsulation and controlled release. The Royal Society of Chemistry, Cambridge, pp. 1-12.

Flamm, G., Glinsmann, W., Kritchevsky, D., Prosky, L. & Roberfroid, M., 2001. Inulin and oligofructose as dietary fiber: A review of the evidence. Critical Reviews in Food Science and Nutrition 41, 353-362.

Fooks, L.J., Fuller, R. & Gibson G.R., 1999. Prebiotics, probiotics and human gut microbiology. International Dairy Journal 9, 53-61.

Franjione J. & Vasishtha N. 1995. The art and science of microencapsulation, Technology Today. Summer 1995.

Frederiksen L., Anton K., van Hoogevest P., Keller H.R., Leueberger H. 1997. Preparation of liposomes encapsulating water-soluble compounds using supercritical carbon dioxide. Journal of Pharmaceutical Sciences 86, 921-928 .

Fuller, R., 2003. Probiotics - what they are and what they do.
http://www.positivehealth.com/permit/Articles/Nutrition/fuller32.htm.

Furrie E., Macfarlane S., Kennedy A., Cummings J.H., Walsh S.V., O'Niell D.A., Macfarlane G.T. 2005. Synbiotic therapy (*Bifidobacterium longum*/Synergy 1) initiates resolution of inflammation in patients with active ulcerative colitis: a randomised controlled pilot trial. Gut 54, 242-249.

Gallaher, D.D. & Khil, J., 1999. The effect of synbiotics on colon carcinogenesis in rats. Journal of Nutrition 129, 1483S-14867S.

Gibbs, B.F., Kermasha, S., Alli, I. & Mulligan, C.N., 1999. Encapsulation in the food industry: a review. International Journal of Food Sciences and Nutrition 50, 213-224.

Gibson, G.R & Fuller, R 2000, 'Aspects of in vitro and in vivo research approaches directed towards identifying probiotics and prebiotics for human use', Journal of Nutrition, 130, 391-395.

Gibson G.R. & Roberfroid M.B. 1995. Dietary modulation of the human colonic microbiota:introducing the concept of prebiotics. Journal of Nutrition 125, 1401-12.

Gibson G.R., Probert H.M., Van Loo J., Rastall R.J., Roberfroid M.B. 2004. Dietary modulation of the human colonic microbiota: updating the concept of prebiotics. Nutrition Research Reviews 17, 259-275.

Gionchetti P., Rizzello F., Venturi A., Brigidi P., Matteuzzi D., Bazzocchi G., Poggioli G., Miglioli M., Campieri M. 2000. Oral bacteriotherapy as maintenance treatment in patients with chronic pouchitis: A double-blind, placebo-controlled trial. Gastroenterology 119, 305-309.

Goldin, B.R., 1998. Health benefits of probiotics. British Journal of Nutrition 20, S202-S207.

Gomes A.M.P., Malcata F.X. 1999. *Bifidobacterium* spp and *Lactobacillus*: biological, biochemical, technological, and therapeutical properties relevant for use as probiotics. Trends in Food science and technology 10, 139-157.

Gorbach S.L. 1997. Health benefits of probiotics. IFT Annual Meeting, Orlando, FL, Abstract 73-1.

Guarner F. & Schaafsma G.J. 1998. Probiotics. International Journal of Food Microbiology 39, 237-238.

Guandalini S., Pensabene L., Zikri M.A., Dias J.A., Casali L.G., Hoekstra H 2000. *Lactobacillus* GG administered in oral rehydration solution to children with acute diarrhea: A multicenter European trial. Journal of Paediatric Gastroenterology and Nutrition 30, 214-216.

Gupta P., Andrew H., Kirschner B.S., Guandalini S. 2000. Is *Lactobacillus* GG helpful in children with Crohn's disease? Results of a preliminary, open-label study. Journal of Paediatric Gastroenterology and Nutrition 31, 453-457.

Hamilton-Miller J.M.T., Shah S., Winkler J.T. 1999. Public health issues arising from microbiological and labelling quality of foods and supplements containing probiotic microorganisms. Public Health Nutrition 2, 223-229.

Hanauer S.B. 2006. Inflammatory bowel disease: Epidemiology, pathogenesis, and therapeutic opportunities. Inflammatory Bowel Diseases 12, S3-S9.

Hansen, L.T., Allan-Wojtas, P.M., Jin, Y.-L. & Paulson, A.T., 2002. Survival of Ca-alginate microencapsulated *Bifidobacterium* spp. in milk and simulated gastrointestinal conditions. Food Microbiology 19, 35-45.

Hargrove R.E. and Alford J.A. 1978. Growth rate and feed efficiency of rats fed yoghurt and other fermented milks. Journal of Dairy Science 61, 11-19.

Harish, K. & Varghese, T., 2006. Probiotics in humans – evidence based review. Calicut Medical Journal 4, e3.

Havenaar R., & Huis int'Veld J.H.J. 1992. Probiotics: a general view. The Lactic Acid Bacteria in Health and Disease (Wood BJB, ed), pp. 209–224. Chapman & Hall, New York.

Heidibach T., Forst P. & Kulozik U. 2009. Microencapsulation pf probiotic cells by means of rennet-gelation of milk-proteins. Food Hydrocolloids 23, 1670-1677.

Helin T., Haahtela S. & Haahtela T. 2002. No effect of oral treatment with an intestinal bacterial strain, *Lactobacillus rhamnosus* (ATCC 53103), on birch-pollen allergy: a placebo-controlled double-blind study. Allergy 57, 243-246

Hénon, F.E., Camaiti, M., Burke, A.L.C., Carbonell, R.G., DeSimone, J.M. & Piacenti, F., 1999. Supercritical CO_2 as a solvent for polymeric stone protective materials. Journal of Supercritical fluids 15, 173-179.

Holgate S.T., 1999. The epidermic of allergy and asthma. Nature 402, B2-B4.

Holzapfel, W.H. & Schillinger, U., 2002. Introduction to pre- and probiotics. Food Research International 35, 109-116.

Hoyos A.B. 1999. Reduced incidence of necrotising enterocolitis associated with enteral administration of *Lactobacillus acidophilus* and *Bifidobacterium infantis* to neonates in an intensive care unit. International Journal of Infectious Diseases 3, 197-202.

Isolauri, E., Arvola, T., Sutas, Y., Moilanen, E. & Salminen, S., 2000. Probiotics in the management of atopic eczema. Clinical and Experimental Allergy 30, 1604-1610.

Jankovic I., Sybesma W., Phothirath P., Ananta E., Mercenier A. 2010. Application of probiotics in food products-challenges and new approaches. Current Opinion in Biotechnology 21, 175-181Johansen H.N., Glitso V., & Knudsen K.E.B. 1996. Influence of extraction solvent and temperature on the quantitative determination of oligosaccharides from plant materials by high-performance liquid chromatography. Journal of Agricultural and Food Chemistry 44, 1470-1474

Johannsen H. & Prescott S.L. 2009. Practical prebiotics, probiotics and synbiotics for allergists: how useful are they? Clinical and experimental allergy 39, 1801-1814.

Kailasapathy, K. & Chin. J., 2000. Survival and therapeutic potential of probiotic organisms with reference to *Lactobacillus acidophilus* and *Bifidobacterium spp.* Immunology and Cell Biology 78, 80-88.

Kailasapathy K. & Rybka S. 1997. *Lactobacillus acidophilus* and *Bifidobacterium* spp.: Their therapeutic potential and survival in yoghurt. The Australian Journal of Dairy Technology 52, 28-35.

Kalai, V., 1996. Probiotic characteristics of Bifidobacteria spp. by in vitro assessment. PhD thesis. Universiti Pitra Malaysia.

Kalliomaki, M., Salminen, S., Arvilomni, H., Kero, P., Koskinen, P. & Isolauri, E., 2001. Probiotics in primary prevention of atopic disease: a randomised placebo-controlled trial. Lancet 357, 1076-1079.

Kalliomaki M., Salminen S., Poussa T., Arvilommi H., Isolauri E. 2003. Probiotics and prevention of atopic disease: 4-year follow-up of a randomised placebo-controlled trial. The Lancet 361, 1869-187.

Kanafani, H. & Mize L., 2002. Process for producing extended shelf life ready-to-use milk compositions containing probiotics. World patent no: WO02102168.

Kießling, G., Schneider, J. & Jahreis, G., 2002. Long-term consumption of fermented dairy products over 6 months increases HDL cholesterol. European Journal of Clinical Nutrition 56, 843-849.

Kim, H.S., Kamara, B.J., Good, I.C. & Enders Jr, G.L., 1988. Method for preparation of stabile microencapsulated lactic acid bacteria. Journal of Industrial Microbiology 9, 253-257.

Kimoto-Nira H., Mizumachi K., Nomura M., Kobayashi M., Fujita Y., Okamoto T., Suzuki I., Tsuji N.M., Kurisaki J., and Ohmomo S. 2007. Review: *Lactococcus* sp. as potential probiotic lactic acid bacteria. Japan Agricultural Research Quarterly 41, 181-189.

Kolida, S, Saulnier, D.M & Gibson, G.R 2006, 'Gastrointestinal Microflora: Probiotics', Advances in Applied Microbiology 59, 187-219.

Kotowska, M., Albrecht, P. & Szajewska, H., 2005. *Saccharomyces boulardii* in the prevention of antibiotic-associated diarrhea in children: a randomized double-blind placebo-controlled trial. Alimentary Pharmacology and Therapeutics 21, 583-590.

Kramer M., Obermajer N., Matijasic B.B., Rogelj I., Kmetec V. 2009. Quantification of live and dead probiotic bacteria in lyophilised product by real-time PCR and by flow cytometry. Applied Genetics and Molecular Biotechnology 84, 1137-1147.

Krasaekoopt W., Bhandari B., Deeth H., 2003. Evaluation of encapsulation techniques   of probiotics for yoghurt. International Dairy Journal, 13, 3-13.

Kunz, A.N., Noel, J.M & Fairchock, M.P 2004, 'Two cases of *Lactobacillus* bacteremia during probiotic treatment of short gut syndrome', Journal of Pediatric Gastro-enterol Nutrition 38, 457-458.

Lacroix C. & Yildirim S. 2007. Fermentation technologies for the production of probiotics with high viability and functionality. Current Opinion in Biotechnology 18, 176-183.

Lahtinen, S.J., Gueimande, M., Ouwehand A. C., Reinikainen, J. P & Salminen, S.J. 2006. Comparison of four methods to enumerate probiotic bifidobacteria in a fermented food product. Food Microbiology 23, 571-577.

Leahy, S.C., Higgins, D.G., Fitzgerald, G.F. & van Sinderen, D., 2005. Getting better with bifidobacteria. Journal of Applied Microbiology 98, 1303-1315.

Lee Y.K and Salminen S. 1995. The coming of age of probiotics. Trends in Food science & Technology 6, 241-245.

Lian, W.-C., Hsiao, H.-C. & Chou, C.-C., 2002. Viability of encapsulated bifidobacteria in simulated gastric juice and bile solution. International Journal of Food Microbiology 2679, 1-9.

Lomax A.R., and Calder P.C. 2009. Prebiotics, immune function, infection and inflammation: a review of the evidence. British Journal of Nutrition 101, 633-658.

Losada, M.A. & Olleros, T., 2002. Towards a healthier diet for the colon: the influence of fructooligosaccharides and lactobacilli on intestinal health. Nutrition Research 22, 71-84.

Lourens-Hattingh A. & Viljoen B. C. 2001. Review: Yoghurt as probiotic carrier food. International Dairy Journal 11, 1-17.

Luchansky, J.B. & Tsai, S., 1999. Probiotic bifidobacterium strain. US Patent no. 5902743.

Lund B., and Edlund C. 2001. Probiotic *Enterococcus faecium* strain is a possible recipient of the vanA gene cluster. Clinical Infectious Diseases 32, 1384-1385.

Madden J.A.J and Hunter O. 2002. A review of the role of gut microflora in irritable bowel syndrome and the effects of probiotics. British Journal of Nutrition 88, S67-S72.

Ma D., Forsythe P., Bienenstock J. 2004. Live *Lactobacillus reuteri* is essential for the inhibitory effect on tumour necrosis alpha-induced interleukin-8 expression. Infection and Immunity 72, 5308-5314.

Mackay, A.D., Taylor, M.D., Kibbler, C.C & Hamilton-Miller, J.M 1999, ' *Lactobacillus endocarditis* caused by a probiotic organism', Clinical Microbial Infections, vol. 5, pp. 290-292.

Mamvura, C. I., Moolman, F. S., Kalombo,L., Hall, A. N. & Thantsha, M. S, Characterisation of the Poly-vinylpyrrolidone)-Poly-(vinylacetate-Co-Crotonic Acid) (PVP:PVAc-CA) interpolymer complex matrix microparticles encapsulating a *Bifidobacterium lactis* Bb12 probiotic Strain. Probiotics & Antimicrobial Proteins(2011) 3:97–102.

Manning, T.S & Gibson, G.R 2004, 'Microbial-gut interactions in health and disease. Prebiotics', *Best* Practice and Research. Clinical Gastroenterology, vol. 18, no. 2, pp. 287-298.

Marteau, P.R., de Vrese, M., Cellier, C.J. & Schreimeir, J., 2001. Protection from gastrointestinal diseases with the use of probiotics[1-3], American Journal of Clinical Nutrition 73, 430S-436S.

Masco L., Huys G., De Brandt E., Temmerman R., Swnings J. 2005. Culture-dependent and culture-independent qualitative analysis of probiotic products claimed to contain bifidobacteria. International Journal of Food Microbiology 102, 221-230.

Matilla-Sandholm, T., Myllärinen, P., Crittenden, R., Mogensen, G., Fondén, R. & Saarela, M., 2002. Technological challenges for future probiotic foods. International Dairy Journal 12, 173-182.

McDonough F., Wells P., Wong N., Hitchins A., Bodewell C. 1983. Role of vitamins and minerals in growth stimulation of rats fed with yoghurt. Federation Proceedings 42, 556-558.

McNaught, C.E. & MacFie, J., 2001. Probiotics in clinical practice: a critical review of evidence. Nutrition Research 21, 343-353.

Meurman J.H and Stamatova I. 2007. Probiotics: contributions to oral health. Oral diseases 13, 443-451.

Mirkin, M.D., 2002. Atopic dermatitis eczema:
http://www.drmirkin.com/morehealth/G108.htm.

Mombelli, B. & Gismondo, M.R., 2000. The use of probiotics in medical practice. International Journal of Antimicrobial Agents 16, 531-536.

Moshashaee S., Bisrat M., Forbes R.T., Nyqvist H., York P. 2000. Supercritical fluid processing of proteins 1: Lysozyme precipitation from organic solution. European Journal of Pharmaceutical Sciences 11, 239-245.

Moolman F. S., Labuschagne P.W., Thantsha M.S., Rolfes H., Cloete T.E. 2006. Encapsulating probiotics with an interpolymer complex in supercritical carbon dioxide. South African Journal of Science 102, 349-354.

Mountzouris K.C., McCartney A.L., and Gibson G.R. 2002. Intestinal microflora of human infants and current trends for its nutritional information: Review. British Journal of Nutrition 87, 405-420.

Mussato S.I. and Mancilha I.M. 2007. Non-digestible oligosaccharides: A review. Carbohydrate polymers 68, 587-597.

Newburg D.S. 2000. Oligosaccharides in human milk and bacterial colonisation. Journal of Paediatric Gastroenterology and Nutrition 30, S8- S17.

Newburg D.S., Ruiz-Palacios G.M.L.,Altaye M., Chaturvedi P., Meinzen-Derr J., de Lourdes Guerrero M., Morrow A.L. 2004. Innate protection conferred by fucosylated oligosaccharides of human milk against diarrhea in breastfed infants. Glycobiology 14, 253-263.

Niro Inc, 2004. http://www.niroinc.com/html/drying/fdspraychem.html.

Nocker A., Mazza A., Masson L., Camper A.K., Brousseau R. 2009. Selective detection of live bacteria combining propidium monoazide sample treatment with microarray technology. Journal of Microbiological Methods 76, 253-261.

Nutraceutix, 2001. Nutraceutix Probiotics. Internet: http://www.nutraceutix.com.

O'Mahony L., McCarthy J., Kelly P., Hurley G., Luo F., Chen K., O'Sullivan G.C., Kiely B., Collins J.K., Shanahan F., Quigley E.M. 2005. *Lactobacillus* and *bifidobacterium* in irritable bowel syndrome: symptom responses and relationship to cytokine profiles. Gastroenterology 128, 541-551.

Orban, J.I & Patterson, J.A., 2000. Modification of the phosphoketolase assay for rapid identification of bifidobacteria. Journal of Microbiological Methods 40, 221-224.

Ouwenhand, A.C., Langstrom, H., Suomalainen, T. & Salminen, S. 2002. Effects of probiotics on constipation, fecal azoreductase activity and fecal mucin content in the elderly. Annals of Nutrition and Metabolism 46, 159-162.

Özer B., Kirmaci H.A., Şenel E., Atamer M., Hayaloğlu A. 2009. Improving the viability of *Bifidobacterium bifidus* BB-12 and *Lactobacillus acidophilus* LA-5 in white-brined cheese by microencapsulation. International Dairy Journal 19, 22-29.

Parracho H., McCartney A.L., & Gibson G.R. 2007. Probiotics and prebiotics in infant nutrition. Proceedings of the Nutrition Society 66, 405-411.

Park, J.K. & Chang, H.N., 2000. Microencapsulation of microbial cells. Biotechnology Advances 18, 303-319.

Park, J., Um, J., Lee, B., Goh, J., Park, S., Kim, W. & Kim, P., 2002. Encapsulated *Bifidobacterium bifidum* potentiates intestinal IgA production. Cellular Immunology 219, 22-27.

Parvez S., Malik K.A., Kang S.A and Kim H.Y. 2006. Probiotics and their fermented food products are beneficial for health. Journal of Applied Microbiology 100, 1171-1185.

Percival, M., 1997. Choosing a probiotic supplement. Clinical Nutrition Insights 6, 1-4.

Petschow B.W and Talbott R.D. 1991. Response of Bifidobacterium species to growth promoters in human and cow milk. Paediatric Research 29, 208-213.

Phillips, C. R. & Poon, Y. N., 1988. Biotechnology Monographs. Immobilization of cells. Volume 5, Springer-Verlag, Germany. pp. 11; 50-64.

Picot A., Lacroix C., 2004. Encapsulation of bifidobacteria in whey protein-based microcapsules and survival in simulated gastrointestinal conditions and in yoghurt. International Dairy Journal, 14, 505-515.

Porubcan, R.S. & Sellars, R.L., 1975. Stabilized dry cultures of lactic acid-producing bacteria. US Patent no. 3897307.

Power D.A., Burton J.P., Chilcott C.N., Dawes P.J., Tagg J.R. 2008. Preliminary investigations of the colonization of upper respiratory tract tissues of infants using a paediatric formulation of the oral probiotic *Streptococcus salivarius* K12. European Journal of Clinical Microbiology and Infectious Diseases 27, 1261-1263.

Prasad J., Gill H., Smart J. and Gopal P.K. 1998. Selection and characterization of *Lactobacillus* and *Bifidobacterium* strains for use as probiotics. International Dairy Journal 8, 993-1002.

Proviva, 2002. Health professionals. Documented beneficial effects. www.proviva.co.uk/hp_doc_ben.htm.

Rattes A.L.R. & Oliveira W.P., 2004. Spray-drying as a method for microparticulate modified release systems preparation. Proceedings of the 14th International Drying Symposium(IDS 2004), Sao Paulo, Brazil, Vol B, pp. 1112-1119.

Ramakrishna S.V. & Prakasham, R.S., 1999. Microbial fermentations with immobilized cells. Current Science 77, 87-100.

Reddy D.S., Hamid R & Rao C.V. 1997. Effect of dietary oligofructose and inulin on colonic preneoplastic aberrant crypt foci inhibition. Carcinogenesis 18, 1371-1374.

Reid, G 2006, 'Safe and efficacious probiotics: what are they?',*Trends in Microbiology*, vol. 14, no. 8, pp. 348-352.

Reid G., Jass J., Sebulsky M.T., McCormick J.K. 2003. Potential uses of probiotics in clinical practice. Clinical Microbiology Reviews 16, 658-672.

Reineccius G. A. 1988. Spray-drying of Food flavours. In Risch, S. J., Reineccius G. A. (eds). Flavor encapsulation. American chemical society, Washington DC. pp. 55-66.

Richardson, D., 1996. Probiotics and product innovation. Nutrition and Food Science 4, 27-33.

Ridlon, J.M., Kang, D.J. & Hylemon, P.B., 2006. Bile salt biotransformations by human intestinal bacteria. Journal of Lipid Research 47, 241-259.

Roberfroid, M. B., 1998. Prebiotics and synbiotics: concepts and nutritional properties. British Journal of Nutrition 80, S197-S202.

Roberfroid, M.B 2000, 'Prebiotics and probiotics: are they functional foods?', *American Journal of Clinical Nutrition*, vol. 7, pp. 1682- 1687.

Rowland I.R., Rumney C.J., Coutts J.T. & Lievense L. 1998. Effect of *Bifidobacterium longum* and inulin on gut bacterial metabolism and carcinogen induced aberrant crypt foci in rats. Carcinogenesis 2, 281-285.

Roy, D 2001, 'Media for the isolation and enumeration of bifidobacteria in dairy products', International Journal of Food Microbiology, 69, 167-182.

Rozada-Sanchez R., Sattur A.P., Thomas K., Pandiella S.S. 2007. Evaluation of *Bifidobacterium* spp. for the production of a potentially probiotic malt-based beverage. Process Biochemistry 43, 848-854.

Ruiz-Moyano S., Martin A., Benito M.J., Nevado F.P., de Guia Cordoba M. 2008. Screening of lactic acid bacteria and bifidobacteria for potential probiotic use in Iberian dry fermented sausages. Meat Science 80, 715-721.

Saarela, M., Mogensen, G., Fondén, R., Mättö, J. & Mattila-Sandholm, T., 2000. Probiotic bacteria: safety, functional and technological properties. Journal of Biotechnology 84, 197-215.

Saikali, J., Picard, C., Freitas, M. & Holt, P., 2004. Fermented milks, probiotic cultures, and colon cancer. Nutrition and Cancer 49, 14-24.

Sakai, K., Mishima, C., Tachiki, T., Kumagai, H. & Tochikura, T., 1987. Mortality of bifidobacteria in boiled yoghurt. Journal of Fermented Technique 65, 215-220.

Sako T., Matsumoto K. and Tanaka R. 1999. Recent progress on research and applications of non-digestible galacto-oligosaccharides. International Dairy Journal 9, 69-80.

Salminen, S., Ouwehand, A.C. & Isolauri, E., 1998a. Clinical applications of probiotic bacteria. International Dairy Journal 8, 563-572.

Salminen, S., Bouley, C., Boutron-Ruault, M.C., Cummings, J.H., Frank, A., Gibson, G.R., Isolauri, E., Moreau, M.C., Roberfroid, M. & Rowland, I., 1998b. Functional food science and gastrointestinal physiology and function. British Journal of Nutrition 80, S147-S171.

Salminen, S, Ouwehand, A, Benno, Y & Lee, Y.K 1999, 'Probiotics: how should they be defined?', Trends in Food Science & Technology 10, 107-110.

Sanders, M.E., 1999. Probiotics. Food Technology 53, 67-77.

Sanders, M.E., Akkermans, L. M.A., Haller, D., Hammerman, C., Heimbach, J., Hörmannsperger, G., Huys, G., Levy, D.D., Lutgendorff, F., Mack, D., Phothirath, P., Solano-Aguilar, G & Vaughan, E., 2010. Safety assessment of probiotics for human use. Gut microbes 1, 164-185.

Sangeetha P.T., Ramesh M.N., Prapulla S.G. 2005. Recent trends in the microbial production, analysis and application of fructooligosaccharides. Trends in Food Science & Technology 16, 442-457.

Sarrade, S., Guizard, C. & Rios, G.M., 2003. New applications of supercritical fluids and supercritical fluid processes in separation. Separation and Purification Technology 32, 57-63.

Saxelin M., Grenov B., Svensson U., Fondén R., Reniero R. and Mattila-Sandholm T., 1999. The technology of probiotics. Trends in Food Science & Technology 10, 387-392

Sazawal S., Hiremath G., Dhinga U., Malik P., Deb S., & Black R.E. 2006. Efficacy of probiotics in prevention of acute diarrhea: A meta-analysis of masked, randomised, placebo-controlled trials. The Lancet Infectious Diseases 6, 374-382.

Schrezenmeir, J. & de Vrese, M., 2001. Probiotics, prebiotics and synbiotics:Approaching a definition. American Journal of Clinical Nutrition 73, 361S-364S.

Scrimshaw T.M., & Murray E.B. 1988. The acceptability of milk and milk products in populations with a high prevalence of lactose intolerance. American Journal of Clinical Nutrition 48, 1079S-1159S.

Sheehan V.M., Sleator R.D., Fitzgerald G.F. and Hill C. 2006. Heterologous expression of Bet1, a betaine uptake system, enhances the stress tolerance of *Lactobacillus salivarius* UCC118. Applied Enviromental Microbiology 72, 2170-2177.

Sheehan V.M., Ross P., and Fitzgerald G.F. 2007. Assessing the acid tolerance and technological robustness of probiotic cultures for fortification in fruit juices. Innovative Food Science and Emerging Technologies 8, 279-284.

Shah N.P. 1993. Effectiveness of dairy products in alleviation of lactose intolerance. Food Australia 45, 268-271.

Shah N.P. 2000. Some beneficial effects of probiotic bacteria. Bioscience Microflora 19, 99-106.

Shah N.P 2002. The exopolysaccharides production by starter cultures and their influence on textural characteristics of fermented milks. Symposium on New Developments in Technology of Fermented Milks. International Dairy Journal, 3rd June, Comwell Scanticon, Kolding, Denmark. Abstract p5.

Shah N.P. 2004. Probiotics and prebiotics. Agrofood Industry HiTech 15, 13-16.

Shah N.P. 2007. Functional cultures and health benefits (Review). International dairy Journal 17, 1262-1277.

Shiel B., McCarthy J., O'Mahony L., Bennett M.W., Ryan P., Fitzgibbon J.J., Kiely B., Collins J.K., Shanahan F. 2004. Is the mucosal route of administration essential for probiotic function? Subcutaneous administration is associated with attenuation of murine colitis and arthritis. Gut 53, 694-700.

Sihvonen, M., Järvenpää, E., Hietaniemi, V. & Huopalahti, R., 1999. Advances in supercritical carbon dioxide technologies. Trends in Food Science and Technology 10, 217-222.

Siuta-Cruce, P. & Goulet, J., 2001. Improving probiotic microorganisms in food systems. Food Technology 55, 36-42.

Sleator R.D. and Hill C. 2007. New frontiers in probiotic research. Letters in Applied Microbiology 46, 143-147.

Stormo, K.E. & Crawford, R.L., 1992. Preparation of encapsulated microbial cells for environmental applications. Applied and Environmental Microbiology 58, 727-730.

Sullivan, Å. & Nord, C.E., 2002. Probiotics in human infections. Journal of Antimicrobial Chemotherapy 50, 625-627.

Sullivan A. & Nord C.E. 2005. Probiotics and gastrointestinal diseases. Journal of Internal Medicine 257, 78-92.

Sultana, K., Godward, G., Reynolds, N., Arumugaswamy, R., Peiris, P. & Kailasapathy, K., 2000. Encapsulation of probiotic bacteria with alginate-starch and evaluation of survival in simulated gastrointestinal conditions and in yoghurt. International Journal of Food Microbiology 62, 47-55.

Talwalkar, A., Kailasapathy, K., Peirs, P. & Arumugaswamy, R., 2001. Application of RBGR- a simple way for screening of oxygen tolerance in probiotic bacteria. International Journal of Food Microbiology 71, 245-248.

Tannock G.W., 2001. Molecular assessment of intestinal microflora. American Journal of Clinical Nutrition 73 (Supplement 2) 410S- 414S.

Taylor, S.A, Steer, T.E. & Gibson, G.R., 1999. Diet bacteria and colonic cancer. Nutrition and Food Science 4, 187-191.

Temmerman R., Pot B., Huys G., Swings J. 2003a. Identification and antibiotic susceptibility of bacterial isolates from probiotic products. International Journal of Food Microbiology 81, 1-10.

Thantsha M.S., Cloete T.E., Moolman F.S., Labuschagne P.W., 2009. Supercritical carbon dioxide interpolymer complexes improve survival of *B. longum* Bb-46 in simulated gastrointestinal fluids. International Journal of Food Microbiology, 129, 88-92.

Theuer, R.C. & Cool, M.B., 1998. Fructan-containing baby food compositions and methods therefore. US Patent no. 5840361.

Touhy, K.M., Probert, H.M., Smejkal, C.W. & Gibson, G.R., 2003. Using probiotics and prebiotics to improve gut health. Drug Discovery Today 8, 692-700.

Vandenplas Y., Nel E., Watermeyer G.A., Walele A., Wittenberg D., Zuckerman M. 2007. Probiotics in infectious diarrhea: are they indicated? A review focusing on *Saccharomyces boulardii*: review. South African Journal of Child Health 1, 116-119.

Vanderhoof J.A. and Young R.J. 2003. Role of probiotics in the management of patients with food allergy. Annals of Allergy, Asthma and Immunology 90, 99-103

Van Loo J., Cummings J., Delzenne N., Englyst H., Franck A., Hopkins M., Kok N., Macfarlane G., Newton D., Quigley M., Roberfroid M., van Vliet T., van den Heuvel E. 1999. Functional food properties of non-digestible oligosaccharides: a consensus report from the ENDO project (DGXII AIRII-CT94-1095). British Journal of Nutrition 81, 121-132.

Vasiljevic T. and Shah N.P. 2008. Probiotics-from Metchnikoff to bioactives. International Dairy Journal 18, 714-728.

Vasishtha, N., 2003. Microencapsulation: Delivering a market advantage. Internet: http//www.preparedfoods.com

Vazquez M.J., Alonso J.L., Dominguez H., Parajo J.C. 2000. Xylooligosaccharides: Manufacture and applications. Trends in Food Science & Technology 11, 387-393.

Veal, D. A., Deere, D., Ferrari, B., Piper, J. & Atfield, PV. 2000. Fluorescence staining and flow cytometry for monitoring microbial cells. Journal of Immunological methods 243, 191-210.

Venter, C.S 2007, 'Prebiotics: an update', Journal of Family Ecology and Consumer Science 35, 17-25.

Vesa, T.H., Marteau, P. & Korpela, R., 2000. Lactose intolerance. Journal of the American College of Nutrition 19, 165S-175S.

Versic, R. J., 1988. Flavor encapsulation: an overview. In Risch, S. J., Reineccius G. A. (eds). Flavor encapsulation. American chemical society, Washington DC. pp. 1-6.

Vidhyalakshmi R., Bhakyaraj R., Subhasree R.S., 2009. Encapsulation "The Future of Probiotics"-A Review. Advances in Biological Research, 3, 96-103.

Villamiel M., Corzo N., Foda M.I., Montes F., Olano A. 2002. Lactulose formation catalysed by alkaline-substituted sepiolites in milk permeate. Food Chemistry 76, 7-11.

Vliagoftis H., Kouranos V.D., Betsi G.I., Falagas M.E. 2008. Probiotics for the treatment of allergic rhinitis and asthma: systemic review of randomized controlled trials. Annals of Allergy and Asthma Immunology 101, 570-579.

Vives-Rego, J., Lebaron, P. & Nebe-von Caron, G. 2000. Current and future applications of flow cytometry in aquatic microbiology. FEMS Microbiology Reviews 24, 429-448.

Voragen A.G.J. 1998. Technological aspects of functional food-related carbohydrates. Trends in Food Science & Technology 9, 328-335.

Wahlqvist, M., 2002. Prebiotics and Probiotics. www.healthyeatingclub.com.

Worthington, J.H., Bolger, J.M. & Rudolph, M.J., 2001. Edible product with live and active probiotics. World patent no. WO0162099.

Zhang L., Li N., Caicedo R., Neu J. 2005. Alive and dead *Lactobacillus rhamnosus* GG decrease tumour necrosis factor-alpha-induced interleukin-8 production in Caco-2 cells. Journal of Nutrition 135, 1752-1756.

Ziemer, C.J. & Gibson, G.R., 1998. An overview of probiotics, prebiotics and synbiotics in the functional food concept: Perspectives and future strategies. International Dairy Journal 8, 473-479.

3

The Impact of Probiotics on the Gastrointestinal Physiology

Erdal Matur and Evren Eraslan
*Department of Physiology, Faculty of Veterinary Medicine,
University of Istanbul, Avcilar, Istanbul
Turkey*

1. Introduction

Researches concerning probiotics were initiated by a Russian scientist named Elie Metchnikoff. He emphasized the importance of *Lactobacillus* species and fermented milk products present in the gastrointestinal tract for a healthy and long life. The term "probiotics" was first introduced in 1953 by Werner Kollath, and he defined probiotics as microbially derived factors that stimulate the growth of other microorganisms. Afterwards, the term "probiotics" was defined by Roy Fuller in 1989 as a live microbial feed supplement which beneficially affects the host by improving its intestinal microbial balance. Fuller's definition emphasizes the requirement of viability for probiotics and introduces the aspect of a beneficial effect on the host. Although, this definition has been widely used by the entire scientific world, according to the currently adopted definition by FAO/WHO, probiotics are: "Live microorganisms confer a health benefit on the host when administered in adequate amounts" (FAO/WHO, 2001).

The most frequently used probiotic microorganisms are Lactobacillus and Bifidobacterium species. However, there are also much more bacteria and some yeast species used as probiotic. Bacteria and yeast species, which are used commonly as probiotic, are listed by Heyman & Menard (2002) as below. *Lactobacillus* species: *L. acidophilus, L. rhamnosus, L. gasseri, L. reuteri, L. bulgaricus, L plantarum, L. johnsonii, L. paracasei, L. casei, L. salivarius, L. lactis.* **Bifidobacterium** species: *B. bifidum, B. longum, B. breve, B. infantis, B. lactis, B. adolescentis.* Other species: *Streptococcus thermophilus, Escherichia coli, Bacillus cereus, Clostridium butyricum, Enterococcus faecalis, Enterococcus faecium.* Yeast: *Saccharomyces boulardii, Saccharomyces cerevisiae,* VSL#3 (four strains of lactobacilli, three strains of bifidobacteria, one strain of *Streptococcus salivarius* sp. *thermophilus*).

There is a mutual interaction between intestinal cells and microorganisms present in the gastrointestinal tract. Commensal microorganisms in the gastrointestinal tract have multidirectional effects on digestion, absorption and barrier function, secretory functions, or postnatal maturation of intestinal mucosa. Furthermore, it has been known that they change gene expression in intestinal cells (Hooper et al., 2001). The changes in the function of intestinal tract (e.g. the increase of motility, or disruption of carbohydrate digestion) also affect bacteria population and colonization.

Probiotics are widely used for the promotion and improvement of health in humans and in animal species. Probiotics have been used as a biologically active substance in a large extend of pathologic conditions ranging from antibiotic-associated or travelers' diarrhea, irritable bowel syndrome (IBS), and lactose intolerance to dental caries, ulcers due to *Helicobacter pylori*, hepatic encephalopathy, intestinal motility disorders and neonatal necrotizing enterocolitis (Deshpande et al., 2011). It has been used as a growth, or production performance promoter in poultry species or farm animals. There are also numerous scientific reports about the interaction between probiotics and immune system. On the other hand, the effects of probiotics on digestive physiology and intestinal tract morphology have not been documented sufficiently. Therefore, the objective of this chapter is to assess the effects of probiotics on gastrointestinal physiology and morphology in human and animal models. The effects of probiotics on digestive and absorptive function of the intestine, expression of brush border enzymes and nutrient transport systems have been investigated in this chapter. The relationship between probiotics and gut motility or transit time of gastrointestinal content has also been highlighted. The effects of probiotics on morphological characteristics and the proliferation capacity of crypt and villus epithelium have been focused and in addition, the effects of probiotic on enteric nervous system have been evaluated. Finally, impact of the probiotics on the physical and functional barrier of gastrointestinal tract has been evaluated in this chapter.

2. The effects of probiotics on intestinal morphology and cell proliferation

To investigate the effects of microorganisms on the development of digestive tract, generally animal models are used. Because, obtaining and examining intestinal mucosal samples of people are technically more difficult. The morphological parameters such as length of villi, depth of crypt, villi/crypt proportion, and surface area of villi are used to investigate the effects of microorganisms on intestinal morphology and cell proliferation. The height of villi and the depth of crypt are considered as the indicators of intestinal functions.

In the comparative studies conducted on germ free and conventional animals it has been determined that microorganisms located to digestive tract during the postnatal period caused to decreased villi length and increased crypt depth in conventional animals i.e. in pig (Willing & Van Kessel, 2007), in rat (Ishikawa et al., 1999) and in birds (Furuse & Okumura, 1994). However, it has been also reported that there is no difference between germ-free and conventional animals regarding development of villi (Sharma et al., 1995). It has been determined that length of villi is higher in gnotobiotic animal models as in germ-free animals compared to conventional animals (Herich et al., 2004). The effects of probiotics have been investigated by inoculating probiotics to germ free animals or supplementing conventional animals with probiotics.

2.1 Villus height

Willing & Van Kessel (2007) have reported that villus height was increased in gnotobiotic piglets inoculated *Lactobacillus fermentum* (monoassociated with *Lactobacillus fermentum*) and Di Giancamillo et al. (2008) also has reported increase in villus height in piglets supplemented with *Pediococcus acidilactici*. Yang et al. (2009) have investigated intestinal tract morphology of mice supplemented orally high, low and moderate doses of *Bifidobacterium adolescentis* BBMN23 and *Bifidobacterium adolescentis* BBMN68 after 2 and 4 weeks of application. Villus height was longer in low dose group compared to those of controls, but moderate and high doses did not affect it after two weeks. However after 4 weeks, villus height increased in all groups supplemented with probiotic. Similarly villus height increase has been reported in studies conducted on birds as an animal model (Samli et al., 2007; Awad et al., 2010).

Effects of the probiotic on villus height may change depending on the species of microorganism or probiotic. For example, villus height in duodenum and ileum increased but did not changed in jejunum of broiler chicks supplemented with *Pediococcus acidlactici* as probiotic (Taheri et al., 2010). On the other hand Günal et al. (2006) reported that villus height of jejunum and ileum increased in broiler chicks applied multi-microbe probiotic product. Segmental differences were also found in comparative studies conducted on germ free and conventional animals. Shirkey et al. (2006) have reported that villus height was the longest in jejunum of pigs supplemented with *Lactobacillus fermentum*. On the other hand Shurson et al. (1990) reported that germ-free pigs had longer ileal and duodenal villi, but shorter jejunal villi compared with their conventional counterparts. *Saccharomyces boulardii* is one of the yeast that has been using as probiotic. It has been determined that there was no significance change in villus height or crypt depth of intestinal biopsy samples obtained from volunteers who were supplemented with *Saccharomyces boulardii* for 14 days (Buts et al., 2002). However, another yeast species (*Saccharomyces cerevisiae*) was reported to increased villus height of ileum in birds (Zhang et al., 2005). Meslin and Sacquet (1984) who investigated microvilli on the surface of enterocytes reported that the microvilli were significantly shorter in all small intestinal regions when the micro flora was present. The decrease in microvillus length (due to the presence of micro flora) in germ free rat, was 5% in the duodenum, 9% in the jejunum and 18% in the ileum. Because increased villus height leads to increased surface area at the same time, digestion and absorption of disaccharides and dipeptides are promoted. In addition, it was indicated that longer villi are correlated with activation of cell mitosis (Samanya & Yamauchy, 2002).

2.2 Crypt depth

The data related to effects of probiotics on crypt depth are inconsistent. Probably there are variations depending on the species, the dose or the application of used probiotic. Yang et al. (2009) have reported that crypt depth decreased in mice supplemented with moderate and high doses of probiotic (*Bifidobacterium adolescentis* BBMN23) for 2 weeks, but on the contrary it was increased in low dose probiotic supplemented group compared to controls. However after 4 weeks of application, increased crypt depth has been reported in moderate and high doses groups. Willing & Van Kessel (2007) have reported that crypt depth was increased in piglets inoculated with *Lactobacillus fermentum* (monoassociated with *Lactobacillus fermentum*) compared to conventional animals. Similarly, increased crypt depth in duodenum, jejunum and ileum of chicks supplemented with *Bacillus subtilis* has been found (Pelicano et al., 2005).

Scharek et al. (2005) have reported that there was no significant change in the crypt depth in proximal jejunum of pigs supplemented with *Enterococcus faecium* 68. Similarly, it has been stated that crypt depth didn't change in duodenum, but decreased in ileum of broiler chicks supplemented with *Lactobacillus sp* (Awad et al., 2009). In addition, it has been reported that crypt depth was not changed in broiler chicks supplemented with *Saccharomyces cerevisiae* yeast (Zhang et al., 2005). Increased crypt depth indicates that both mucosal secretion (Chiou et al., 1996) and cell turnover are high (Yason et al., 1987).

2.3 Villus height/crypt depth ratio

In studies conducted on germ free animals it has been determined that the villus height/crypt depth ratio is higher in germ free animals than conventional animals (Heneghan et al., 1984). Awad et al. (2010) have reported that villus height to crypt depth ratio increased in duodenum and ileum of chicks supplemented with *Lactobacillus* sp. Similarly, supplementation of multi-microbe probiotic product has been reported to cause increased villus height to crypt depth ratio in duodenum and ileum (Kim et al., 2011). It has been indicated that, increased villus height to crypt depth ratio are directly correlated with an increased epithelial turnover (Fan et al., 1997). Therefore, it may be concluded that bacteria used as probiotic positively affect development of intestinal epithelia.

2.4 Villus surface area

The effects of probiotics on villus surface area may change depending on the segment which bacteria colonized. For example, jejunum villus surface area increased, but duodenum or ileum surface area did not affected in chicks supplemented with probiotic containing *Lactobacillus acidophilus, Lactobacillus casei, Bifidobacterium bifidum,* and *Enterococcus faecium* species (Smirnov et al., 2005). Similarly Samanya and Yamauchy (2002) have reported that *Bacillus subtilis natto* increased villus surface dose dependently but this increase varied between different segments. Increased surface area allows for increased intestinal absorptive area. Increased absorptive area is useful because digested nutrients pass into the villi through diffusion, so effectiveness of diffusion increases.

2.5 Cell proliferation, migration and turnover

Proliferation, migration, number and apoptosis of cells in intestinal tract are affected by secreted molecules or fermented products of microorganisms in digestive tract.

It has been determined that cell count and mitotic index in intestinal villus and crypt was higher in gnotobiotic rats mono-associated with *Lactobacillus rhamnousus* GG compared to germ-free or conventional animals (Banasaz et al., 2002). Probiotics both increase cells in intestinal mucosa and affect the migration of cells in crypt to the tip of villus. Canonici et al. (2011) have revealed by *in vitro* and *in vivo* studies that *Saccharomyces boulardii* accelerates migration of intestinal enterocytes through crypt-villus axis by activating α2β1 integrin collagen receptor. Because of this effect, *Saccharomyces boulardii* accelerates the repair of intestinal epithelium damage.

Results related to the effects of probiotics on the proliferation of intestinal epithelium cells are controversial. Mogilner et al. (2007) have reported that *Lactobacillus* GG' did not affect proliferation of enterocytes in rats with short bowel syndrome. Similarly, it has been reported that *Saccharomyces boulardii* did not affect proliferation of enterocytes (Canonici et al., 2011). However Ichikawa et al. (1999) have suggested that *Clostridium butyricum* and *Lactobacillus casei* had tropic effect on digestive tract by enhancing proliferation of intestinal epithelial cells. It has been reported that probiotics increased the production of short-chain fatty acids (SCFA) (Sakata et al., 1999). Investigators have suggested that proliferative effects of probiotics on intestinal epithelial cells are based on the probiotic induced increased SCFA production. In the same way, Di Giancamillo et al. (2008) have reported that enterocyte proliferation increased in piglets supplemented with *Pediococcus acidilactici*.

Mogilner et al. (2007) have reported that there was a decrease in enterocyte death via apoptosis in rats with short bowel syndrome supplemented with *Lactobacillus* GG.

It has been suggested that bacteria used as probiotic affect functions and counts of the goblet cells in intestinal mucosa other than enterocytes. Because the mucus secreted by goblet cells is one of the factors composing intestinal barrier, it has significance on the prevention of pathogen invasion in digestive tract.

Gauffin Cano et al. (2002) reported an increase in the number of goblet cells after the administration of the probiotic strain *Lactobacillus casei* CRL 431 in a malnourished mouse model. In addition there is ample evidence that intestinal microbiota affect goblet cell dynamics, including mucus secretion and composition either directly by the secretion of bioactive factors or indirectly by the activation of host immune cells (Sharma et al., 1995).

3. The effect of probiotics on the motility of the gastrointestinal tract

Either gastrointestinal motility or the kinetic of its content is one of the most important variations providing gastrointestinal tract's comfort. The changes in motility can make symptoms varying from constipation to diarrhea come into being (Ohashi & Ushida, 2009). The interest to probiotics, due to their motility regulatory effects, is rising in functional gastrointestinal disorders.

The influence of microorganisms on intestinal motility was reported for the first time by Abraham and Bishop. These researchers observed that both small and large intestinal transit time and gastric emptying decreased in germ-free animals (Abraham & Bishop, 1967). Husebye et al. (1994) detected that phase-3 intervals in migrating motor complex (MMC) in germ-free animals were extended. In addition, they noticed that the motility became normal when specific pathogen free bacteria were inoculated in these animals' intestines. They also noticed that the motility of intestines became normal when probiotics were inoculated instead of doing so with commensal bacteria.

Actually gastrointestinal motility and microorganisms in the tracts are mutually influencing each other. The presence or the absence of the motility affects microorganisms' colonization and also the motility is being altered in case the microorganisms are lacking. Both migrating motor complex in stomach and the one way peristaltic movements in small intestine influence the colonization in the area (Quigley, 2011). Thus the decrease of intestinal motility causes small intestinal bacterial overgrowth (SIBO).

In addition to commensal bacteria in gastrointestinal tract, those used as probiotic were also detected to be influencing the motility (Williams et al., 2010). Diverse researches related to the subject in both human and animal models were conducted. Massi et al. (2006), observed *in vitro* the influence of probiotics on motility in ileum and proximal colon segments isolated from guinea pigs. They realized that *Lactobacillus* and cytoplasmic extract obtained from *Bifidobacterium* caused a contraction in ileum and a relaxation in proximal colon. They claimed that the extract mentioned above does not exert its effect via muscarinic receptors since its effect was not inhibited by atropine. Yet, its mechanism is not fully elucidated so far (Waller et al., 2011).

The motility-probiotic relationship in humans was both in healthy individuals and in case of different diseases evaluated despite of technical difficulties. Indrio et al. (2008) who observed the connection between gastric emptying and the probiotics determined that gastric emptying time in infants being given *Lactobacillus reuteri* was significantly rapid compared to those in placebo group. Cherbut et al. (1997) noticed that the motility of terminal colon rises while sleeping in humans supplemented with *Lactobacillus casei*. Marteau et al. (2002) reported *Bifidobacterium lactus* strain DN 173010 to reduce colonic transit time in healthy female individuals. Waller et al. (2011) explained that whole gut transit time (WGTT) decreased in a dose-dependent manner in male and females obtaining different doses of *Bifidobacterium lactis* HN019 during 14 days.

Indrio et al. (2009) observing electrical activity that forms motility reported that the percentage of propagation (the electric activity turning into peristaltic movement) was higher in infants to which *Lactobacillus reuteri* was given compared to those in placebo group.

Lots of diseases such as irritable bowel syndrome (IBS) causing gastrointestinal dysfunction, also influence digestive tract motility or its motor activity. Probiotics are used in treatment of motoric function disorders seen in such diseases' post infective periods. For example post infective period hyper contractility was observed to be present in digestive tract of mice infected with *Trchinella spiralis*. It has been observed that the hyper contractility in mice given *Lactobacillus paracasei* NCC2461 specifically weakened (Verdu et al., 2004). In the same way delayed gastric emptying was observed in mice infected via *Helicobacter pylori*. Gastric functions were detected to be normalized in the same mice following probiotic treatment with *Lactobacillus rhamnosus* R0011 and *Lactobacillus helvaticus* R0052 (Verdu et al., 2008). Agrawal et al. (2009) reported that both colonic and orocecal transit were accelerated when fermented milk product containing *Bifidobactreium lactis* DN-173010 were given to patients suffering from irritable bowel syndrome presented with abdominal distension and constipation and also that this was making the case symptoms' influences to be diminished. Intestinal transit time was detected to be lengthened in diseases representing with digestive tract functional disorders such as IBS. Even the mechanism that lies beneath is not fully elucidated; it was estimated to be related to the imbalance in intestinal micro flora due to the illness itself.

The effects of probiotics on intestinal tract are being influenced by diverse factors. The motility in intestinal tract was acclaimed to be possibly specific to the type of the probiotic used (Husebye et al., 2001). Either the physiologic situation of the human or the animal is another factor affecting the motility. For example it was detected that in elderly people, *Bifidobacterium* DN 173010 reduces oro-fecal transit time while the same bacteria accelerates only colonic transit time in healthy volunteers. In addition, its effects in males were established to differ from that in females (Meance et al., 2001).

3.1 The mechanism of action

The mechanism lying beneath the effects of probiotics on motility are not fully elucidated. Yet the probable influence mechanisms can be divided into three headlines; 1) Products secreted by bacteria or final products formed at the end of fermentation 2) Influence of microorganisms on intestinal neuroendocrine factors 3) Influence of mediators secreted due to gastrointestinal tract's immune reaction (Barbara et al., 2005).

The stimulation of colonic motility via the rise of fecal bacterial mass, the stimulated cholecystokinin and deconjugated or dehydroxylated bile salts is considered to be a part of other mechanisms. Some probiotics such as *Bifidiobacteium lactis* HN019 stimulate the production of lactic acid bacteria in the environment. As a consequence of lactic acid bacteria production, WGTT time decreases while peristaltic accelerates owing to the reduction of the intestinal content pH (Salminen et al., 1997).

A high number of gas occurring due to the digestion of indigested carbohydrates by colonic microbiota influences intestinal motility. Yet different influences may occur in motility related to the gas type formed. For example, when methane producing bacteria in intestinal flora multiplies, compared to the effects of those releasing hydrogen, intestinal transit time increases, motor activity is directly inhibited, and on the contrary non propulsive and segmental contractions increase (Pimentel et al., 2006).

Short chain fatty acid (SCFA) appearing as an outcome of carbohydrate or lipid fermentation by probiotics is one of the most important final products influencing gastrointestinal motility. Cherbut et al. (1997) observing the influence of SCFA on motility detected that SCFA showed contractile activity via enteric cholinergic reflex in low concentrations (0.1 to 10 mmol/L). Nevertheless this was also detected to be a temporary effect. SCFA in high concentrations (100 mmol/L) was observed to inhibit colonic contraction (Sakata, 1987). McManus et al. (2002) reported that SCFA inhibits peristaltic activity while it stimulates the tonic activity in the large intestine of dogs. It exerts this effect by influencing Ca^{+2} influx to gastrointestinal smooth muscle cells. Besides colonic motility SCFA was also determined to influence upper part of digestive tract, to cause relaxation in both lower esophageal sphincter and proximal stomach and also it decreases gastric emptying time. It was explained that it showed this effect via hormonal way with the use of polypeptide YY (Labayen et al., 2001).

In addition, probiotics affect the motility in an indirect way by influencing some inflammatory mediators' expression occurring during the disease that alters gastrointestinal tract functions. For example, *Lactobacillus paracasei* weaken the hyper contractility rising in the post infective period of diseases by increasing the expression of COX-2 being one of the inflammatory mediators (Verdu et al., 2004). Mediators such as TGF-β and prostaglandin E(2) released during gastrointestinal diseases damage both enteric nervous system and interstitial cells of cajal. Disorders in the motility occur since the neuronal structures mentioned above regulate intestinal tract motility. Probiotics given in post infective period normalize the motility as they accelerate the healing of damaged cells in enteric nervous system (Indrio et al., 2008).

4. Effects of probiotics on pancreatic digestive enzymes

There is only limited research on the effects of probiotics on pancreatic digestive enzymes such as amylase, lipase, trypsin, chymotrypsin, although there are few publication related to effects of probiotics on mucosal digestive enzymes. The relation between microorganisms of intestinal tract and pancreatic enzymes has been investigated in some studies using germ-free animals. It has been indicated that the bacterial status altered preferentially the exocrine pancreatic function. The specific activities of amylase, trypsin and carboxypeptidase-A were lower in germ-free than in conventional rats (Lhoste et al., 1996). How microorganisms in digestive tract affect secretion of pancreatic enzymes has not been determined. However hormones which stimulate enzyme secretion in pancreas such as enteroglucagon, gastrin or pancreatic polypeptide have been reported to be lower in germ-free animals compared to conventional animals (Goodlad et al., 1989). Decreased pancreatic enzymes in germ-free animals may be explained by this report. Moreover the cecal micro flora may also affect the pancreas via its metabolites. In fact, SCFA can stimulate amylase release from the rat pancreas directly (Ohbo et al., 1996).

Matur et al. (2007) have been reported that chymotrypsin levels decreased but amylase, lipase and trypsin levels did not changed in pancreas of broiler chicks which were supplemented with *Enterrococcius facium* NCIMB10415. In addition, intestinal tract enzyme activities were reported to be lower in animals supplemented with probiotics than those of control animals in the same study. The researchers have suggested that the relevant probiotics may affect the biosynthesis of pancreatic enzymes or their secretion to small intestines, although the mechanism underlying this effect has not been fully elucidated yet.

Microorganisms in digestive tract may also affect digestive enzyme activities indirectly. Drouault et al. (2002) have reported that *Lactobacillus lactis* produces lipase and this lipase ameliorated steatorrhea in pigs fed on high lipid meal.

4.1 Probiotic application in diseases related to digestive enzyme deficiencies

Sucrase deficiency, also known as sucrase-isomaltase deficiency, is the most common disaccharidase deficiency in human. It is a genetic disorder and causes to malabsorption of sucrose in diet and consequently to accumulation of hydrogen in the colon, swelling, diarrhea and abdominal cramps (Rolfe, 2000). *Saccharomyces cerevisiae* expresses significant sucrase and some isomaltase activity, and it has been proposed to improve malabsorption in patients with sucrase-isomaltase deficiency (Harms et al., 1987). Similarly Treem et al. (1993) have reported that the liquid preparation which is a by-product of the manufacture of baker's yeast reduced breath hydrogen excretion in patients with congenital sucrase-isomaltase deficiency that were given a sucrose load and allowed most patients to consume a sucrose-containing diet.

4.2 Lactase deficiency

Lactase insufficiency means that the concentration of the lactose cleaving enzyme β-galactosidase, also called lactase, in the brush border membrane of the mucosa of the small intestine is too small. Lactase deficiency is a very common condition characterized with lactose malabsorption in the intestinal mucosa. High concentrations of lactase enzyme are physiologically present in neonates. In the post weaning period, an irreversible reduction of its activity occurs in human (Montalto et al., 2006), and in mammalian animal species (Batchelor et al., 2011). Secondary lactase deficiency can be seen any condition that damages the small intestinal epithelial cells or significantly increases the gastrointestinal transit time. Thus, secondary hypolactasia is transient and reversible (Montalto et al., 2006).

It has been observed that patients with lactose maldigestion had higher lactose tolerance when eating fermented dairy products such as yogurt and could easily digest them compared to milk. There are two mechanisms lying beneath this situation. First, β-galactosidase is released from bacteria in yogurt after digested by bile acids. Second, delaying gastric emptying and slowing intestinal transit times prolong the action of residual β-galactosidase in the small intestine and decrease the osmotic load of the lactose (Marteau et al., 2001). Ojetti et al. (2010) were investigated hydrogen breath excretion and gastrointestinal symptoms as indicators of lactose intolerance in patients. They have reported that hydrogen excretion decreased and clinical symptoms improved in the group given *Lactobacillus reuteri* compared to those of placebo group. De Vrese et al. (2001) tested whether live bacteria in the fermented or non-fermented milk product are a prerequisite for enhanced lactose cleavage by microbial β-galactosidase. They found that lactose digestion in lactose malabsorbers and gastrointestinal well-being can be significantly improved if a milk product contains active microbial β-galactosidase. The bacteria need not to be alive but intact cell walls are required to act as a mechanical protection of the enzyme during gastric passage.

5. The effect of probiotics on the absorptive function of the intestine

5.1 Sodium and chloride absorptions

It has been determined that two carrier proteins play a role in the sodium absorption; "sodium hydrogen exchanger-2" (NHE-2) and NHE-3 which are the members of "solute carrier family-9" (SLC9) (Malakooti et al., 2011). While NHE-2 is expressed mostly in colon, NHE-3 is expressed mainly in ileum (Dudeja et al., 1996). The carrier proteins "down regulated in adenoma" (DRA) and putative anion transporter-1 (PAT-1) from SLC26 gene family have a role in chloride absorption. While PAT-1 is mainly expressed in small intestines, DRA is more expressed in colon than small intestines (Wang et al., 2002).

Probiotics such as *Lactobacillus* are used as a treatment support in diseases especially characterized by fluid loss in children. It has been determined that probiotics reduce sodium chloride and fluid loss in these diseases (Raheja et al., 2010). Furthermore it has been reported that *Saccharomyces boulardii* increases chloride net absorption from jejunum and descending colon *in vitro* (Krammer & Karbash, 1993).

To investigate the molecular mechanisms underlying the effects of probiotics on electrolyte and water absorption from intestinal tract, some *in vivo* and *in vitro* studies have been carried on. Human colon adenocarcinoma cell (Caco-2) has been used extensively as a model cell *in vitro* experiments subjected intestinal epithelium. Borthakur et al. (2008) reported that DRA activity increased in Caco-2 cells after short term *Lactobacillus acidophilus* application and this will cause chloride absorption eventually. *Lactobacillus acidophilus* was reported to cause this effect by increasing DRA expression in apical membranes of epithelial cells. However, it has been determined that total DRA amount in the cell did not changed, only DRA expression on the surface increased and this effect was caused via phosphatidyl-inositol 3-kinase pathway. It has been also considered that some soluble substances secreted by *Lactobacillus acidophilus* revealed this effect.

Bacteria present in the intestines are consistently interacting with epithelial cells. Therefore, it has been determined that, while *Lactobacillus acidophilus* increase DRA mRNA expression in epithelial cells of colon by transcriptional mechanisms, it is not effective in jejunum and ileum during its long-term applications. DRA is primary chloride transporter in colon, therefore significance of probiotics in chloride and water absorption has been proved (Binder & Mehta, 1989; Raheja et al., 2009). There is a limited knowledge on the molecular mechanisms underlying the effects of probiotics on sodium absorption. It is well known that probiotics produce short chain fatty acids. The short chain fatty acids increase the expression of NHE-3 which plays a main role in the absorption of sodium from ileum (Kiela et al., 2007).

5.2 Na$^+$-coupled glucose absorption

Glucose is absorbed from intestinal brush border membrane by mainly sodium-dependent glucose co-transporters 1 (SGLT-1) and glucose transporter 2 (GLUT-2) (Shimizu et al., 2000). Absorption rate of the intestinal glucose depends on the SGLT-1 affinity and density in the membrane. High affinity SGLT-1 is primary transporter for glucose absorption.

It has been reported that sodium coupled glucose absorption increased in small intestines of pigs treated with *Saccharomyces boulardii* or *Bacillus cereus var. toyoi* (Breves et al., 2000). It has been also determined that *Enterococcus faecium* NCIMB 10415 used as a probiotic caused an increase in intestinal transport and barrier function and glucose absorption (Lodeman et al., 2006). Similarly, sodium coupled D-glucose absorption increase has been reported in rats orally applied *Saccharomyces boulardii* (Buts et al., 1999).

The mechanism underlying the sodium coupled glucose absorption increasing effect of probiotics in intestinal epithelium cells has not been fully defined. However it has been suggested that specific and non-specific mechanisms may be effective. It may be a non-specific reason such as an increase in the absorptive surface or in affinity of transporters to substrates due to probiotics. On the other hand Rooj et al. (2010) have reported that supernatant obtained from lactobacilli increased the glucose transport in Caco-2 cells non-genomically and undefined metabolites produced by the probiotic caused this effect. This researchers have suggested that the metabolites produced by the probiotic cause to expression of cytosolic transporters in brush border membranes of enterocytes or to activation of transporters which were already in the membrane.

Although it has been suggested that probiotics affect intestinal glucose transport by non-genomic responses, SGLT-1 expression increases in rats applied *Saccharomyces boulardii* (Buts, 2009). Therefore, it is considered that the probiotics may be effective by changing gene expression via transcriptional or post translational mechanisms.

5.3 Calcium absorption

It has been reported that probiotics increase the calcium absorption from intestinal tract. However mechanisms underlying the increasing absorption are not fully elucidated and more than one mechanism may be considered (Gilman et al., 2006). Fermentation products occurred as a result of probiotics' activity may increase the absorption surface by accelerating proliferation in enterocytes (Scholz-Ahrens at al., 2007). Furthermore short chained fatty acids and the other products produced by the bacteria decrease the pH of intestines microenvironment. Therefore, calcium solubility increases and this may be related to increased calcium absorption (Gilman et al., 2006; Scholz-Ahrens at al., 2007). Tang et al.

(2007) reported that fermenting calcium-fortified soymilk with some *Lactobacillus* species can potentially enhance the calcium bioavailability.

Brassart & Yey (1998) have determined that 7 *Lactobacillus* species, which were tested *in vitro*, increased the transepithelial calcium transport in Caco-2 monolayer cells. Gilman & Cashman (2006) have reported that the transepithelial calcium transport did not change in Caco-2 monolayer cells treated by *Lactobacillus salivatorius* (UCC 118) and *Bifidobacterium infantis* (UCC 35624), however UCC 118 increased calcium uptake after 24 hours. Although the differences between the results of these studies have not exactly clarified, it has been suggested that the differences may be due to the different adheration of used bacteria to epithelial cells (Gilman & Cashman, 2006). Intestinal calcium absorption increasing effect of probiotics may be also related to increased expression of calcium channels in intestinal mucosa. Vinderola et al. (2007) observed that supernatant from milk fermented by *Lactobacillus helveticus* R389 enhanced expression of TRPV6 channels in the duodenum. Enhanced expression Ca^{+2} channels indicate an improved capacity for dietary Ca^{+2} uptake.

5.4 The effects of probiotics on cholesterol absorption

Cholesterol entered the body via food or re-absorbed from the bile secretion to the blood, is primary factor for heart and vascular diseases. Hypercholesterolemia is one of the most significant risk factor for the cardio-vascular diseases. It has been determined that various probiotic species decrease the serum cholesterol levels in human (Larkin et al., 2009), experimental animals (Park et al., 2007) or farm animals (Özcan et al., 2003; Strompfova et al., 2006). However hypocholesterolemic effect of probiotics depends on the species of the bacteria. This hypocholesterolemic effect has been suggested to be caused by more than one mechanism. For example lactic acid bacteria exert hypocholesterolemic effect by assimilating endogenous or exogenous originated cholesterol in intestinal tract or deconjugating bile acids (Gilliland et al., 1990). In addition, it has been reported that cholesterol and free bile acids bound to the cellular surface of microorganism or co-precipitate with free bile acids by probiotics (Guo & Zhang, 2010).

The recent researches have revealed that probiotics affect gene expression of carrier proteins which are responsible for cholesterol absorption. The protein called Niemann-Pick C1-like 1 (NPC1L1) which is abundantly expressed on the surface of enterocytes, plays a key role on the absorption of cholesterol from intestines. Reduction or inhibition of expression levels of this protein leads to a decrease in plasma cholesterol levels. The probiotic *Lactobacillus acidophilus* (American type culture collection) ATCC 4356 reduced NPCIL-1 gene expression and inhibited the cellular uptake of micellar cholesterol in Caco-2 cells. Soluble effector molecules secreted by ATCC 4356 were shown to be responsible for the decrease in NPC1L-1. Furthermore, ATCC 4356 mediated this effect partly through the liver X receptors (LXR) (Huang & Zheng, 2010).

6. Probiotics and enteric nervous system

Enteric nervous system (ENS), which is located in the wall of the digestive tract, is a neural network called as second brain that is consisted of sensory neurons, motor neurons, inter neurons and glial cells. It regulates complicated reflexes, motility and secretory functions of digestive tract. Although it is connected to central nervous system, ENS can regulate the function of its target organ without input from the central nervous system (CNS) (Gershon, 2005).

There is a mutual communication between CNS and microorganisms in the digestive tract. The central nervous system affects microorganisms by chancing motility, secretion, and permeability of digestive tract or via various mediators that are secreted by neuro-endocrine cells (Barbara et al., 2005). Microorganisms in the digestive tract affect functions of ENS and CNS via direct or indirect mechanisms. Microorganisms both affect development of sensory and motor neurons and induce plasticity.

Microorganisms in intestines communicate with nervous system via epithelial cells, various receptors or cells in lamina propria. Enterochromaffin cells play a key role in this communication. They function such as a transducer and provide a link between intestinal lumen and ENS (Indrio & Neu, 2011).

Effects of microorganisms in intestinal tract on nervous system occur via more than one mechanism. They affect development of sensory and motor neurons in gut by secreted substances or fermented products. For example SCFA, which is a fermented product of microorganisms in digestive tract, may affect motor activity in digestive tract (Soret et al., 2010). Furthermore, certain mediators secreted by immune cells which are activated by microorganisms in intestinal tract are effective on the regulation of ENS. Because, enteric neurons have receptors which are responsive to immune cells secreted mediators. For example, secretion of substances such as histamine, interleukin-6, leukotrienes, 5-hydroxytryptamine, platelet activating factor, mast cell proteases, adenosine, interleukin-1β, prostaglandins as a result of stimulation of mast cells affect functions of ENS by connecting to the receptors on the neurons of ENS (Wood, 2007).

Bacteria including probiotics can be considered as a chemical factory producing biologically active substance such as neurotransmitters and neuromodulators (Wang et al., 2010). It has been determined that *Lactobacillus* and *Bifidobacterium* produce GABA, *Escherichia, Bacillus* and *Saccharomyces* produce norepinephrine, *Candida, Streptococcus, Escherichia* and *Enterococcus* produce serotonin, *Bacillus* produce dopamine, *Lactobacillus* produce acetylcholine (Lyt, 2011).

It has been determined that *Lactobacillus reuteri* increases the excitability of myenteric AH cells in rats by inhibiting calcium dependent potassium channels (Kunze et al., 2009). The same researches have also reported that activity of ENS was inhibited as a result of the effect of *Lactobacillus reuteri* on AH cells (Whang et al., 2010). Because ENS depresses intestines motility, inhibition of ENS causes an increase in motility.

Probiotics reveal their effects by changing neuro-chemical characteristics of enteric neurons. Kamm et al. (2004) have reported that the numbers of neurons containing calbidin, which is a multiple calcium binding protein, decreased in jejunum of pigs supplemented with *Sacharomyces boulardii*. Similarly Giancamillo et al. (2010) have reported that the density of galaninergic and calcitonin gene-related peptide (CGRP) positive neurons increased in submucosal plexus of ileum of *Pediococcus acidilactici* treated pigs. Galanin is effective on peristaltic activity, secretion, blood flow and eating behaviors, and CGRP is effective on the modulation of sensory functions and the regulation of activity of smooth muscle. Furthermore, the same researchers have determined that density of glial cells in ileums' inner and outer sub mucosal plexus was increased in *Pediococcus acidilactici* treated pigs.

Probiotics have been used in the treatments of neuromotoric and sensory functional disorders of digestive tract since their effects on ENS have been revealed. For example, it has been reported that functional disorders such as delayed gastric emptying, increased visceral perception and abnormal feeding pattern which occurs in mice due to *Helikobacter* infection, were treated by supplementation of *Lactobacillus rhamnosus* R0011 and *Lactobacillus helveticus* R0052 (Verdu et al., 2008).

Probiotics in digestive tract affect central nervous system by both ENS and parasympathetic fibers that innervates digestive tract. However this effect is probably species specific. For example, *Lactobacillus reuteri* changes mRNA expressions of $GABA_A$ and $GABA_B$ receptors in central nervous system. The changes in these receptors have found to be related with anxious and depressive-like behaviors (Cryan & O'Mahony, 2011). Similarly it has been reported that *Bifidobacterium longum* has anxiolytic effect and decreases the excitability of ENS (Bercik et al., 2011).

7. The effect of probiotics on the intestinal barrier functions

Intestinal barrier is a morphologic and physiologic structure placed between tissues and intestinal lumen which is known as external environment and it ensures continuing of events such as absorption and secretion between them. Intestinal lumen consists of microclimate on epithelial cells and lamina propria under epithelium. It regulates nutrients absorption, water and ion fluxes, and represents the first defensive barrier against toxins and enteric pathogens. Intestinal barrier consists of internal and external layers; the internal layer includes intestinal epithelial cells and tight junctions (TJ), the external layer includes bacteria and a mucus layer (Catalioto et al., 2011).

The intestinal epithelium is formed by a monolayer epithelial cells, the spaces between epithelial cells is sealed by tight junctions. Tight junctions are specific structures comprised of transmembrane proteins. Microclimate consists of unstirred water layer, glycocalyx, and mucus layer. Lamina propria is a layer existed under epithelial cells. In this layer there are cells of innate and acquired immunity secreting immunoglobulins and cytokines which are substantial for intestinal barrier.

Proper intestinal barrier function is essential for maintaining optimal health and balance throughout the body. The epithelium of the intestinal mucosa prevents the passage of commensal and pathogenic microorganisms. Therefore, it is the first line of defense against luminal antigens and toxins. An impairment of this intestinal barrier is critical for pathogenesis of several diseases such as inflammatory bowel disease, celiac disease (Chichlowski et al., 2008) and atopic dermatitis (Rosenfeldt et al., 2004).

Development of physical and functional intestinal barrier begins during embryonic period. In human, enterocytes appear in intestinal mucosa at 8th weeks, and TJ appear at 10th weeks of pregnancy. Functional immune barrier becomes functional after the formation of panet cells at 12th weeks. In this period, panet cells produce antimicrobial defensins and lysozymes. Mucins, which start to be expressed at 6.5th weeks of pregnancy and increase in time, constitute functional barrier. Although the development of intestinal barrier begins at prenatal period, it continues through postnatal period (Patel & Lin, 2010). Because, intestinal barrier is not yet fully developed in preterm infants, aberrant inflammatory and apoptotic responses to bacteria may occur. When premature infants treated with probiotics, bacteria used as probiotic easily pass lamina propria and trigger immune reaction there.

It has been determined by *in vivo* and *in vitro* studies that probiotics strengthen intestinal barrier. This effect occurs through species specific various mechanisms. These mechanisms are the inhibition of apoptosis of epithelial cells, the regulation of TJ proteins expression and the distribution, prevention of attachments of pathogens to mucosa, and the regulation of mucus secretion.

7.1 Tight junction protein expression

The intestinal bacteria or probiotics change the expression and distribution of TJ proteins (Mennigen & Bruewe, 2009). Several studies investigated the effects of different probiotics on TJ protein expression and distribution under pathological conditions. Occludin is an integral plasma-membrane protein located at the TJs. Zonula occludens-1 (ZO-1) is a peripheral membrane protein and it is found to be associated with the cytoplasmic surfaces of TJs (Gottardi et al., 1996). Probiotic bacteria *Streptococcus thermophilus* and *Lactobacillus acidophilus* prevent the reduction in phosphorylation of occludin and zonula occludens-1 (ZO-1) caused by enteroinvasive *Escherichia coli* (EIEC) infection (Resta-Lenert & Barrett, 2003). Re-distribution of ZO-1 protein has been observed after epithelial cells were treated by a pathologic bacterium *Salmonella dublin*. However, treatment of epithelial cells with multi-microbe probiotic product VSL#3 prevented the redistribution of ZO-1 (Ng et al., 2009).

7.2 Epithelial adherence and pathogen exclusion

Many intestinal bacteria can adhere to the outer mucus layer to form a biofilm on their surface (Guarner & Malageda, 2003). This is an important mechanism for intestinal barrier. Three different situations in favor of the host and against pathogens should be considered. One of them is exclusion of pathogens by probiotics competitively. The second is the prevention of pathogen adhesion. And the third is displacement of adhered pathogen. Sherman et al. (2005) have reported that *Lactobacillus rhamnosus* and *acidophilus* could adhere to intestinal epithelial cells *in vitro* and pre-treatment of these probiotic strains reduced the binding of EPEC and EHEC. Additionally, *Lactobacillus* strains can directly compete with other pathogens, such as *Salmonella* species, for binding sites on human mucins or Caco-2 cell surfaces. It has been observed that the mentioned probiotics can also displace bound pathogens, although more slowly and to a lesser extent (Lee et al., 2003). There is a competition between pathogens and probiotics for sources of nutrients as well as a competition for adherence to mucosa or displacement from mucosa. This competition is useful for exclusion of pathogens and for strengthening intestinal barrier.

7.3 Mucus secretion

It has been reported by *in vivo* and *in vitro* studies that certain bacteria contribute to strengthen mucosal barrier by increasing mucus secretion. Mattar et al. (2002) reported that *Lactobacillus casei* GG increased mucin expression in the human intestinal cell lines Caco-2 (MUC2) and HT29 (MUC2 and MUC3), thus blocking pathogenic *Escherichia coli* invasion and adherence. Additionally, Otte & Podolsky (2004) observed that VSL#3 increased expression of MUC2, MUC3 in HT29 cells. Probiotics induce this mucus expression increasing effect by modifying gene expressions. For example, it has been observed that MUC2 and MUC3 mRNA expressions were increased after incubation of epithelial cells with *Lactobacillus plantarum* 299v (Mack et al., 1999). Similarly Caballero-Franco et al. (2007) have reported that basal luminal mucin content increased by 60% in Wistar rats that were orally administered the probiotic mixture VSL#3 on a daily basis for seven days. In addition, they exposed isolated rat colonic loops to the VSL#3 probiotic formula, which significantly stimulated colonic mucin (MUC) secretion and MUC2 gene.

Probiotics also contributes to strengthening of intestinal barrier with some mechanisms other than above mentioned ones. For example, Polyphosphate (poly-P) is produced by probiotics and it is a bioactive molecule that induced cytoprotective heat shock protein through activation of the integrin–p38 mitogen-activated protein kinase pathway, and it prevents oxidant-induced intestinal barrier weakening. Furthermore, poly-P ameliorated epithelial injury (Segawa et al., 2011). It has been reported that multi-microbe probiotic product VSL#3 normalized monolayer permeability and conductance in stimulated tissues, thus strengthened barrier integrity (Madsen et al., 2001). It has been determined that *Lactobacillus rhamnousus* GG prevented cytokine induced apoptosis in young adult mouse colon cell model (YAMC) and human colonic epithelial carcinoma cell line (HT29) (Yan & Polk, 2002).

8. References

Abrams, G.D. & Bishop, I.E. (1967). Effect of the normal microbial flora on gastrointestinal motility. *Proc Soc Exp Biol Med*, Vol. 126, pp. (301-304).

Agrawal, A., Houghton, L.A., Morris, J., Reilly, B., Guyonnet, D., Goupil Feuillerat, N., Schlumberger, A., Jakob, S. & Whorwell, PJ. (2009). Clinical trial: the effects of a fermented milk product containing Bifidobacterium lactis DN-173 010 on abdominal distension and gastrointestinal transit in irritable bowel syndrome with constipation. *Aliment Pharmacol Ther*, Vol. 29, No. 1, pp. (104-114).

Awad, W.A., Ghareeb, K. & Böhm, J. (2010). Effect of addition of a probiotic micro-organism to broiler diet on intestinal mucosal architecture and electrophysiological parameters. *J Anim Physiol Anim Nutr*, Vol. 94, No. 4, pp. (486-94).

Awad, W.A., Ghareeb, K., Abdel-Raheem, S. & Böhm, J. (2009). Effects of dietary inclusion of probiotic and synbiotic on growth performance, organ weights, and intestinal histomorphology of broiler chickens. *Poult Sci*, Vol. 88, No. 1, pp. (49-56).

Banasaz, M., Norin, E., Holma, R. & Midtvedt, T. (2002). Increased enterocyte production in gnotobiotic rats mono-associated with Lactobacillus rhamnosus GG. *Appl Environ Microbiol*, Vol. 68, No. 6, pp.(3031-3034).

Barbara, G., Stanghellini, V., Brandi, G., Cremon, C., Di Nardo, G., De Giorgio, R. & Corinaldesi, R. (2005). Interactions between commensal bacteria and gut sensorimotor function in health and disease. *Am J Gastroenterol*, Vol. 100, No. 11, pp. (2560-8).

Batchelor, D.J., Al-Rammahi, M., Moran, A.W., Brand, J.G., Li, X., Haskins, M., German, A.J. & Shirazi-Beechey, S.P. (2011). Sodium/glucose cotransporter-1, sweet receptor, and disaccharidase expression in the intestine of the domestic dog and cat: two species of different dietary habit. *Am J Physiol Regul Integr Comp Physiol,* Vol. 300, No. 1, pp. (67–75).

Bercik, P., Park, A.J., Sinclair, D., Khoshdel, A., Lu, J., Huang, X., Deng, Y., Blennerhassett, P.A., Fahnestock, M., Moine, D., Berger, B., Huizinga, J.D., Kunze, W., McLean, P.G., Bergonzelli, G.E., Collins, S.M. & Verdu, E.F. (2011). The anxiolytic effect of Bifidobacterium longum NCC3001 involves vagal pathways for gut-brain communication. *Neurogastroenterol Motil,* doi: 10.1111/j.1365-2982.2011.01796.x.

Binder, H.J. & Mehta, P. (1989). Short-chain fatty acids stimulate active sodium and chloride absorption in vitro in the rat distal colon. *Gastroenterology,* Vol. 96, pp. (989–996).

Borthakur, A., Gill, R.K., Tyagi, S., Koutsouris, A., Alrefai, W.A., Hecht, G.A., Ramaswamy, K. & Dudeja, P.K. (2008). The Probiotic Lactobacillus acidophilus Stimulates Chloride/ Hydroxyl Exchange Activity in Human Intestinal Epithelial Cells. *J Nutr,* Vol. 138, No. 7, pp. (1355-1359).

Brassart, D. & Vey, E. (1998). Patient Cooperation Treaty. WO99/021-70.

Breves, G., Faul, K., Schröder, B., Holst, H., Caspary, W.F. & Stein, J. (2000). Application of the colon-simulation technique for studying the effects of Saccharomyces boulardii on basic parameters of porcine cecal microbial metabolism disturbed by clindamycin. *Digestion.* Vol 61, No. 3, pp. (193-200).

Buts, J.P. (2009). Twenty-Five Years of Research on Saccharomyces boulardii Trophic Effects: Updates and Perspectives. *Digestive Diseases and Sciences,*Vol. 54, No. 1, pp. (15-18).

Buts, J.P., De Keyser, N., Marandi, S., Hermans, D., Sokal, E.M., Chae, Y.H., Lambotte, L., Chanteux, H. & Tulkens, P.M. (1999). Saccharomyces boulardii upgrades cellular adaptation after proximal enterectomy in rats. *Gut,* Vol. 45, No. 1, pp. (89-96).

Buts, J.P., De Keyser, N., Stilmant, C., Sokal, E. & Marandi, S. (2002). Saccharomyces boulardii enhances N-terminal peptide hydrolysis in suckling rat small intestine by endoluminal release of a zinc-binding metalloprotease. *Pediatr Res,* Vol. 51, No. 4, pp. (528-34).

Caballero-Franco, C., Keller, K., De Simone, C. & Chadee, K. (2007). The VSL#3 probiotic formula induces mucin gene expression and secretion in colonic epithelial cells. *Am J Physiol Gastrointest Liver Physiol,* Vol. 292, No. 1, pp. (G315-232).

Canonici, A., Siret, C., Pellegrino, E., Pontier-Bres, R., Pouyet, L., Montero, M.P., Colin, C., Czerucka, D., Rigot, V. & André, F. (2011). Saccharomyces boulardii improves intestinal cell restitution through activation of the $\alpha2\beta1$ integrin collagen receptor. *PLoS One,* Vol. 31, No. 6(3), pp. (e18427).

Catalioto, R.M., Maggi, C.A. & Giuliani, S. (2011). Intestinal epithelial barrier dysfunction in disease and possible therapeutical interventions. *Curr Med Chem,* Vol. 18, No. 3, pp. (398-426).

Cherbut, C., Aube, A.C., Blottiere, H.M. & Galmiche, J.P. (1997). Effects of short-chain fatty acids on gastrointestinal motility. *Scandinavian journal of gastroenterology,* Vol. 222, pp. (58–61).

Chichlowski, M. & Hale, L.P. (2008). Bacterial-mucosal interactions in inflammatory bowel disease--an alliance gone bad. *Am J Physiol Gastrointest Liver Physiol,* Vol. 662, No. 295, pp. (G1139-G1149).

Chiou, P.W.S., Lu, T.W. Hsu, J.C. & Yu, B. (1996). Effect of different sources of fiber on the intestinal morphology of domestic geese. Asian Australas. *Journal of Animal Science,* Vol. 4, pp. (539–550).

Cryan, J.F. & O'Mahony, S.M. (2011). The microbiome-gut-brain axis: from bowel to behavior. *Neurogastroenterol Motil*, Vol. 23, No. 3, pp. (187-92).

de Vrese, M., Stegelmann, A., Richter, B., Fenselau, S., Laue, C. & Schrezenmeir, J. (2001). Probiotics--compensation for lactase insufficiency. *Am J Clin Nutr*, Vol. 73, No. 2 Suppl, pp. (421S-429S).

Deshpande, G., Rao, S. & Patole, S. (2011). Progress in the field of probiotics: year 2011. *Current Opinion in Gastroenterology*, Vol. 27, No.1, pp. (13-18).

Di Giancamillo, A., Vitari, F., Savoini, G., Bontempo, V., Bersani, C., Dell'Orto, V. & Domeneghini, C. (2008). Effects of orally administered probiotic Pediococcus acidilactici on the small and large intestine of weaning piglets. A qualitative and quantitative micro-anatomical study. *Histol Histopathol*, Vol. 23, No. 6, pp. (651-64).

Di Giancamillo, A., Vitari, F., Bosi, G., Savoini, G. & Domeneghini, C. (2010). The chemical code of porcine enteric neurons and the number of enteric glial cells are altered by dietary probiotics. *Neurogastroenterol Motil*, Vol. 22, No. 9, pp. (e271-8).

Drouault, S., Juste, C., Marteau, P., Renault, P. & Corthier, G. (2002). Oral treatment with Lactococcus lactis expressing Staphylococcus hyicus lipase enhances lipid digestion in pigs with induced pancreatic insufficiency. *Appl Environ Microbiol*, Vol. 68, No. 6, pp. (3166-8).

Dudeja, P.K., Rao, D.D., Syed, I., Joshi, V., Dahdal, R.Y., Gardner, C., Risk, M.C., Schmidt, L., Bavishi, D. & Kim, K. E. (1996). Intestinal distribution of human Na+/H+ exchanger isoforms NHE-1, NHE-2, and NHE-3 mRNA. *Am. J. Physiol*, Vol. 271, pp. (G483–G493).

Fan, Y.K., Croom, J., Christensen, V.L., Black, B.L., Bird, A.R., Daniel, L.R., Mcbride, B.W. & Eisen, E.J. (1997). Jejunal glucose uptake and oxygen consumption in turkey poults selected for rapid growth. *Poult Sci*, Vol. 76, No. 12, pp. (1738-45).

FAO/WHO (2001). Report of a Joint FAO/WHO Expert Consultation on Evaluation of Health and Nutritional Properties of Probiotics in Food Including Powder Milk with Live Lactic Acid Bacteria, (October 2001).

Furuse, M. & Okumura, J. (1994). Nutritional and physiological characteristics in germ-free chickens. Comp Biochem Physiol A Physiol. Vol. 109, No.3, pp. (547-56).

Gauffin, C.P., Agüero, G. & Perdigon, G. (2002). Adjuvant effects of Lactobacillus casei added to a renutrition diet in a malnourished mouse model. *Biocell*, Vol. 26, No. 1, pp. (35-48).

Gershon, M.D. (2005). Nerves, reflexes, and the enteric nervous system: pathogenesis of the irritable bowel syndrome. *Journal of Clinical Gastroenterology*, Vol. 39, pp. (S184–S193).

Gilliland, S.E. & Walker, D.K. (1990). Factors to consider when selecting a culture of Lactobacillus acidophilus as a dietary adjunct to produce a hypocholesterolemic effect in humans. *J Dairy Sci*, Vol. 73, No. 4, pp. (905–11).

Gilman, J. & Cashman, K.D. (2006). The effect of probiotic bacteria on transepithelial calcium transport and calcium uptake in human intestinal-like Caco-2 cells. *Curr Issues Intest Microbiol*, Vol. 7, No. 1, pp. (1-5).

Goodlad, R.A., Ratcliffe, B., Fordham, J.P., Ghatei, M.A., Domin, J., Bloom, S.R. & Wright, N.A. (1996). Influence of caecal microflora and of two dietary protein levels on the adaptation of the exocrine pancreas: comparative study in germ-free and conventional rats. *Br J Nutr*, Vol. 75, No. 3, pp. (433-44).

Gottardi, C.J., Arpin, M., Fanning, A.S. & Louvard, D. (1996). The junction-associated protein, zonula occludens-1, localizes to the nucleus before the maturation and during the remodeling of cell-cell contacts. *Proc Natl Acad Sci U S A*, Vol. 93, No. 20, pp. (10779-84).

Guarner, F. & Malagelada, J.R. (2003). Gut flora in healt and disease. *Lancet*, Vol. 361, pp. (512-519).

Gunal, M., Yayli, G., Kaya, O., Karahan N. & Sulak, O. (2006). The Effects of Antibiotic Growth Promoter, Probiotic or Organic Acid Supplementation on Performance, Intestinal Microflora and Tissue of Broilers. *International Journal of Poultry Science*, Vol. 5, No. 2, pp. (149-155).

Guo, C. & Zhang, L. (2010). Cholesterol-lowering effects of probiotics--a review. *Wei Sheng Wu Xue Bao*, Vol. 50, No. 12, pp. (590-9).

Harms, H.K., Bertele-Harms, R.M. & Bruer-Kleis, D. (1987). Enzyme-substitution therapy with the yeast Saccharomyces cerevisiae in congenital sucrase-isomaltase deficiency. N Engl J Med, Vol. 316, No. 21, pp. (1306-9).

Heneghan, J.B. (1984). Physiology of the alimentary tract, In: *The Germ-free Animal in Biomedical Research*, ME Coates & BE Gustafsson, pp. (169-191), Laboratory Animals Lt, London.

Herich, R., Levkut, M., Bomba, A., Gancarcíková, S. & Nemcová, R. (2004). Differences in the development of the small intestine between gnotobiotic and conventionally bred piglets. *Berl Munch Tierarztl Wochenschr*, Vol.117, No. 1-2, pp. (46-51).

Heyman, M. & Ménard, S. (2002). Probiotic microorganisms: how they affect intestinal Pathophysiology. *Cellular and Molecular Life Sciences*, Vol. 59, pp. (1-15).

Hooper, L.V. & Gordon J.I. (2001). Commensal Host-Bacterial Relationships in the Gut. *Science*, Vol. 292, No. 5519, pp. (1115-1118).

Huang, Y. & Zheng, Y. (2010). The probiotic Lactobacillus acidophilus reduces cholesterol absorption through the down-regulation of Niemann-Pick C1-like 1 in Caco-2 cells. *Br J Nutr*, Vol. 103,No. 4, pp. (473-478).

Husebye, E., Hellström, P.M. & Midtvedt, T. (1994). Intestinal microflora stimulates myoelectric activity of rat small intestine by promoting cyclic initiation and aboral propagation of migrating myoelectric complex. *Dig Dis Sci*, Vol. 39, No. 5, pp. (946-56).

Husebye, E., Hellström, P.M., Sundler, F., Chen, J. & Midtvedt, T. (2001). Influence of microbial species on small intestinal myoelectric activity and transit in germ-free rats. *Am J Physiol Gastrointest Liver Physiol*, Vol. 280, No. 3, pp. (G368-80).

Ichikawa, H., Kuroiwa, T., Inagaki, A., Shineha, R., Nishihira, T., Satomi, S. & Sakata, T. (1999). Probiotic bacteria stimulate gut epithelial cell proliferation in rat. *Digestive Diseases and Sciences*, Vol. 44, No. 10, pp. (2119-2123).

Indrio, F. & Neu, J. (2011). The intestinal microbiome of infants and the use of probiotics. *Curr Opin Pediatr*, Vol. 23, No. 2, pp. (145-50).

Indrio, F., Riezzo, G., Raimondi, F., Bisceglia, M. & Francavilla, R. (2008). The Effects of Probiotics on Feeding Tolerance, Bowel Habits, and Gastrointestinal Motility in Preterm Newborns. *J Pediatr*, Vol. 152, pp. (801-806).

Indrio, F., Riezzo, G., Raimondi, F., Bisceglia, M., Cavallo, L. & Francavilla, R. (2009). Effects of probiotic and prebiotic on gastrointestinal motility in newborns. *Physiol Pharmacol*, Vol. 60 (Suppl 6), pp. (27-31).

Kamm, K., Hoppe, S., Breves, G., Schröder, B. & Schemann, M. (2004). Effects of the probiotic yeast Saccharomyces boulardii on the neurochemistry of myenteric neurones in pig jejunum. *Neurogastroenterol Motil*, Vol.16, No.1, pp. (53-60).

Kiela, P.R., Kuscuoglu, N., Midura, A.J., Midura-Kiela, M.T., Larmonier, C.B., Lipko, M. & Ghishan, F.K. (2007). Molecular mechanism of rat NHE3 gene promoter regulation by sodium butyrate. *Am J Physiol Cell Physiol*, Vol. 293, No. 1, pp. (C64-74).

Kim, J.S., Ingale, S.L., Kim, Y.W., Kim, K.H., Sen, S., Ryu, M.H., Lohakare, J.D., Kwon, I.K. & Chae, B.J. (2011). Effect of supplementation of multi-microbe probiotic product on growth performance, apparent digestibility, cecal microbiota and small intestinal morphology of broilers. *J Anim Physiol Anim Nutr (Berl)*, doi: 10.1111/j.1439-0396.2011.01187.x.

Krammer, M. & Karbach, U. (1993). Antidiarrheal action of the yeast Saccharomyces boulardii in the rat small and large intestine by stimulating chloride absorption. *Zeitschrift fur Gastroenterologie*, Vol. 31(Suppl 4), pp. (73–77).

Kunze, W.A., Mao, Y.K., Wang, B., Huizinga, J.D., Ma, X., Forsythe, P. & Bienenstock, J. (2009). Lactobacillus reuteri enhances excitability of colonic AH neurons by inhibiting calcium-dependent potassium channel opening. *J Cell Mol Med*, Vol. 13, No. 8B, pp. (2261-70).

Labayen, I., Forga, L., González, A., Lenoir-Wijnkoop, I., Nutr, R. & Martínez, J.A. (2001). Relationship between lactose digestion, gastrointestinal transit time and symptoms in lactose malabsorbers after dairy consumption. *Aliment Pharmacol Ther*, Vol. 15, No. 4, pp. (543-9).

Larkin, T.A., Astheimer, L.B. & Price, W.E. (2009). Dietary combination of soy with a probiotic or prebiotic food significantly reduces total and LDL cholesterol in mildly hypercholesterolaemic subjects. *Eur J Clin Nutr*, Vol. 63, No. 2, pp. (238-45).

Lee, Y.K., Puong, K.Y., Ouwehand, A.C. & Salminen, S. (2003). Displacement of bacterial 819 pathogens from mucus and Caco-2 cell surface by lactobacilli. *J Med Microbiol*, Vol. 52(Pt 10), pp. (925-930).

Lhoste, E.F., Catala, I., Fiszlewicz, M., Gueugneau, A.M., Popot, F., Vaissade, P., Corring, T. & Szylit, O. (1996). Influence of caecal microflora and of two dietary protein levels on the adaptation of the exocrine pancreas: comparative study in germ-free and conventional rats. *Br J Nutr*, Vol. 75, No. 3, pp. (433-44).

Lodemann, U., Hübener, K., Jansen, N. & Martens, H. (2006). Effects of Enterococcus faecium NCIMB 10415 as probiotic supplement on intestinal transport and barrier function of piglets. *Arch Anim Nutr*, Vol. 60, No. 1, pp. (35-48).

Lyt, M. (2011). Probiotics function mechanistically as delivery vehicles for neuroactive compounds: Microbial endocrinology in the design and use of probiotics. *Bioessays*, Vol. 33, pp. (574–581).

Mack, D.R., Michail, S., Wei, S., McDougall, L. & Hollingsworth, M.A. (1999). Probiotics inhibit enteropathogenic E. coli adherence in vitro by inducing intestinal mucin gene expression. *Am J Physiol*, Vol. 276(4 Pt 1), pp. (G941- 950).

Madsen, K., Cornish, A., Soper, P., McKaigney, C., Jijon, H., Yachimec, C., Doyle, J., Jewell, L. & De Simone, C. (2001). Probiotic bacteria enhance murine and human intestinal ephitelial barrier function. *Gastroenterology*, Vol. 121, No. 3, pp. (580-591).

Malakooti, J., Saksena, S., Gill, K.R. & Dudeja, P.K. (2011). Transcriptional regulation of the intestinal luminal Na+ and Cl− transporter. *Biochem J*, Vol. (435), pp. (313–325).

Marteau, P., Cuillerier, E., Meance, S., Gerhardt, M.F., Myara, A., Bouvier, M., Bouley, C., Tondu, F., Bommelaer, G. & Grimaud, J.C. (2002). Bifidobacterium animalis strain DN-173 010 shortens the colonic transit time in healthy women: a double-blind, randomized, controlled study. *Aliment Pharmacol Ther*, Vol. 16, No. 3, pp. (587-93).

Marteau, P.R., de Vrese, M., Cellier, C.J. & Schrezenmeir, J. (2001). Protection from gastrointestinal diseases with the use of probiotics. *Am J Clin Nutr*, Vol. 73(2 Suppl), pp. (430S-436S).

Massi, M., Ioan, P., Budriesi, R., Chiarini, A., Vitali, B., Lammers, K.M., Gionchetti, P., Campieri, M., Lembo, A. & Brigidi, P. (2006). Effects of probiotic bacteria on gastrointestinal motility in guinea-pig isolated tissue. *World J Gastroenterol*, Vol. 12, No. 37, pp. (5987-94).

Mattar, A.F., Teitelbaum, D.H., Drongowski, R.A., Yongyi, F., Harmon, C.M. & Coran, A.G. (2002). Probiotics up-regulate MUC-2 mucin gene expression in a Caco-2 cell-culture model. *Pediatr Surg Int*, Vol. 18, pp. (586–590).

Matur, E., Cotelioglu, U., Arslan, M., Ergül, E., Akyazi, I. & Eraslan E. (2007): The effects of Enterococcus faecium NCIMB10415 on the development of pancreas and small intestine and on activity of pancreatic digestive enzymes in broiler chickens. *Archiv Für Geflugelkunde*, Vol. 71, pp. (162-168).

Mcmanus, C.M., Michel, K.E., Simon, D.M. & Washabau, R.J. (2002). Effect of short-chain fatty acids on contraction of smooth muscle in the canine colon. *Am J Vet Res*, Vol. 63, No. 2, pp. (295-300).

Meance, S., Cayuela, C., Turchet, P., Raimondi, A., Lucas, C. & Antoine, J.M. (2001). A fermented milk with a bifidobacterium probiotic strain DN-173 010 shortened oro-fecal gut transit time in elderly. *Microb Ecol Health Dis*, Vol. 13, pp. (217–22).

Mennigen, R. & Bruewe, M. (2009). Effect of Probiotics on Intestinal Barrier Function Molecular Structure and Function of the Tight Junction. *Ann NY Acad Sci*, Vol. 1165, pp. (183–189).

Meslin, J.C. & Sacquet, E. (1984).Effects of microflora on the dimensions of enterocyte microvilli in the rat. *Reprod Nutr Dev*, Vol. 24, No. 3, pp. (307-314).

Mogilner, J.G., Srugo, I., Lurie, M., Shaoul, R., Coran, A.G., Shiloni, E. & Sukhotnik, I. (2007). Effect of probiotics on intestinal regrowth and bacterial translocation after massive small bowel resection in a rat. *J Pediatr Surg*, Vol. 42, No. 8, pp. (1365-71).

Montalto, M., Curigliano, V., Santoro, L., Vastola, M., Cammarota, G., Manna, R., Gasbarrini, A. & Gasbarrini, G. (2006). Management and treatment of lactose malabsorption. *World J Gastroenterol*, Vol. 12, No. 2, (187-91).

Ng, S.C., Hart, A.L., Kamm, M.A., Stagg, A.J. & Knight, S.C. (2009). Mechanisms of action of probiotic: Recent Advances. *Imflamatuar Bowel disease*, Vol. 15, No. 2, pp. (300-10).

Ohashi, Y. & Ushida, K. (2009). Health-beneficial effects of probiotics: Its mode of action. *Animal Science journal*, Vol. 80, pp. (361-371).

Ohbo, M., Katoh, K. & Sasaki, Y. (1996). Effects of saturated fatty acids on amylase release from exocrine pancreatic segments of sheep, rats, hamsters, field voles and mice. *J Comp Physiol B*, Vol.166, No.5, pp (305-309).

Ojetti,V.G., Gigante, M., Gabrielli, M.E., Ainora, A., Mannocci, E.C., Lauritano, G. & Gasbarrini, A. (2010). The effect of oral supplementation with Lactobacillus reuteri or tilactase in lactose intolerant patients: randomized trial. *Eur Rev Med Pharmacol Sci*, Vol. 14, No. 3, pp. (163-170).

Otte, J.M. & Podolsky, D.K. (2004). Functional modulation of enterocytes by gram-positive and gram-negative microorganisms. *Am J Physiol Gastrointest Liver Physiol*, Vol. 286, pp. (G613–G626).

Özcan, M., Arslan, M., Matur, E., Çötelioğlu, Ü., Akyazi İ., & Eraslan. E. (2003). The Effects of Enterococcus faecium Cernelle 68 (SF 68) on Output Properties and Some Hematological Parameters In Broilers. *Medycyna Wet*, Vol. 59, pp. (496–500).

Park, Y.H., Kim, J.G., Shin, Y.W., Kim, S.H. & Whang, K.Y. (2007). Effect of dietary inclusion of Lactobacillus acidophilus ATCC 43121 on cholesterol metabolism in rats. *J Microbiol Biotechnol*, Vol. 17, No. 4, pp. (655-62).

Patel, R.M. & Lin, P.W. (2010). Developmental biology of gut-probiotic interaction. *Gut microbes*, Vol. 1, No. 3, pp. (186-195).

Pelicano, E.R.L., Souza, P.A., Souza, H.B.A., Figueiredo, D.F., Boiago, M.M., Carvalho, S.R. & Bordon, V.F. (2005). Intestinal Mucosa Development in Broiler Chickens Fed Natural Growth Promoters. *Brazilian Journal of Poultry Science*, Vol. 7, No. 4, pp. (221- 229).

Pimentel, M., Lin, H.C., Enayati, P., van den Burg, B., Lee, H.R., Chen, J.H., Park, S., Kong, Y. & Conklin, J. (2006). Methane, a gas produced by enteric bacteria, slows intestinal transit and augments small intestinal contractile activity. *Am J Physiol Gastrointest Liver Physiol*, Vol. 290, No. 6, pp. (G1089-95).

Quigley, E.M. (2011). Gut microbiota and the role of probiotics in therapy. *Curr Opin Pharmacol*, Vol. 11, pp. (1-11).

Raheja, G., Borthakur, A., Singh, V., Gill, R.K., Alrefai, W.A., Malakooti, J., Ramaswamy, K. & Dudeja, P.K. (2010). Mechanisms underlying upregulation of intestinal electrolyte absorption by probiotics. *Genes Nutr*, Vol. 5 (Suppl 1), pp. (S25–S100).

Raheja, G., Singh, V., Ma, K., Boumendjel, R., Borthakur, A., Gill, R.K., Saksena, S., Alrefai, W.A., Ramaswamy, K. & Dudeja, P.K. (2010). Lactobacillus acidophilus stimulates the expression of SLC26A3 via a transcriptional mechanism. *Am J Physiol Gastrointest Liver Physiol*, Vol. 298, No. 3, pp. (G395-401).

Resta-Lenert, S. & Barrett, K.E. (2003). Live probiotics protect intestinal epithelial cells from the effects of infection with enteroinvasive Escherichia coli (EIEC). *Gut*, Vol. 52, pp. (988–997).

Rolfe, R.D. (2000). The role of probiotic cultures in the control of gastrointestinal health. *J Nutr*, Vol. 130(2S Suppl), pp. (396S-402S).

Rooj, A.K., Kimura, Y. & Buddington, R.K. (2010). Metabolites produced by probiotic Lactobacilli rapidly increase glucose uptake by Caco-2 cells. *BMC Microbiol*, 10:16.

Rosenfeldt, V., Benfeldt, E., Valerius, H.N., Pærregaard, A. & Michaelsen, K.F. (2004). Effect of probiotics on gastrointestinal symptoms and small intestinal permeability in children with atopic dermatitis. *J Pediatr*, Vol. 145, No. 5, pp. (612-6).

Sakata, T. (1987). Stimulatory effect of short-chain fatty acids on epithelial cell proliferation in the rat intestine: a possible explanation for trophic effects of fermentable fibre, gut microbes and luminal trophic factors. Br J Nutr, Vol. 58, No.1, pp. (95-103).

Sakata, T., Kojima, T., Fujieda, M., Miyakozawa, M., Takahashi, M. & Ushida K. (1999). Probiotic preparations dose-dependently increase net production rates of organic acids and decrease that of ammonia by pig cecal bacteria in batch culture. Dig Dis Sci, Vol. 44, No. 7, pp. (1485-1493).

Salminen, S. & Salminen, E. (1997). Lactulose, lactic acid bacteria, intestinal microecology and mucosal protection. Scand J Gastroenterol Suppl, Vol. 222, pp. (45-8).

Samanya, M. & Yamauchi, K.E. (2002). Histological alterations of intestinal villi in chickens fed dried Bacillus subtilis var. natto. *Comp Biochem Physiol A Mol Integr Physiol*, Vol. 133, No. 1, pp. (95-104).

Samli, H.E., Senkoylu, N., Koc, F., Kanter, M. & Agma, A. (2007). Effects of Enterococcus faecium and dried whey on broiler performance, gut histomorphology and intestinal microbiota. *Arch Anim Nutr*, Vol. 61, No. 1, pp. (42-9).

Scharek, L., Guth, J., Reiter, K., Weyrauch, K.D., Taras, D., Schwerk, P., Schierack, P., Schmidt, M.F., Wieler, L.H. & Tedin, K. (2005). Influence of a probiotic Enterococcus faecium strain on development of the immune system of sows and piglets. *Vet Immunol Immunopathol*, Vol. 105, No. 1-2, pp. (151-61).

Scholz-Ahrens, K. E., Ade, P., Marten, B., Weber, P., Timm, W., Açil, Y., Glüer, C.C. & Schrezenmeir, J. (2007). Prebiotics, Probiotics, and Synbiotics Affect Mineral Absorption, Bone Mineral Content, and Bone Structure. *J Nutr*, Vol. 137, pp. (838S-846S).

Segawa, S., Fujiya, M., Konishi, H., Ueno, N., Kobayashi, N., Shigyo, T., & Kohgo, Y. (2011). Probiotic-derived polyphosphate enhances the epithelial barrier function and maintains intestinal homeostasis through integrin-P 38 MAPK pathway. *PLoS One*, Vol. 6, No. 8, pp. (e23278).

Sharma, R., Schumacher, U., Ronaasen, V. & Coates, M . (1995). Rat intestinal mucosal responses to a microbial flora and different diets. *Gut*, Vol. 36, pp. (209-214).

Sherman, P.M., Johnson-Henry, K.C., Yeung, H.P., Ngo, P.S.C., Goulet, J. & Tompkins, T.A. (2005). Probiotics reduce enterohemorrhagic Escherichia coli O157:H7-and enteropathogenic E. coli O127:H6-induced changes in polarized T84 epithelial cell monolayers by reducing bacterial adhesion and cytoskeletal rearrangements. *Infect Immun*, Vol. 73, pp. (5183-5188).

Shimizu, M., Kobayashi, Y., Suzuki, M., Satsu, H. & Miyamoto, Y. (2000). Regulation of intestinal glucose transport by tea catechins. *Biofactors*, Vol. 13, No. 1-4, pp. (61-5).

Shirkey, T.W., Siggers, R.H., Goldade, B.G., Marshall, J.K., Drew, M.D., Laarveld, B. & Van Kessel, A.G. (2006). Effects of commensal bacteria on intestinal morphology and expression of proinflammatory cytokines in the gnotobiotic pig. *Exp Biol Med (Maywood)*, Vol. 231, No. 8, pp. (1333-1345).

Shurson, G.C., Ku, P.K., Waxler, G.L., Yokoyama, M.T. & Miller, E.R. (1990). Physiological relationships between microbiological status and dietary copper levels in the pig. *J Anim Sci*, Vol. 68,No. 4, pp. (1061-71).

Smirnov, A., Perez, R., Amit-Romach, E., Sklan, D. & Uni, Z. (2005). Mucin dynamics and microbial populations in chicken small intestine are changed by dietary probiotic and antibiotic growth promoter supplementation. *J Nutr*, Vol. 135, No. 2, pp. (187-92).

Soret, R., Chevalier, J., De Coppet, P., Poupeau, G., Derkinderen, P., Segain, J.P. & Neunlist, M. (2010). Short-chain fatty acids regulate the enteric neurons and control gastrointestinal motility in rats. *Gastroenterology*, Vol. 138, No. 5, pp. (1772-82).

Strompfova, V., Marcináková, M., Simonová, M., Gancarcíková, S., Jonecová, Z., Scirankova, L., Koscová, J., Buleca, V., Cobanová, K. & Lauková, A. (2006). Enterococcus faecium EK13--an enterocin a-producing strain with probiotic character and its effect in piglets. *Anaerobe*, Vol. 12, No. 5-6, pp. (242-8).

Taheri, H.R., Moravej, H., Malakzadegan, A., Tabandeh, F., Zaghari, M., Shivazad, M. & Adibmoradi, M . (2010). Efficacy of Pediococcus acidlactici-based probiotic intestinal Coliforms and villus height, serum cholesterol level and performance of broiler. *African Journal of Biotechnology*, Vol. 9, No. 44, pp. (7564-7567).

Tang, A.L., Shah, N.P., Wilcox, G., Walker, K.Z., Stojanovska, L. (2007). Fermentation of Calcium-Fortified Soymilk with *Lactobacillus*: Effects on Calcium Solubility, Isoflavone Conversion, and Production of Organic Acids. *Journal of Food Science*, Vol. 72, No. 9, pp. (M431–M436).

Treem, W.R., Ahsan, N., Sullivan, B., Rossi, T., Holmes, R., Fitzgerald, J., Proujansky, R., Hyams, J. (1993). Evaluation of liquid yeast-derived sucrase enzyme replacement in patients with sucrase-isomaltase deficiency. *Gastroenterology*, Vol. 105, No. 4, pp. (1061-8).

Verdu, E.F., Bercík, P., Bergonzelli, G.E., Huang, X.X., Blennerhasset, P., Rochat, F., Fiaux, M., Mansourian, R., Corthésy-Theulaz, I. & Collins, S.M. (2004). Lactobacillus paracasei normalizes muscle hypercontractility in a murine model of postinfective gut dysfunction. *Gastroenterology*, Vol. 127, No. 3, pp. (826-37).

Verdu, E.F., Bercik, P., Huang, X.X., Lu, J., Al-Mutawaly, N., Sakai, H., Tompkins, T.A., Croitoru, K., Tsuchida, E., Perdue, M. & Collins, S.M. (2008). The role of luminal factors in the recovery of gastric function and behavioral changes after chronic Helicobacter pylori infection. *Am J Physiol Gastrointest Liver Physiol*, Vol. 295, No. 4, pp. (G664-70).

Vinderola, G., Matar, C. & Perdigón, G. (2007). Milk fermentation products of L. helveticus R389 activate calcineurin as a signal to promote gut mucosal immunity. *BMC Immunology*, 8:19.

Waller, P.A., Gopal, P.K., Leyer, G.J., Ouwehand, A.C., Reifer, C., Stewart, M.E. & Miller, L.E. (2011). Dose-response effect of Bifidobacterium lactis HN019 on whole gut transit time and functional gastrointestinal symptoms in adults. *Scand J Gastroenterol*, Vol. 46, No. 9, pp. (1057-64).

Wang, B., Mao, Y.K., Diorio, C., Pasyk, M., Wu, R.Y., Bienenstock, J. & Kunze, W.A. (2010). Luminal administration ex vivo of a live Lactobacillus species moderates mouse jejunal motility within minutes *FASEB J*, Vol. 24, No. 10, pp. (4078-88).

Wang, B., Mao, Y.K., Diorio, C., Wang, L., Huizinga, J.D., Bienenstock, J. & Kunze, W. (2010). Lactobacillus reuteri ingestion and IK(Ca) channel blockade have similar effects on rat colon motility and myenteric neurones. *Neurogastroenterol Motil*, Vol. 22, No. 1, pp. (98-107).

Wang, Z., Petrovic, S., Mann, E. and Soleimani, M. (2002) Identification of an apical Cl−/HCO3 − exchanger in the small intestine. *Am J Physiol Gastrointest Liver Physiol*, Vol. 282, pp. (G573–G579).

Williams, M.D., Ha, C.Y. & Ciorba, M.A. (2010). Probiotics as therapy in gastroenterology: a study of physician opinions and recommendations. *Clin Gastroenterol*, Vol. 44, No. 9, pp. (631-6).

Willing, B.P. & Van Kessel, A.G. (2007). Enterocyte proliferation and apoptosis in the caudal small intestine is influenced by the composition of colonizing commensal bacteria in the neonatal gnotobiotic pig. *Journal Of Animal Science*, Vol. 85, No. 12, pp (3256-66).

Wood, J.D. (2007). Effects of Bacteria on the Enteric Nervous System: Implications for the Irritable Bowel Syndrome. *Journal of Clinical Gastroenterology*, Vol. 41, No. 1, pp. (S7-S19).

Yan, F. & Polk, D.B. (2002). Probiotic bacterium prevents cytokine-induced apoptosis in intestinal epithelial cells. *J Biol Chem*, Vol. 277, No. 52, pp. (50959-65).

Yang, H., Liu, A., Zhang, M., Ibrahim, S.A., Pang, Z., Leng, X. & Ren, F. (2009). Oral administration of live Bifidobacterium substrains isolated from centenarians enhances intestinal function in mice. *Curr Microbiol*, Vol. 59, No. 4, pp. (439-445).

Yason, C.V., Summers, B.A. & Schat, K.A. (1987). Pathogenesis of rotavirus infection in various age groups of chickens and turkeys: pathology. *American Journal of Veterinary Research*, Vol. 6, pp. (927–93).

Zhang, A.W., Lee, B.D., Lee, S.K., Lee, K.W., An, G.H., Song, K.B. & Lee, C.H. (2005). Effects of yeast (Saccharomyces cerevisiae) cell components on growth performance, meat quality, and ileal mucosa development of broiler chicks. *Poult Sci*, Vol. 84, No. 7, pp. (1015-21).

4

The Benefits of Probiotics in Human and Animal Nutrition

Camila Boaventura, Rafael Azevedo, Ana Uetanabaro,
Jacques Nicoli and Luis Gustavo Braga
Universidade Estadual de Santa Cruz
Brazil

1. Introduction

At birth, the gastrointestinal tract of any animals is sterile, and it is rapidly colonized by bacteria from the mother and the environment. This colonization by the gut microbiota plays an important role in intestinal tract maturation of newborn (in terms of anatomy, digestive physiology, and immunology) (Hooper 2004). After this colonization, considering healthy human individuals, the gastrointestinal tract harbors 10 or more times as many microbes than there are eukaryotic cells (10^{14} viable cells for indigenous microbiota/10^{13} body cells).These microorganisms, altogether weighing approximately 1.5 kg, can be considered as a complementary major organ, responsible for three main functions: colonization resistance, immunomodulation, and nutritional contribution (Hayashi et al., 2002; Zoetendal et al., 2011). Colonization resistance inhibits the installation of exogenous microorganisms as well as the uncontrolled multiplication of microorganisms belonging to the indigenous microbiota. Immunomodulation maintains the immune system under a watchful state, which permits a faster but adequate response in the case of infectious aggression. Nutritional contribution furnishes complementary sources of vitamins, enzymes, and energy substrates (volatile fatty acids).

Unfortunately, several factors can disturb both the initial colonization and posterior maintenance of the gut microbiota, leading to a microbial ecosystem with beneficial functions transitorily or irreversibly less efficient. As examples, the type of delivery (cesarean or natural) or the reduction of mother-child contacts (premature baby in an incubator or in an intensive care unit) interfere with the supply of microorganisms necessary for post-natal colonization. Additionally, the alimentation (breast- or formula-fed) and the ingestion of antibacterial drugs may be other factors that modify the normal sequence of colonization (Harmsen et al., 2000; Bonnemaison et al., 2003; Westerbeek et al., 2006; Chen et al., 2007). Once installed, the beneficial functions of the microbiota are very powerful but also fragile and can be disturbed by ingestion of drugs (especially antibiotics), drastic changes in diet or stress. In view of what was presented above, the importance of a correct initial colonization and a subsequent preservation of the gut microbiota is evident to obtain optimal functions from this microbial ecosystem. When disturbances of the indigenous microbiota functions are forecasted or installed, you should think about the possibility of compensating failures of these functions. In this sense, probiotics can be considered as biotherapeutics to be used in microbial ecosystems during the installation phase (colonization of the newborn), or with installed (treatment) or forecasted disturbances (prophylaxis).

Probiotics have been defined in a joint meeting of the Food and Agriculture Organization/World Health Organization as "live microorganisms which when administered in adequate amounts confer a benefit to host health" (WHO / FAO, 2002). The objective of its use is to install, enhance or compensate the functions of the indigenous microbiota inhabiting the digestive tract or other body surfaces. The suggestion of using fermented food to obtain some benefits for the health is not new. It was mentioned in the Persian version of the Old Testament (Genesis 18:8) that "Abraham attributed his longevity to the consumption of sour milk." Later in 76 BC Pline, a Roman historian, recommended the use of fermented milk products for the treatment of gastroenteritis (Schrezenmeir & de Vres, 2001). However, a scientific approach, recognizing the beneficial role of certain microorganisms has been only applied in the first decades of the twentieth century with the suggestion of the use of *Lactobacillus* (Elie Metchnikoff attributing the longevity of Bulgarian populations to the yogurt consumption in 1907), *Bifidobacterium* (Henri Tissier observing a higher presence of bifidobacteria in the feces of healthy breast-fed children in 1906) and *Saccharomyces boulardii* (Henri Boulard noting the use of a tropical fruit colonized by this yeast to treat diarrhea by local populations in Eastern Orient during a cholera outbreak in 1920) to prevent or treat gastrointestinal disorders (Shortt, 1999). The probiotics most often used at the moment are bacteria producing lactic acid (*Lactobacillus, Bifidobacterium*) and yeasts (*Saccharomyces boulardii*).

Many health benefits have been related to human and animal intake of probiotic. Several studies have supplied clinical evidences of the benefits generated by probiotics, as for example in diarrhea treatment (Billooet al., 2006; De Vrese & Marteau, 2007), lactose intolerance (He et al., 2008), irritable bowel syndrome (De Vrese et al., 2001; Nagala & Routray, 2011), allergies (Jain et al., 2010), cancer (Chen et al., 2009) and hypercholesterolemia (Baroutkoub, 2010). According to recent meta-analysis based on well conducted clinical trials with probiotics, a clear protective effect was evident, which did not vary significantly between products containing *S. boulardii, Lactobacillus rhamnosus* GG, *L. acidophilus, L. bulgaricus, L. casei, Bifidobacterium longum, B. bifidum* var. *infantis* and *B. animalis* var. *lactis* (Sazawal et al., 2006).

Probiotics have also received special attention by animal nutrition researchers who search for alternatives to the use of traditional growth promoters (antibiotics). Therefore, the use of probiotics is seen more and more as an alternative to the use of antibiotics in animal production, and many scientific works show the beneficial effects of supplementation with probiotic strains in diets fed to chicken, swine, cattle and fish (Veizaj-Delia, 2010; Soleimani et al., 2010; Ignatova, 2009; Aly et al., 2008). Therefore, this chapter will approach action mechanisms and the effects on health of probiotics for human and animal use.

1.1 Mechanisms of action

The potential mechanisms by which probiotic agents might exert their protective effect include: antagonism by the production of substances that inhibit or kill the pathogen (Servin, 2004); competition with the pathogen for adhesion sites or nutritional sources

(Servin & Coconnier, 2003; Momose et al., 2008); immunomodulation of the host (Ezendam et al, 2006); and inactivation of microbial toxin (Brandão et al., 1998). Other mechanisms by which probiotics may exert protection is through a recuperation of mucosal barrier function when disturbed (Penna et al., 2008), trapping pathogens on their surface (Martins et al, 2010; Martins et al, 2011) and stimulating mucus production (Caballero-Franco et al., 2007).

According to De Vrese & Marteau (2007), mechanism and efficiency of probiotic effect depend mainly on the interactions between probiotic microorganisms and microbiota of the host or with imunocompetent cell of the intestinal mucous.

Althought they had not been completely elucidated, the classical mechanisms of action of bacteria used as probiotics are described as: i) competition for bound sites: also known as "competitive exclusion", where bacteria of probiotics are linked to the bound site in the intestinal mucosa, making a physical barrier, impeding the bound by pathogenic bacteria; ii) production of anti-bacterial substances: bacteria of probiotics synthetize compounds as for example bacteriocins, hydrogen peroxide, which has antibacterial action, mainly in relation to pathogenic bacteria, in addition to the production of organic acid which reduced pH in the gastrointestinal tract, preventing growth of many pathogens and development of certain species of *Lactobacillus*; iii) competition for nutrients: shortage of available nutrients which can be used by pathogenic bacteria is a limiting factor for their maintenance; iv) stimulus to the immune system: some bacteria of the probiotics are directly linked to the stimuli of immune response by increasing antibodies production, activation of macrophages, T cells proliferation and interferon production (Fuller, 1992; Jin et al., 1997).

Action mechanism of yeasts still needs studies for their evidencing. A probable mechanism of action of yeast is related to total (*in vitro*) or partial inhibition of pathogenic microorganisms. Dead yeasts contain in their walls important quantities of polysaccharides and proteins able to act positively in the immune system and on nutrient absorption. Moreover, yeasts produce nutritive metabolites in the digestive tract which increase animal performance, in addition of having minerals (Mn, Co, Zn) and vitamins (A, B_{12}, D_3) which improve action of beneficial microorganisms (Hill et al., 2006).

Although some mechanisms had been suggested on the action of probiotics, they are not completely clarified, but it is known that they inhibit growth of pathogenic microorganism by producing antimicrobial compounds; they compete with pathogens for adhesion sites and nutrients; and they model immune system of the host (Oelschlaeger, 2010). In the present, a more complete view on the possible mechanisms of action are been studied, based mainly on the manipulation of normal microbiota.

The composition of human microbiota has about 10 - 100 trillion members and varies within the gut and among individuals (Zoetendal et al., 2011; Hayashi et al., 2002). These members belong mainly to the dominant bacteria, but there are also representatives from Archaea (Eckburg et al., 2003), Eukarya, and viruses, including bacteriophages (Breitbart et al., 2003). Intestinal microbiota plays a fundamental role in maintaining immune homeostasis which, in other words, involves minimizing the adverse health effects of intestinal microbiota, such as shifts in microbial community structure, changes in the diet of the host or overt pathogenic challenge (Hooper & Macpherson, 2010).

According to Sonnenburg, et al. (2006) some evidences show that by manipulating the microbiota with probiotics could influence the host health and probiotic bacteria could be used as a therapeutic strategy to improve human health. The precise mechanisms influencing the crosstalk between the microbe and the host are still unclear but there are evidences suggesting that bacteria in the gut could modulate the functioning of the immune system at systemic and mucosal levels (Ng et al., 2009).

2. Effect of probiotics on human health

2.1 Probiotic selection

Requirements that a probiotic organism should meet are the following: resistance to gastric acidity, resistance to bile and pancreatic enzymes; adherence to intestinal mucosa cells; colonization capacity; keep itself alive for a long time during transportation, storage, so they can effectively colonize the host; production of antimicrobial substances against pathogenic bacteria and absence of translocation (Capriles et al., 2005).

For a microorganism be used as a probiotic, it is necessary its isolation, characterization and assessments which will prove its probiotic efficiency (Figure 1).

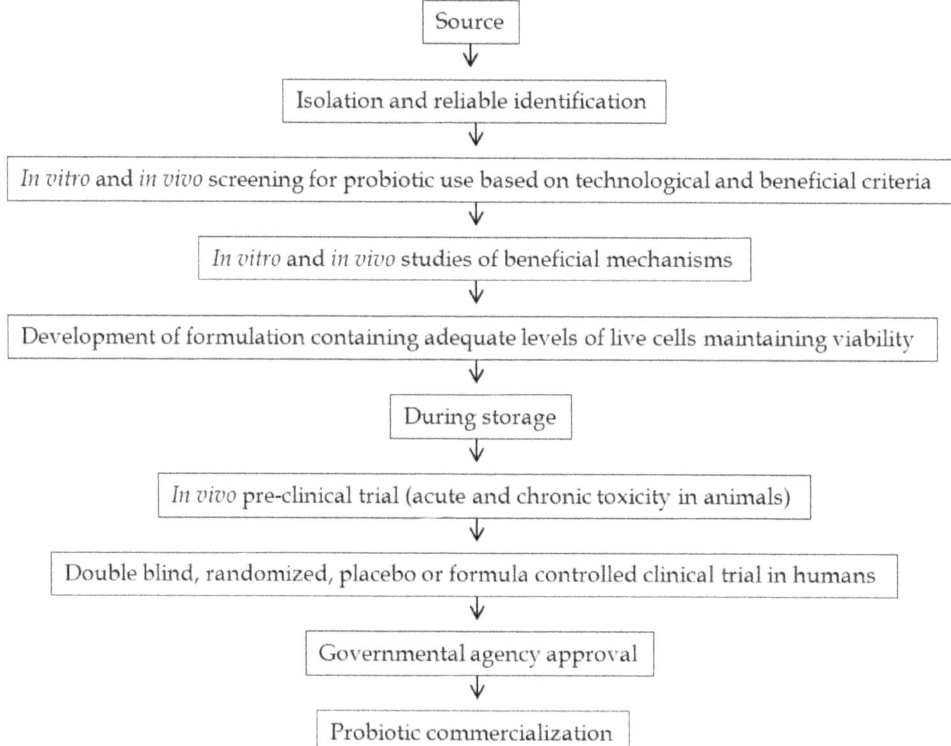

Fig. 1. Probiotic selection chart.

Firstly, a microorganism source have to be selected (for example: digestive tract of health animals or other niches such as flowers, decomposing fruits). Then, the microorganisms which are intended to work with are isolated and identified through selective culture media.

Afterwards, a new culture is prepared only with the target colonies for *in vivo* assessment (pathogen inhibition, target species pathogenicity; resistance to host conditions; among others). If there are no restriction to the use of the target species, experiments with in vivo supplementation at big and small scale are carried out to check if there are real benefits to the host. Finally, the probiotic which presented significant satisfactory results can be commercially produced and used.

2.2 Prevention or reduction of diarrhea symptoms

One of the main applications of probiotic microorganisms is at preventing or in the treatment of gastrointestinal disturbances. In a clinical trial carried out with children hospitalized for acute rotavirus diarrhea, three treatments were assessed. The first group of children received oral rehydration therapy plus placebo; the second group was submitted to oral rehydration plus *Saccharomyces boulardii* treatment and the third group received oral rehydration and a compound containing *Lactobacillus acidophilus*, *Lactobacillus rhamnosus*, *Bifidobacterium longum* e *Saccharomyces boulardii*. Mean duration of diarrhea was shorter for the children who received the treatment with *Saccharomyces boulardii* strain (58 hours) and for the children who received the compound with for different microorganism strains (60 hours), when compared to the control group (84.5 hours) (Grandy et al., 2010). In Brazil, a double-blind, placebo controlled trial showed that protection against diarrhea (32.2% reduction in diarrhea during the first year of life) was obtained by oral inoculation with a single dose of plasmid-free human *Escherichia coli* EMO soon after birth (Figueiredo et al., 2001).

Treatment with antibiotics can cause an unbalance in the indigenous microbiota, increasing concentration of pathogenic microorganisms and toxin production, promoting diarrhea symptoms (Vasiljevic & Shah, 2008). A significant effect was observed in a study carried out with patients who presented diarrhea caused by antibiotics, in which intake of a probiotic drink containing *L. casei*, *L. bulgaricus* e *S. thermophilus* reduced the incidence of diarrhea (Hickson et al., 2007). In a double-blind, formula controlled trial performed in Brazil, a milk lyophilized formulation supplemented with *B. bifidum* and *S. thermophilus* was compared with another without supplementation for the prevention of antibiotic-associated diarrhea in children 6 to 36 months old. The authors observed a significant reduction of diarrhea frequency in children treated with the probiotic formula (16% of 80 patients) when compared to the control group (31% of 77 patients) (Corrêa et al., 2005). In another double-blind, placebo controlled trial also performed in Brazil, the treatment with a lyophilized preparation of *S. boulardii* in children with acute diarrhea was evaluated and a reduction in duration of rotavirus diarrhea was observed in the group treated with the probiotic yeast (Corrêa et al., 2011). Other examples of clinical trials related to prevention or shortening of diarrhea symptoms by using probiotics are summarized in Table 1.

2.3 Irritable bowel syndrome

Irritable bowel syndrome is a diseased characterized by abdominal pain, diarrhea, constipation and mucus secretion along with feces (Vahedi et al., 2010). Although many physiopathology factors had been correlated to the cause of this disease, in the last years, researchers have considered feed intolerance and unbalance of intestinal microbiota as the main factors responsible for symptoms of the irritable bowel syndrome. Probiotics are a

Author (year)	Assessed probiotic	Results
Figueiredo et al. (2001)	*Escherichia coli* EMO	Protection against diarrhea during the first year of life was obtained by oral inoculation of *Escherichia coli* EMO soon after birth
Billoo et al. (2006)	*Saccharomyces boulardii*	The use of *S. boulardii* reduced frequency and duration of acute diarrhea in children
Giralt et al. (2007)	*Lactobacillus casei* DN-114 001	*L. casei* DN-114 001 did not reduced radiation-induced diarrhea incidence
Corrêa et al. (2005)	*Bifidobacterium bifidum* + *Streptococcus thermophilus*	Use of lyophilized milk supplemented with *Bifidobacterium* and *Streptococcus* reduced antibiotic-associated diarrhea in hospitalized infants
Beausoleil et al. (2007)	*Lactobacillus acidophilus* + *Lactobacillus casei*	Addition of *Lactobacillus* strains in the fermented milk was effective in the prevention of antibiotic-associated diarrhea

Table 1. Clinical trials on the use of probiotics in the treatment of diaheia

good alternative for the treatment of this syndrome inasmuch as the use of probiotic may lead to an unbalance of intestinal microbiota, making the carrier more susceptible to the disease (Rolfe, 2000).

Nagala & Routray (2010) studied the effect of a probiotic supplement containing *Lactobacillus acidophilus*, *Bifidobacterium bifidum*, *B. longum* and *B. lactis*, on patients with irritable bowel syndrome. It was observed a significant improvement after two months of the treatment, with 84% of the patients showing improvement in abdominal pain, 73.9% in bloating, 88% in flatulence, 90.9% in diarrhea and 86.9% in constipation.

2.4 Bowel inflammatory disease

Inflammatory bowel disease involves two subtypes: ulcerative colitis and Crohn's disease. Ulcerative colitis is determined by a continuous inflammation, which starts in the rectum and it is restricted to colon, whereas inflammation from Crohn's disease can occur in any region of the gastrointestinal tract (Bousvaros et al., 2007; Mack, 2011).

The non-pathogenical strain *E. coli* Nissle 1917 showed to be efficient in the Crohn's disese maintenance therapy. This microorganism was able to adhere to intestinal epithelial cells in addition to its inhibitory effect observed against pathogenic strains isolated from patients with the disease (Boudeau et al., 2003).

A study conducted by Furrie et al. (2005) pointed the efficiency of *Bifidobacterium longum* associated to inulin-oligofructose prebiotic in the treatment of ulcerative colitis. The treatment resulted in an improvement of the full clinical appearance in patients who received this therapy.

2.5 Hypercholesterolemia

Saturated fat rich diets can increase serum cholesterol rates, which is one of the main risk factor for cardiovascular disease (Vasiljevic & Shah, 2008). Many studies have been carried out on the hypocholesterolemic activity of non-pathogenic bacteria through mechanism of hydrolysis of biliar salt (Pereira et al., 2003; Noriega et al., 2006; Parvez et al., 2006; Nguyen et al., 2007).

Baroutkoub et al. (2010) observed that consumption of probiotic yogurt with *Lactobacillus acidophilus* and *Bifidobacteria* cepas by people with hypercholesterolemia resulted in the reduction of total cholesterol and LDL (Low Density Lipoproteins: it is believed they are the harmful class to human beings) and in the increase of good cholesterol, HDL (High Density Lipoproteins: it is believed that they are able to absorb cholesterol crystals which are deposited in arteries/veins wall, therefore delaying arteriosclerotic process) in the blood.

Despite the great number of studies, reduction of serum cholesterol effect by probiotics is not considered an established effect, yet. Thus, new clinical trials controlled by placebo should be carried out to prove the efficiency of those microorganisms.

2.6 Cancer control

The fight against cancer is one of the biggest challenges faced by humanity. According to some authors, consumption of probiotic-supplemented products can prevent and even suppress tumor growth. According to Ma et al. (2010), *Bacillus polyfermenticus* was able to suppress in vitro and in vivo growth of cancer cells, suggesting that such microorganism can be used to prevent colon cancer development. Probiotic strains of *E. faecium* RM11 and *L. fermentum* RM28, isolated from fermented-milk were also shown to have antiproliferative properties against colon cancer cells, suggesting that such microorganisms can be used as an alternative to colon cancer (Thirabunyanon et al., 2009).

It was observed in volunteer subjects who received *Lactobacillus rhamnosus* LC705 and *Propionibacterium freudenreichii* a reduction of intestinal absorption of aflatoxin B1, a toxin correlated to the high liver cancer index. Therefore, probiotic supplementation can be effective in preventing development of liver cancer and other types of cancer caused by environmental factors (El-Nezami et al., 2006).

2.7 Allergy

Probiotics are able to reduce *in vitro* various inflammatory cytokines and intestinal permeability, which are effects considered beneficial in allergic conditions. In addition, gut microbiota of atopic patients seems quite different, with an increase in clostridia and a decrease of bifidobacteria when compared to microbiota of non-atopic individuals. Studies have been performed to evaluate the effectiveness of probiotics in food allergy, atopic eczema and rhinitis (Michail et al., 2006).

The administration of *Lactobacillus* GG in pregnant women, nursing mothers and babies in the first months of life was associated with a decrease in the occurrence of topic eczema in children at risk of developing allergies compared to a placebo group at the end of a year of life (Kalliomäki et al., 2003). Another two controlled studies showed improvement of atopic dermatitis in children after use of *L. rhamnosus* and *L. reuteri*, and children with atopic eczema and allergy to cow's milk responded more effectively to a hydrolyzed formula supplemented with *Lactobacillus* GG (Majamaa et al., 1997; Rosenfeldt et al., 2003). These results are promising for the use of probiotics in allergies, but more studies are needed to confirm this property.

3. Probiotics for animal use

The use of growth promoters permit to improve animal performance. Initially, a great variety of antibiotic function substances, particularly penicillin and tetraclines, were used to improve performance of birds, swines and cattle. The use of antibiotics as feed additive showed great benefices to animal production, mainly expressed in an improvement of weight gain and feed conversion. Antibiotics were used for many years, but they are being banned from animal production activities especially because of risks presented by resistant bacteria, which can result in problems to animal and human health. Therefore, probiotics are receiving special attention by animal nutrition researchers, who search for alternatives to the traditional use of growth promoters.

Probiotics have been incorporated through diets, with the objective to keep intestinal microbiota balance of animals, preventing digestive tract diseases, improving feed digestibility, leading to a greater use of nutrients and improving animal performance (Fuller, 1992).

Overall, effects of probiotic addition tend to be more outstanding in inadequate production conditions or in stress conditions, in which microbiota are unbalanced, especially in young animals. The most commonly highlighted factors among those previously cited are: temperature below or above thermal comfort zone; presence of pathogens; deficient sanitary conditions; management stressing conditions; change in feeding; weaning; transportation; high stock density; post-antibiotics treatment; sudden environment change. Regarding the results obtained in experiments with probiotics, those can be affected by factors as for example: type of probiotic microorganism; method and administered amount; host condition; intestinal microbiota condition; age of the animal.

3.1 Probiotic in aquaculture

Probiotics in aquatic organisms can act similarly to terrestrial animals. However, the relationship between aquatic animals and cultivation environment is much more complex than that involving terrestrial animals. Because of this closer relationship between animal and cultivation environment, the traditional definition of probiotics is insufficient for aquaculture. Therefore, Verschuere et al. (2000) suggest a broader definition: "it is a microbial supplement with living microorganisms, with beneficial effects on the host, by modifying its microbial community associated with the host or its cultivation environment, by ensuring improved use of the artificial feed or its nutritional value, by enhancing the host response towards diseases and by improving the quality of its ambient environment."

Microorganisms in the aquatic environment are in direct contact with the outer part of the animals, as for example gills and with the supplied feed, with easy access to the digestive tract of the animal. Among those microorganism present in the aquatic environment are the potentially pathogenic ones, which are opportunists, that is, they take advantage of some stress situation of the animal (high density, deficient feeding), causing infections, which can worse animal performance and even death. *Vibrio* sp., *Plesiomonas shigelloides*, in addition to *Aeromonas* sp. are the main agents causing death in aquaculture, and they can also cause feed infections in human beings. Thus, the objective of using probiotics by aquatic organisms is not only the direct beneficial to the animal but also its effect in the environment (Verschuere et al., 2000).

The interaction between environment and host in an aquatic environment is complex. Microorganism in the water influence host intestinal microbiota and vice-versa. Makridis et al. (2000) showed that supply of the bacteria strains through the feed and direct in the cultivation water, in turbot (*Scophthalmus maximus*) larvae incubators, promoted their maintenance in the environment, and they also promoted colonization of the digestive tract of the larvae.

Changes in the salinity, temperature, dissolved oxygen variations, alter conditions of the environment, which are propitious to different organism, with consequent changes in the dominant species, which may lead to a efficacy loss of the product. Thus, addition of a probiotic into the cultivation water must be constant, because the medium conditions undergo periodical changes. So, when choosing the pro biot to be used in aquaculture, variety of the microorganism present in the medium must be taken into account.

Intensive cultivation systems use high stock densities, among other stressing factors (for example: management), which result in low growth rates and feeding efficiency, a fragility in the immune system, making those animals susceptible to the presence of opportunist pathogens present in the cultivation environment. Thus, the effect of the probiotics on the immune system has led to a great number of studies with results beneficial to the health of aquatic organisms, although the way they act have not been clarified, yet. Gram et al. (1999) showed that the use of *Pseudomonas fluorescens* AH2 as probiotic, reduced mortality of rainbow trout (*Oncorhynchus mykiss*) juveniles exposed to *Vibrio anguillarum*. The joint administration of *Lactobacillus fructivorans* and *Lactobacillus plantarum* through live or dry feeding promoted colonization in intestine of *sea bream* (*Spaurus aurata*) larvae and the reduction of animal mortality during larva culture and nursery (Carnevali et al., 2004). Kumar et al. (2006) observed a greater survival in *Labeo rohita* carp fed *Bacillus subtilis*, submitted to intraperitoneal injection with *Aeromonas hydrophila*.

Regarding cultivated shrimp, bacterial illness are considered the greatest mortality cause in larvae. The administration of a bacterium mixture (*Bacillus* sp. e *Vibrio* sp.) influenced positively survival and presented protection effect against *Vibrio harveyi* and the white spot virus (Balcázar et al., 2006). In the clam *Argopecten purpuratus*, an *Alteromonas haloplanktis*, able to reduce larva mortality when submitted to challenge with *Vibrio anguillarum*, was isolated (Riquelme et al., 1996).

Probiotics can also be used to promote growth in aquatic organisms, either by a direct help in nutrient absorption or by supplying them. Lara-Flores et al. (2003) concluded that the use of *Saccharomyces cerevisiae* yeast as probiotic for Nile tilapia (*Oreochromis niloticus*) alevino as growth promoter, resulted in a greater growth and feed efficiency, suggesting that yeast is a proper growth promoter in the tilapia farming. Lin et al. (2004) used *Bacillus* sp. in the diet of shrimp *Litopenaeus vannamei* improving feed digestibility indices. Ziaei-Nejad et al. (2006) added probiotic *Bacillus* sp. in the cultivation of shrimp *Fenneropenaeus indicus* larvae and observed that in addition to the increase of survival, there was an increase in the activity of enzymes lipase, protease and amylase in the digestive tract of shrimp, which may stimulate the better use of the artificial feed.

However, addition of probiotics *Bacillus subtilis* at different doses (2.5; 5.0 and 10 g kg⁻¹ of diet) in diets for bullfrog (*Lithobates catesbeianus*) with initial weight of 3.13g did not improve weight gain, apparent feed conversion and survival when compared to control treatment (without addition of probiotic), but the immunostimulatory effect was evidenced through the increase of phagocytic capacity in the animals (França et al., 2008).

Another aspect of using probiotics in aquaculture is the improvement of the water quality in culture ponds. Reduction on nitrogen and phosphate compounds in the water used in *Litopenaeus vannamei* shrimp cultivation was observed when commercial probiotics were added into the water (Wang et al., 2005). Similarly, it was observed an improvement in the water used for cultivation of *Penaeus monodon* shrimp when *Bacillus* sp. was used as probiotic (Dalmin et al., 2001).

The conditions in which animal are submitted during cultivation can influence directly efficiency of probiotics. Thus, when they are not submitted to stressing situations, the obtained results many times do not show significant effect of probiotics on animal performance, so, more scientific studies should be conducted to know better interactions between those factors with the animals.

3.2 Probiotics in poultry production

The objective of using probiotics in poultry production is to improve performance in broiler chickens and to increase egg production in laying hens in addition to reduce intestinal colonization by pathogens as *Salmonella* sp. the main genus of bacteria identified in gastrointestinal tract of birds are: *Bacillus, Bifidobacterium, Clostridium, Enterobacter, Lactobacillus, Fusobacterium, Escherichia, Enterococcus* and *Streptococcus*.

The starting point in the use of probiotics in birds was set by Nurmi & Rantala (1973), who observed that when intestinal content of the healthy adult birds were orally administrated to birds at one day of age, it changed their sensitivity to *Salmonella* sp. in poultry production, manners of probiotic administration to birds more commonly observed are: by the feeds, by drinking water, by pulverization on the birds, inoculation via cloaca or in embryonated eggs (*in ovo*), among others, and the manner of administration has effect on intestinal colonization capacity.

Except if submitted to stress situation, bacteria which colonize gastrointestinal tract of the birds since their birth, tend to remain there for the rest of their lives. Therefore, *in ovo* inoculation is an aspect of using probiotics for birds. *In ovo* inoculation of probiotics

Lactobacillus casei, *Lactobacillus plantarum* and *Enterococcus faecium* at 10^6 UFC egg^{-1}, at 16 days of incubation and the performance of challenge of chicks at one day of age via stomach with 13.6×10^6 UFC mL^{-1} of *Salmonella enteritidis*, improved performance of animals fed probiotics when compared to control treatment (Leandro et al., 2004). Moreover, in the same experiment, authors observed that from 7 to 21 days of age, *Salmonella* sp. was identified only in challenged animals which were not fed probiotic. It is suggested that probiotic avoided bacterium colonization in the gastrointestinal tract of the birds.

In chicks emerging from incubators, pH concentration and the presence of volatile fatty acids, which are one of the main protection barriers of the animal organism, are not sufficiently chemically to avoid that pathogens enter in their organism. Moreover, the small variety of the birds' intestinal microbiota in this phase is considered as a limiting factor for the digestion and for the possibility of intestinal colonization by enteric pathogens. Thus, probiotic supplementation seems to be a beneficial action for the animal performance and health of birds from commercial incubators.

An efficient immune response is related to the presence of immunomodulaters in the diet, which will act by reducing immune stress and then reducing nutrient mobilization to activities which are not related with production (meat or eggs), permitting in addition to a greater survival in stress situations, the non-harmful effect on animal performance.

The use of yeast *Saccharomyces boulardii* in the diet for broiler chickens reduced the level of *Salmonella* sp. from 53.3% to 40.0% at stress conditions in transportation to slaughter (Line et al., 1998). The used of yeast *Saccharomyces cerevisiae* var. *chromium* reduced negative effects of caloric stress on broiler chickens (Guo & Liu, 1997).

The results of studies with probiotics in poultry production have been showed to be rather contradictory regarding to its efficiency. Not always are positive results observed by using probiotics. Those vary with age of the animal, type of probiotic used, viability of the microorganisms, storage conditions, level and manner of administration, in addition to the low challenge in relation to the experimental condition concerned to sanity, management and other stressful conditions. Some researchers have stated that the addition of probiotics into the diet did not improve animal performance in broiler chickens. Estrada et al. (2001) observed that the administration of *Bifidobacterium bifidum* did not alter significantly animal growth. But, according to Zulkifli et al. (2000), even by observing an increase in the feed intake, there was no reduction in feed efficiency in broiler chickens when *Lactobacillus* sp. was administered in the diet.

On the other hand, several studies have shown extremely interesting results on adition of probiotics into diets for broiler chickens. The addition of *Bacillus subtilis* into the diet increased weight gain and feed conversion (Fritts et al., 2000). The addition of *Lactobacillus* increased weight gain and improved feed conversion of supplemented animals (Kalavathi et al., 2003). The use of yeast *Saccharomyces boulardii* in *Salmonella enteritidis* infected broiler chickens improved feed efficiency by 10% when compared to control treatment, and by 12% in animals supplemented with *Bacillus cereus* var. toyoii (Gil de los Santos, 2004).

Concerning to carcass quality of broiler chickens, the beneficial effect of probiotic use was also observed. The addition of *Lactobacillus acidophilus* e *Streptococcus faecium* reduced plasma protein concentration, levels of total cholesterol and HDL in addition to an increase in the protein content of probiotic supplemented animals (Pietras, 2001).

3.3 Probiotics in swine farming

The bacteria usually found in the gastrointestinal tract of swine are: Bacteroides rumnicola, B. uniformis, B. succinogenes, Butyruvibrio fibrisalvens, Clostridium perfringens, Escherichia coli, Eubacterium aerofaciens, Lactobacillus acidophilus, L. casei, L. fermentum, Peptostreptococcus productis, Selenomonas ruminantium, Streptococcus salivarius and the yeast found are: Saccharomyces cerevisiae and Candida sp. (Russel, 1979).

By evaluating the balance between beneficial and pathogenic bacteria in the intestinal epithelium of swines in normal conditions, Robinson et al. (1984) found *Lactobacillus acidophilus* in 11.9%, *Streptococcus faecium* in 54,4% and *Escherichia coli* in less than 1%. When there were intestinal disorders, reduction of *L. acidophilus* and *S. faecium* up to 6% was observed, resulting in an increase of *E. coli* to 14%.

Regarding microbiota in the gastrointestinal tract, it is found two critical moments in the swine farming, which are birth and weaning. Piglets are born without microbiological contamination, but in a short time, gastrointestinal tract is mostly colonized by *Lactobacillus*, *Bifidobacterium* and *Bacteroides*, and less by potentially pathogenic organism as for example *Escherichia coli*, *Enterococcus*, *Clostridium* and *Staphylococcus*. After weaning, there is a drop in lactic bacteria population, so population of pathogenic organism increases (for example: *E. coli*). These pathogenic microorganisms can be adhered to the intestinal epithelium, then they multiply, unbalancing intestinal microbiota, causing post-weaning diarrhea.

Administration of *Lactobacillus* sp. as probiotic for piglets during a six-week period increased its presence in the intestine and reduced *Pseudomonas* sp. and *Clostridium perfringens*, in addition to reduce intestinal pH, although effect on weight gain and apparent feed conversion had not been observed, compared to the control group (Tereda et al., 1994). Likewise, administration of probiotic for sows from the end of gestation to the end of lactation will be able to stabilize intestinal microbiota of the female, establishing a favorable microbiota in piglets in suckling. This fact was evidenced by Alexopoulos et al. (2004).

Conditions of microbial unbalance during stress create a favorable condition for fixation of pathogenic microorganisms, leading to structural changes, as for example shortening of villi. This reduction results in a smaller absorption area, lower production of enzymes and nutrient transportation, predisposing animals to poor absorption, a possible dehydration and conditions of enteric infections. Upon this aspect, results obtained with the use of probiotics for swines are very contradictory. Pollman & Bandick (1984) reported that animals fed *Lactobacillus* based products did not present difference on small intestine morphology when challenged by *E. coli*. But, Jonsson & Henningsson (1991) did not observe probiotic effect on the size of the villus. Kritas et al. (2006) observed less incidence of diarrhea in piglets supplemented with *Bacillus subtilis* and *Bacillus licheniformis* during suckling and post-weaning. However, Utiyama et al. (2006) did not observe any benefic effect of supplementation with *Bacillus subtilis* and *Bacillus licheniformis* in diets for weaned piglets under diarrhea control when compared to the ones which were not fed probiotic.

Those differences can come from factors as for example: genetics of the animals, species of the microorganisms used in the product; the used dose; environment temperature and sanitary condition of the swine farm inasmuch as many experiments evaluate the use of probiotics in low sanitary challenge conditions. In addition to a good sanitary quality, those conditions must provide no stress for the animals and balanced microbial community, probiotics and even antibiotics used at subclinical dose will have little or any effect on animal performance. However, it is difficult that an animal will not suffer from stress or will live in an environment free of pathogenic microorganisms in the exiting commercial production nowadays.

Regarding animal performance, Roth & Kirchgessener (1988) observed improvement in weight gain, feed intake and feed conversion when using *Bacillus toyoii* based probiotic in diets for piglets. Cristani et al. (1999) observed an improved of up to 8% in feed conversion of piglets in the nursery phase, when bacteria *Lactobacillus acidophilus* was administered in the diet. Those results can be related to enzymatic production of probiotics with improve nutrient digestion by lactase and galactosidase production, which hydrolyzes lactose, permitting its absorption. The use of a probiotic congaing *Bacillus licheniformis* and endospore of *Bacillus subtilis* increased feed intake, reduced weight loss and reduced the interval between weaning and estrus in sows (Alexopoulos et al., 2004). In the same study, it was observed in piglets from those sows, an average of 0.38 kg more than the control group.

3.4 Probiotics for ruminants

From the possible effects observed with the addition of probiotics for ruminants, it stands out: increase in the number of bacteria in the rumen; increase in rumen digestion of cellulose, increasing nutrient availability for production process, improving use efficiency of roughage, in addition of stimulating greater dry matter ingestion; competitive exclusion in the intestine, resulting in a reduction of bacteria which cause diarrhea; production of bacteriocine; acting as immunostimulants.

Yeasts are used in ruminant feeding with the objective of increasing dry matter digestibility, especially neutral detergent fiber and acid detergent fiber (Kamalamma et al., 1996). Yeast supplementation increases the number of bacteria in the rumen, particularly cellulosic bacteria. Growth factor supply (for example: vitamins), removal of oxygen by *Saccharomyces* (rumen content is essentially anaerobic), buffer effect and reduction in the number of protozoan are some of the factors associated to this response (Callaway & Martin, 1997).

Among the several species of bacteria present in the rumen, cellulose bacteria, essential for ruminant nutrition for cellulose digestion, stands out. Another important function of the microbiota in the rumen is the production of complex B vitamins. Fermentative activities and qualitative content of microorganisms in the rumen can vary and decrease according to the diet and stressing situations as well. In the modern agriculture, cattle are constantly submitted to stressing factors as for example frequent management in the barn, vaccinations, identification, castration, contention, artificial insemination, confinement, and so on. Therefore, it can be concluded that depression in rumen microbiota, resulting from stress, will reduce feed digestibility, vitamin synthesis, resulting in growth and milk production.

Because increase of genetic potential of the animals it becomes more and more necessary the development of diets with greater genetic and protein content jointed with adequacy of fibrous fraction, which is important in rumen health. Therefore, the inclusion of grains into the diet favors growth of bacteria as *Streptococcus bovis*, which is lactate producer, causing reduction in the rumen pH. Submitting cattle to diet with high percentage of concentrate may result in rumen fermentation detriment. Therefore, addition of products which are able to keep or change rumen fermentation pattern, maintaining animal health, has become an important strategy in the feeding of those animals.

Ruminants have a differential in their digestive organ which confers to them a great capacity of digesting fibrous feedstuff. However, this capacity of converting fibrous feed into meat due to an inadequate feeding management, for example, can be poorly efficient. Thus, nutrition of those animals should search optimization of rumen fermentation, improving nutrient digestibility with a consequent better animal performance.

As it was previously mentioned for other species, positive effect of probiotics in animal nutrition are not always evidenced due to differences in sanitary conditions and different types of diets used as well. However, when this happens, increase in productivity parameters and improvement in the sanitary status are observed (Breul, 1998).

Krehbiel et al. (2003) observed that there was a smaller incidence of diarrhea when feeding bezeras with *Streptococcus* and *Lactobacillus acidophilus*, compared to animals which were not fed probiotic. In the work of Bechman et al., (1977), it was demonstrated that administration of *Lactobacillus acidophilus* for dairy calves improved feed conversion and reduced diarrhea incidence. Zhao et al. (1998) also observed that the possibility of reduction in the detection of *Escherichia coli* in probiotic supplemented animals.

According to Martin (1998), direct supplementation of microbial additive can improve ruminant production up to 8%. By analyzing results from several trials on confinement, Krehbiel et al. (2003) observe an increase in daily weight gain of 2.5 to 5.0% in addition to improving feed efficiency of 2% in animals supplemented with probiotics in the diet.

The use of high concentrate content diets results in increase of disturbances related to rumen fermentation, as for example bloat and acidosis. Mir & Mir (1994) observed that the audition of *Saccharomyces cerevisiae* into grain high content diets resulted in less occurrence of acute rumen acidosis in supplemented cattle compared to the control, suggesting that yeast promoted the use of lactate in the rumen. Administration of *Saccharomyces cerevisiae* for cattle submitted to a rapid fermentable diet improved daily weight gain in comparison to a diet without yeast (Agazzi et al., 2009) and improved digestion of low quality neutral detergent fiber in ruminants (Sommart et al., 1993).

Regarding to the reproductive system, it is observed that uterine pathologies during puerperal period are responsible for the reduction in reproductive efficiency in cows. Colonization by *Lactobacillus* is considered the first microbiologic barrier against pathogen infection in the genital tract (Ocaña et al., 1999). Thus, addition of those microorganisms as probiotics may improve reproductive efficiency of those animals, either by lactic acid production which reduced vaginal pH or by competition for nutrients and adhesion site in the vaginal epithelium.

3.5 Use of probiotics in other animals

3.5.1 Rabits

In rabbits, the occurrence of digestive disorders associated to feeding changes has risen mortality indices in the period close to weaning. So, the use of probiotics has been an alternative in this phase because it favors improvement of digestive tract conditions by action on beneficial microbiota able to improve sanitary and physiologic status of the animal. Michelan et al. (2002) used probiotic Calsporin® (based upon endospores of *Bacillus subtilis*) for growing rabbits, evaluating digestibility of diets and their intestinal morphometry. The presence of probiotic did not influence nutrient digestibility neither morphometric traits of jejune. Hollister et al. (1989) observed an improvement in apparent feed conversion, in addition to mortality reduction caused by enteritis in growing rabbits supplemented with Lacto-Sacc® (probiotic constituted by *Lactobacillus acidophilus, Streptococcus faecium, Saccharomyces cerevisae*, and fermentation residues of *Aspergillus orizae* and *Aspergillus niger*). Moreover, the use of Lacto-Sacc® improved crude fiber digestibility (Yamani et al., 1992) by weaned White New Zealand rabbits. However, Lambertini et al. (1990) did not observe any influence of probiotic composed of *Bacillus subtilis* on the performance of growing rabbits.

3.5.2 Equines

According to Frape (1998), the use of probiotics stimulates intestinal biota growth and improves digestibility of crude fiber and crude protein. The main sources of fiber on composition of diets for equines are grass or legume hays. Legume hays normally presented greater nutritional value when compared to grass hay, however, they are more expensive and more difficult to be produced. So, the use of probiotics increases efficiency of grass hay use. But, results from the use of probiotics with this aim are not conclusive, yet. Morgan et al. (2007), evaluating addition of yeast in low and high quality Russel Bermuda grass hay diets observed an increase in crude protein and neutral detergent fiber digestibility only in the low quality diets, although neutral detergent fiber digestibility had not presented improvement. Likewise, Hill et al. (2006) observed increase in crude protein apparent digestibility for equines fed diets with high proportion of roughage:concentrate (80:20) supplemented with yeast. Increase in crude protein digestibility may be due to microbial activity in the large intestine which favored nitrogen compounds digestibility. By contrasting with those results, Moura et al. (2009) did not observe any improvement in total dry matter digestibility in foal fed grass and concentrate, yeast supplemented. Moore & Newman (1993), supplementing foals with yeast, observed maintenance of the highest values of pH in the large intestine. According to these authors, reduction in pH below 6.5 affect cellulose bacteria therefore it affects fiber digestion and help to prevent colic and laminitis.

The use of yeast in diets for mare during gestation and lactation resulted in greater contents of crude protein, sugar, total lipids and proteins in the milk, and beneficial effects were also observed in the foals of those mares (Glade, 1991).

3.5.3 Dogs

Kosaza (1989) reports that in cases of acute diarrhea in dogs, treatment with *Bifidobacterium pseudolongum* was positive. Swanson et al. (2002) observed that administration of *Lactobacillus acidophilus* increased digestibility of dry matter, organic matter and crude protein. However, Biourgue et al. (1998) observed no improvement regarding digestibility of dry matter, protein, lipids and energy.

4. Conclusions

The use of probiotics for the prevention and / or treatment of gastrointestinal disorders have a strong theoretical justification, based on the beneficial functions of the indigenous microbiota, fundamental for maturation and health of the digestive ecosystem. However, a number of issues need to be resolved before general guidelines regarding the use of probiotics can be given. Basic research must provide more detailed data on the mechanisms of probiotic action on the molecular level, after which coordinated rigorously conducted clinical trials must be undertaken to find the probiotic strain and dosage with optimal results for each clinical situation. It is unlikely that one strain or probiotic combination will be sufficient for all purposes. At the moment, the heterogeneity of probiotic clinical trials hampers interpretation – in particular the diversity of probiotic strains, dosing regimens and forms of administration used and the varied patient groups recruited in the available studies makes interpretation difficult. Concluding, more biological and well controlled clinical trials must be carried out for a more precise understanding of both the mechanisms underlying the probiotic action and the complex gastrointestinal ecosystem with which probiotics are expected to interact.

5. References

Agazzi, A., Invernizzi, G., Ferroni, M., Fanelli, A. & Savoini, G. (2009). Effects of live yeast (*Saccharomyces cerevisiae*) administration on apparent digestibility of horses. *Italian Journal of Animal Science*, Vol. 8, Suppl. 2, pp. 685-687, ISSN 1594-4077

Alexopoulos, C., Georgoulakis, I., Tzivara, A., Kritas, S., Siochu, A. & Kyriakis, S. (2004). Field evaluation of the efficacy of a probiotic containing *Bacillus licheniformis* and *Bacillus subtilis* spores, on the health status and performance of sows and their litters. *Journal of Physiology and Animal Nutrition*, Vol. 88, No. 1, pp. 381–392, ISSN 0931-2439

Balcázar, J., De Blas, I., Zarzuela-Ruiz, I., Cunningham, M., Vendrell, D. & Músquiz, J. (2006). The role of probiotics in aquaculture. *Veterinary Microbiology*, Vol. 114, No. 1, pp. 173-186, ISSN 0378-1135

Baroutkoub, A., Mehdi, R., Beglarian, R., Hassan, J., Zahra, S., Mohammad, M. & Mohammad hadi, E. (2010). Effects of probiotic yoghurt consumption on the serumcholesterol levels in hypercholestromic cases in Shiraz, Southern Iran. *Scientific Research and Essays*, Vol. 5, No.16, pp. 2206-2209, ISSN 1992-2248

Beausoleil, M., Fortier, N., Guenette, S., L'Ecuyer, A., Savoie, M., Franco, M., Lachaine, J. & Weiss, K. (2007). Effect of a fermented milk combining lactobacillus acidophilus Cl1285 and *Lactobacillus casei* in the prevention of antibiotic-associated diarrhea: A randomized, double-blind, placebo-controlled trial. *The Canadian Journal of Gastroenterology*, Vol. 21, No.11, pp. 732-736, ISSN 0835-7900

Bechman, T., Chambers, J. & Cunningham, M. (1977). Influence of *Lactobacillus acidophilus* on performance of young dairy calves. *Journal of Dairy Science*, Vol. 60, Suppl. 1, pp. 74, (Abstract), ISSN 0022-0302

Billoo, A., Memon, M., Khaskheli, S., Murtaza, G., Iqbal, K., Shekhani, M. & Siddiqi, A. (2006). Role of a probiotic (*Saccharomyces boulardii*) in managementand prevention of diarrhea. *World Journal of Gastroenterology*, Vol.12, pp. 4557-4560, ISSN 1007-9327

Biourge, V., Vallet, C., Levesque, A., Sergheraert, R., Chevalier, S. & Roberton, J. (1998). The use of probiotics in the diet of dogs. *The Journal of Nutrition*, Vol. 128, No. 12, pp. 2730-2732, ISSN 1760-4788

Bonnemaison, E., Lanotte, P., Cantagrel, S., Thionois, S., Quentin, R., Chamboux, C. & Laugier, J. (2003). Comparison of fecal flora following administration of two antibiotic protocols for suspected maternofetal infection. *Biology of the Neonate*, Vol. 84, No. 4, pp. 304-310, ISSN 0006-3126

Bousvaros, A., Antonioli, D., Colletti, R., Dubinsky, M., Glickman, J., Gold, B., Griffiths, A., Jevon, G., Higuchi, L., Hyams, J., Kirschner, B., Kugathasan, S., Baldassano, R. & Russo, P. (2007). Differentiating ulcerative colitis from Crohn disease in children and young adults: report of a working group of the North American Society for Pediatric Gastroenterology, Hepatology and Nutrition and the Crohn's and Colitis Foundation of America. *Journal of Pediatric Gastroenterology and Nutrition*, Vol. 44, No. 5, pp. 653–674, ISSN 1536-4801

Brandão, R., Castro, I., Bambirra, E., Amaral, S., Fietto, L., Tropia, M., Neves, M., Santos, R., Gomes, N., & Nicoli, J. (1998). Intracellular signal triggered by cholera toxin in *Saccharomyces boulardii* and *Saccharomyces cerevisiae*. *Applied and Environmental Microbiology*, Vol. 64, No. 2, pp. 564-568, ISSN 1098-5336

Breitbart, M. et al. (2003). Metagenomic analyses of an uncultured viral community from human feces. *The Journal of Bacteriology*, No. 185, pp. 6220-6223, ISSN 1098-5530

Breul, S. (1998). Les probiotiques en alimentation animale. *Medicine et Chirurgie Digestives*, Vol. 27, No. 3, pp. 85-93, ISSN 0047-6412

Caballero-Franco, C., Keller, K., De Simone, C. & Chadee, K. (2007). The VSL#3 probiotic formula induces mucin gene expression and secretion in colonic cells. Gastrointestinal and Liver Physiology, Vol. 292, No. 1, pp. 315–322, ISSN 1522-1547

Callaway, E. & Martin, S. (1997). Effects of a *Saccharomyces cerevisiae* culture on ruminal bacteria that utilize lactate and digest cellulose. *Journal of Dairy Science*, Vol. 80, No. 9, pp. 2035-2044, ISSN 0022-0302

Capriles, V., Silva, K. & Fisberg, M. (2005). Prebióticos, probióticos e simbióticos: Nova tendência no mercado de alimentos funcionais. *Revista Nutrição Brasil*, Vol. 4, No. 6, pp. 327-335, ISSN 1677-0234

Carnevali, O., Zamponi, M., Sulpizio, R., Rollo, A., Nardi, M., Orpianesi, C., Silvi, S., Caggiano, M., Polzonetti, A. & Cresci, A. (2004). Administration of probiotic strain to improve sea bream wellness during development. *Aquaculture International*, Vol. 12, No. 4-5, pp. 377-386, ISSN 1573-143X

Chen, J., Cai, W. & Feng, Y. (2007). Development of intestinal bifidobacteria and lactobacilli in breast-fed neonates. *Clinical Nutrition*, Vol. 26, No. 5, pp. 559-566 ISSN 0261-5614

Chen, X., Fruehauf, J., Goldsmith, J., Xu, H., Katchar, K., Koon, H., Zhao, D., Kokkotou, E., Pothoulakis, C. & Kelly, C. (2009). *Saccharomyces boulardii* Inhibits EGF Receptor Signaling and Intestinal Tumor Growth in Apc(min) mice. *Gastroenterology*, Vol. 137, No. 3, pp. 914 –923, ISSN 0016-5085

Corrêa, N., Péret Filho, L., Penna, F., Lima, F. & Nicoli, J. (2005). A randomized formula controlled trial of *Bifidobacterium lactis* and *Streptococcus thermophilus* for prevention of antibiotic-associated associated diarrhea in infants. *Journal of Clinical Gastroenterology*, Vol. 39, No. 5, pp. 385-389, ISSN 1539-2031

Corrêa, N., Penna, F., Lima, F., Nicoli, J. & Péret Filho, L. (2011). Treatment of acute diarrhea with *Saccharomyces boulardii* in infants: a double-blind, randomized, placebo controlled trial. *Journal of Pediatric Gastroenterology and Nutrition*, (Ahead of Print) DOI:10.1097/MPG.0b013e31822b7ab0, ISSN 1536-4801

Cristani, J., White, C. & Sabino, N. (1999). Efeitos do uso do *Lactobacillus acidophilus* como aditivo alimentar na produção de suínos. In: *Congresso Brasileiro de Veterinários Especialistas em Suínos*, 9., pp. 433-434, CD-ROOM

Dalmin, G., Kathiresan, K. & Purushothaman, A. (2001). Effect of probiotics on bacterial population and health status of shrimp in culture pond ecosystem. *Indian Journal of Experimental Biology*, Vol. 39, No. 9, pp. 939-942, ISSN 0019-5189

De Vrese, M., Stegelmann, A., Richter, B., Fenselau, S., Laue, C. & Schrezenmeir, J. (2001). Probiotics-compensation for lactase insufficiency. *The American Journal of Clinical Nutrition*. Vol. 73, Suppl. 2, pp. 421–429, ISSN 1938-3207

DeVrese, M. & Marteau, P. (2007). Probiotics and Prebiotics: Effects on Diarrhea. *The Journal of Nutrition*. Vol.137, No. 3, pp. 803-811, ISSN 1541-6100

Dutta, P., Mitra, U., Dutta, S., Rajendran, K., Saha, T. & Chatterjee, M. (2011). Randomised controlled clinical trial of *Lactobacillus sporogenes* (*Bacillus coagulans*), used as probiotic in clinical practice, onacute watery diarrhoea in children. *Tropical Medicine and International Health*, Vol. 16, No. 5, pp. 555–561, ISSN 1360-2276

Eckburg, P., Lepp, P. & Relman, D. (2003). Archaea and their potential role in human disease. *Infection and Immunity*, Vol. 71, pp. 591–596, ISSN 0019-9567

El-Nezami, H., Polychronaki, N., Ma, J., Zhu, H., Ling, W., Salminen, E., Juvonen, R., Salminen, S., Poussa, T. & Mykkanen, H. (2006). Probiotic supplementation reduces a biomarker for increased risk ofliver cancer in young men from Southern China. *The American Journal of Clinical Nutrition*, Vol. 83, pp. 1199–203, ISSN 1938-3207

Estrada, A., Wilkie, D. & Drew, M. (2001). Administration of *Bifidobacterium bifidum* to chicken broilers reduces the number of carcass condemnations for cellulitis at the abattoir. *Journal of Applied Poultry Research*, Vol. 10, No. 4, pp. 329-334, ISSN 1537-0437

Ezendam, J. & van Loveren, H. (2006). Probiotics: immunomodulation and evaluation of safety and efficacy. *Nutrition Reviews*, Vol. 64, No. 1, pp. 1-14 ISSN 1753-4887

FAO/WHO. Report of a joint FAO/WHO expert consultation on evaluation of health and nutritional properties of probiotics in food including powder milk with live lactic acid bacteria. Córdoba, Argentina, 2001.

Figueiredo, P., Vieira, E., Nicoli, J., Nardi, R., Raibaud, P., Duval-Iflah, Y. & Penna, F. (2001). Influence of oral inoculation with plasmid-free human *Escherichia coli* on the frequency of diarrhea during the first year of life in human newborns. *Journal of Pediatric Gastroenterology and Nutrition*, Vol. 33, No. 1, pp. 70-74, ISSN 1536-4801

França, F., Dias, D., Teixeira, P., Marcantônio, A., De Stéfani, M., Antonucci, A., Rocha, G., Ranzani-Paiva, M. & Ferreira, C. (2008). Efeito do probiótico *Bacillus subtilis* no crescimento, sobrevivência e fisiologia de rãs-touro (*Rana catesbeiana*). *Boletim do Instituto de Pesca*, Vol. 34, No. 3, pp. 403-412, ISSN 1678-2305

Frape, D. (1998). *Equine Nutrition and Feeding* (2nd edition), Blackwell Science, ISBN 9780632053032, United States of America: 1998. 404 pp.

Fritts, C., Kersey, J., Motl, M., Kroger, E., Yan, F., Si, J., Jiang, Q., Campos, M., Waldroup, A. & Waldroup, P. (2000). *Bacillus subtilis* C-3102 (Calsporin) improves live performance and microbiological status of broiler chickens. *Journal of Applied Poultry Research*, Vol. 9, No. 2, pp. 149-155, ISSN 1537-0437

Fuller, R. (1989). Probiotics in man and animals. *Journal of Applied Bacteriology*, Vol. 66, pp. 365-378, ISSN 1365-2672

Fuller, R. (1992). Problems and prospects. In: *Probiotics – The scientific basis*, Fuller, R. pp. 377-386, Chapman & Hall, ISBN 0412408503, London

Furrie, E., Macfarlane, S., Kennedy, A., Cummings, J., Walsh, S., O'Neil, D. & Macfarlane, G. (2005). Synbiotic therapy (Bifido bacteriumlongum/Synergy 1) initiates resolution of inflammation in patients with activeulcerative colitis: a randomised controlled pilot trial. Gut; Vol. 54, pp. 242–249, ISSN 1468-3288

Gao, X., Mubasher, M., Fang, C., Reifer, C., & Miller, L. (2010). Dose – Response Efficacy of a Proprietary Probiotic Formula of Lactobacillus acidophilus CL1285 and *Lactobacillus casei* LBC80R for Antibiotic-Associated Diarrhea and *Clostridium difficile* -Associated Diarrhea Prophylaxis in Adult Patients, *The American Journal of Gastroenterology*, Vol. 105, pp.1636–1641, ISSN 0002-9270

Gil de los Santos, J., Storch, O. & Gil-Turnes, C. (2005). *Bacillus cereus* var. toyoii and *Saccharomyces boulardii* increased feed efficiency in broilers infected with *Salmonella enteritidis*. *British Poultry Science*, Vol. 46, No. 4, pp. 494-497, ISSN 0007-1668

Glade, M. (1991). Dietary yeast culture supplementation of mares during late gestation and early lactation. 2. Effects on milk production, milk composition, weight gain and linear growth of nursling foals. *Journal of Equine Veterinary Science.* Vol. 11, No. 2, pp. 89-95, ISSN 0737-0806

Gram, L., Melchiorsen, J., Spanggard, B., Huber, I. & Nielsen, T. (1999). Inhibition of *Vibrio anguillarum* by *Pseudomonas fluorescens* AH2, a possible probiotic treatment of fish. *Applied and Environmental Microbiology*, Vol. 65, No. 3, pp. 969-973, ISSN 1098-5336

Grandy, G., Medina, M., Soria, R., Terán, C. &, Araya, M.(2010). Probiotics in the treatment ofacute rotavirus diarrhoea. A randomized, double-blind, controlled trial using twodifferent probiotic preparations in Bolivian children. *BMC Infectious Diseases*, Vol. 10, No. 253, pp. 1-7, ISSN 1471-2334

Guo, Y. & Liu, C. (1997). Impact of heat stress in broiler chicks and effect of supplemental yeast chromium. *Biotehnologija u Srocarstvu*, Vol. 13, No. 3-4, pp. 171-176, ISSN 0353-6289

Harmsen, H., Wildeboer-Veloo, A., Raangs, G., Wagendorp, A., Klijin, N., Bindels, J. & Welling, G. (2000). Analysis of intestinal flora development in breast-fed and formula-fed infants by using molecular identification and detection methods. *Journal of Pediatric Gastroenterology and Nutrition*, Vol. 30, No. 1, pp. 61-67, ISSN 1536-4801

Hayashi, H., Sakamoto, M. & Benno, Y. (2002). Phylogenetic analysis of the human gut microbiota using 16S rDNA clone libraries and strictly anaerobic culture-based methods. *Microbiology and Immunology.* Vol. 46, pp. 535–548, ISSN 1348-0421

He, T., Priebe, M., Zhong, Y., Huang, C., Harmsen, H., Raangs, G., Antoine, J., Wellingand, G. & Vonk, R. (2008). Effects of yogurt and bifidobacteria supplementation onthe colonic microbiota in lactose-intolerant subjects. *Journal of Applied Microbiology*, Vol. 104, pp. 595–604, ISSN 1364-5072

Hickson M, D'Souza AL, Muthu N, Thomas R RogersTrust, Want,S., Rajkumar, C. & Bulpitt, C. (2007). Use of probiotic Lactobacillus preparation to prevent diarrhoea associated with antibiotics: randomised doubleblind placebo controlled trial. *British Medical Journal*, Vol. 335, No. 7610, pp. 80, ISSN 0959-8138

Hill, J., Tracey, S., Willis, M., Jones, L. & Ellis, A. (2006). Yeast culture in equine nutrition and physiology. In: *Proceedings of Alltech's Annual Symposium*, 17., 31.08.2011, Available from: http://eNo.engormix.com/MA-equines/nutrition/articles/yeast-culture-equine-nutrition-t279/p0.htm

Hollister, A., Cheeke, P., Robinson, K. & Patton, M. (1989). Effects of water-administered probiotics and acidifiers on growth, feed conversion and enteritis mortality of weanling rabbits. *Journal of Applied Rabbit Research*, Vol. 12, No. 4, pp. 143-147, ISSN 0738-9760

Hooper, L. (2004). Bacterial contributions to mammalian gut development. Trends in Microbiology, Vol. 12, No. 3, pp. 129–134, ISSN 0966-842X

Hooper, L. & Macpherson, A. (2010). Immune adaptations that maintain homeostasis with the intestinal microbiota. *Nature Reviews – Immunology*, Vol.10, pp. ISSN 1474-1733

Ignatova, M., Sredkova, V. & Marasheva, V. (2009). Effect of dietary inclusion of probiotic on chickens performance and some blood. *Biotechnology in Animal Husbandry*, Vol. 25, No. 5-6, pp.1079-1085, ISSN 1450-9156

J. Boudeau, Glasser, A., Julien, S., Colombel, J. & Darfeuille-Michaud, A. (2003). Inhibitory effect of probiotic Escherichia coli strain Nissle 1917on adhesion to and invasion of intestinal epithelial cellsby adherent–invasive E. coli strains isolated from patients with Crohn's disease. *Alimentary Pharmacology Therapeutics*. Vol. 18, pp. 45–56, ISSN 0269-2813

Jain, S., Yadav, H., Sinha, P., Kapila, S., Naito, Y. & Marotta, F. (2010) Anti-allergic effects of probiotic Dahi through modulation of the gut immune system. *Turkish Journal of Gastroenterology*. Vol. 21, No. 3, pp. 244-250, ISSN 1300-4948

Jin, L., Ho, Y., Abdullah, N. & Jalaludin, S. (1997). Probiotics in poultry: modes of action. *World's Poultry Science Journal*, Vol. 53, No. 4, pp. 351-368, ISSN 0043-9339

Jonsson, E. & Henningsson, S. (1991). Establishment in the piglet gut of lactobacilli capable of degrading mixed-linked beta-glucans. *Journal Applied Bacteriology*, Vol. 70, No. 6, pp. 512-516, ISSN 1364-5072

Kalavathy, R., Abdullah, N., Jalaludin, S. & Ho, Y. (2003). Effects of Lactobacillus cultures on growth performance, abdominal fat deposition, serum lipids and weight of organs of broiler chickens. *British Poultry Science*, Vol. 44, No. 1, pp. 139-144, ISSN 0007-1668

Kalliomaki, M., Salminen, S., Poussa, T., Arvilommi, H. & Isolauri, E. (2003). Probiotics and prevention of atopic disease: 4-year follow-up of a randomised placebo-controlled trial. *The Lancet*, Vol. 361, No. 9372, pp. 1869-1871, ISSN 0140-6736

Kamalamma, Krishnamoorty, U. & Krishnappa, P. (1996). Effect of feeding yeast culture (Yea-sacc[1026]) on rumen fermentation in vitro and production performance in crossbred dairy cows. *Animal Feed Science Technology*, Vol. 57, No. 3, pp. 247-256, ISSN 0377-8401

Kozasa, M. (1989). Probiotics for animal use in Japan. *Revue Scientifique et Technique de l'Ofisse International des Epizooties*, Vol. 8, No. 2, pp. 517-531, ISSN 0253-1933

Krehbiel, C., Rust, S., Zhang, G. & Gilliland, S. (2003). Bacterial direct-fed microbials in ruminant diets: performance response and mode of action. *Journal of Animal Science*, Vol. 81, No. 14, Suppl. 2, pp. 120-132, ISSN 1525-3163

Kritas, S., Alexopoulos, C. & Kyriakis, S. (2006). The effect of an EU-registered probiotic on the health status and performance of sows and their litters. In: *3° Congresso Latino-americano de Suinocultura*, pp. 737-740, CD-ROOM

Kumar, R., Mukherjee, S., Prasad, K. & Pal, A. (2006). Evaluation of *Bacillus subtilis* as a probiotic to indian major carp *Labeo rohita* (Ham.). *Aquaculture Research*, Vol. 37, No. 12, pp. 1215-1221, ISSN 1355-557X

Lambertini, L., Zaguini, G. & Dammacco, D. (1990). Risultati acquisiti com l'impiego di *Bacillus subtilis* in mangini per conigli. *Rivista di Coniglicoltura*, Vol. 1, No. 5, pp. 29-32, ISSN 0010-5929

Lara-Flores, M., Olvea-Novoa, M., Guzman-Mendez, B. & López-Madrid, W. (2003). Use of the bacteria *Streptococcus faecium* and *Lactobacillus acidophilus*, and the yeast *Saccharomyces cerevisiae* as growth promoters in Nile tilapia (*Oreochromis niloticus*). *Aquaculture*, Vol. 216, No. 1-4, pp. 193-201, ISSN 0044-8486

Leandro, N., Oliveira, A., Andrade, M., Stringhini, J., Andrade, L., Chaves, L.S. & Silva, T. (2004). Efeito de probiótico inoculado via ovo sobre o desempenho e colonização do TGI por *Salmonella enteritidis* de pintos desafiados. In: *41ª Reunião Anual da Sociedade Brasileira de Zootecnia*, 31.08.2011, Available from http://www.sbz.org.br/visualizar.php?idiom=pt&artigo=13752

Lin, H., Guo, Z., Yang, Y., Zheng, W. & LI, Z. (2004). Effect of dietary probiotics on apparent digestibility coefficients of nutrients of white shrimp *Litopenaeus vannamei* Boone. *Aquaculture Research*, Vol. 35, No. 15, pp. 1441-1447, ISSN 1355-557X

Line, E., Bailey, S., Cox, N., Stern, N. & Tompkins, T. (1998). Effect of yeast-supplemented feed on *Salmonella* and *Compylobacter* populations in broilers. *Poultry Science*, Vol. 77, No. 3, pp. 405-410, ISSN 0032-5791

Ma, E., Choi, Y., Choi, J., Rhee, S. & EunokIm. (2010). The anticancer effect of probiotic Bacillus polyfermenticuson human colon cancer cells is mediated through ErbB2and ErbB3. *Inhibition International Journal of Cancer*, Vol. 127, pp. 780–790, ISSN 1097-0215

Mack, D. (2011). Probiotics in inflammatory bowel diseases and associated conditions. *Nutrients*, Vol. 3, pp. 245-264, ISSN 2072-6643

Majamaa, H. & Isolauri, E. (1997). Probiotics: a novel approach in the management of food allergy. *Journal of Allergy and Clinical Immunology*, Vol. 99, No. 2, pp. 179-185, ISSN 0091-6749

Makridis, P., Fjellheim, A., Skjermo, J. & Vadstein, O. (2000). Colonization of the gut in first feeding turbot by bacterial strains added to the water or biencapusated in rotifers. *Aquaculture International*, Vol. 8, No. 5, pp. 367-380, ISSN 1573-143X

Martin, S. (1998). Manipulation of ruminal fermentation with organic acids: a review. *Journal of Animal Science*, Vol. 76, No. 12, pp. 3123-3132, ISSN 1525-3163

Martins, F., Elian, S., Vieira, A., Tiago, F., Martins, A., Silva, F., Souza, E., Sousa, L., Araujo, H., Pimenta, P., Bonjardim, C., Arantes, R., Teixeira, M. & Nicoli, J. (2011). Oral treatment with *Saccharomyces cerevisiae* strain UFMG 905 modulates immune responses and interferes with signal pathways involved in the activation of inflammation in a murine model of typhoid fever. *International Journal of Medical Microbiology*, Vol. 301, No. 4, pp. 359-364, ISSN 1438-4221

Martins, F., Dalmasso, G., Arantes, M., Doye, A., Lemichez, E., Lagadec, P., Imbert, V., Peyron, J., Rampal, P., Nicoli, J. & Czerucka, D. Interaction of *Saccharomyces boulardii* with *Salmonella enterica* serovar Typhimurium protects mice and modifies T84 cell response to the infection. *Plos One*, Vol. 5, No. 1, e8925, 2010, ISSN 1932-6203

Michail, S., Sylvester, F., Fuchs, G. & Issenman, R. (2006). North American Society for Pediatric Gastroenterology, Hepatology, and Nutrition (NASPGHAN) Nutrition Report Committee. Clinical efficacy of probiotics: review of the evidence with focus on children. *Journal of Pediatric Gastroenterology and Nutrition*, Vol. 43, No. 4, pp. 550-557, ISSN 1536-4801

Michelan, A., Scapinello, C., Natali, M., Furlan, A., Sakaguti, E., Faria, H., Santolin, M. & Hernandes, A. (2002). Utilização de probiótico, ácido orgânico e antibiótico em dietas para coelhos em crescimento: ensaio de digestibilidade, avaliação da morfometria intestinal e desempenho. *Revista Brasileira de Zootecnia*, Vol. 31, No. 6, pp. 2227-2237, ISSN 1516-3598

Mir, Z. & Mir, P. (1994). Effect of the addition of live yeast (*Saccharomyces cerevisiae*) on growth and carcass quality of steers fed high-forage or high-grain diets and on feed digestibility and in situ degradability. *Journal of Animal Science*, Vol. 72, No. 3, pp. 537-545, ISSN 1525-3163

Momose, Y., Hirayama, K. & Itoh, K. (2008) Competition for proline between indigenous *Escherichia coli* and *E. coli* O157:H7 in gnotobiotic mice associated with infant intestinal microbiota and its contribution to the colonization resistance against *E. coli* O157:H7. *Antonie van Leeuwenhoek. Journal of Microbiology*, Vol. 94, pp. 165-171, ISSN 1572-9699

Moore, B. & Newman, K. (1993). Influence of feeding yeast culture (Yea-Sacc) on cecum and colon pH of the equine. *Journal of Animal Science*, Vol. 71, No. 1, pp. 261 (Abstract), ISSN 1525-3163

Morgan, L., Coverdale J., Froetschel, M. & Yoon, I. (2007). Effect of yeast culture supplementation on digestibility of varying forage quality in mature horses. *Journal of Equine Veterinary Science*, Vol. 27, No. 6, pp. 260-265, ISSN 0737-0806

Moura, R., Saliba, E., Almeida, F., Lana, A., Silva, V. & Rezende, A. (2009). Feed efficiency in Mangalarga Marchador foals fed diet supplemented with probiotics or phytase. *Revista Brasileira de Zootecnia*, Vol. 38, No. 6, pp. 1045-1050, ISSN 1516-3598

Nagala, M. & Routray, M. (2011). Clinical case study—multispecies probiotic supplement minimizes symptoms of irritable Bowel Syndrome. *US Gastroenterology & Hepatology Review*. Vol.7, pp. 36-37, ISSN 1758-3934

Ng, S., Hart, A., Kamm, M., Stagg, A. & Knight, S. (2009). Mechanisms of Action of Probiotics: Recent Advances. *Inflammatory Bowel Diseases*, Vol. 15, No. 2, pp.300-310 ISSN 1536-4844

Nguyen, T., Kang, J. & Lee, M. (2007). Characterization of Lactobacillus plantarum PH04, a potential probiotic bacterium with cholesterol-lowering effects. *International Journal of Food Microbiology*, Vol. 113, No. 3, pp. 358-361, ISSN 0168-1605

Noriega, L., Cuevas, I., Margolles, A. & Reyes-Gavilán, C. (2006). Deconjugation and bile salts hydrolase activity by Bifido bacterium strains with acquired resistance to bile. *International Dairy Journal*, Vol.16, pp. 850–855, ISSN 0958-6946

Nurmi, E. & Rantala, M. (1973). New aspects of *Salmonella* infection in broiler production. *Nature*, Vol. 241, No. 1, pp. 210-211, ISSN 0028-0836

Ocaña, V., Holgado, A. & Nader-Macias, M. (1999). Characterization of a bacteriocin-like substance produced by a vaginal *Lactobacillus salvaricus* strain. *Applied and Environmental Microbiology*, Vol. 65, No. 12, pp. 5631-5635, ISSN 1098-5336

Oelschlaeger, T. (2010). Mechanisms of probiotic actions – A review. *International Journal of Medical Microbiology*. Vol. 300, pp. 57-62, ISSN 1438-4221

Parker, R.B. (1974). Probiotics, the other half of the antimicrobial story. *Animal Nutrition and Health*, Vol.29, pp.4-8, ISSN 0003-3553

Parvez, S., Kim, H., Lee, H. & Kim, D. (2006). Bile salt hydrolase and cholesterol removal effect by Bifidobacterium bifidum NRRL 1976S. *World Journal of Microbiology & Biotechnology*, Vol. 22, pp. 455-459, ISSN 1573-0972

Penna, F., Peret, L., Vieira, L. & Nicoli, J. (2008). Probiotics and mucosal barrier in children. *Current Opinion in Clinical Nutrition and Metabolic Care*, 11: 640-644, ISSN 1473-6519

Pereira, D., McCartney, A. & Gibson, G. (2003). An In Vitro Study of the Probiotic Potential of a Bile-Salt-Hydrolyzing Lactobacillus fermentum Strain, and Determination of ItsCholesterol-Lowering Properties. *Applied and Environmental Microbiology*, Vol. 69, No. 8, pp. 4743–4752, ISSN 0099-2240

Pietras, M. (2001). The effect of probiotics on selected blood and meat parameters of broiler chickens. *Journal of Animal and Feed Sciences*, Vol. 10, No. 2, pp. 297-302, Suppl.2, ISSN 1230-1388

Pollman, D. & Bandyck, C. (1984). Stability of viable lactobacillus products. *Animal Feed Science and Technology*, Vol. 11, No. 4, pp. 261-267, ISSN 0377-8401

Regadera, J., Verges, R., Romero, J., Fuente, I., Biete, A., Villori, J., Cobo, J. & Guarner, F. (2008). Effects of probiotic *Lactobacillus casei* DN-114 001 in prevention ofradiation-induced diarrhea: results from multicenter, randomized,placebo-controlled nutritional trialjordi giraltInt. *International Journal of Radiation Oncology - Biology - Physics*, Vol.71, No .4, pp.1213–1219, ISSN 0360-3016

Riquelme, C., Hayashida, G., Araya, R., Uchida, A., Satomi, M. & Ishida, Y. (1996). Isolation of a native bacterial strain from the scallop *Argopecten purpuratus* with inhibitory effects against pathogenic vibrios. *Journal of Shellfish Research*, Vol. 15, No. 2, pp. 369–374, ISSN 0730-8000

Robinson, J., Whipp, S., Bucklin, J. & Allison, M. (1984). Characterization of predominant bacteria from the colons of normal and dysenteric pigs. *Applied and Environmental Microbiology*, Vol. 48, No. 5, pp. 964-969, ISSN 1098-5336

Rolfe, R. (2000). The role of probiotic cultures in the control of gastrointestinal health. *The Journal Nutrition*, Vol. 130, pp. 396–402, ISSN 0899- 9007

Rosenfeldt, V., Benfeldt, E., Nielsen, S., Michaelsen, K., Jeppesen, D., Valerius, N. & Paerregaar, A. (2003). Effect of probiotic Lactobacillus strains in children with atopic dermatitis. *Journal of Allergy and Clinical Immunology*, Vol. 111, No. 2, pp. 389-95, ISSN 0091-6749

Roth, F. & Kirchgessner, M. (1988). Nutritive effects of toyocerin. 1 Piglet feeding. *Landwirtschaftliche Forschung*, Vol. 41, No. 1-2, pp. 58-62, ISSN 0023-8147

Russel, E. (1979). Types and distribution of anaerobic bacteria in the large intestine of pigs. *Applied and Environmental Microbiology*, Vol. 37, No. 2, pp. 187-193, ISSN 1098-5336

Sazawal, S., Hiremath, G., Dhingra, U., Malik, P., Deb, S. & Black, R. (2006) Efficacy of probiotics in prevention of acute diarrhoea: a meta-analysis of masked, randomised, placebo-controlled trials. *The Lancet Infectious Diseases*, Vol.6, pp. 374-382, ISSN 1474-4457

Schrezenmeir, J. & de Vrese, M. (2001) Probiotics, prebiotics, and synbiotics – approaching a definition. *The American Journal of Clinical Nutrition*, Vol. 73, pp. 361S-364S, ISSN , ISSN 1938-3207

Servin, L. & Coconnier, M. (2003) Adhesion of probiotic strains to the intestinal mucosa and interaction with pathogens. *Best Practice & Research Clinical Gastroenterology*, Vol. 17, pp.741–754, ISSN 1521-6918

Servin, A. (2004) Antagonistic activities of lactobacilli and bifidobacteria against microbial pathogens. *Microbiology Reviews*, Vol. 28, pp.405–440, ISSN 0168-6445

Shortt, C. (1999) The probiotic century: historical and current perspectives. *Trends in Food Science & Technology*, Vol. 10, pp. 411-417, ISSN 0924-2244

Soleimani, N., Kermanshahi, R., Yakhchali, B.& Sattari, T. (2010). Antagonistic activity of probiotic lactobacilli against *Staphylococcus aureus* isolated from bovine mastitis. *African Journal of Microbiology Research*. Vol. 4, No .20, pp. 2169-2173, ISSN 1996-0808

Sommart, K., Wanapat, M., Wongsrikeao, W. & Ngarmsak, S. (1993). Effects of yeast culture and protein levels on ruminal fermentation, intake, digestibility and performance in ruminants fed straw based diets. *Journal of Animal Science*, Champaign, Vol. 71, Suppl.1, pp. 281, ISSN 1525-3163

Sonnenburg, J., Chen, C. & Gordon, J. (2006). Genomic and metabolic studies of the impact of probiotics on a model gut symbiont and host. PLoS Biol 4(12): e413. DOI: 10.1371/journal.pbio.0040413

Swanson, K., Grieshop, C., Flickinger, E., Bauer, L., Wolf, B., Chow, J., Garleb, K. & Williams, J. (2002). Fructooligosaccharides and *Lactobacillus acidophilus* modify bowel function and protein catabolites excreted by healthy humans. *The Journal of Nutrition*, Vol. 132, No. 10, pp. 3042-3050, ISSN 1760-4788

Tereda, A., Hara, H., Li, T., Ichikawa, H., Nishi, J. & Ko, S. (1994). Effect of a microbial preparation on fecal flora and fecal metabolic products of pigs. *Animal Science and Technology*, Vol. 65, No. 9, pp. 806-814, ISSN 0918-2365

Thirabunyanon, M., Boonprasom, P. & Niamsup, P. (2009). Probiotic potential of lactic acid bacteria isolated from fermented dairy milks on antiproliferation of colon cancer cells. *Biotechnology Letters*, Vol. 31, pp. 571–576, ISSN 1573-6776

Utiyama, C., Oetting, L., Giani, P., Ruiz, U. & Miyada, V. (2006). Efeitos de antimicrobianos, prebióticos, probióticos e extratos vegetais sobre a microbiota intestinal, a frequência de diarreia e o desempenho de leitões recém-desmamados. *Revista Brasileira de Zootecnia*, Vol. 35, No. 6, pp. 2359-2367, ISSN 1516-3598

Vahedi, H., Ansari, R., Mir-Nasseri, M. & Jafari, E. (2010). Irritable Bowel Syndrome: A Review Article. *Middle East Journal of Digestive Diseases*. Vol. 2, No. 2, ISSN 2008-5249

Vasiljevic, T & Shah, N. (2008). Probiotics— from Metchnikoff to bioactives. *International Dairy Journal*, Vol. 18, pp. 714– 728, ISSN 0958-6946

Veizaj-Delia, E., Piub, T., Lekajc, P. & Tafaj, M. (2010). Using combined probiotic to improve growth performance of weanedpiglets on extensive farm conditions. *Livestock Science*, Vol.134, pp. 249–251, ISSN 1871-1413

Verschuere, L., Rombaut, G., Sorgeloos, P. & Verstraete, W. (2000). Probiotic bacteria as biological control agents in aquaculture. *Microbiology and Molecular Biology Review*, Vol. 64, No. 4, pp. 655–671, ISSN 1098-5557

Wang, Y., Xu, Z. & Xia, M. (2005). The effectiveness of commercial probiotics in Northern White Shrimp *Penaeus vannamei* ponds. *Fisheries Science*, Vol. 71, No. 5, pp. 1034-1039, ISSN 0919-9268

Westerbeek, E., van der Berg, A., Lafeber, H., Knol, J., Fetter, W. & van Elburg, R. (2006) The intestinal bacterial colonization in preterm infants: a review of the literature. *Clininical Nutrional*, Vol. 25, pp. 361-368, ISSN 1532-1983

WHO/FAO. Joint World Health Organization/Food and Agricultural Organization Working Group. (2002). *Guidelines for the Evaluation of Probiotics in Food*, London, Ontario, Canada

Yamani, K., Ibrahim, H. & Rashwan, A. (1992). Effects of a pelleted diet supplemented with probiotic (Lacto-Sacc) and water supplemented with a combination of probiotic and acidifier (Acid Pak-4-Way) on digestibility, growth, carcass and physiological aspects of weanling New Zealand White rabbits. *Journal of Applied Rabbit Research*, Vol. 15, No. 1, pp. 1087-1100, ISSN 0738-9760

Zhao, T., Doyle, M., Harmon, B., Brown, C., Mueller, P. & Parks, A. (1998). Reduction of carriage of enterohemorrhagic *Escherichia coli* O157:H7 in cattle by inoculation with probiotic bacteria. *Journal of Clinical Microbiology*, Vol. 36, No. 3, pp. 641-647, ISSN 0095-1137

Ziaei-Nejad, S., Rezaei, M., Takami, G., Lovett, D., Mirvaghefi, A. & Shakouri, M. (2006). The effect of *Bacillus* sppp. bacteria used as probiotics on digestive enzyme activity, survival and growth in the Indian white shrimp *Fenneropenaeus indicus. Aquaculture*, Vol. 252, No. 2-4, pp. 516-524, ISSN 0044-8486

Zoetendal, E., Akkermans, A., Akkermans-van Vliet, W., de Visser, J. & de Vos, W. (2001). The host genotype affects the bacterial community in the human gastronintestinal tract. *Microbial Ecology in Health and Disease*, Vol.13, pp. 129–134, ISSN 1651-2235

Zulkifli, I., Abdullah, N., Azrin, N. & Ho, Y. (2000). Growth performance and immune response of two commercial broiler strains fed diets containing Lactobacillus cultures and oxytetracycline under heat stress conditions. *British Poultry Science*, Vol. 41, No. 5, pp. 593-597, ISSN 0007-1668

5

Gut Microbiota in Disease Diagnostics

Knut Rudi[1,2,3] and Morten Isaksen[1]
[1]*Genetic Analysis AS, OSLO*
[2]*The Norwegian University for Life Sciences, Ås*
[3]*Hedmark University College, Hamar*
Norway

1. Introduction

A substantial amount of scientific documentation is mounting for the significance of the gastrointestinal microbiota (gut or GI microbiota) on human health. In addition to the obvious connection between the gut microbiota and inflammation in the colon (leading to IBD, IBS and possibly colon cancer), recent articles have highlighted the not-so-obvious connection between the gut microbiota and the brain (Heijtz et al., 2011)) and cardiovascular system (Wang et al., 2011).

Despite several major breakthrough discoveries of the importance of the gut microbiota in human health, this information has not yet been transformed into diagnostic or therapeutic approaches. A major bottleneck in the gut microbiota diagnostics is the reproducibility and throughput of the analytical approaches used.

Since we do not know the growth conditions for most gut bacteria, traditional cultivation based analysis of bacteria cannot be used for a comprehensive overview of the gut microbiota. Currently, quantitative PCR are quite extensively being used to detect the presence of specific pathogens. However, since the gut microbiota is complex and contains hundreds of different microbes, such technology does not hold the promise to be used as a general analysis tool to monitor changes in the gut microbiota that affect health conditions. The current focus in human gut microbiota screenings are based on explorative deep sequencing. It is expected that it will take considerable time and further development before sequencing of the gut microbiota could become a routine diagnostic tool. However, since the human gut microbiota is getting more thoroughly characterized, it is time to look for more targeted approaches rather than the current explorative screenings.

The most widely applied targeted approach to describe microbial diversity are by probes targeting the gene encoding 16S ribosomal RNA. This gene is ancient, universally distributed and comprise highly conserved sequence domains interspersed with more variable regions (Woese, 1987). The conserved regions provide information for classification of higher taxa, while the variable regions can be used for differentiation between closely related species. An average bacterial 16S rRNA molecule has a length of approximately 1 500 nucleotides, making it experimentally manageable by e.g. PCR amplification.

The first step in 16S rRNA gene microbiota analyses is to purify DNA from all bacteria present in a sample without introducing bias due to e.g. differential lysis or recovery. Subsequent to DNA purification, all bacterial 16S rRNA genes in the samples are amplified using primers targeting generally conserved regions in the 16S rRNA gene. The ratio between 16S rRNA gene copies for different bacteria is (in theory) conserved during the PCR amplification process.

Currently the most widely used approach to analyze 16S rRNA gene diversity is through next generation sequencing (Kunin et al 2010). The depth of the information that can be obtained form such sequencing efforts are dependent on the number of reads that are being done.

An alternative approach is the use of high-density microarrays based on 16S rRNA sequence variations. These approaches are explorative, and intended for discovery rather than diagnostics. A major challenge with traditional 16S rRNA gene microarrays is probe specificity, and cross-reactivity between closely related species (Cox et al 2010). For microarrays, this challenge has recently been addressed by tilling probes covering the variable region of the 16S rRNA gene (Rajilic-Stojanovic et al 2009). The principle by tilling is that a large number of overlapping probes cover the region of interest, with the combined probe signals providing a relatively good signal-to-noise ratio. Both for next generation sequencing and microarray analysis, a comprehensive data analysis of the information is required in order to obtain interpretable results.

A more direct approach for characterizing the gut microbiota is the use of highly specific single nucleotide primer extension (SNuPE) probes (Eggesbo et al 2011).The high specificity of the SNuPE assay is obtained by DNA polymerase based incorporation of a labeled dideoxynucleotide (Syvanen et al 1990). The SNuPE probes are constructed so that the probes hybridize adjacent to discriminative gene positions. If the target bacterium is present, a labeled dideoxynucleotide is incorporated by the polymerase.

A technology platform have been developed that can readily be applied to analyze the gut microbiota based on the SNuPE principle. The method – called GA-map™ (Genetic Analysis' Microbiota Analysis Platform) - has already demonstrated its usefulness in applications for assessing various disease states based on analysis of the composition of the gut microbiota.

Here, we discuss the possibility of using a novel comprehensive targeted approach for quantifying the inhabitants of the human gut microbiota in disease diagnostics.

2. Requirements for a gut microbiota test

The general requirements for a gut microbiota test is (i) simple sample collection, (ii) comprehensive, (iii) reproducible, (iv) high-throughput and (v) affordable. In addition, the test must deliver results that can be interpreted and be relevant to disease.

There are still major challenges with all these requirements. Most methods developed for research are actually not well documented, and promises far more than the methods in reality can deliver. A current example of this is the emergence of the next generation sequencing approaches. For instance, it is now being realized that these techniques inflate diversity measures (Kunin et al 2010). New software tools have been developed to reduce this inflation of diversity, but it is still uncertain if the number of different Operational Taxonomic Units (OTUs) obtained by next generation sequencing techniques gives a correct representation of the actual number of different bacteria present in the sample.

Perhaps the largest challenge in gut microbiota diagnostics is the establishment of the correlation between microbiota patterns and disease. Since the characterization of the gut microbiota is in its infancy, there are not many diseases that have actually been characterized with respect to specific dysbiosis of the gut microbiota. Furthermore, since the analysis represent patterns rather than single bacteria, new diagnostic principles must also be implemented.

Diagnostic approaches related to dysbiosis of the gut microbiota have until now been dominated by culture dependent techniques which only detect a minor portion of the true diversity. Doctors used to such techniques may find it challenging to adapt knowledge about non-cultivable bacteria in their diagnostics because that would include bacteria that they are not familiar with.

We have for instance found that the clostridal family Lachnospiraceae is the most stable and dominant phylogroup in the human gut (Sekelja et al., 2011).This phylogroup has been overlooked by the traditional cultivation dependent techniques, probably because it is strictly anaerobic and that it has special growth requirements that are difficult to simulate on plates.

3. Function vs phylogeny of gut bacteria

A long standing debate is how well functionality of bacteria in the gut correlates to phylogeny. There are recent reports suggesting that the function of gut bacteria is a relatively stable feature, while the microbiota composition is unstable (Turnbaugh et al., 2009).

Although functions cannot directly be deduced from the gut microbiota 16S rRNA gene analyses, correlations between gut microbiota phylogenetic composition and function can be established. We have recently addressed this issue by mapping functions onto a phylogenetic map as illustrated in Figure 1. As seen in this figure, there are good correlations between functions and phylogeny, with different functions being clustered in different phylogroups.

The take home message from this analysis is that the phylogenetic framework can be used to deduce the probability of functions in the gut microbiota, and aid in identifying functions through other targeted approaches. Still, however, our knowledge about the correlations between function and phylogeny is limited. The current major genomic sequencing efforts will aid in these investigations. It will be particularly interesting to determine which functions follow a phylogenetic distribution pattern, and which do not.

For genes located on mobile elements, such as those encoding antibiotic resistance, an important aspect would be to determine the host range of the mobile elements. For instance, given that there are antibiotic resistance genes present on mobile elements in the commensal microbiota with a host range that include pathogens, there will be a severe risk that the antibiotic resistance genes can be transferred to the pathogen.

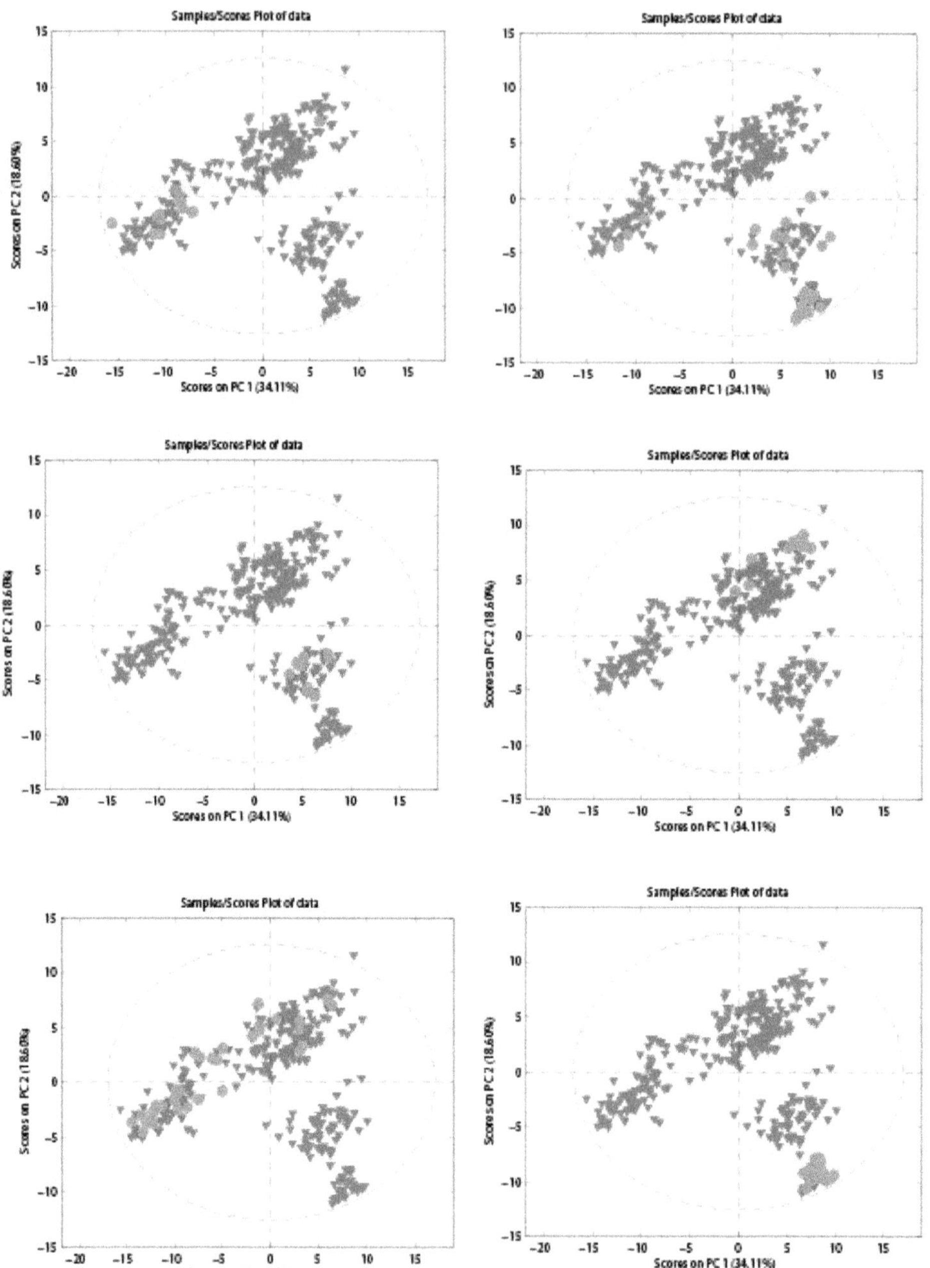

Fig. 1. Properties of gut bacteria in a phylogenetic framework. The PCA biplots represent the 16S rRNA phylogenetic relatedness between the bacteria, while the green circles represent different functions for the different panels. The six panels represent six different functional groups.

4. Diseases with established correlation to the gut microbiota

Necrotizing enterocolitis (NEC) (Wang et al 2009) and inflammatory bowels disease (IBD) (Frank et al 2007, Nell et al 2010) are two diseases that have a recognized established link to the gut microbiota.

NEC is a severe disease affecting preterm infants with a high mortality. About 10% of infants with a birth weight below 1500 g develop NEC, with mortality rate is as high as 30%. It has been suggested that this disease is associated with a reduced diversity of the gut microbiota (Wang et al 2009). Both due to the impact of the test, and because the preterm infant gut microbiota is relatively simple, NEC is an attractive target for developing a human gut microbiota test.

IBD represents a collection of diseases associated with gut inflammation. It has two main sub forms: Crohn's Disease (CD) and Ulcerative colitis (UC). Disturbance of the normally stable GI microbiota are predicted to adversely affect the health of the host (Frank, et al., 2007). Studies of experimental animal models of IBD reveal that germ-free animals show few signs of inflammation; experimental colitis is exhibited only when the animal is exposed to natural microbial communities. Likewise human studies have shown a response of IBD patients to antibiotic and probiotic treatment (Hecht, 2008). In CD patients inflammation most commonly appears in the gut locations where bacterial concentrations are high. Furthermore, diversion of the fecal stream from the lumen is associated with improvement of the inflammation, indicating a role for bacteria in the IBD pathogenesis (Baker, Love, & Ferguson, 2009). Taken together, there are relatively good evidence for a correlation between IBD and the gut microbiota.

5. Diseases with suspected correlation to gut microbiota

There is a very wide range of diseases that have been suggested correlated to the gut microbiota. Among these are diabetes, cardiovascular diseases, rheumatism, metabolic syndrome and obesity (Wang et al. 2011, Wen et al., 2008, Ley et al., 2006). Common for most of these diseases is the correlation to some form of underlying inflammation. Thus, imbalance in the gut microbiota could be a common underlying factor that triggers inflammation. Still, detailed knowledge is lacking about such potential correlations.

Future knowledge building with respect to microbiota composition could open new diagnostic possibilities for these diseases, which all have major impacts on human health. Gut microbiota diagnostics may also help in understanding the etiology of the disease, which potentially could help in developing therapeutic approaches.

The perhaps most surprising correlation to the gut microbiota are cardiovascular disease (Wang et al. 2011). There were relatively strong correlations between microbial metabolites and atherosclerotic disease. Gut microbiota diagnostic in this field could potentially have major impacts on human health.

6. Gut micobiota diagnostic for diffuse conditions

Major diseases with more diffuse symptoms such as irritable bowels disease (IBS) (Salonen et al 2010) and depression (Maes et al 2009) could be targets for development of future diagnostics. These are diseases representing enormous burden and costs to society. If these diseases can be linked to some kind of gut microbiota disorders, then there may also be potential for intervention and treatment.

Discomfort such as abdominal pain, flatulence and bloating affect our everyday life. It has recently been shown correlation between these discomforts and specific gut bacteria (Jalanka-Tuovinen et al., 2011). Although not life threatening, the quality of life can be severely reduced by these discomforts. Diagnosis of the gut microbiota could potentially help in dietary interventions.

Although the severity of IBS is not pronounced, 10% - 20% of people in the Western world suffer from this (Maxion-Bergemann et al 2001). Therefore, a diagnostics for this condition could have major impact, given the potential for advice that would increase the quality of life through reducing discomforts.

7. Stratification of patients with respect to gut microbiota in clinical trials

It has recently been discovered that the gut microbiota plays a major role in the human metabolome (Nicholson et al 2005), and that the effects of drugs can be dependent on the gut microbiota (Clayton et al 2009). Combined with recent evidence that the human microbiome may consist of only three enterotypes (Arumugam et al 2011), diagnostics of such enterotypes is expected to provide important information with respect clinical trials. Enterotypes represent clusters of bacteria with a high frequency of co-occurrence, suggesting different states of the microbiota with different functionalities. There are several evidences for gut microbiota metabolism of important drugs, such as drugs against Alzheimer (Pieper et al., 2009)

Combined with the enterotype knowledge we believe that stratification will be a highly interesting field for gut microbiota diagnostics. This will be in line with the recent developments of personalized drugs –drugs adapted to individuals. Clearly, a major part of defining an individual would be the composition of gut microbiota. Information about the gut microbiota may therefore help to increase the success rate of clinical trials.

8. Manipulation of gut microbiota with pro- and prebiotics

The diet plays a major role in stratifying the gut microbiota (Muegge, 2011). This gives promise for food related gut microbiota perturbations. Manipulation of the gut microbiota through the diet is an old concept, either through probiotic live bacteria, or through prebiotic oligosaccharides.

Even though there is a range of products on the marked, there have been challenges in documenting the effect of these products. Diagnostic products that will help in substantiating the potential health claims would be of great benefit to the food industry. A main reason for the lack of documentation could actually be the lack of proper tools to describe the microbiota, rather than that the products have no effect.

Given proper documentation, the marked for pro- and prebiotics is very large. In particular, documentation that can be used in marketing would have a high commercial value. New diagnostic approaches could also potentially enable the discovery of new pro- and prebiotic products.

9. GA-map tecnology platform in gut microbiota diagnostics

The GA-map platform has given rise to a pipeline of assays for analysis of disease based on the microbiota composition. This platform includes a DNA purification module, a module for probe design, a patent protected approach for the actual gut microbiota screening, in addition to a diagnostic database. The GA-map assay will help to utilize information in the gut microbiota for diagnostic purposes.

An outline of the GA-map platform for gut microbiota diagnostics is illustrated in Figure 2. The platform can be used to assess health conditions of individuals based on the composition of the gut microbiota. In addition, it can serve both the the pharmaceutical industry and governmental health authorities in epidemiological population screenings and clinical trials. In addition, the technology can be used for early detection of undesirable conditions in the gut that can be corrected before the illnesses are manifested. The core aspects of the technology was developed and patented at the University of Oslo in 1998 (US patent # 6 617 138 Nucleic Acids Detection Methods). The technology has since then been refined at Nofima Mat (Matforsk). Currently the technology is patented worldwide and Genetic Analysis AS has been set up to commercialize the technology.

A high throughput analysis platform based on this technology will make it possible to gain greater understanding of the relationship between the composition of the gut microbiota and health, as well as being used as a diagnostic and prognostic tool in the future.

9.1 GA-map array

Probe labeling is based on the minisequencing principle, where a DNA polymerase extends the probe with a single labeled dideoxy nucleotide (Syvannen et al., 1990). In the GA-map assay several probes are labeled simultaneously, with the detection by reverse hybridization to the complementary strands spotted on to a solid phase (Vebo et al., 2011). This process is illustrated in Figure 3. The probes are constructed so that the probes hybridize adjacent to discriminative gene positions. If the target bacterium is present then a labeled dideoxynucleotide is incorporated by the polymerase. This is illustrated in Figure 3A. The solid phase (i.e. microarray or beads) is used to separate the probes by hybridization to their respective complementary sequences attached to the solid phase, which is illustrated in Figure 3B (exemplified by an array).

9.2 Probe design

There are several steps in the GA-map array process that can lead to wrong patterns if the probes are not properly designed. The probes may bind to the wrong target, and be labeled that way. Furthermore, the probes may be labeled by using itself as a target, or another probe as target. Finally, the probes may bind to the wrong spots on the array. Successful application of the GA-map assay requires therefore the application of a probe design software that takes into account many of the potentially unwanted reactions mentioned above, leading to false results.

The probe design is based on a novel way of bacterial classification based on 16S rRNA gene sequences. Rather than classifying bacteria by traditional phylogenetic tree-based approaches, the bacteria are classified in a coordinate system (Rudi et al., 2006). The benefit of this approach is both that very large numbers of bacteria can be analyzed, and that phylogroups are easily identified for probe design. This is illustrated in Figure 4.

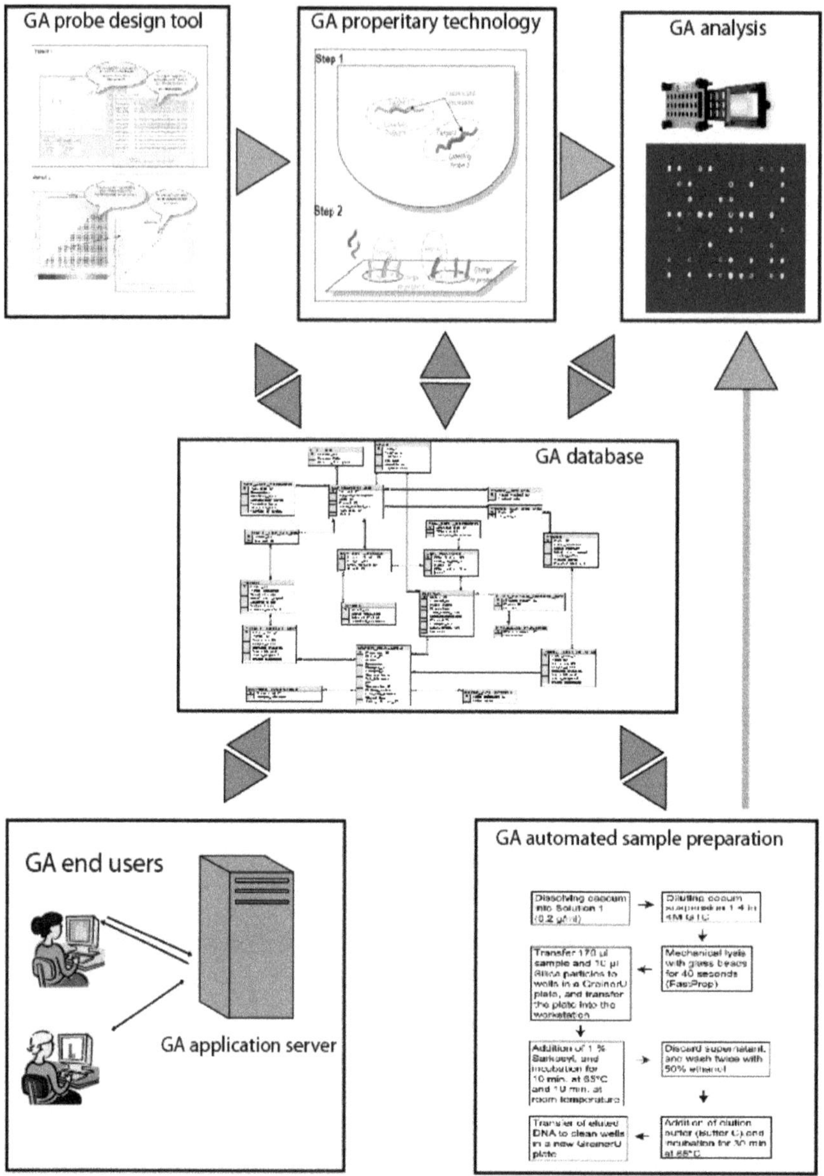

Fig. 2. GA pipeline. This figure illustrates the GA core technology and pipeline. Based on signatures in the 16S rRNA gene sequences GA probes are designed and evaluated *in silico* using the GA probe design tool. The GA analysis involves automated sample preparation combined with array hybridization . The whole information flow is stored in the GA database including the information about sample preparation and storage. The results to the end user are in the form of a direct description of the microbiota with respect to consequences for health and disease. Using this proprietary GA technology, a GA array is obtained, giving a specific "fingerprint" of each persons gut microbiota.

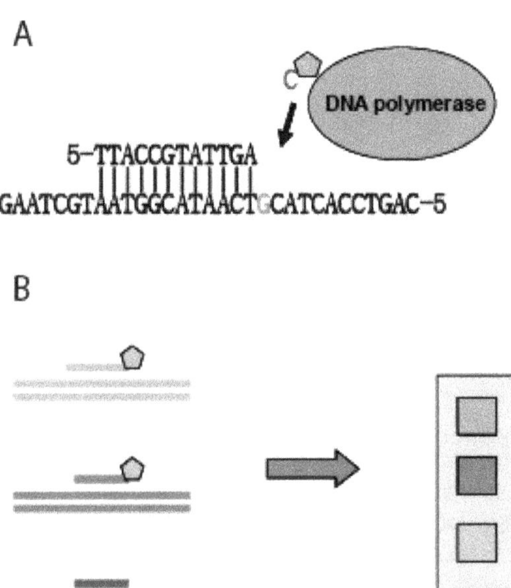

Fig. 3. Schematic outline of the GA map assay(A) Illustration of the SNuPE principle. An unlabelled probe hybridizes adjacent to a discriminative guanine on the complementary DNA strand. A DNA polymerase single-base extends the probe with a labeled cytosine dideoxy nucleotide. (B) Illustration of array hybridization of SNuPE labeled probes. Three probes are illustrated by green - , red – and blue bars. The green and the red probe are labeled. The probes are hybridized to their complementary sequences on an array as illustrated with the squares. The green and red probes will give a signal on the array due to the label, while the blue probe will not give a signal since it is not labeled.

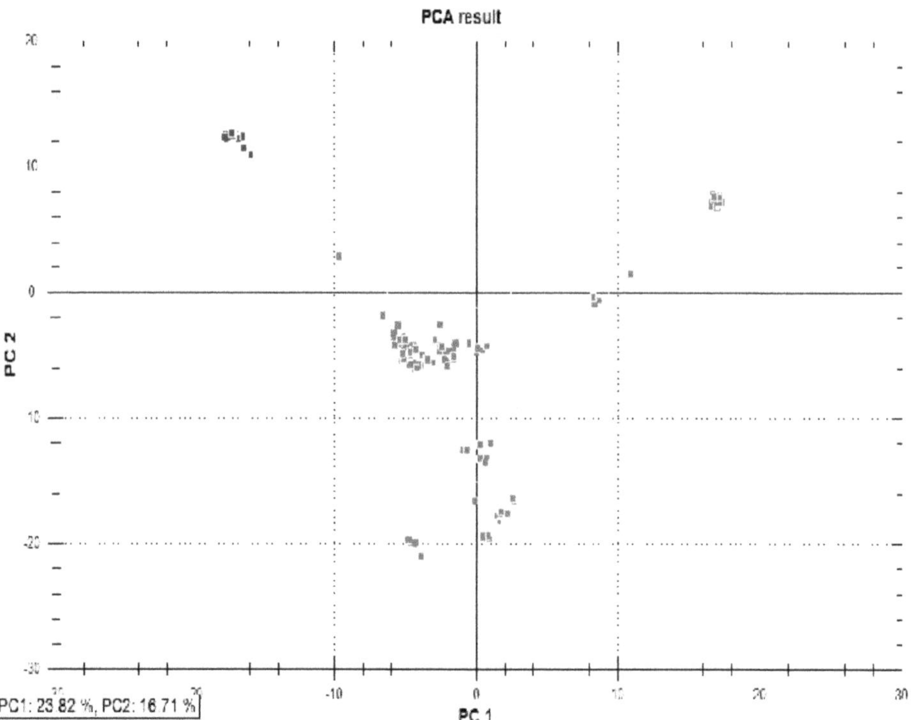

Fig. 4. Illustration of coordinate based classification of bacteria related to IBD. Each point in the plot represent a 16S rRNA gene sequence from a single bacterium. The distances between the points reflect the relatedness between the bacteria. For illustration, the points labeled green are target organisms for probe design, while those labeled red are non-target organisms.

After a set of probes have been constructed, the probes are evaluated with respect to if they will self-label (Figure 5A), whether they can cross-label (Figure 5B), or whether they will bind to a wrong spot on the array (Figure 6C). This bioinformatics evaluation is crucial for the successful construction of functional probe-set based on the GA-map technology (Vebo et al., 2011).

Validation of probes constructed with the probe design software have shown a high success rate (Vebo et al., 2011). Prior to the development of the software, probes were identified manually from multiple sequence alignments. The conclusion from the manual constructions, however, was that these probes did not perform satisfactory, and that there were too many considerations when performing this probe construction to make it possible to do manually.

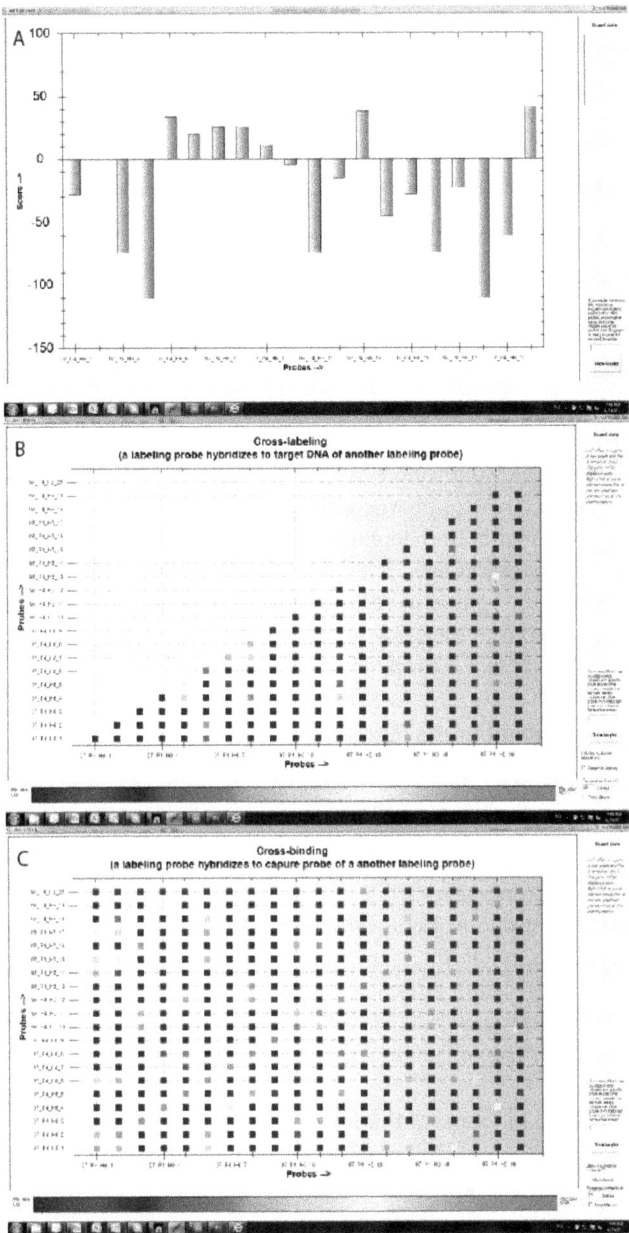

Fig. 5. Illustration of steps in probe evaluation. (A) The first step is to evaluate whether the probe will self label. A high value here indicates a high risk of self labeling. (B) The next step is to evaluate the potential of cross-labeling. A color code is used to illustrate the risk of cross-labeling. High values indicate high risk. (C) The final evaluation is whether the probe will bind to the right spot on the array. The red diagonal line indicates correct hybridization, while red squares outside the diagonal would indicate wrong hybridization.

9.3 Application of the GA-map array to describe the temporal development of the gut microbiota in infants

We have evaluated the recently developed GA-map infant microarray as a high throughput assay for screening of the gut microbiota. We analyzed 216 faecal samples collected from a cohort of 47 infants from 1 day until 2 years of age. To test the predictive ability of the assay we asked the question whether we could predict the age of the infants based on the microarray data.

The Prevention of Allergy Among Children in Trondheim (PACT) study is a large population based intervention study in Norway focused on childhood allergy (Oyen et al., 2006). The samples included here is a subset from the PACT study. Mechanical lysis was used for cell disruption, and an automated magnetic bead-based method was used for DNA purification. The approach is previously described by Skånseng et al. (2006)

We experienced that the primer pairs commonly used for amplification of the full-length 16S rRNA gene showed poor amplification of bifidobacteria. To circumvent this problem we developed a novel primer pair to obtain a near full-length 16S rRNA universal amplicon. The amplicon was evaluated both theoretically based on sequences in the RDP II database, and experimentally for bacterial species expected in the infant gut. We found that all the currently known infant gut bacteria were amplified with this new, optimized primer pair. A primer pair that is able to representably amplify the 16S rRNA gene from all the bacteria present in the sample is critical for proper analysis of the sample.

9.3.1 Temporal development of the infant gut microbiota

Based on signals from the GA-map array we determined the temporal development of the gut microbiota in the infants. These results are pressented in Figure 6.

The prevalence data showed that proteobacteria and lactobacilli reached a maximum between one month and one year, while the bacteroides subgroup containing B. fragilis reached a maximum after one to two years. Surprisingly, we found a high prevalence of bifidobacteria for infants older than one month. This is in contrast to another recent microarray screening of the infant gut microbiota, where they found that bifidobacteria were underrepressented (Palmer et al., 2007). This demsontrates the importance of using an optimal primer pair in the amplification of the 16S rRNA gene.

9.3.2 Modelling age as a function of the microbiota composition

We used the temporal information in the gut microbiota to determine if it is possible to describe age as a function of the composition. This was done using generalized additive models (GAM).

The following function was derived:

$$age = \quad s(E.coli) + s(Clostridium) + s(Staphylococcus) \\ + s(Bif.breve) + s(Bacteroides.dorei.vulg.theta.frag.)$$

The functions s to the data are shown in Figure 7.

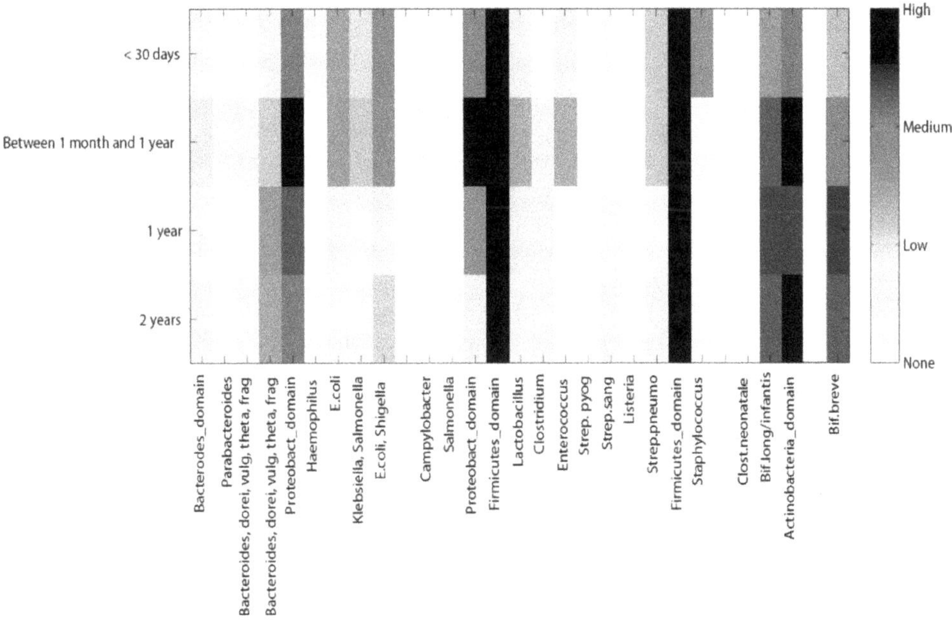

Fig. 6. The prevalence of the G-map bacteria was determined within age groups. The color code indicates the prevalence from absent (white) to present in all samples (black).

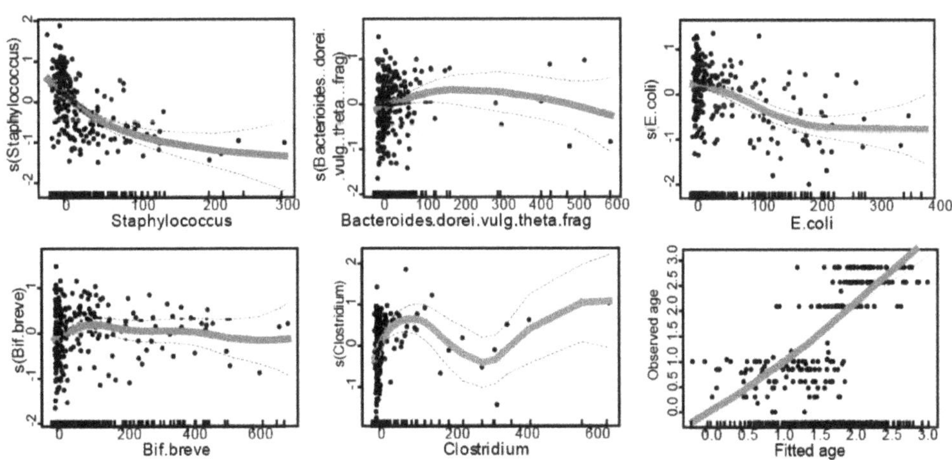

Fig. 7. Bacteria which are important for age prediction. For each bacterium the age contribution is a function of probe signal. Adding all the age contributions gives the predicted age (see function above). The final panel shows a regression between the observed and predicted ages for all the samples in our data.

High E. coli and staphylococci abundance predict an early age, while for the bacteroidetes and B. breve a medium abundance predicts a high age (Fig. 7 B and D). However, very high abundance predicts an early age. The Clostridium probe, on the other hand, shows a complex association with age.

Figure 7 shows that the age can be modelled with high accuracy from the microbiota composition.We found that the observed and modelled age gave a squared regression coefficient of 0.6. These results show that the development of the human gut microbiota is very structured with age, and that it can be predicted. The consequence is that it could potentially be possible to determine the normal development of the microbiota in infants, and use deviations from the normal pattern in identifying disorders. For instance, from our results we can conclude that high levels of staphylococcus for older children would clearly indicate some kind of deviation form the normal development, and indicate some kind of diseased state.

9.4 Application and development of the GA-map assay for diagnostic purposes

We are currently adapting the GA-map assay for detection of the human adult core microbiota, as defined by (Arumugam, et al., 2011). This will enable an assay for the normal gut microbiota, and in identifying the gut microbiota enterotypes. We foresee that, in addition to disease-specific diagnosis, such an assay could potentially be valuable for the pharmacutical industry in population stratification in clinical trials. This tool could also be used by the food industry to determine whether their pro- prebiotic products have an impact on the normal gut microbiota.

9.4.1 IBD

Diagnostic of IBD is an important target for the GA-map assay since there are established correlations between gut microbiota composition and disease. The intention with the assay would be early detection of IBD, and potentially in the following up of IBD treatments. Alternatively, it can be used to rule out IBD from IBS patients. In the future, given a causal relation between gut bacteria and IBD, knowledge about the microbial composition could be used in disease treatment. Preliminary data using a very limited probe-set illustrates that it should be possible to develop IBD diagnostics using the GA-map technology (Frøyland, 2010). The assay is currently being refined by the addition of more probes, and through validations on clinical material. Since we are using feces and not mucosal samples in our analysis we were surprised to obtain the relatively high specificity for CD.

9.4.2 NEC

The GA-map assay is also currently being evaluated for the analysis of NEC. NEC is a very severe disease where rapid and precise diagnostics are crucial. As for IDB there are already established correlations between gut microbiota and the disease. Furthermore, for this disease there are currently no good diagnostic approaches. Preliminary data show promise for separation NEC samples from that of controls. The aim is to further improve the assay and model in order to develop a prognostic assay for NEC development. Such a test would be of great help for pediatricians and neonatologists working with pre-term infants as a guide in treatment regimes.

	CD patients	Control patients
Diagnosed as CD	35	28
Diagnosed as non-CD	25	77
Total number of patients	60	105
	Sensitivity	Specificity
	58,3%	73,3%

Table 1. Single probe GA-map diagnostics of CD (Frøyland, 2010)

9.4.3 Test for assessing health condition of individuals

Many medical doctors find that an analysis of a patients gut microbiota is helpful in obtaining a more complete picture of the condition of the patient, and thus determining the disease state and best treatment. Several such tests exists in the marketplace. The GA-map technology is positioned to become a very powerful test for this purpose, with its complex probe selection and high through-put capabilities.

The general process for the application of the GA-map assay for diagnostic purposes is illustrated in Figure 8.

After implementation of the pilot diagnostic assays, new approaches and diseases will be implemented under the GA-map umbrella. There will also be a transformation over time towards decentralized analyses.

10. Future directions of gut microbiota diagnostics

There is currently a major focus on exploring the gut microbiota. This is mainly done through the application of explorative techniques such as next generation sequencing. The next phase will be the validation where the discoveries are validated using targeted techniques such as microarray analyses or quantitative PCR. The final phase will be to identify correlations between microbiota and disease that will give some added value

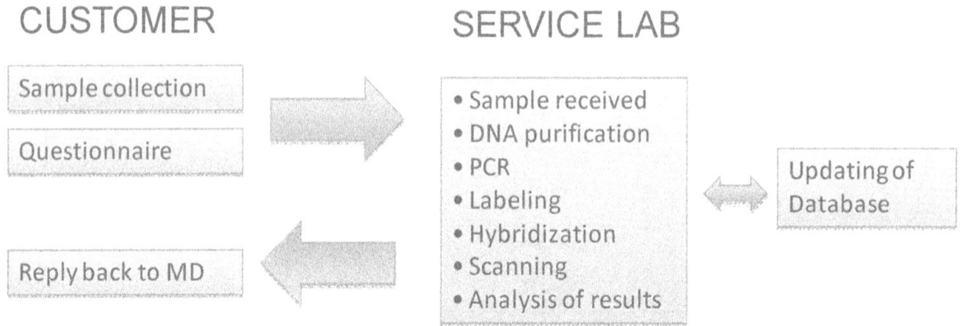

Fig. 8. Illustration of the GA-map diagnostic procedure. The GA-map assay will initially be offered through centralized service labs. A database covering relationships between profiles and disease will constantly be updated based on accumulated information, and a web-based interface with the customers will be available.

through diagnostics. This would open up for various applications of tests for profiling the gut microbiota in disease management.

As the importance of the gut microbiota on health becomes more established and recognized, profiling the composition of the gut microbiota will become an important diagnostic and prognostic tool in the future. This will give an additional window for health professionals to assess the conditions of the patient.

As technology advances and miniaturization and sophisticated Point-of-Care devises are being developed, such comprehensive tests will become easier to perform and more affordable. We see at least three areas where such a test would be applied in health care in the future:

1. **Disease specific diagnostics**

As discussed in this paper, certain health conditions are related to imbalance in the gut microbiota. A test that can correlate imbalances in the gut microbiota to specific health conditions will have a value as a diagnostic and prognostic tool. Furthermore, such tests could also act as a general help for physicians in determining the best treatment for patients.

2. **Personalized medicine**

Understanding how different bacteria in the gut influences the metabolism of drugs and foodstuff, leads to a more personalized, tailor-made drug treatment regime. Since it is generally recognized that the composition of the gut microbiota has a profound effect on health as well as how foodstuff and drugs are metabolized, a profiling of the gut microbiota would constitute an important aspect of the personalized medicine approach. It is expected that personal medicine would lead to more effective treatments, as well as cost-saving on healthcare budget due to optimizing the drug treatment for each person.

3. **Deviations from each individuals normal flora**

The search for a common core gut microbiota has revealed that each individual has a unique and fairly stable microbiota, at least in adults. Therefore, each individual's own microbiota may be the best control for that person. This calls for routine checks where deviations from its own "normal" core microbiota will be evaluated. Such a test would also include other genetic and physical markers, which combined would give a status of the individual's health condition.

With future technical development we believe the next generation gut microbiota diagnostic will integrate phylogeny and functionality of the gut microbiota. A functionality that is particularly relevant is antibiotic resistance. There is currently a major fear for the development of multi-resistant pathogens, and that the current treatment regimes with broad-spectrum antibiotics will eradicate beneficial bacteria. In this regard targeted narrow spectrum antibiotics could be the solution. Narrow-spectrum antibiotics, however, would require better diagnostics of the actual disease causing organisms. Therefore, a profiling of the gut microbiota may be essential prior to administration of such narrow antibiotics to ensure optimal treatment.

Another aim in treatment of gut microbiota disorders is to restore the diseased gut microbiota towards the healthy state. This could be done either through tailor-made administration of probiotics, prebiotics and antibiotics, or a combination of these substances. Another approach would be to transplant the gut microbiota from close relatives or samples from the same individual collected before disease occurs. Such an approach would resemble what is currently done for treatment of *Clostridium difficile* infections where the gut microbiota is transplanted from relatives.

11. Conclusions

As more data are being generated, the importance of the gut microbiota on health will become more recognized. The advancement in characterizing the composition of the gut microbiota in humans paves the way for new and better health treatments. The techniques used for exploring the gut microbiota and characterizing the functions of the microbiota, may not necessarily be the same techniques used to diagnose and monitor treatment of gut health related diseases. The GA-map assay is a promising tool for the development of gut microbiota diagnostics in routine applications. Such assays has the potential to be set up as a high through-put service, and can also be incorporated into smaller Point-of-Care devices, opening up new, exciting applications to health management. A comprehensive and rapid characterization of the gut microbiota will be part of the tool-box physicians will use in the future to improve diagnosis and treatments of patients.

12. Acknowledgments

The work was supported by Genetic Analysis and the Norwegian Research council through the grant 192940. We would like to thank all the employees at Genetic Analysis, and our collaborators that have contributed in the detailed experimental setups.

13. References

Arumugam M, Raes J, Pelletier E, Le Paslier D, Yamada T, Mende DR *et al* (2011). Enterotypes of the human gut microbiome. *Nature* advance online publication.

Clayton TA, Baker D, Lindon JC, Everett JR, Nicholson JK (2009). Pharmacometabonomic identification of a significant host-microbiome metabolic interaction affecting human drug metabolism. *Proceedings of the National Academy of Sciences* 106: 14728-14733.

Cox MJ, Huang YJ, Fujimura KE, Liu JT, McKean M, Boushey HA *et al* (2010). *Lactobacillus casei* Abundance Is Associated with Profound Shifts in the Infant Gut Microbiome. *PLoS ONE* 5: e8745.

Eggesbo M, Moen B, Peddada S, Baird D, Rugtveit J, Midtvedt T *et al* (2011). Development of gut microbiota in infants not exposed to medical interventions. *APMIS* 119: 17-35.

Frank DN, St. Amand AL, Feldman RA, Boedeker EC, Harpaz N, Pace NR (2007). Molecular-phylogenetic characterization of microbial community imbalances in human inflammatory bowel diseases. *Proceedings of the National Academy of Sciences* 104: 13780-13785.

Frøyland C (2010), Diagnostics of Inflammatory Bowel Disease using Fecal Microbiota Master Thesis, Høgskolen i Hedemark, Norway

Heijtz, R.D., Wang, S., Anuar, F., Qian, Y., Bjorkholm, B., Samuelsson, A., Hibberd, M.L., Forssberg, H. and Pettersson, S. (2011) Normal gut microbiota modulates brain development and behavior. Proceedings of the National Academy of Sciences of the United States of America 108, 3047-3052.

Kunin V, Engelbrektson A, Ochman H, Hugenholtz P (2010). Wrinkles in the rare biosphere: pyrosequencing errors can lead to artificial inflation of diversity estimates. *Environmental microbiology* 12: 118-123.

Maes M, Yirmiya R, Noraberg J, Brene S, Hibbeln J, Perini G *et al* (2009). The inflammatory & neurodegenerative (I&ND) hypothesis of depression: leads for future research and new drug developments in depression. *Metabolic Brain Disease* 24: 27-53.

Ley, R.E., Turnbaugh, P.J., Klein, S. and Gordon, J.I. (2006) Microbial ecology: human gut microbes associated with obesity. Nature 444, 1022-1023.

Maxion-Bergemann, S., Thielecke, F., Abel, F. & Bergemann, R (2006). Costs of irritable bowel syndrome in the UK and US. Pharmacoeconomics 24(1), 21-37

Muegge, B.D., Kuczynski, J., Knights, D., Clemente, J.C., González, A., Fontana, L., Henrissat, B., Knight, R. and Gordon, J.I. (2011) Diet Drives Convergence in Gut

Microbiome Functions Across Mammalian Phylogeny and Within Humans. Science (New York, NY 332, 970-974..

Nell S, Suerbaum S, Josenhans C (2010). The impact of the microbiota on the pathogenesis of IBD: lessons from mouse infection models. *Nat Rev Micro* 8: 564-577.

Nicholson JK, Holmes E, Wilson ID (2005). Gut microorganisms, mammalian metabolism and personalized health care. *Nature reviews* 3: 431-438.

Oien, T., Storro, O. and Johnsen, R. (2006) Intestinal microbiota and its effect on the immune system--a nested case-cohort study on prevention of atopy among small children in Trondheim: the IMPACT study. Contemporary clinical trials 27, 389-395.

Palmer, C., Bik, E.M., DiGiulio, D.B., Relman, D.A. and Brown, P.O. (2007) Development of the Human Infant Intestinal Microbiota. PLoS Biology 5, e177

Pieper, I.A. and Bertau, M. (2010) Predictive tools for the evaluation of microbial effects on drugs during gastrointestinal passage. *Expert Opinion on Drug Metabolism & Toxicology* 6, 747-760.

Rajilic-Stojanovic M, Heilig HG, Molenaar D, Kajander K, Surakka A, Smidt H *et al* (2009). Development and application of the human intestinal tract chip, a phylogenetic microarray: analysis of universally conserved phylotypes in the abundant microbiota of young and elderly adults. *Environmental microbiology.*

Rudi, K., Zimonja, M. and Naes, T. (2006) Alignment-independent bilinear multivariate modelling (AIBIMM) for global analyses of 16S rRNA gene phylogeny. *International journal of systematic and evolutionary microbiology* 56, 1565-1575

Salonen A, de Vos WM, Palva A (2010). Gastrointestinal microbiota in irritable bowel syndrome: present state and perspectives. *Microbiology (Reading, England)* 156: 3205-3215.

Sekelja, M., Berget, I., Naes, T. and Rudi, K. (2011) Unveiling an abundant core microbiota in the human adult colon by a phylogroup-independent searching approach. *Isme Journal* 5, 519-531.

Skanseng, B., Kaldhusdal, M. and Rudi, K. (2006) Comparison of chicken gut colonisation by the pathogens Campylobacter jejuni and Clostridium perfringens by real-time quantitative PCR. Mol Cell Probes.

Syvanen AC, Aalto-Setala K, Harju L, Kontula K, Soderlund H (1990). A primer-guided nucleotide incorporation assay in the genotyping of apolipoprotein E. *Genomics* 8: 684-692.

Turnbaugh, P.J., Hamady, M., Yatsunenko, T., Cantarel, B.L., Duncan, A., Ley, R.E., Sogin, M.L., Jones, W.J., Roe, B.A., Affourtit, J.P., Egholm, M., Henrissat, B., Heath, A.C., Knight, R. and Gordon, J.I. (2009) A core gut microbiome in obese and lean twins. *Nature* 457, 480-484. A potential challenge would therefore be to use pylogenetic markers to predict functions in the gut microbiota.

Vebo, H.C., Sekelja, M., Nestestog, R., Storro, O., Johnsen, R., Oien, T. and Rudi, K. (2011) Temporal development of the infant gut microbiota in IgE sensitized and non-sensitized children determined by the GA-map infant array. Clin Vaccine Immunol..

Wang Y, Hoenig JD, Malin KJ, Qamar S, Petrof EO, Sun J *et al* (2009). 16S rRNA gene-based analysis of fecal microbiota from preterm infants with and without necrotizing enterocolitis. *Isme J* 3: 944-954.

Wang, Z., Klipfell, E., Bennett, B.J., Koeth, R., Levison, B.S., DuGar, B., *et al.* (2011) Gut flora metabolism of phosphatidylcholine promotes cardiovascular disease. Nature 472, 57-63.

Wen, L., Ley, R.E., Volchkov, P.Y., Stranges, P.B., Avanesyan, L., Stonebraker, A.C., Hu, C., Wong, F.S., Szot, G.L., Bluestone, J.A., Gordon, J.I. and Chervonsky, A.V. (2008) Innate immunity and intestinal microbiota in the development of Type 1 diabetes. Nature.

6

Delivery of Probiotic Microorganisms into Gastrointestinal Tract by Food Products

Amir Mohammad Mortazavian[1],
Reza Mohammadi[2] and Sara Sohrabvandi[1]
*[1]Department of Food Science and Technology,
National Nutrition and Food Technology Research Institute,
Faculty of Nutrition Sciences and Food Technology,
Shahid Beheshti University of Medical Sciences, Tehran
[2]Students Research Committee, Department of Food Science and Technology,
National Nutrition and Food Technology Research Institute,
Faculty of Nutrition Sciences and Food Technology,
Shahid Beheshti University of Medical Sciences, Tehran
Iran*

1. Introduction

The health of gastrointestinal tract affects by numerous factors and probiotics are of the most important. There are two main ways to increase the population of viable probiotic bacteria within the human body: 1) adequate daily nutrition as well as avoiding factors and stresses lead to decrease in probiotics *in vivo* viable population, and 2) ingestion of high viable population of probiotics. The common, widespread and popular method to ingest high viable population of probiotics is via food products consumption. Probiotic food products are regarded as an important group of 'functional foods'.

Today, there is a strong increase in the consumption of probiotic bacteria using food products, mainly probiotic dairy products. Also, recently, many probiotic non-dairy products have been developed. Therefore, the manufacture of dairy- and nondairy products containing probiotic bacteria is an important issue with industrial and commercial consequences and many products of this kind are available in the world market.

Viability of probiotic bacteria (the number of viable and active cells per g or mL of probiotic food products at the time of consumption) is the most critical value for these products because it determines their healthful efficiency. Therefore, it is important to ensure a high survival rate of the probiotic bacteria during production as well as during the storage time. Many complicated and inter-related factors influence the viability of probiotic microorganisms in each food product during production and storage. Apart from the viability of probiotics in products until the time of consumption, their survival in food matrices after exposure to gastrointestinal tract (GIT) conditions is crucial. They must arrive viable and active to different parts of intestine, adhere and colonize. Some factors affect viability of probiotics during delivery into the intestine while they are enclosed in food matrices. In this chapter, the concept of ingestion and delivery of probiotic microorganisms via food products are discussed.

2. Probiotic food products

Probiotic microorganisms are available in three different types for direct or indirect human consumption: 1) culture concentrate to be added to a food (dried or deep-freeze form) for industrial or home uses, 2) food products (fermented or non-fermented), and 3) dietary supplements (drug products in powder, capsule or tablet forms) (Tannis, 2008). Consumption of probiotic cells via food products are the most popular and widespread way.

Worldwide, the demand for consumption of functional foods is growing rapidly due to the increased awareness of the consumers from the impact of food on health. For example, in the year 2000, the world-wide market of functional foods generated US$ 33 billion, in 2005, this total was US$ 73.5 billion, and was US$ 167 billion in 2010 (Granato et al., 2010). Functional foods are those that contain chemical/microbial components that may affect beneficially one or more target functions in the body, beyond adequate nutritional effects, in a way that is relevant to either the state of well-being and health or the reduction of the risk of a disease (Diplock et al., 1999). Probiotic food products are classified in the category of functional foods and represent a significant part of this market that probiotic foods comprise between 60 and 70% of the total functional food market (Holzapfel, 2006).

During the past three decades, significant attention has been paid to dairy products containing probiotic bacteria such as fermented milks, ice cream, various types of cheese, baby-food, milk powder, frozen dairy desserts, whey-based beverages, sour cream, butter milk, normal and flavored liquid milk, and concentrated milk. Also, recently, many non-dairy products such as vegetarian-based products, cereal-based products, fruit juice, soya-based products, oat-based desserts, confectionary products, breakfast cereals and baby foods) and baby foods have been developed. Causes for this ongoing trend are demands provide by vegetarianism, high prevalence of lactose intolerance in many populations around the world, and providing variety and development in probiotic food products (Granato et al., 2010; Mortazavian et al., 2011). Dairy products have the largest probiotic food market share. Today, a total of 78% of current probiotic sales in the world are delivered through yogurt (Cargill, 2009). Therefore, still, the manufacture of dairy products containing probiotic bacteria is an important issue with industrial and commercial consequences. Table 1 represents some types of probiotic products available in the world market (dairy and nondairy products). Figure 1 indicates qualitative aspects of probiotic food products.

3. Probiotic microorganisms used in food products

It is clear that the right selection and application of a probiotic strains in food materials exhibits fundamental impacts on qualitative aspects of final products, namely safety (related to the mentioned strains), health benefits (related to probiotics), sensory attributes and even, the price. Therefore, selecting the adequate probiotic strains is the first prerequisite for designing a specific probiotic food product. The incorporation of incorrectly identified probiotic bacteria in functional food products clearly has public health implications, by undermining the efficiency of probiotics and by affecting public confidence in functional foods (Huys et al., 2006). Thus, the use of adequate tools to provide proper strain identification for legal and good manufacturing practices and to track probiotics during food production as well as during their intestinal transit are strictly necessary (Lee and Salminen, 2009).

Dairy products	Reference	Non dairy products	Reference
Regular full-fat yogurts	Aryana and Mcgrew (2007)	Vegetable-based drinks	Lambo et al. (2005)
Iranian yogurt drink (Doogh)	Mortazavian et al. 2008	Fermented banana	Tsen et al. (2009)
Acidophilus milk drink	Itsaranuwat et al. (2003)	Tomato-based drink	Yoon et al. (2004)
Stirred fruit yogurts	Kailasapathy et al. (2008)	Many dried fruits	Betoret et al. (2003)
Dairy fermented beverage	Shobharani and Agrawal (2009)	Green coconut water	Prado et al. (2008a)
Whey-protein-based drinks	Dalev et al. (2006)	Peanut milk	Mustafa et al. (2009)
Synbiotic acidophilus milk	Amiri et al. (2008)	Cranberry, pineapple, and orange juices	Sheehan et al. (2007)
Cheddar cheese	Ong and Shah (2009)	Ginger juice	Chen et al. (2008)
Feta cheese	Kailasapathy and Masondole (2005)	Grape and passion fruit juices	Saarela et al. (2006)
Cheese from caprine mil	Kalavrouzioti et al. (2005)	Cabbage juice	Yoon et al. (2006)
Semi-hard reduced-fat cheese	Thage et al. (2005)	Carrot juice	Nazzaro et al. (2008)
White-brined cheese	Yilmaztekin et al. (2004)	Noni juice	Wang et al. (2009)
Minas Fresco cheese	Souza and Saad (2009)	Onion	Roberts and Kidd (2005)
Cottage cheese	Blanchette et al. (1996)	Nonfermented fruit juice beverages	Renuka et al. (2009)
Canestrato Pugliese hard cheese	Corbo et al. (2001)	Nonfermented soy-based frozen desserts	Heenan et al. (2005)
Argentine Fresco cheese	Vinderola et al. (2000b)	Fermented soymilk drink	Donkor et al. (2007)
Goat semi-solid cheese	Gomes and Malcata (1999)	Soy-based stirred yogurt	Saris et al. (2003)
Manufacture of Turkish Beyaz cheese	Kilic et al. (2009)	Rice-based yogurt	Helland et al. (2005)
Iranian White-brined cheese	Ghoddusi and Robinson (1996)	Oat-based drink	Angelov et al. (2006)
White-brined cheese	özer et al. (2008)	Oat-based products	Martensson et al. (2002)
Minas fresh cheese	Souza and Saad (2008)	Oat-bran pudding	Blandino et al. (2003)
Synbiotic ice cream	Homayouni et al. (2008)	Fermented maize beverage	McMaste et al. (2005)
Fermented goat's milk	Mart´ın-Diana et al. (2003)	Wheat fermented probiotic beverages	Blandino et al. (2003)
Probiotic ice cream	Kailasapathy and Sultana (2003)	Malt-based drink	Kedia et al. (2007)
Low-fat ice cream	Haynes and Playne (2002) Akalin and Erisir (2008)	Millet or sorghum flour fermented probiotic beverage	Muianja et al (2003)

Dairy products	Reference	Non dairy products	Reference
Mango soy fortified probiotic yogurt	Kaur et al (2009)	Starch-saccharified probiotic drink	Oi and KIitabatake (2003)
Frozen yogurt	Davidson et al. (2000)	Meat products	Rouhi et al. (2010)
Frozen synbiotic dessert		Tempeh (base on soybean)	Feng et al. (2005)
Acidophilus butter	Gomes and Malcata (1999)	Chocolate	Possemiers et al. (2010)
Traditional Greek yogurt	Maragkoudakisa et al. (2006)		
Frozen dairy dessert	Shah and Ravula (2000)		
Corn milk yogurt	Supavititpatana et al. (2008)		
High pressure-homogenized probiotic fermented milk	Patrignani et al. (2009)		
Banana-based yogurt	Sousa et al. (2007)		
Mango soy fortified probiotic yogurt	Kaur et al. (2009)		
Yog-ice cream	El-Nagar et al. (2002)		

Table 1. Some types of probiotic products available in the world market (dairy and non dairy products)

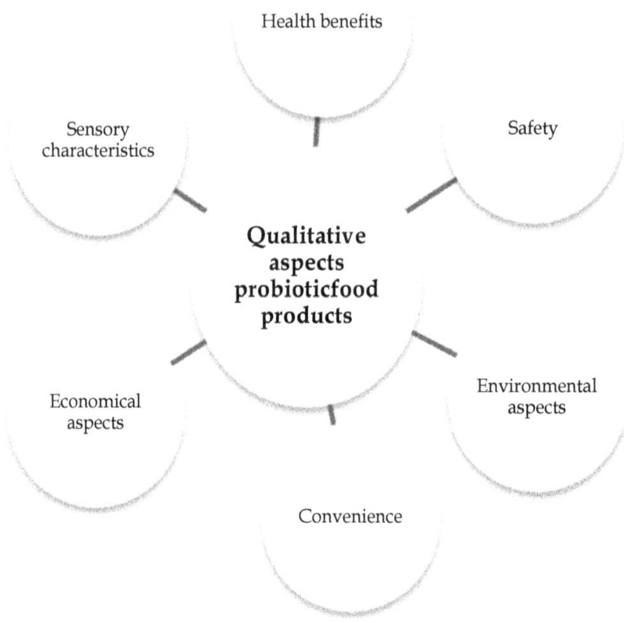

Fig. 1. Qualitative aspects of probiotic food products.

Many of the bacteria used in probiotic preparations (bifidobacteria and lactic acid bacteria) have been isolated from human fecal samples to maximize the likelihood of compatibility with the human gut microflora and improve their chances of survival (Andersson et al., 2001). Microorganisms isolated from fermented nondairy foods have shown these abilities in *in vitro* studies (Rivera-Espinoza and Gallardo-Navarro, 2010). Probiotic organisms are predominantly bacteria selected from the genera *Lactobacillus* and *Bifidobacterium*, which are normal constituents of the human intestinal microbiota. However, species belonging to the genera *Lactococcus, Enterococcus, Saccharomyces* and *Propionibacterium* are also considered as probiotic due to their health-promoting effects (Blandino et al., 2003; Rivera-Espinoza and Gallardo-Navarro, 2010; Sanders and Huis Veld, 1999; Vinderola and Reinheimer, 2003). A primary reason for this is that both these genera are dominant inhabitants of their respective niches in the intestine (*Lactobacillus* in the small intestine and *Bifidobacterium* in the large intestine) and both have a long history of safe use and are considered as GRAS (generally regarded as safe). Of the lactobacilli, *L. acidophilus* is by far the most widely used probiotic as it has a long history of research and use. As *L. acidophilus* is one of the predominant organisms in the intestinal tract of breast-fed babies, it quickly took the place of *L. bulgaricus* as the probiotic of choice in the U.S. (O'Sullivan 2006). It, therefore, has almost 100 years of use in human diets. Of the bifidobacteria, *B. longum* is particularly dominant in human intestines (Perdigon et al., 2003), It is a highly recommend *Bifidobacterium* species in commercial human probiotics (Sanders, 2006). *Bifidobacterium lactis* (*Bifidobacterium animalis* ssp. *lactis*) is a very commonly used probiotic, although it is not a normal human inhabitant. It was first isolated in 1997 from fermented milk by Meile et al. (1997) and was noted to have a higher tolerance to oxygen and other detrimental environmental conditions (generally, higher adaptation to food conditions) than other bifidobacteria (Cai et al., 2000; Ventura and Zink, 2002). The changes that occurred in *B. lactis* during its adaptation to fermentation conditions make it a very resilient strain that can remain viable during processing and storage longer than other bifidobacteria. Mentioned practical reasons contribute to its popularity. These adaptations, however, would not give it a competitive edge in the intestine as the most competitive strains lose unwanted traits in a natural environment. Although this would limit the full potential of *B. lactis*, it still has the potential for many positives during its transient passage through the intestine (O'Sullivan, 2006).

While emphasizing the importance of strain-specificity of technological attributes of probiotics, some generalizations can still be made on the robustness of probiotic organisms. Generally, lactobacilli are more robust than bifidobacteria (Erkkilä et al., 2001; Mättö et al., 2006; Ross et al., 2005). There is a wider range of probiotic *Lactobacillus* species that are technologically suitable for food applications than bifidobacteria (Lee and Salminen, 2009). They are resistant to low pH, have native association with traditional fermented foods, and have adaptation to milk and other food substrates.

A significant proportion of the commercialized probiotic bacterial species was originally selected on the basis of their technological stability (e.g., viability during food processing and storage), survival during intestinal transit, and health benefits on consumers. Good probiotic strains have demonstrated health and safety data from randomized, controlled clinical trials (Lee and Salminen, 2009; Ventura and Perozzi, 2011).

4. Viability of probiotics in food products

Improving the viability of probiotic bacteria in different food products (especially fermented products) until the time of consumption has been the subject of hundreds of studies. Viability of probiotic microorganisms, namely, the number of viable and active cells per g or mL of probiotic food products at the moment of consumption is the most critical value of these products, because determines their medicinal efficacy (Khorbekandi et al., 2011; Tamime et al., 2005). Therefore, in order to maintain consumer confidence in probiotic products, it is important to ensure a high survival rate of the bacteria during the production of product as well as over the product shelf life (Saxelin et al., 1999). Although there is no world-wide agreement on the minimum of viable probiotic cells per gram or milliliter of probiotic product, generally, the concentrations of 10^6 and 10^7-10^8 cfu mL^{-1} (cfu g^{-1}), respectively, have been accepted as the minimum and satisfactory levels. It has also stated that probiotic products should be consumed regularly with an approximate amount of 100 g d^{-1} in order to deliver about 10^9 viable cells into the intestine (Karimi et al., 2011; Mohammadi et al., 2011; Vinderola et al., 2000a).

In order to have a positive effect in the intestinal tract some specific requirements regarding food products should be fulfilled. First, probiotics need to resist the manufacturing process; second, they should remain viable during the storage period in the commercial products until the end of the shelf-life. Many factors influence the viability of probiotic microorganisms in food products during production and storage periods. The main mentioned factors are: pH, titrable acidity, molecular oxygen, redox potential, hydrogen peroxide, bacteriocins, short chain fatty acids, flavoring agents, microbial competitions, packaging materials and packaging conditions, rate and proportion of inoculation, step-wise/stage-wise fermentation, micro-encapsulation, milk solid non-fat content, supplementation of milk with nutrients, heat treatment of milk, incubation temperature, storage temperature, carbonation, addition of salt, sugar and sweeteners, cooling rate of the product and scale of production. Figure 2 implies main factors affecting viability of probiotics in food products. These factors are discussed below:

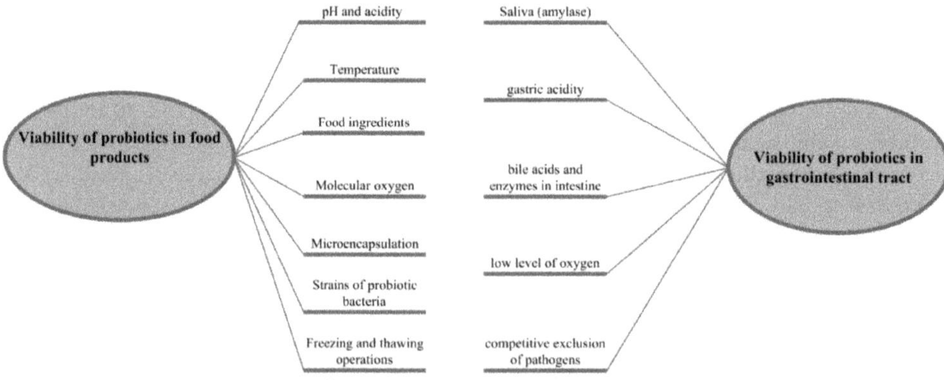

Fig. 2. Main factors affecting the viability of probiotic food products and during delivery through gastrointestinal tract.

4.1 Strains of probiotic bacteria

Care must be taken in selecting the most appropriate strain for a particular food application. Indeed, the first step in incorporating a probiotic into a food is identifying compatibilities between the attributes of the selected strains and the food production steps, food matrix and storage conditions. Selection of probiotic strains used in food products should be according to both the criteria of compatibility with and resistance to the product and *in vivo* conditions in order to increase the viability of the probiotic bacterial strains (Korbekandi et al., 2011). The tolerance of probiotics both to the product and to the internal conditions of the living consumer is strain-dependent (strain-specific). Suitable probiotic strains are those enable to maintain their survival and stability during commercial production of products as well as during the storage period (Godward et al., 2000; Talwalker and Kailasapathy, 2004). Furthermore, high viable survival rate during delivery through the gastrointestinal tract is necessary to allow enough live cell arrival to the human intestine. Therefore, selection of resistant probiotic strains against production, storage and gastrointestinal tract condition is of prime importance. Researchers have indicated that the survival of bacteria against harsh conditions in food products such as pH, titrable acidity, oxygen toxicity, freezing and low temperatures and storage temperatures are species- and strain-specific (Godward et al., 2000; Kailasapathy and Sultana, 2003; Ravula and Shah, 1998; Takahashi et al., 2007; Tamim et al., 2005).

Selected probiotic strains should also results in adequate sensory characteristics of final product. Some studies have shown that flavor is the first indicator with respect to the choice of a food, followed by considerations with respect to health (Mohammadi and mortazavian, 2011; Tuorila and Cardello, 2002). Consumers are not interested in consuming a functional food if the added ingredients confer disagreeable flavors on the product, even if this results in advantages with respect to their health. Therefore, a pleasant aroma and taste profiles are of importance in the formulation of probiotic functional foods and is strain-dependent. The metabolism of the probiotic cultures can result in the production of components that may contribute negatively to the taste and aroma of the product, such as acetic acid produced by *Bifidobacterium* spp. during fermentation and over storage period. Figure 3 shows main criteria for selection of probiotic strains in food products.

4.2 pH and titrable acidity

pH and titrable acidity of probiotic products considerably affect cell survival of probiotic microorganisms (Mortazavian et al., 2010). Low pH is of the most important factor that restricts the growth and stability of probiotic bacteria in fermented products. Hydrogen ions damage probiotic cells via disrupting mass transfer through the cell membranes and acidic starvation of the cells (Mortazavianand and Sohrabvandi, 2006). Very low pH ranges in fermented milks might cause an increase in the concentration of undissociated organic acids in them and, as a result, enhances the bacteriocidal effect of these acids. The aforementioned effect of organic acids arises from their lipophilic nature. They can be transferred through the microbial cells and dissociate within them, changing the intracellular pH. Also, organic acids might bind to various intracellular compounds. Both of these phenomena disturb cell metabolism (Korbekandi et al., 2011).

The optimum pH for growth of *Lactobacillus acidophilus* is 5.5-6.0, but for bifidobacteria this range is 6.0 –7.0 (De Vuyst, 2000). In food products, lactobacilli are able to grow and survive

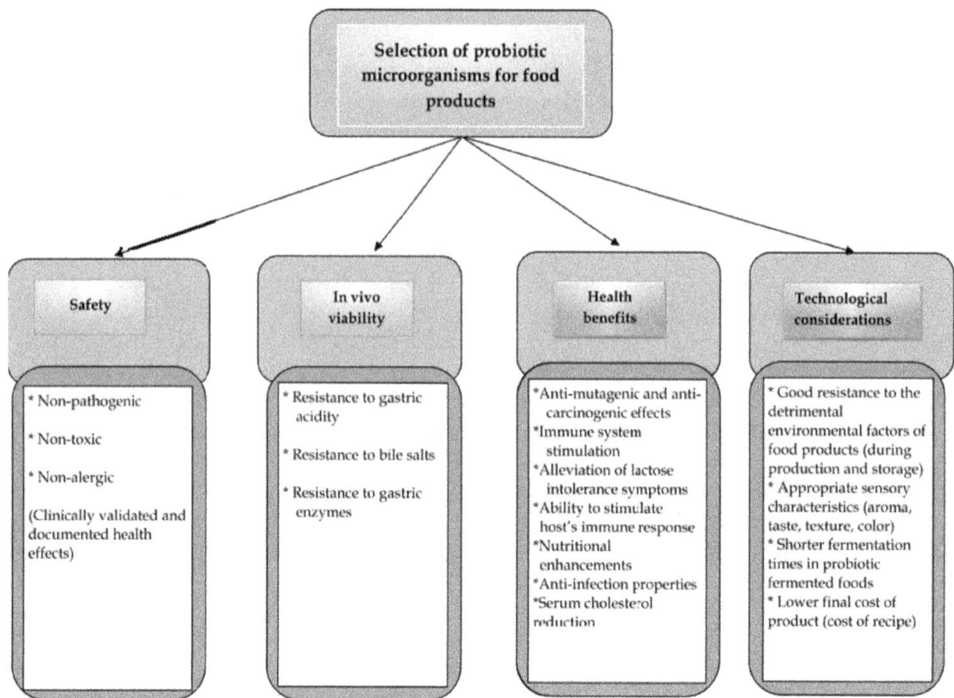

Fig. 3. Main criteria for selection of probiotic strains in food products.

in fermented milks and yogurts with pH values between 3.7 and 4.3 (Boylston, 2004). Bifidobacteria tend to be less acid tolerant, with most species surviving poorly in fermented products at pH levels below 4.6 (Boylston, 2004; Lee and Salminen, 2009; Ross et al., 2005). The tolerance of *Bifidobacterium* spp. to acidic conditions is strain-specific. The best survivability of bifidobacteria have been observed in *B. longum* in the presence of acidic conditions and bile salts, and for *B. lactis* (*B. animalis* ssp. *lactis*) in fermented milks conditions (korbekandi et al., 201; Tamim et al., 2005).

Survival in low pH beverages such as fruit juices (pH 3.5-4.5) possesses a significant challenge to probiotic survival. Researchers have reported that cell viability depends of the strains used, the characteristics of the substrate, the oxygen content and the final acidity and the concentration of lactic acid and acetic acid of the product (Shah, 2001). According to Sheehan et al., (2007), when adding *Lactobacillus* and *Bifidobacterium* orange, pineapple and cranberry juice, extensive differences regarding their acid resistance were observed. All of the strains screened survived for longer in orange and pineapple juice compared to cranberry. *L. casei*, *L. rhamnosus* and *L. paracasei* display a great robustness surviving at levels above 7.0 log cfu/ml in orange juice and above 6.0 log cfu ml[-1] in pineapple juice for at least 12 weeks (Rivera-Espinoza and Gallardo-Navarro, 2010).

4.3 Molecular oxygen

Lactobacilli are aerotolerant or anaerobic, and strictly fermentative, while bifidobacteria are strictly anaerobic and saccharoclastic (Holzapfel et al., 2001; De Vuyst, 2000). Therefore, molecular oxygen is detrimental to probiotic growth and survival. However, the degree of oxygen sensitivity varies considerably between different species and strains (Kawasaki et al., 2006). In general, lactobacilli, which are mostly microaerophilic, are more tolerant of oxygen than bifidobacteria, to the point where oxygen levels are rarely an important consideration in maintaining the survival of lactobacilli (Lee and Salminen, 2009). Oxygen content and redox potential have been shown to be important factors for the viability of bifidobacteria especially during the storage period. Oxygen affects probiotic cultures in three ways. Firstly, it is directly toxic to some cells; secondly, in the presence of oxygen, certain cultures, especially *L. delbrueckii* ssp. *bulgaricus* produces peroxide (especially in dairy products), which is toxic to probiotic cells particularly *L. acidophilus*; and thirdly, free radicals produced from the oxidation of components (e.g., fats) are toxic to probiotic cells (Korbekandi et al., 2011; Tamim et al., 2005).

Several methods have been used to decrease oxygen content. The most important ones are accomplishing fermentation under vacuum (for fermented products), using vacuum packaging, using packaging materials with low permeability to oxygen, adding antioxidants and oxygen scavengers to milk (such as ascorbic acid), and controlling the production process in such a way that minimum dissolved oxygen entered into product (Dave and Shah 1997; Korbekandi et al 2011; Shah, 2000; Talwalkar and Kailasapathy, 2003; Talwalkar et al., 2004).

4.4 Food ingredients

The compatibility of probiotics with other ingredients within food formulations can have a significant impact on bacterial survival. Interactions between probiotics and other ingredients can be protective, neutral, or detrimental to probiotic stability (Lee and Salminen, 2009; Mattila-Sandholm et al., 2002). The main affective food ingredients are mentioned as follows:

4.4.1 Food additives

Food additives used in the food industry could significantly affect the growth and viability of probiotic bacteria (e.g. *L. acidophilus*, *L. casei*, *L. paracasei*, *L. rhamnosus* and bifidobacteria) and starter cultures (e.g. *S. thermophilus*, *L. delbrueckii* ssp. *Bulgaricus*, *Lactococcus lactis* and *Saccharomyces* spp.) used for fermented and nonfermented products (Vinderola et al., 2002). These additives include salts (NaCl and KCl), sugars (sucrose and lactose), sweeteners (acesulfame and aspartame), aroma compounds (diacetyl, acetaldehyde and acetoin), natural colorings for fermented milks (red, yellow and orange colorings), flavoring agents (strawberry, vanilla, peach and banana essences), flavoring–coloring agents (strawberry, vanilla and peach), nisin (a polypeptide-type antibiotic produced by *L. lactis* which is active against spore- forming bacteria and could be used as a natural preservative in addition to lactic acid), natamycin, lysozyme and nitrate (Vinderola et al., 2002). Elevated levels of ingredients can inhibit probiotics during storage (Arihara et al., 1998; Boylston et al., 2004; Kourkoutas et al., 2006; Lee and Salminen, 2009).

4.4.2 Growth and protective factors

Probiotic lactobacilli and, in particular, bifidobacteria grow poorly in milk due to lack of non-protein nitrogen (free amino acids and small peptides) and some vitamins, as well as to their slow activity of β-galactosidase (Korbekandi et al., 2011). A good and common method to compensate for slow growth is to fortify milk with different growth factors (consumed by probiotics as nutrients) and/or growth promoters (which improve viability of probiotics but not as a direct nutrient) such as casein, whey protein hydrolysates, L-cysteine, yeast extract, glucose, vitamins, minerals and antioxidant. These supplements have significant positive effects on the survival of probiotic microorganisms (Mohammadi et al., 2011).

The addition of L-cysteine, whey protein concentrate, acid casein hydrolysate and tryptone improved the viability of *L. acidophilus* and bifidobacteria by providing growth factors as these probiotic bacteria lack proteolytic activity (Dave and Shah, 1998). Protein derivatives promote probiotic survival due to several reasons; namely, their nutritional value for the cells, reducing redox potential of the media as well as increasing buffering capacity of the media (which results in a smaller decrease in pH) (Dave and Shah, 1998; Mortazavian et al., 2010). It should be pointed out that effects of milk proteins on the viability of probiotics depends on various factors such as the type of the strains used, specifications of the milk protein derivative added, inoculation conditions and formulation of the product. It has been reported that casein and whey protein hydrolysate enhanced the acidification rate of *S. thermophilus* and reduced the growth rate of probiotic organisms (*L. acidophilus* La-5 and *L. rhamnosus* Lr-35) in fermented milks during the manufacturing stages, although the survival of the latter bacteria was improved after storage (Lucas et al., 2004).

Prebiotics are non–viable and non-digestible (or minimally digestible) food ingredients which are metabolized selectively by beneficial intestinal bacteria and enhance their growth and/or activity. They are mostly sugar-like compounds (oligosaccharides) comprising between two and ten monomers that largely resist digestion by pancreatic and brush border enzymes. The term "synbiotic" is used to describe products that contain both probiotics and prebiotics (Nobakhti et al., 2009). These compounds (such as fructooligosaccharides and galactooligosaccharides) can have suitable effect on retention of probiotics viability (especially bifidobacteria) in food products as well as in gastrointestinal tract (Gibson et al., 2004; Mizota, 1996; Mohammadi et al., 2011; Rycroft, 2001).

The food matrix, itself, can be protective. An example is cheese, where the anaerobic environment, high fat content and buffering capacity of the matrix helps to protect the probiotic cells both in the product and during intestinal transit (Boylston et al., 2004; Lee and Salminen, 2009). In contrast to liquid foods, the solid matrices in food products, such as the gel structure in yogurt or cheese, support probiotic cells by reducing their exposure to detrimental factors (e.g., hydrogen ions and organic acids) (Karimi et al., 2011; Mohammadi and Mortazavian, 2011). These matrices can act as a barrier (by physically and chemically binding hydrogen ions and organic acids (Korbekandi et al., 2011). Increasing the buffering capacity of milk would stimulate growth and activity of probiotics in fermented milks. It leads to higher viability of probiotics in dairy fermented products as well as in the gastrointestinal tract due to the maintenance of pH at higher values. Also, the pH of the products with higher buffering capacity declines slowly during refrigerated storage and results in a greater survival of probiotic cells. Moreover, by absorbing hydrogen ions into the dry matter of product matrix (such as proteins), the amounts of undissociated organic acids are increased, resulting in the reduction of bacteriocidic effect of these compounds on probiotics (Mortazavian et al., 2011; korbekandi et al., 2011; Heydari 2011).

4.5 Temperature

The temperature at which probiotic organisms grow is important in food applications where fermentation is required. Also, storage temperature exhibits considerably important role. Fermentation temperature is one of the most important factors affecting the qualitative parameters of probiotic fermented milks, including the viability of probiotic microorganisms and fermentation time (incubation time). The optimum temperature for growth of most probiotics is between 37°C and 43°C (Boylston et al., 2004; Doleyres and Lacroix 2005; Lee and Salminen, 2009). Although the growth of *L. acidophilus* may occur at temperatures as high as 45 °C, the optimum growth occurs within 40-42°C. The optimum growth temperature for bifidobacteria is 37-41°C (Korbekandi et al., 2011). Species of bifidobacteria isolated from the human intestinal tract such as *B. longum* (infantis), *B. breve*, *B. bifidum*, and *B. adolescentis* have optimum growth temperatures in the range of 36–38°C, whereas *B. animalis* ssp. *lactis* can grow at higher temperatures of 41–43°C (Crittenden, 2004; Doleyres and Lacroix 2005; Lee and Salminen, 2009).

Temperature is also a critical factor influencing probiotic survival during storage period. Probiotic food products usually, should be stored at a refrigerated temperature, preferably 4-5°C. The storage temperature of probiotic food products affects the viability of the probiotics via effects of temperature on the cells survival, the type and concentration of metabolites formed between starter bacteria and probiotics in fermented products. Mortazavian et al. (2007a) found that storage in ABY-type culture (*L. acidophilus*, *B. lactis* and yogurt bacteria) at 2°C for 20 days resulted in the highest viability of *L. acidophilus* LA-5, whereas, for *Bifidobacterium lactis* BB-12, the highest viability was obtained when yogurt was stored at 8°C (Mortazavian et al., 2007b). Low resistance of bifidobacteria cells to low refrigeration temperatures (2°C or less) has been proven (Kailasapathy and Rybka, 1997; Korbekandi et al., 2011). In general, in ABY-type culture, storage of the product at 4-5°C appears to result in greatest viability of both probiotics, i.e., *L. acidophilus* and bifidobacteria (Mortazavian et al., 2008). During processing, temperatures above 45–50°C will be detrimental to probiotic survival. The higher the temperature, the shorter the time period of exposure required to severely decrease the numbers of viable bacteria, ranging from hours or minutes at 45–55°C to seconds at higher temperatures. It is obvious that probiotics should be added downstream of heating/cooking/pasteurization processes in food manufacture (Lee and Salminen, 2009). Freezing temperatures can also affect viability of probiotics. This is discussed in the next section.

4.6 Freezing and thawing operations

Probiotics can survive well over long shelf lives in products such as frozen yogurts and ice cream. During the freezing process, the cells of probiotics can be lethally injured by damaging their cell walls or their cell membranes caused by mechanical stresses of the ice crystals formed in the external medium or inside the cells, by temperature decrease chock to the cells and cold injuries, by condensation of solutes (those are detrimental to probiotic cells) in the extracellular/intracellular media, or by dehydration of the cells. All mentioned factors cause reduction or interruption of vital metabolic activities of the cells that are necessary for their live (Akin et al., 2007; Davies and Obafemi, 1985; Gill 2006; Jay et al., 2005). The size of the ice crystals increases with decrease in freezing rate and larger intracellular ice crystals causes greater damage to the cells (Gill, 2006; Jay et al., 2005). Therefore, rapid freezing after inoculating with the probiotic microorganisms contributes to the good maintenance of the populations of these microorganisms in the product (Mohammadi et al., 2011).

Probiotic cells are subjected to some chemical stresses during melting (freeze-thaw) of the frozen products which can cause mortality to them. On one hand, the cells are exposed to osmotic effects (Jay et al., 2005). On the other hand, the high concentrations of detrimental factors such as hydrogen ions, organic acids, oxygen and other poisoning components to probiotic cells in melting media, associated with freezing concentration, are the factors having a great effect on viability loss of probiotics. pH has been found to exhibit a crucial role in this regard.

4.7 Drying process

Powdered foods have much longer shelf life at an ambient temperature. Drying can be achieved by different methods such as freeze drying, spray drying, microwave drying and vacuum drying. Spray drying could be achieved at a lower cost compared with other techniques. However, spray drying could lead to a loss of viability of the probiotic cells due to encountering them to several stresses including high temperature, dehydration, osmotic pressure, gradual increase in detrimental compounds during drying and mechanical stress (shearing). Also, concentration of dissolved oxygen might also increase in dried products which could be toxic to bifidobacteria (Korbekandi et al 2011; Rybka and Kailasapathy, 1997). In the spray drying method, the most critical parameters affecting survival of bifidobacteria are the type of atomization, air pressure, and the outlet temperature (Champagne and Møllgaard, 2008). Freeze drying is the best process for maintaining the viability of the bacterial cells used for preparing starter culture cells. However, its cost-effectiveness should be evaluated before usage.

4.8 Microencapsulation

Microencapsulation, as one of the new and efficient methods, has recently been under especial consideration and investigation. From microbiological point of view, microencapsulation can be defined as the process of entrapment/enclosure of microorganisms cells by means of coating them with proper hydrocolloid(s) in order to segregate the cells from the surrounding environment; in a way that results in appropriate cell release in the intestinal medium (Krasaekoopt et al., 2003; Mortazavian et al., 2007b, 2008; Picot and Lacroix, 2003; Sultana et al., 2000). Microencapsulation of probiotic cells has been shown to preserve them from detrimental environmental factors such as low pH and high acidity (Wenrong and Griffiths, 2000), bile salts (Lee and Heo, 2000), cold shocks induced by the process conditions such as deep freezing and freeze drying (Shah and Rarvula, 2000), molecular oxygen in case of obligatory anaerobic microorganisms (Sunohara et al., 1995), heat shocks caused by process conditions such as spray drying, bacteriophages (Steenson et al., 1987) and chemical antimicrobial agents (Sultana et al., 2000). In addition, other advantages such as increase improvement and stabilization of sensory properties (Gomes and Malcata, 1999) and immobilization of the cells for their homogeneous distribution throughout the product (Krasaekoopt et al., 2003) can also be achieved by this process.

This process has been recently used as an efficient method for improving the viability of probiotic bacteria in fermented milk drinks, fermented frozen dairy desserts, ice cream and juices (Adhikari et al., 2000; Krasaekoopt et al., 2004; 2005; Kailasapathy, 2006; Mohammadi et al., 2011), and simulated gastrointestinal tract (Hansen et al., 2002; Korbekandi et al., 2011; Lee and Heo, 2000; Krasaekoopt et al., 2004; Mortazavian et al., 2008; Sultana et al., 2000; Wenrong and Griffiths, 2000). Encapsulated probiotic organisms, when incorporated into fermented frozen dairy desserts, showed an improved viability of >10^5 cfu g^{-1} in the product compared to counts of <10^3 cfu g^{-1} when non-encapsulated organisms were used (Mortazavian et al., 2010 ; Shah and Ravula 2004). Studies suggest that, micro-encapsulation of free probiotic cells can increase their viability by ≥2 log cycles in fermented milks during a refrigerated storage period. As mentioned earlier, in fermented milk drinks with pH values of less than 4.2, free cells of *L. acidophilus* LA-5 lost their viability to less than 10^6 cfu mL^{-1} after 1 week; and in the case of *Bifidobacterium lactis* BB-12, a similar loss occurred after 2 weeks of storage. For encapsulated cells, viable population of *L. acidophilus* and bifidobacteria remained higher than 10^5 and 10^6 cfu mL^{-1} after 42 days of refrigerated storage, and counts of free probiotic free cells were not detected and 10^2 cfu mL^{-1}, respectively (Mortazavian et al., 2008).

4.9 Packaging materials and conditions

The packaging of probiotic food products influences the oxygen permeability into the product, and as a result, affects the viability of bifidobacteria, *L. acidophilus* and other probiotic species during the storage period. Several aspects of food packaging materials including the type of the packaging materials (Glass and plastic) their thickness, and the application of active/intelligent packaging systems could influence survival of probiotic bacteria (Korbekandi et al., 2011). In general, two important points are worth mentioning. Firstly, apart from the packaging materials, the temperature and relative humidity of the atmosphere are the key factors affecting oxygen permeability. Secondly, besides the efficiency of packaging, the economic aspect should also be taken into account (the price of packaging materials as well as the price of packaging machines) because they can significantly influence the final price of products and their sale volumes.

5. Viability of probiotics in food products during delivery through gastrointestinal tract

The gastrointestinal tract (GIT) with its diverse and concentrated microbial population (at birth 10^{14} cfu g^{-1} and between 400 and 500 species) is one of the key organs of the human body, and it is in fact an ecosystem of highest complexity that mediates numerous interactions with the chemical (and nutritional) environment. The gastrointestinal tract starts in mouth, travels through the stomach, intestines and ends at the anus. In each section of the gastrointestinal tract, different types and quantities of microbes are found. The average adult carries about four pounds of microbes in their intestinal tract (Tannis, 2008). Nonetheless, diversity at a division level is among the lowest (Bäckhead et al., 2005) and the lactobacilli and bifidobacteria comprise less than 5% of the total microbiota (Lay et al., 2005; Lee and Salminen, 2009).

Probiotics targeting the intestine clearly encounter the greatest hurdles in order to be delivered to their targeted site. The main factors to be considered that influence the viability of food-containing probiotics in GIT conditions are: 1) Food matrix, 2) very low pH in the stomach, 3) bile salts and gastro-enzymes in the small intestine, 4) Lysozyme in saliva, and 5) colonic environments (competitions with other microorganisms including pathogens).

The effect of food matrix on the intestinal survival of probiotic bacteria is insufficiently studied. Rochet et al. (2008) did not see any difference in the faecal level of B. animalis strain, when 6×10^{10}– 2×10^{11} cfu g^{-1} were administered in fermented milk or in freeze-dried form, but the food matrix improved significantly the survival of *L. plantarum* MF1298 (Klingberg and Budde, 2006) and *L. rhamnosus* GG (Saxelin et al., 1993), when lower doses (6×10^9 cfu and 1–2×10^9 cfu, respectively) were used (Saxelin et al., 2010). Fresh dairy products are the most common product forms of probiotic delivery, but ripened cheeses have also been successfully tested as a carrier matrix. Data from Saxelin et al. (2003) showed an increased recovery of *L. rhamnosus* in human stools resulting from the following delivery matrices: powder<juice or fermented milk<unfermented milk<cheese. The appropriate protecting effect of cheese matrix toward probitic cells can be attributed to its dense matrix, high buffering capacity and relatively high fat content (Gardiner et al., 1999; Karimi et al., 2011). The buffering ability of the food matrix is arguably a critical factor. But the presence of a fermentable carbohydrate also improves a culture's ability to survive a simulated gastric environment (Corcoran et al., 2005). In this regard, the carbohydrate provides the cell with the ability to produce ATP, which is required for pumping out acid from the cytoplasm. Not surprisingly, the fibre/carbohydrate content of the food matrix strongly affects the stability of probiotic bacteria during storage in a fruit juice (Saarela et al., 2006; Farnworth and Champagne, 2010).

Among the hurdles and stressful conditions against safe transition of probiotic cells to the intestine, harsh acid conditions in stomach and the bile substances in the duodenum (The first part of the small intestine) are the most important (Lee and Salminen, 2009). The first barrier that bacteria must overcome is the very low pH values of the stomach with values ranging from 1 to 3 and mean exposure times of 90 min. Into the duodenum the pH value rises to 6–6.5, but bile salts are poured from the gallbladder to reach concentrations ranging from 1.5 to 2% during the first hour of digestion and decreasing afterwards to 0.3% w/v or lower (Noriega et al., 2004). The residence period in the small intestine until 50% emptying oscillate between 2.5 and 3 h and the transit through the colon could take up to 40 h (Camilleri et al., 1989). Even when product formulation procedures that ensure viability during production and storage have been used as described above, the live bacteria must survive transit of the upper GIT. Ethics, cost, and complexity of tests prevent the testing of foods containing probiotics using human feeding trials. *In vitro* tests, using models of the GIT, can be used to provide data about the ability of bacteria to survive the harsh conditions of the upper GIT. Several pH values and bile concentrations are tested for variable times in order to determine the survival of the strain(s) under test. Many studies that have used test-tube experiments to simulate the acidic conditions in the stomach, and exposure to bile salts and digestive enzymes that occur in the small intestine have been reported (Boza et al., 2004; Horaczek and Viernstein, 2004; Farnworth and Champagne, 2010; Pascual et al., 1999). De Smet et al., (1995) indicated that a concentration of 0.3% bile salts is critical for the screening of human probiotics, and this ability was associated to the presence of bile salt hydrolase activity. Nevertheless, Schmidt et al., (2001) showed that at least in lactobacilli, bile salt resistance could not be correlated to the presence of this enzyme. The study performed by Floch et al. (1972) indicated that conjugated bile acids are less inhibitory than free bile acids (cholic and deoxycholic) toward intestinal aerobic and anaerobic bacteria (Rivera-Espinoza and Gallardo-Navarro, 2010). The results of viability obtained are strain dependent and, in general, bifidobacteria strains are less tolerant to acidic conditions than lactobacilli, whereas the first seems to be more tolerant to bile challenge (Lee and Salminen, 2009). The recovered strains were intrinsically resistant to acid gastric conditions (pH 2.0) and also showed good tolerance to high concentrations of bile salts and NaCl. This cross-resistance between low pH and bile salts was previously described in bile-adapted strains (Noriega et al 2004). It is known that exposure to one stress can induce a response that protects cells against multiple stresses (Duwat et al 2000). As the stress response is already induced at that stage, it may be capable of surviving the bile in the duodenum. This is pertinent as many candidate isolates may be overlooked if they do not display direct resistance to bile, when in reality the ability to induce sufficient tolerance is all that is required (O'Sullivan, 2006).

The development of intestinal microbiota is of major importance for the health of newborns. Especially lysozyme present in human milk may affect colonization of newborn intestinal tract by specific bifidobacterial strains. Lysozyme is an antimicrobial enzyme (EC 3.2.1.17) found in tears, saliva, human milk, mucus, neutrophil granules and egg white (Field, 2005). It hydrolyses the β-(1,4) linkage between N-acetylglucosamine and N-acetylmuramic acid in bacterial cell wall and Gram-positive bacteria are more susceptible to lysozyme than Gram-negative bacteria. The effect of saliva on the intestinal survival of probiotic bacteria is insufficiently studied. The resistance to lysozyme at 25–35 mg L^{-1} was recommended as a criterion for the selection of a lactic acid bacterial strain suitable for use in milk industry (Guglielmonti et al., 2007). The resistance to lysozyme at 25–35 mg L^{-1} was recommended as a criterion for the selection of a lactic acid bacterial strain suitable for use in milk industry (Guglielmonti et al., 2007). According to findings, the tolerance of probiotics to lysozyme is strain-dependent (Rada et al., 2010). Bifidobacteria naturally occur within the whole intestinal tract from oral cavity to large intestine. Lysozyme is naturally present in saliva and other biological fluids (tear fluid). Hence, the interaction of inhabitant bifidobacteria or bifidobacteria-containing food products and lysozyme is inevitably occurred. The salivary lysozyme may also interact with other probiotic bacteria and can vary from 17 to 181 µg mL^{-1} (Koh et al., 2004). Some bifidobacteria seems to be also completely lysozyme-resistant (Rada et al., 2010). Therefore, being resistance to lysozyme is a criterion for the selection of new probiotic bifidobacterial strains. Figure 3 represents main factors affecting viability of probiotics during transition through the GIT.

6. Conclusion

Probiotic functional foods, one of the largest markets of functional foods, represent a huge growth potential for the food industry and may be explored through the development of innovative ingredients, processes, and products. Therefore, the process of producing and manufacturing probiotic functional foods should have standardized protocols and quality control procedures. Safety and functional efficiency of the probiotic food products in the body and technological characteristics (viability, sensory properties, economic aspects and physicochemical and rheological characteristics) has been under special attention in recent years and many achievements in mentioned aspects have been attained. To provide health benefits related to probiotic organisms, maintaining viable counts of each probiotic strain in gram or milliliter of probiotic products above a minimum standard level (e.g., 10^6 cfu mL^{-1})

until the time of consumption is quite important. Adding probiotics to food products holds many challenges, such as biorelationships among the starter bacteria, pH, organic acids, molecular oxygen, freezing and thawing operations, additives such as sodium chloride, sugar, anti-microbial preservatives. Therefore, a wide range of research has been focused on optimization of formulation and processing as well as packaging of probiotic food products in order to increase the viability of probiotic cells in them until the time of consumption. However, a high viable population of probiotic bacteria in food products at the time of consumption does not guarantee the same survival rate after the arrival of the cells in the intestine. Probiotics targeting the intestine clearly encounter the greatest hurdles in order to be delivered to their targeted site. The biggest hurdles are the acid conditions of the stomach, the bile in the duodenum and competitive exclusion of pathogens. Therefore, clinical studies as well as simulated gastrointestinal tract investigations, should be integrated to the technological research.

7. References

Adhikari, K; Mustapha, A; Grun, I. U. & Fernando, L. (2000). Viability of microencapsulated bifidobacteria in set yogurt during refrigerated storage. J Dairy Sci 83: 1946-1951

Akalin. A.S. and D. Erisir (2008). Effects of inulin and oligofructose on the rheological characteristics and probiotic culture survival in low-fat probiotic ice cream. J Food Sci 73:184–188.

Akin. M. B., M. S. Akin and Z. Kirmaci (2007). Effects of inulin and sugar levels on the viability of yogurt and probiotic bacteria and the physical and sensory characteristics in probiotic ice cream. Food Chem 104:93–99

Amiri, Z. R., P. Khandelwal, B. R. Aruna and N. Sahebjamnia (2008). Optimization of process parameters for preparation of synbiotic acidophilus milk via selected probiotics and prebiotics using artificial neural network. J Biotechnol 136:460

Andersson, H., N.G. Asp, A. Bruce, S. Roos, T. Wadstrom and A. E. Wold (2001). Health effects of probiotics and prebiotics. A literature review on human studies. Scand J Nutr/Naringsforskning 45: 58–75

Angelov, A., V. Gotcheva, R. Kuncheva and T. Hrstozova (2006). Development of a new oat-based probiotic drink. Int J Food Microbiol 112:75–80

Arihara, K., H. Ota, M. Itoh, Y. Kondo, T. Sameshima, H. Yamanaka, M. Akimoto, S. Kanai and T. Miki (1998). Lactobacillus acidophilus group lactic acid bacteria applied to meat fermentation. J. Food Sci 63: 544-547.

Aryana, K. J. and P. Mcgrew (2007). Quality attributes of yogurt with *Lactobacillus casei* and various prebiotics. LWT-Food Sci Technol 40:1808–14

Bäckhead, F., R. E. Ley, J. L. Sonnenburg, D. A. Peterson and J.I. Gordon (2005). Host-bacterial mutualism in the human intestine. Science 307: 1915–1919

Betoret, N., L. Puente, M. J. Diaz, M. J. Pagan, M. J. Garcia and M. L. Gras (2003). Development of probioticenriched dried fruits by vacuum impregnation. J Food Engr 56:273–277

Blanchette, L., D. Roy. G. Belanger and S. F. Gauthier (1996). Production of cottage cheese using dressing fermented by bifidobacteria. J Dairy Sci 79:8–15

Blandino, A., M. E. Al-Aseeri, S. S. Pandiella, D. Cantero and C. Webb (2003). Review: Cereal-based fermented foods and beverages. Food Res Int 36: 527–543.

Blandino, A., M. E. Al-Aseeri, S.S. Pandiella, D. Cantero and C Webb (2003). Cereal-based fermented foods and beverages. Food Res Int 36:527–43

Boylston, T. D., C. G. Vinderola, H. B. Ghoddusi and J. A. Reinheimer (2004) Incorporation of bifidobacteria into cheeses: challenges and rewards. Int Dairy J 14: 375–387

Boza, Y., D. Barbi and A. R. P. Scamparini (2004). Survival of Beijerinckia sp. microencapsulated in carbohydrates by spray-drying. J Microencapsul 21: 15–24

Cai, Y. M., M. Matsumoto, and Y Benno. (2000). *Bifidobacterium lactis* is a subjective synonym of *Bifidobacterium animalis* (Mitsuoka 1969; Scardovi and Trovatelli 1974). Microbiol Immunol 44: 815–820

Camilleri, M., L. J. Colemont, S. F. Phillips, M. L. Brown, G. M. Thomforde, N. Chapman, and A. R. Zinsmeister (1989). Human gastric emptying and colonic filling of solids characterized by a new method. Am. J. Physiol. Gastrointest. Liver Physiol 257: 284–290

Cargill. 2009. Cargill beverage concepts will address consumer demands for health, taste and texture at IFT 2008. Available from: http://www.cargill.com/news-center/news-releases/ 2008/NA3007612.jsp. Accessed Jul 20, 2009.

Champagne, C. P and H. Møllgaard (2008). Production of Probiotic Cultures and Their Addition in Fermented Foods. In R. F. Edward (Eds.), Handbook of Fermented Functional Foods (2 edition). United States of America: CRC Press, Taylor & Francis Group.

Chen, I. N. C. C., C. Y. Wang and T. L. Chang (2008). Lactic fermentation and antioxidant activity of Zingiberaceae plants in Taiwan. Int J Food Sci Nutr 22:1–10

Corbo, M. R., M. Albenzio, M. De Angelis, A. Sevi and M. Gobbetti (2001). Microbiological and biochemical properties of Canestrato Pugliese hard cheese supplemented with bifidobacteria. J Dairy Sci 84:551–61.

Corcoran, B. M., C. Stanton, G. F. Fitzgerald and R. P. Ross (2005). Survival of probiotic lactobacilli in acidic environments is enhanced in the presence of metabolizable sugars. Applied Environ Microbiol 71:3060–3067

Crittenden, R (2004). An update on probiotic Bifidobacteria. Salminen S., A. von Wright and Ouwerhand A(eds). Lactic Acid Bacteria: Microbiological and Functional Aspects. Marcel Dekker, New York, 125–157.

Dalev, D., M. Bielecka, A. Troszynska, S. Ziajka and Lamparski (2006). Sensory quality of new probiotic beverages based on cheese whey and soy preparation. Pol J Food Nutr Sci 15:65–70

Dave, R. I. and N. P. Shah (1997). Effectiveness of ascorbic acid as an oxygen scavenger in improving viability of probiotic bacteria in yoghurts made with commercial starter cultures. Int Dairy J 7: 435-43

Dave, R.I. and N.P. Shah (1998). Ingredient supplementation effects on viability of probiotic bacteria in yogurt. J Dairy Sci 81:2804–2816

Davidson, R. H., S. E. Duncan, C. R. Hackney, W. N. Eigel and J.W. Boling (2000). Probiotic culture surival and implications in fermented frozen yogurt characteristics. J Dairy Sci 83:666–73

Davies, R. and A Obafemi (1985) Response of micro-organisms to freeze-thaw stress. In: Robinson RK (ed) Microbiology of frozen foods, Elsevier Applied Science Publishers, London U.K pp, 83–107.

De Smet, I., L.Van Hoorde, M. Van de Woestyne, H. Christiaens and W. Verstraete (1995). Significance of bile salt hydrolytic activities of lactobacilli. J Appl Bacteriol 79: 292–301

De Vuyst, L. (2000). Technology Aspects Related to the Application of Functional Starter Cultures. Food Tech Biotech 38: 105–12

Diplock, A.T., P. J. Aggett, M. Ashwell, F. Bornet, E. B. Fern and M. B. Robrrfroid (1999). Scientific concepts of functional food in Europe: Consensus document. Br J Nutr 81: 11–27.

Doleyres, Y. and C. Lacroix (2005). Technologies with free and immobilised cells for probiotic bifidobacteria production and protection. Int Dairy J 15: 973–988

Donkor, O. N., A. Henriksson, T. Vasiljevic and N. P. Shah (2007) a-Galactosidase and proteolytic activities of selected probiotic and dairy cultures in fermented soymilk. Food Chem 104:10–20

Duwat, P., B. Cesselin, S. Sourice and A. Gruss (2000). *Lactococcus lactis*, a bacterial model for stress responses and survival. Int J Food Microbiol 55: 83–86

El-Nagar, G., G. Clowes, C. M. Tudorica and V. Kuri (2002) Rheological quality and stability of yog-ice cream with added inulin. Int J Dairy Technol 55:89–93

Erkkilä S., M. L. Suihko, S. Eerola, E. Petäjä and T. Mattila-Sandholm (2001). Dry sausage fermented by Lactobacillus rhamnosus strains. Int J Food Microbiol 64: 205–210

Farnworth E. R. and C.Champagne (2010). Production of Probiotic Cultures and Their Incorporation into Foods. In: Watson R. R and V. R. Preedy (Eds) Bioactive Foods in Promoting Health: Probiotics and Prebiotics. Elsevier, Oxford, UK. Pp 2-18

Feng, X. M., A. R. B. Eriksson and J. Schnurer (2005). Growth of lactic acid bacteria and Rhizopus oligosporus during barley tempeh. Int J Food Microbiol 104:249–256

Field, C.J (2005). The immunological components of human milk and their effect on immune development in infants. J Nutr 135:1-4

Floch, M. H., H. J. Binder, B. Filburn and W. Gershengoren (1972). The effect of bile acids on intestinal microflora. Am J Clin Nutr 25:1418–1426

Gardiner G, Ross RP, Stanton C, Lynch PB, Collins JK, Fitzgerald G (1999) Evaluation of Cheddar cheese as a food carrier for delivery of a probiotic strain to the gastrointestinal tract. J Dairy Sci 82:1379–1387

Ghoddusi, H. B. and R. K. Robinson (1996). The test of time. Dairy Indust Int 61:25–28

Gibson, G. R., B. Rabiu, C. E. Rycroft and R.A. Rastall (2004) Trans-Galactooligosaccharides as Prebiotics. In: Shortt, C., J.O. Brien (eds) Handbook of Functional Dairy Products, CRC Press LLC USA pp.91-109

Gill,C. O. (2006). Microbiology of frozen foods. In: Da-Wen Boca S (ed) Handbook of frozen food processing and packaging . CRC Press Ranton pp. 85-100

Godward, G., K .Sultana, K. Kailasapathy, P. Peiris, R. Arumugaswamy and N. Reynolds (2000) The importance of strain selection on the viability of probiotic bacteria in dairy foods. Milchwissenschaft 55:441-445

Gomes, A. M. P. and F. X. Malcata (1999). *Bifidobacterium* spp. and *Lactobacillus acidophilus*: biological, biochemical, technological and therapeutical properties relevant for use as probiotics. Trends Food Sci Technol 10:139–57

Granato, D., G. F. Branco, A. G. Cruz, J.A.F.Faria and F. Nazzaro (2010). Functional foods and nondairy probiotic food development: Trends, Concepts and products. Compr Rev Food Sci Food Saf. 9: 292–302.

of probiotic fermented milk containing *Lactobacillus paracasei* and *Lactobacillus acidophilus*. J Dairy Res 76:74–82

Perdigon, G., M. Locascio, M. Medici, A. P. D. Holgado and G. Oliver (2003). Interaction of bifidobacteria with the gut and their influence in the immune function. *Biocell 27:* 1–9

Pico, A. and C. Lacroix (2003). Effect of micronization on viability and thermotolerance of probiotic freeze-dried cultures. Int Dairy J 13:455-462

Possemiers, S., M. Marzorati, W. Verstraete and T. V. de Wiele (2010). Bacteria and chocolate: A successful combination for probiotic delivery Int J Food Microbiol 141: 97–103

Prado, F. C., J. L Parada, J. C. Carvalho, C. R. Soccol (2008). Isolation and characterization of lactic acid bacteria from green coconut microbiota for us in non-dairy probiotic beverage. In: 18th International Congress of Chemical and Process Engineering. Proceedings: 18th ICCPE. Praga: CHISA 2008. CD. p 1–2

Rada V., Splichal I.., Rockova S., Grmanova M., Vlkova E (2010). Susceptibility of bifidobacteria to lysozyme as a possible selection criterion for probiotic bifidobacterial strains. Biotechnol Lett 32:451–455

Ravula, R. R and N. P. Shah (1998). Effect of acid casein hydrolyzates and cysteine on the viability of yogurt and probiotic bacteria in fermented frozen dairy desserts. Aust J Dairy Technol 53:174–179

Renuka. B., S. G. Kulkarni, P. Vijayanand, S. G. Prapulla (2009). Fructooligosaccharide fortification of selected fruit juice beverages: effect on the quality characteristics. LWT-Food Sci Technol 43:1031–3

Rivera-Espinoza, Y. and Y. Gallardo-Navarro (2010). Non-dairy probiotic products. Food Microbiology 27: 1-11

Roberts, J.S. and D. R. Kidd (2005) Lactic acid fermentation of onions. Food Sci Technol 38:2185–90

Rochet, V., L. Rigottier-Gois, A. Ledaire, C. Andrieux, M. Sutren, S. Rabot, A. Mogenet, J. Bresson, S. Cools, C. Picard, N. Goupil-Feuillerat and J.Doré (2008). Survival of Bifidobacterium animalis DN-173 010 in the faecal microbiota after administration in lyophilised form or in fermented product - a randomised study in healthy adults. J Molecular Microbiol Biotechnol 14:128–136

Ross, R. P., C. Desmond, G. F. Fitzgerald and C. Stanton (2005). Overcoming the technological hurdles in the development of probiotic foods. J Appl Microbiol 98: 1410–1417

Rouhi, M. and A. M. Mortazavian (2010). Probiotic fermented Sausage: Viability of probiotic microorganisms and sensory characteristics. Cri Rev Food Sci Nutr. In press.

Rybka, S and K. Kailasapathy (1997) Effect of freeze drying and storage on the microbiological and physical properties of AB-yoghurt. Milchwissenschaft 52:390–394

Rycroft, C. E., M. R. Jones, G. R. Gibson and R. A. Rastall (2001) A comparative in vitro evaluation of the fermentation properties of prebiotic oligosaccharides. J Appl Microbiol 91:878–887

Saarela, M., I .Virkajarvi and H. L. Alakomi (2006). Stability and functionality of freeze-dried probiotic Bifidobacterium cells during storage in juice and milk. Int Dairy J 16: 1477–1482

Sanders, M and J. Huis in't Veld (1999). Bringing a probiotic-containing functional food to the market: microbiological, product, regulatory and labeling issues. Antonie van Leeuwenhoek 76: 293–315.

Sanders, M. E (2006).Summary of probiotic activities of Bifidobacterium lactis HN019. J Clin Gastroenterol 40: 776–783

Saris, P. E. J., S. Beasley and H. Tourila (2003). Fermented soymilk with a monoculture of *Lactococcus lactis*. Int J Food Microbiol 81:159–62

Saxelin, B., U. Grenov, R. Svensson, R. Fonden, T. Reniero and T. Mattila-andholm (1999). The technology of probiotics. Trends Food Sci Technol 10:387–392

Saxelin, M., A. Lassig, H. Karjalainen, S. Tynkkynen, A. Surakka, H. Vapaatalo, S. Järvenpää, R. Korpela, M. Mutanen, K. Hatakka (2010). Persistence of probiotic strains in the gastrointestinal tract when administered as capsules, yoghurt, or cheese. Int J Food Microbiol 144: 293–300

Saxelin, M., M. Ahokas and S. Salminen (1993). Dose response on the faecal colonization of Lactobacillus strain GG administered in two different formulations. Microbial Ecology in Health and Disease 6: 119–122

Saxelin, M., R. Korpela and A. Mayra-Makinen (2003). Introduction: classifying functional dairy products. In T. Mattila-Sandholm and M. Saarela, (Eds.) Functional Dairy Products: Vol. 1 (pp. 1–15). Boca Raton, FL: CRC Press,Woodhead Publishing Ltd.

Schmidt, E. J., J. S. Boswell, J. P. Walsh, M. M. Schellenberg, T.W. Winter, C. Li, C.W. Allman and P.V Savage (2001). Activities of cholic acid-derived antimicrobial agents against multidrug-resistant bacteria. J Antimicrob Chemother 47: 671–674

Shah, N. P (2000). Probiotic bacteria: selective enumeration and survival in dairy foods. J Dairy Sci 83: 894–907

Shah, N. P (2001). Functional foods from probiotics and prebiotics. Food Technol 55: 46–53

Shah, N.P. and R. Ravula (2000) Microencapsulation of probiotic bacteria and their survival in frozen fermented dairy desserts. Aust J Dairy Technol 55:139-144

Shah, N.P. and R. Ravula (2004). Selling the cells in desserts. Dairy Indus Int 69:31-32

Sheehan, V.M., P. Ross and G. F. Fitzgerald (2007). Assessing the acid tolerance and the technological robustness of probiotic cultures for fortification in fruit juices. Innovative Food Sci Emerg Technol 8:279–284

Shobharani, P. and R. Agrawal (2009). Supplementation of adjuvants for increasing the nutritive value and cell viability of probiotic fermented milk beverage. Int J Food Sci Nutr 60:70-83

Sousa. R. C. S., R. A. Lira, F. C. Oliveira, D. O. Santos and O. A. P. Sierra (2007). Desenvolvimento e aceitac,˜ao sensory de iogurte probi´otico light de banana. In: Proceedings of IX Encontro Regional Sul de Ciencia e Tecnologia de Alimentos. Curitiba, Brazil: Anais do IX ERSCTA. p 549–553

Souza, C. H. B. and S. M. I. Saad (2009). Viability of *Lactobacillus acidophilus* La-5 added solely or in co-culture with a yogurt starter culture and implications on physico-chemical and related properties of Minas fresh cheese during storage. LWT-Food Sci Technol 42:633–640

Steenson, L. R., T. R. Klaenhammer and H. E. Swaisgood (1987). Calcium alginate-immobilized cultures of lactic streptococci are protected from attack by lytic bacteriophage. J Dairy Sci 70:1121-1127

Sultana, K., G. Godward, N. Reynolds, R. Arumugaswamy, P. Peiris and K. Kailasapathy (2000). Encapsulation of probiotic bacteria with alginate-starch and evaluation of survival in simulated gastrointestinal conditions and in yoghurt. Int J Food Microbiol 62:47-55

Sunohara, H., T. Ohno, N. Shibata and K. Seki (1995). Process for producing capsule and capsule obtained thereby. US Patent 5:478-570

Supavititpatana, P., T. I. Wirjantoro, A. Apichartsrangkoon and P. Raviyan (2008). Addition of gelatin enhanced gelation of corn–milk yogurt. Food Chem 106:211–216

Takahashi. N., J. Z. Xiao, K .Miyaji, and K Iwatsuki (2007). H+-ATPase in the acid tolerance of *Bifidobacterium longum*. Milchwissenschaft 62:151-153

Talwalkar, A. and K. Kailasapathy (2003). Metabolic and biochemical responses of probiotic bacteria to oxygen. J Dairy Sci 86: 2537-46

Talwalkar, A. I. and K. A. Kailasapathy (2004). The role of oxygen in the viability of probiotic bacteria with reference to *L. acido*philus and *Bifidobacterium* spp. Curr Iss Intest Microbiol 5:1-8

Talwalkar, A., C. W. Miller, K. Kailasapathy and M. H. Nguyen (2004). Effect of packaging materials and dissolved oxygen on the survival of probiotic bacteria in yoghurt. Int J Food Sci Technol 39: 605-11

Tamime, A. Y., M. Saarela, A. K. Sondergaard, V. V. Mistry, and N. P. Shah (2005) Production and maintenance of viability of probiotic microorganisms in dairy products. In: Tamime AY (ed) Probiotic Dairy Products, Blackwell Publishing Ltd, Uk, pp. 39-72

Tannis, A. (2008). Probiotic rescue: how you can use probiotics to fight cholesterol, cancer superbugs, digestive complaints and more, John Wiley & Sons Canada, Ltd P:269

Thage, B.V., M. L. Broe, M. H. Petersen, M. A. Petersen, M. A. Bennedsen and Y. Ardö (2005). Aroma development in semi-hard reduced-fat cheese inoculated with *Lactobacillus paracasei* strains with different aminotransferase profiles. Int Dairy J 15:795–805.

Tsen J. H., Y. P. Lin and V.A. King (2004). Fermentation of banana media by using k-carrageenan immobilized *Lactobacillus acidophilus*. Int J Food Microbiol 91:215–20

Tuorila, H. and A. V Cardello (2002). Consumer responses to an off flavour in juice in the presence of specific health claims. Food Qual Pref 13: 561–569

Ventura M. and G. Perozzi (2011). Introduction to the special issue "Probiotic bacteria and human gut microbiota" Genes Nutr 6:203–204

Ventura, M. and R. Zink (2002) Rapid identification, differentiation, and proposed new taxonomic classification of *Bifidobacterium lactis*. Appl Environ Microbiol 68: 6429–6434

Vinderola, C. G. and J. A. Reinheimer (2003). Lactic acid bacteria: a comparative *"in vitro"* study of probiotic characteristics and biological barrier resistance. Food Res Int 36: 895–904

Vinderola, C. G., G. A. Costa, S. Regenhardt and J. A. Reinheimer (2002). Influence of compounds associated with fermented dairy products on the growth of lactic acid starter and probiotic bacteria. Int Dairy J 12:579-89.

Vinderola, C. G., W. Prosello, T. D. Ghiberto and J. A. Reinheimer (2000a). Viability of probiotic (*Bifidobacterium, Lactobacillus acidophilus and Lactobacillus casei*) and non probiotic microflora in Argentinean fresco cheese. J Dairy Sci 83:1905–1911

Vinderola, C.G., N. Bailo, J. A. Reinheimer (2000b). Survival of probiotic microflora in Argentinian yoghurts during refrigerated storage. Food Res Int 33:97–102

Wang, C., C. C. Ng, W. Tzeng and Y. T. Shyu (2009). Probiotic potential of noni juice fermented with lactic acid bacteria and bifidobacteria. Int J Food Sci Nutr 1:1–9

Wenrong, S. and M.W. Griffiths (2000). Survival of bifidobacteria in yogurt and simulated gastric juice following immobilization in gellan-xanthan beads. Int J Food Microbiol 61:17-26

Yilmaztekin, M., B. H. özer and F. Atasoy (2004). Survival of *Lactobacillus acidophilus* La-5 and *Bifidobacterium bifidum* BB-02 in white-brined cheese. Int J Food Sci Nutr 55:53–60

Yoon, K. Y., E. E. Woodamns and Y. D. Hang (2004). Probiotication of tomato juice by lactic acid bacteria. J Microbiol 42:315-8

Yoon, K.Y., E.E. Woodamns and Y.D. Hang (2006). Production of probiotic cabbage juice by lactic acid bacteria. Biores Technol 9:1427–30

Pathomechanism and Management of the Upper Gastrointestinal Tract Disorders

7

Chronic NSAIDs Therapy and Upper Gastrointestinal Tract – Mechanism of Injury, Mucosal Defense, Risk Factors for Complication Development and Clinical Management

Francesco Azzaroli*, Andrea Lisotti,
Claudio Calvanese, Laura Turco and Giuseppe Mazzella
*Department of Clinical Medicine,
St. Orsola-Malpighi Hospital,
University of Bologna, Bologna
Italy*

1. Introduction

Non steroidal anti-inflammatory drugs (NSAIDs) are the most prescribed medications worldwide because of their analgesic and anti-inflammatory properties. In fact, NSAIDs are generally prescribed for pain management in musculoskeletal or osteoarticolar pathologies and for rheumatic diseases, very common diseases in the general population.

About twenty million US patients were prescribed NSAIDs every year. Although NSAIDs are generally well tolerated, chronic therapy is responsible for a significant morbidity and mortality rate; in fact, the incidence of GI events is significantly higher (about four fold) in patients receiving NSAIDs chronic therapy (Shaheen et al., 2006; Lawrence et al., 1998).

NSAIDs and aspirin present a favorable benefit profile in relief from pain, inflammation reduction and contribute to lower the risk of cancer, as demonstrated by some epidemiologic and clinical studies showing a reduced incidence of colon cancer in patients receiving low-dose aspirin (Din et al., 2010; Rothwell et al., 2010; Elwood et al., 2009).

Moreover, low-dose aspirin therapy induce a significant reduction in cardiovascular (CV) and cerebrovascular events and effectively lower the rate of deaths in patients with cardiovascular risk factors and previous CV events. On the other hand, adverse gastrointestinal events related to NSAIDs therapy occur in a little but significant amount of patients, resulting in an important morbidity and mortality; world mortality secondary to NSAIDs therapy has been estimated to be similar to that caused by HIV-related complications (Abraham et al., 2005; Laine et al., 2010). For example, in the US more than

---

* Corresponding Author

100.000 patients were admitted every year for NSAIDs related adverse events, resulting in about 15000 deaths (Weil et al., 2000; Ofman et al., 2002).

Non-selective NSAIDs (nsNSAID) inhibit both cyclooxigenase-1 (COX1) and cyclooxigenase-2 (COX2). These two enzyme have different roles in the cell and, in particular, COX1 mediates prostaglandin (PG) secretion which is one of the upper GI protective mechanisms. That is why, with the aim of reducing NSAIDs related upper GI toxicity, selective COX2 inhibitors (coxibs) were developed in the last decade. Coxibs weakly inhibit COX1 and a reduced relative risk of developing upper GI injury was demonstrated in clinical trials in patients receiving coxibs.

2. Epidemiology

The incidence of peptic ulcer disease is tightly related to epidemiological changes in environmental factors, reflecting aging, prevalence of *Helicobacter pylori* infection and use of NSAIDs.

Non-steroidal anti-inflammatory drugs (NSAIDs) are estimated to be the most prescribed therapy worldwide (Clinard, 2001); unfortunately, chronic NSAIDs therapy may induce upper gastrointestinal injury, leading to symptoms such as dyspepsia, chest pain or heartburn or severe complications (i.e. gastroduodenal ulcers bleeding or perforation).

The incidence of GI injuries is significantly higher (about four fold) in patients receiving NSAIDs chronic therapy and 1-2.5 clinically significant adverse events were recorded for 100 patients treated/year; it was estimated that 20-40% of patients receiving chronic NSAIDs therapy present endoscopic finding of gastroduodenal mucosal injury (MacDonald, 1997; Ramey, 2005; Targownik 2006; Taha, 1996). All these evidences, lead to an increased mortality of patients receiving NSAIDs.

Moreover, these adverse event rates, resulting from observational studies, refer to general population receiving NSAIDs; when clinical studies evaluate high-risk categories, the relative risk for upper GI events significantly increase. Therefore, the available guidelines identify these high-risk categories of patients and try to outline possible specific management strategies for each category (Anon, 2000; Lanza, 2009; Moens, 2004; MacLean 2001).

Different guidelines identify various risk factors for the development of upper GI injury under NSAIDs therapy: age, previous history of an upper GI event, the need of high-dose NSAIDs, Helicobacter pylori infection, use of antiplatelet agents, use of warfarin or other anticoagulant agents, corticosteroids, selective serotonin re-uptake inhibitors (SSRI), and alendronate (Langman 1994; Garcia Rodriguez 1994; Papatheodoridis, 2006; Huang, 2002). On the other hand, GI risk factors in patients receiving coxibs are not well defined, with a significant lack of data: only a previous history of peptic disease or ulcer bleeding, presence of *Helicobacter pylori* infection and concomitant assumption of antiplatelet agents are considered independent risk factors (Lanas, 2005).

In order to minimize NSAID-related events, evidence-based guidelines suggest to prescribe coxibs or a gastroprotective agent combined to a nsNSAID to high risk patients (Lanza, 2009).

The first drug registered as a gastroprotective agent, in patients receiving NSAID, was misoprostol, a PG analogue. Clinical studies assessed the efficacy of misoprostol in reducing the onset of gastroduodenal injuries in patients receiving chronic NSAIDs therapy; however, misoprostolis poorly tolerable. Effective doses of misoprostol induce dyspepsia and are often associated to development of diarrhea and abdominal pain/bloating while low doses do not induce side effects but are ineffective as gastroprotection (Lanza, 1989; Targownik, 2008).

Other recent and effective therapies were developed in order to reduce upper GI symptoms and prevent complications: histamine-2 receptor antagonists (H2RAs) and proton pump inhibitors (PPI) have both demonstrated efficacy in NSAID-related GI side effects (Hawkey, 2005; Hooper, 2004; Rostom, 2002; Scheiman, 2006).

During chronic NSAIDs therapy, a significant amount of patients present with dyspeptic symptoms; however, development of GI symptoms is not predictive for development of NSAID-related injury (gastropathy or ulcers). Moreover, about 60% of patients with endoscopic findings of NSAID-related injury do not present GI symptoms until bleeding or perforation occur. Finally, only 10% of NSAID-related injury become symptomatic for hemorrhage (Somerville, 1986).

Pathophysiology of NSAIDs peptic ulceration: Defense and injury mechanisms

Defense mechanisms

The gastroduodenal mucosa is continuously exposed to endogenous (HCl, pepsin and bile acids) and exogenous (drugs, alcohol and bacteria) noxious agents; therefore, upper GI tract is characterized by a complex biological defense system, in order to prevent and heal any injury.

Pre-epithelial, epithelial and post-epithelial defenses were together involved in this complex mechanism preventing mucosal injury and maintaining integrity. The *pre-epithelial defense* level consists of mucus and a bicarbonate barrier, secreted by upper GI epithelial cells. Mucus is composed by water (95%), lipids (fatty acids and phospholipids) and glycoproteins (mucin), and constitutes an hydrophobic layer preventing ions and molecules (eg. pepsine) passage. Bicarbonate, directly secreted into the mucus layer, forms a high pH gradient (6-7) able to neutralize lumen acidity even when pH falls below 2. The *epithelial defense* layer is constituted by a continuous layer of GI epithelial surface cells linked to each other by tight junctions, these complexes constitute an hydrophobic barrier limiting the diffusion of hydrogen ions and water-soluble agents through the mucosa; moreover, hydrogen ions that enter into the epithelial cells can be removed by basolateral ion pumps (i.e. Na^+/H^+ and a Cl^-/HCO_3^- exchanger). Minimal mucosal injury can be rapidly recovered thanks to the migration of the nearest healthy cells able to close the mucosal gap, a phenomenon known as *rapid restitution*. This event involves several growth factors such as *epidermal growth factor (EGF), transforming growth factor alpha (TGFa) and fibroblast growth factor (FGF)*. Rapid restitution involves only cell migration not cell division so that only minor mucosal defects can be healed; large peptic lesions requires cellular proliferation and neoangiogenesis *(regeneration)*. The rich vascular system that underlies the mucosa represents the *post-epithelial defense* mechanism. Blood flow continuously provides bicarbonate to neutralize the acids released and supplies nutrients and oxygen essential for cells metabolism while taking away all the toxic catabolites produced. (Malfertheiner, 2009; Laine, 2008).

GI injury occur when the caustic acid-peptic factors on gastrointestinal lumen overwhelm all three components of epithelial defense or when those mechanisms are impaired.

Injury mechanisms

NSAID-induced upper GI injury result from both topical damage and systemic effects mainly related to COX inhibition. *Topical injury* is a direct consequence of the chemical proprieties of these drugs. NSAIDs are weak acids that remain in non-ionized lipophilic form in the highly acid gastric environment. This condition promote the NSAIDs migration through the hydrophobic cell membrane into the cell where, because of the neutral pH, they get trapped inside in an ionized form (ion trapping). The resulting hydrogen ions are responsible of cellular toxicity; oxidative phosphorylation is compromised with impaired mithocondrial energy production, reduced cellular integrity and increased permeability. All these changes, lead to retrodiffusion of H+ and pepsin with consequent amplification of cellular toxicity (Sostres C., 2010).

Topical injury was once thought to be the main mechanism of NSAID-induced damage, but it is now clear that most of the NSAID-related gastrointestinal injuries come from their systemic effects; NSAID-related inhibition of GI mucosal cyclooxygenase, regardless of the drug administration modality, could lead to clinically significant GI toxicity.

Cyclooxigenase converts arachidonic acid into active prostaglandins (PGs); in humans (at least) two isozymes of COX were described, COX-1 and COX-2 (Wallace et al., 2000). These two isoforms present different characteristics of expression in human cells and substrates: COX-1 is almost ubiquitary and necessary for cellular homeostasis (gastric protection, vascular regulation, platelet aggregating effect and kidney function), while COX-2 is expressed in cells exposed to inflammatory signals (cytokines or chemokines) or growth factors.

Gastric cells COX-1 is the rate-limiting enzyme in PGs biosynthesis; these molecules guarantee the mucosal coating protection from the caustic action of acid and pepsin in many ways. First of all, PGs reduce gastric acid secretion and stimulate the production of glycoprotein (mucin), bicarbonate and phospholipid by epithelial cells. Moreover, PGs guarantee mucosal blood flow and oxygen delivery through vasodilatation, promote epithelial cells migration towards the luminal surface during restitution and finally enhance cells proliferation (Brzozowski, 2008; Sostres, 2010).

Most of nsNSAIDs inhibit both COX-1 and COX-2, leading to a strong impairment of gastric PG biosynthesis; therefore, in the last decades, research interest was focused on the development of new molecules with a COX-2 selective inhibitory effect, in order to obtain an effective anti-inflammatory effect and preserve PG-mediated gastrointestinal mucosal protection. (Malfertheiner, 2009; Laine, 2008).

First trials evaluating coxibs GI safety profile (Laine, 1999) were very promising; rofecoxib appeared to be safer than ibuprofen with a reported GI event rate similar to that observed in the placebo group.

However, the initial enthusiasm secondary to coxibs' GI safety was put in perspective because of the evidence of serious CV side effects (hypertension, edema, hearth failure and acute coronary syndrome) that, in some cases, brought to their withdrawal from the market (rofecoxib, precoxib and valdecoxib). Coxibs, when given at clinically effective doses, present a significantly reduced but still effective COX-1 inhibitory effect leading to a blockade of gastrointestinal mucosal COX-1-dependent PGs production: therefore, coxibs significantly reduce, but do not completely abolish, the risk of gastrointestinal events. Moreover, as observed with nsNSAIDs other than naproxen, coxibs increase CV risk because of their pro-aggregating action; the selective inhibition of COX-2 create a disequilibrium between endothelial synthesis of PGs (mostly COX-2 dependent) and the platelets TxA2 synthesis (COX-1 dependent), with relative increased activity of the latter (Antman, 2005). Coxibs are now strongly contraindicated in patients with CV disease (Abraham, 2010; Bhatt, 2008). Finally, the evidences that COX-2 is considerably expressed in the proliferating zone of gastric mucosa undergoing mucosal repair or regeneration during ulcer healing, suggest that COX-2, although being of lesser significance in resting conditions, possess a crucial role in processes of mucosal repair and ulcer healing (Brzozowski, 2008).

The impairment of mucosal microcirculation should be considered one of the most important mechanism of damage that results from NSAIDs consumption. It originate both from the PGs inhibited biosynthesis and, at the same time, from the phlogosis that brings to leukocytes recruitment, activation and endothelial-adherence. An answer to this key source of mucosal injury has been found in nitric oxide (NO). Thanks to NO vasodilatatory activity mucosal defense mechanisms, including mucus/alkaline secretion and inhibition of leukocytes activation, result enhanced. CINODs (COX-inhibiting NO-donating drugs), a new class of anti-inflammatory compounds putting its conceptual basis on the protective action of NO, appear to preserve their anti-inflammatory proprieties with a greater gastrointestinal safety (Brzozowski, 2008). Several CINODs are currently being tested in clinical trials, the most advanced of which regards naproxcinod (NO-naproxen, nitronaproxen) that is in phase III trials for the treatment of osteoarthritis.

Aspirin

Acetylsalicylic acid (ASA), the first molecule studied for its anti-inflammatory properties, presents various effects; the mechanisms underlying these effects appear to be related to the doses: low doses (< 80 mg/day) induce an acetylation of cyclooxygenase-1 in an irreversible way, leading to antithrombotic effect; medium doses (650 mg - 4 g/day) block prostaglandin production through an inhibition of both COX-1 and COX-2; higher doses (> 4g/day) induce an anti-inflammatory effect through both a cyclooxygenase-dependent and a COX-independent way (Lauer, 2002). Most of aspirin effects, like non-salicylate NSAIDs, are mediated by inhibition of cyclooxigenase active site of PGH2 (prostaglandin synthase H2).

Aspirin acts through an irreversible inhibition of both COX isoenzymes, impairing PG production. Inhibition of COX-1 is about 10-fold greater than COX-2 ones; on this basis, the dose necessary to achieve an anti-inflammatory effect is significantly higher than antiplatelet dose and GI toxic dose.

Moreover, aspirin inhibits (although not completely) the expression of iNOS (inducible Nitric Oxide Synthase) independently from COX-inhibition; this effect leads to an impaired production of nitric oxide, a molecule responsible for inflammatory response, host defenses and tissue healing process. This partial COX-independent suppression of NO production lead to a synergistic anti-inflammatory effect (coupled with COX inhibition) induced by ASA, but also to a synergistic GI toxic effect with both nsNSAIDs and coxibs.

Moreover, aspirin GI toxicity, is worsened by its topic injury due to the rapid absorption of this drug from the stomach (low PKa) that result in an enhanced local gastric toxicity.

Finally, the use of acetylsalicylic acid, even if prescribed at low doses, seems to abolish the GI safety profile of coxibs. Although the use of a COX-2 selective inhibitors could lead to a significant decrease in GI adverse events, when coxibs are prescribed together with aspirin the overall GI toxicity appear to be similar to that observed with standard NSAIDs (Silverstein, 2000).

Role of *Helicobacter pylori* infection

Although GI injury (peptic ulcers or erosive gastropathy) is the most frequently observed side effects in patients on chronic NSAIDs therapy, presence of *Hp* infection is the most common cause of peptic disease in patients not on NSAIDs therapy. It was estimated that chronic *Hp* infection was present in about 50% of the population worldwide; however, only a little amount of these patients (5-10%) will develop GI injuries. Risk factors for development of Hp-related peptic ulcers are not well understood; however, different histological pattern of gastritis, change in acid secretion, the presence of duodenal gastric metaplasia, ulcerogenic bacterial strains and host genetic factors are all involved. For example, the relative risk to present peptic ulceration is increased in patients infected by the CagA-positive bacterial strain (Pilotto, 1997; Covacci, 1993; Li, 1999; van Doorn, 1998; Garcia Rodriguez, 1994; Huang, 2002).

3. Management of NSAIDs therapy

In order to reduce the incidence of GI complications among patients receiving chronic NSAIDs therapy, various management strategies were developed (prevention strategy, identify and treat modifiable risk factors, use of gastroprotective agents, use of "low-risk" NSAIDs)

General prevention strategies

Prevention strategies have to be followed by all patients receiving long-term NSAIDs therapy; crucial point is to stratify patient's risk (both gastrointestinal and cardiovascular).

Some general rules have to be kept in mind by physicians who prescribe NSAIDs: use the "safer" NSAID at the lowest effective dose and for the shortest period of time (see Table 1 for relative GI toxicity of NSAIDs); when possible, prescribe anti-dolorific drugs other than NSAIDs (i.e. acetaminophen, tramadol or codeine). Avoid concomitant therapy, when possible, with antiplatelet agents, anticoagulants or corticosteroids; suggest to the patients to avoid physical (and psycological) stress and reduce (or avoid) smoke and/or alcohol assumption (Lanza et al., 2009).

Prescription of selective COX2 inhibitors

The anti-dolorific, anti-inflammatory and chemo-preventive effects of NSAIDs are mediated by inhibition of COX. The development of an NSAID selectiveely inhibiting the COX-2 isoform was reached in order to avoid NSAID-related GI toxicity. Coxibs appear to be 200 to 300-fold more selective for COX-2 than COX-1.

The active effects of coxibs are similar to those observed with nsNSAIDs but with a better GI safety profile (based on the reduced inhibition on COX-1 dependent prostaglandins secretion in upper GI tract). However, these benefits are balanced with the well reported increased CV risk observed in long-term users; the registration trials of coxibs (rofecoxib and

Drug	Dose	RR
Acetaminophen	< 2000 mg	1.2
	2000 – 3900 mg	1.2
	> 4000 mg	1.0
Ibuprofen	< 1200 mg	1.1
	1200 – 1799 mg	1.8
	> 1800 mg	4.6
Diclofenac	< 75 mg	2.2
	75 – 149 mg	3.2
	> 150 mg	12.2
Piroxicam	< 10 mg	9.0
	10 – 19 mg	12.0
	> 20 mg	79.0

Table 1. Dose-dependent risk for Upper GI bleeding (Acetaminophen and ns-NSAIDs)
Dose-dependent risk for Upper GI bleeding (Acetaminophen and ns-NSAIDs)

subsequently valdecoxib) reported an alarming increase of CV events (congestive heart failure, polmunary edema and myocardial infarction), leading to withdrawal from market of both drugs (Juni et al., 2004; Abraham et al., 2007).

Currently, this new drug generation accounts for about 33% prescription (60% of the relative healthcare expenditure). Initially, a completely safe profile of coxibs was speculated based on preclinical and clinical trial, even for high risk patients (Skelly and Hawkey, 2002). However, these benefit effects were initially demonstrated only in patients without GI risk factors. The incidence of GI events in patients with one or more risk factors was similar in those receiving coxibs or nsNSAIDs (Silverstein et al., 2000; Bombardier et al., 2000; Skelly and Hawkey, 2002; Farkouh et al., 2004).

Clinical trials demonstrated that coxibs have a reduced relative risk of development of peptic ulcers and other GI complications (Hooper et al.,2004); in fact, a significant reduction in ulcers found on endoscopy studies (about 4-fold reduction) was observed (FitzGerald and Patrono, 2001),. High doses of coxibs (rofecocix or celecoxib) allow an approximately 50% reduction in the incidence of GI injury when compared to nsNSAIDs (Bombardier et al., 2000). Coxibs present a reduced but not abolished GI toxicity when compared to nsNSAIDs. For example, patients receiving Rofecoxib present an increased risk for peptic ulcer bleeding when compared to patients receiving placebo (0.88 vs. 0.18 clinically significant events registered/year; relative risk 4.9) (Lanas et al., 2007).

Moreover, coxibs do not show advantages over nsNSAIDs in healing ulcers in patients with recent bleeding, because they inhibit the natural healing process of peptic ulcers (Perini et al., 2003).

In addition, clinical evidences showed that all GI benefits of coxibs disappear in patients receiving also low-dose aspirin (i.e. for CV primary prevention) (Schnitzer et al., 2004; Farkouh et al., 2004). Moreover, when coxibs are used in combination to antiplatelet agents other than low-dose aspirin (i.e. clopidogrel and ticlopidine), the relative risk of upper GI bleeding was similar to patients receiving aspirin alone or nsNSAIDs. Finally, the combination of coxibs to low dose aspirin appears to attenuate its CV protective effects.

Recently, a large prospective trial, was conducted in order to assess the safety profile of celecoxib compared to a combination regimen of a non-selective NSAID plus PPI (omeprazole plus diclofenac) (Chan et al., 2010); results of this randomized controlled trial, enrolling more than 4400 patients, demonstrated a reduced risk of GI adverse events of COX-2 selective treatment when compared to a nsNSAID plus a PPI regimen.

Based on clinical trial experience (Chan et al., 2007), co-therapy with coxibs plus PPIs could be considered in those patients with exceptionally high risk of peptic ulcer disease (eg recent NSAID-related ulcer bleeding) in order to significantly reduce the risk of development of GI injury or re-bleeding.

In conclusion, use of coxibs is a valuable strategy to minimize upper GI events; however, because of the increased CV risk and the reduced GI benefit in patients receiving antiplatelet agents, the use of these drugs have to be carefully evaluated in some high-risk categories of patients (i.e. older patients on low-dose aspirin regimen for primary CV prevention, patients with previous CV events or with CV risk factors, etc.); for a detailed discussion, see the specific section in this chapter.

Clear indications for COX-2 selective inhibitors prescription are (Lanza et al., 2009; Jawad, 2001):

- Prolonged use of nsNSAIDs at the highest dose
- Age > 65 years
- Previous history of peptic ulcer disease
- Co-treatment with corticosteroids or anticoagulants

Prescription of gastroprotective agents

The understanding of mechanisms underlying the pathogenesis of peptic ulcer disease lead, in the last decades, to significant development in gastroprotective treatments:

- Prostaglandin analogues (misoprostol) were demonstrated effective in prevention of NSAID-induced ulcers (while no role in healing ulcers was demonstrated)
- Anti-secretory drugs (H2RAs and PPIs) demonstrated their pivotal role in peptic ulcers disease preventing, healing and maintaining of remission
- Antacids, like sucralfate and bismuth salts have no proven efficacy in healing NSAID-related peptic ulcer
- Antibiotic therapy and bismuth-containing compounds were recognized as indicated in patients with HP-positive ulcer disease (even if related to NSAIDs)

Prostaglandins (PG) inhibit histamine-induced cAMP generation in parietal cells, leading to a significant reduction in acid secretion. Prostaglandin analogues are indicated mostly for the prevention of NSAID-related GI injury because there are no clearly demonstrated effect on ulcer healing. The only available PG analogue registered for NSAID-related peptic ulcer disease is misoprostol (Donnely et al., 2000; Silverstein et al., 2005). However, the use of misoprostol is limited by its low tolerability. PG analogues, in a dose-dependent manner, induce diarrhea associated to abdominal pain and bloating; in order to minimize these side effects, misoprostol should be started at the lowest dose (100 mcg x 3 daily) and, if tolerated, increased to 800mcg/day.

H2RAs (i.e. ranitidine, cimetidine) induce acid suppression through the blockade of histamine H2 receptors in gastric parietal cells, while *PPIs* (i.e. omeprazole, lansoprazole, esomeprazole, pantoprazole and rabeprazole) act on the H+/K+ ATPase pump, localized on parietal cell lumen inducing an irreversible inhibition (Kitchingman et al., 1989).

PPIs appear to be more effective in preventing and healing NSAID-related ulcers (better duodenal than gastric ones) than high-doses of H2RAs because of the long-lasting inhibition of parietal cells acid secretion (standard H2RA doses are not effective in preventing GI injury) (Taha et al., 1996). Moreover, H2RA treatment could be "complicated" by phenomenon of tolerance which is not always observed, but could significantly reduce H2RA-induced acid suppression. Although the tolerance phenomenon is not observed in patients receiving PPIs, a rapid metabolization in some patients (rapid acetylators) may reduce PPI efficacy. Therefore, standard PPI therapy may sometimes not be sufficient to heal ulcers or treat NSAID-relate dyspepsia and in those cases an higher dose or a different PPI may be needed.

Finally, on the basis of the incomplete gastroprotective effect of H2RAs and the significant reduction in PPIs' cost, there is no reason to prescribe H2RAs for gastroprotection in patients receiving chronic NSAID therapy; since H2RAs could mask warning symptoms of peptic ulcer disease (Singh and Rosen Ramey, 1998) their use should be limited to patients with NSAID-related dyspepsia unresponsive to PPI and with a negative upper GI endoscopy.

Table 2 summarizes key-points regarding PPI gastroprotective effects.

Evidences on PPI gastroprotection
- reduced risk of NSAID-related upper GI injuries
- effective in preventing ulcer complications
- strongly recommended in patients with high GI risk
- comparable to coxibs in high-risk patients
- superior to Coxibs in reducing and preventing NSAID-related dyspepsia
- effective in prevention of upper GI events in patients receiving antiplatelet agents
- effective in healing and preventing upper GI ulcers in patients on chronic NSAID therapy

Table 2. Evidences on PPI gastroprotection

Antacids (containing aluminium or magnesium) are not clearly effective in preventing or healing NSAID-related ulcers and their potential healing mechanism appear to be unrelated to acid inhibition (i.e. promotion of angiogenesis, binding bile acids, suppressing *Hp* growth): *sucralfate* increase angiogenesis and tissue repair leading to prevention of mucosal injury; *bismuth salts* act through the inhibition of peptic activity.

4. Management of specific populations

Management strategies are designed to reduce the incidence of GI complications and take into account patient's overall risk and specific NSAID-related risk factors. Most guidelines describe specific strategies for high-risk categories of patients; designed to significantly reduce side effects (both general and gastrointestinal) and the number needed to treat (NNT) to achieve the endpoints (reduction in GI events). These strategies often involve the prescription of a gastroprotecive agent (PPIs), reduction of nsNSAIDs dose and the change to selective COX-2 inhibitors.

Management of low-risk patients

Most guidelines do not suggest gastroprotective strategies for low-risk patients. Physicians prescribing NSAIDs to low-risk patients (less than 65 years, no comorbidity, no concomitant antiplatelet, anticoagulants or corticosteroids and no previous history of NSAID-related GI complications) should follow the general suggestions for GI complications reduction (eg. prescribe the lowest effective dose and avoid drugs with high GI toxicity).

However, even in patients without risk factors, two clinical trials demonstrated a significant reduction of GI events (detection of asymptomatic ulceration and bleeding) in patients receiving coxibs compared to those on nsNSAIDs (Bombardier et al., 2000; Silverstein et al., 2000); these evidences suggest that the low-risk category of patients could become a "no-risk" one, if well managed.

Patient with history of peptic ulcer disease

Epidemiological and retrospective studies identified a past episode of peptic ulcer as a risk factor for development of GI events in patients receiving chronic NSAID therapy; moreover, both *Hp* positive and negative patients present an increased relative risk of complications (Rockal et al., 1995). In order to reduce the risk of GI injury, the switch to a coxib was evaluated in patients with a past history of ulcer disease; both rofecoxib and celecoxib demonstrated their efficacy in reduction of GI events (from 8.8/100 patient/year with non selective NSAID to 2 with rofecoxib) (Laine, 2001). Therefore, in patients with a previous history of peptic ulcer disease, the switch to a selective COX-2 inhibitor could be considered a practical and cost-effective strategy.

Although switching to a coxib induces a significant risk reduction, in these patients there is still a high residual risk of development of GI complications (10 events per 100 patients treated/year in VIGOR study) (Bombardier et al., 2000). In this setting, the combination therapy of a PPI to a standard NSAID appears to be more appropriate than a coxib alone; clinical studies demonstrated that combination with omeprazole induces a significant reduction in ulcer development both in patients with previous ulceration and perforation when compared to patients receiving a COX-2 selective inhibitors (rofecoxib) or monotherapy with ns-NSAID (ibuprofen) [Cullen et al., 1998; Hawkey et al., 1998). After this first evidence, PPIs other than omeprazole (both lansoprazole, pantoprazole and esomeprazole) demonstrated a similar efficacy (Yeomans et al., 1998; Hawkey et al., 1998; Agrawal et al., 2000) in preventing NSAID-related bleeding (a mean reduction of at least four-fould).

Subsequently, in patients with previous GI complications, usually considered to be at exceptionally high risk of GI events, a combined treatment of a coxib with a PPI was proposed in order to reduce GI toxicity. This strategy was evaluated in a RCT comparing the combination therapy of celecoxib plus PPI to celecoxib plus placebo in *Hp* negative patients who presented an upper GI bleeding. The addiction of a PPI to a COX-2 selective inhibitor

was demonstrated effective for prevention of ulcer re-bleeding (13-month incidence of 0%
vs. 8.9% in patients treated with celecoxib alone) and considered the best treatment
management in the very high risk group of patients (Chan et al., 2007).

Patients requiring high-doses NSAIDs

When physicians have to prescribe high NSAID doses, there is a significant increase in the
relative risk of development of GI complications (about three-fold).(Henry et al., 1996;
Langman et al., 1994). In those cases, pharmacological and clinical evidences demonstrated
that coxibs are safer than nsNSAIDs with a similar anti-inflammatory and analgesic effects.
However, high-doses of coxibs show an overall increased risk of adverse events (both CV
and related to fluid retention) and this should be taken into account in each single case to
balance the risk/benefit ratio..

Helicobacter pylori positive

Large population-based studies and meta-analysis demonstrated that *Hp* infection induce a
two-fold increase in the risk of developing peptic complications in patients receiving
NSAIDs (Chan et al., 2002; Vergara et al., 2005). Moreover, also in patients receiving coxibs,
H pylori remain a risk factor for development of GI ulcers and bleeding (Bombardier et al.,
2000). Systematic reviews and meta-analysis (Chan, 1997; Chan 2002; Vergara 2005)
confirmed the efficacy of *Hp* eradication in preventing upper GI complications in patients on
chronic NSAIDs therapy, even though treating *Helicobacter pylori* does not completely
abolish the risk of bleeding in high risk patients (Chan, 2001). Therefore, even though it is
often underestimated in general clinical practice, a test-and-treat strategy is mandatory in
patients who require long-term NSAIDs therapy (Gabriel, 1991; Wolfe, 1999; Sauerbaum,
2002; Barkin, 1998; Laine, 2002; Chan, 2002; Laine, 1992; Hawkey, 1998; Loeb, 1992;
Aalykke,.1999; Cullen, 1997).

Patients on corticosteroids

Corticosteroids have a synergistic effect with NSAID, magnifying their GI toxicity, and an
intrinsic gastrolesive potential effect, specially in patients with multiple concurrent diseases;
the risk of ulcer development is increased both in patients receiving NSAIDs and in non-
NSAID users. A correct strategy, for the management of patients who need both
corticosteroids and NSAIDs was suggested by post-hoc analysis of large clinical trials,
showing that prescription of coxibs seems to reduce the risk of GI complications.

When prescribing NSAIDs to patients requiring high-doses of corticosteroids, a
management strategy able to guarantee a reduced GI risk seems to be the choice of a coxib
coupled by gastroprotection with a PPI; however, specific data in this setting are lacking
(Holvoet et al., 1991; Hochain et al., 1995; Laine et al., 2010; Weil et al., 2000).

Use of anticoagulant agents or patients affected by coagulopathy

Co-prescription of anticoagulants and NSAIDs induce a significant increase in GI events and
bleeding (both clinically manifest and occult); consequently, in these patients NSAID
prescription should be considered a contraindication. Although there is a lack of specific
data, in those patients when necessary, the co-prescription of a selective COX-2 inhibitor
plus a PPI have to be considered in order to reduce the high risk of bleeding and the high
morbidity and mortality that goes with it.

5. Management of NSAID prescription and gastroprotective strategies in patients with both CV and GI risk factors

The greatest intellectual and clinical challenge in the area of NSAID-induced GI injury is the management of patients with both gastrointestinal and cardiovascular disease; a tight correlation between GI bleeding and CV disease (and related treatment) is well recognized (Hallas et al., 2006). Most of these events appear to be related to antiplatelet and/or anticoagulant agents prescribed in those patients (Pearson et al., 2002; McQuaid and Laine, 2006; Derry and Loke, 2000; Peters et al., 2003). Even though, in epidemiologic studies, presence of CV disease appear to be an independent risk factor for ulcer bleeding, not related to aspirin and anticoagulant agents use (Weil et al., 2000).

For a complete discussion of the pathogenesis of NSAID-related (including aspirin) GI injury see specific section of this chapter. However, both NSAIDs and ASA through topic and systemic effects induce mucosal injury.

Clopidogrel, through a specific inhibition of platelet aggregation, play a pivotal role in impairment of ulcer healing process; in fact, platelet aggregation and angiogenesis are both critical for healing of GI injuries. Therefore, even if clopidogrel may not be the primary cause of gastroduodenal injury, its related impairment of mucosal healing and angiogenesis could lead to clinically significant ulceration in the presence of other co-factors (eg. excessive acid exposure, other drugs or *Hp*) (Ma et al., 2001).

Patients with CV co-morbidities, requiring NSAIDs for their anti-inflammatory or analgesic effects (i.e. rheumatoid arthritis, muscle-skeletal disease, etc.) present an increased GI risk and are exposed to an increased rate of systemic hypertension secondary to NSAIDs or coxibs use (Lanas et al., 2000; Antman, 2005). The management of these patients is based on the assessment of the risk/benefit ratio of every drug prescribed. In patients on secondary prophylaxis for myocardial infarction or cerebrovascular event, prescription of antiplatelet agents (aspirin or clopidogrel or both) is mandatory and also some high-risk CV patients would benefit from a low-dose aspirin prophylaxis; in such cases, especially in those with GI risk factors, the prescription of a gastroprotective agent appear to be useful and effective in reducing adverse events.

It has be kept in mind that, coxibs and nsNSAIDs might be associated with an increased risk of acute cardiovascular events, and that co-administration of an NSAID (ibuprofen) and aspirin reduce the antiplatelet effects and consequently the prophylactic efficacy. Data are lacking about the consequences of co-administration of coxibs and aspirin on cardioprotection.

Finally, in this setting, presence of CV co-morbidities or assumption of prophylactic low-dose aspirin should be considered a contraindication for NSAIDs prescription; in those case in which appear necessary, general prescription strategies designed to reduce the adverse events rate have to be kept in mind (see specific section in this chapter).

Gastroprotective strategies in patients with CV disease

When a physician approaches a patient who need NSAID therapy with CV and GI disease, there are some considerations to take in mind in order to reduce adverse events related to co-morbidities:

- Aspirin induce a 2- to 4-fold increase in risk of development of GI injury with a dose-dependent effect; therefore <80 mg/day should be preferred coupled to gastroprotection.
- When prescription of low dose of aspirin is associated to NSAIDs a gastroprotective strategy should be offered.
- PPIs are demonstrated as the most effective gastroprotective agents in patients receiving both NSAIDs and aspirin (Lai et al., 2002)
- When aspirin or clopidogrel (or both) are prescribed together with anticoagulant agents (heparin, fractionated heparin or oral anticoagulant) a significant increase in upper GI bleeding risk is observed. Combination of antiplatelet and anticoagulant agent must be prescribed only with a clear indication (vascular, valvular or arrhythmic). In order to reduce the overall bleeding risk (both extracranial and intracranial) when warfarin is co-administered to aspirin, INR must be < 2.5 (Andreotti et al., 2006; Zhurram et al., 2006).
- In high-risk patients, ASA and non-ASA antiplatelet agents (ticlopidine and clopidogrel) present similar bleeding risk, therefore, switching aspirin to clopidogrel do not reduce GI events (Chan et al., 2005).

Gastroprotective strategies in patients receiving clopidogrel

Dual anti-platelet therapy (low-dose aspirin plus clopidogrel), prescribed to patients for secondary prevention of acute coronary syndrome or undergoing coronary stent implantation, is effective in preventing stent thrombosis and reducing the risk of re-infarction, but significantly increase the risk of GI bleeding. The relative risk increase to about 2.5-fold in patients receiving clopidogrel or ASA, when compared to patients not on antiplatelet agents (Ibanez et al., 2006; van Hecken et al., 1998; Delaney et al., 2007). Use of clopidogrel in aspirin-taking patients synergistically increase the risk of bleeding (2- to 3-fold) and the mean blood loss in case of haemorrhage (Yusuf et al., 2001; Connoly et al., 2009). Dual antiplatelet agents are not indicated for CV primary prevention because of the observed low reduction in CV events and significant increase in severe GI bleeding.

Clopidogrel, as discussed above, does not induce ulceration of upper GI tract, but impairs natural healing process (through inhibition of platelet attivation and aggregation) and increases bleeding from preexisting lesions (induced by other causes). As in NSAID-related GI bleeding, acid suppression could favors the healing process and stabilization of thrombi thereby reducing the rate of complications from upper GI injury (Ma et al., 2001).

Acid suppressive therapy (both H2RAs and PPIs) demonstrated its efficacy in reduction of bleeding risk related to antiplatelet therapy. H2RAs appear to be able to reduce the rate of GI adverse events in patients receiving low-dose aspirin (3.8% in famotidine-receivers vs. 23.5% of placebo ones) (Taha et al., 2009) while no reduction was found in those treated with clopidogrel (Lanas et al., 2007). PPIs resulted to be more effective than H2RAs in reducing upper GI events in a cohort of patients receiving both aspirin and clopidogrel (OR:0.04 of PPI-receiving vs 0.43 of H2RA-receiving) (Ng et al., 2008).

After the evidence of the positive effects of PPI prescription in reducing GI adverse events among clopidogrel-receiving patients, some observational studies suggested the presence of a possible interaction between clopidogrel and PPI determining a reduced antiplatelet effect (Ho et al., 2009; Juurlink et al., 2009). Moreover, in vitro studies (assessing platelet activation/activity as a surrogate marker of antiplatelet effect) confirmed this hypothesis of interaction.

Clopidogrel and PPIs (mostly omeprazole) share a common metabolic pathway: clopidogrel is a pro-drug, whose bioavailability is dependent from intestinal absorption (ABCB1-dependent) and liver metabolism (through cytochrome P-450 pathway). Clopidogrel 2-step activation in the liver is secondary to CYP2C19 and CYP3A activity. Most of the PPIs available (omeprazole, lansoprazole and rabeprazole) share the same hepatic pathway through CYP2C19 (Li et al., 2004). Among PPIs, pantoprazole is the only that do not significantly inhibit hepatic CYP2C19 at therapeutic doses, because it is mostly metabolized through CYP3A4 pathway, while the other PPIs available present a lower interaction with this isoenzyme (Ishizaki and Horay, 1999).

Co-prescription of clopidogrel and PPIs may result in a competition of CYP2C19 metabolism, with reduced transformation of clopidogrel in its active form (Roden and Stein, 2009). This hypothesized impairment was additionally supported by the finding of genetic polymorphisms associated in CYP2C19 activity (Mega et al., 2009; Singh et al. 2010; Ma et al., 2010; Tiroch et al., 2010) and with a reduced antiplatelet activity and a worse clinical outcome (CV adverse events and re-infarction). Early clinical prospective studies in humans demonstrated a negative effect of omeprazole on surrogate clinical endpoints (ex vivo platelet assay, vasodilatator-stimulated phosphoprotein VASP) while other PPIs (pantoprazole and esomeprazole) did not (Gilard et al., 2008; Cuisset et al., 2009; O'Donoghue et al., 2009; Siller-Matula et al., 2009).

Based on conflicting data emerging from observational studies biased by non uniform prescription behaviours (eg. PPIs could be prescribed mainly to high-risk patients), a randomized controlled trial was designed enrolling patients receiving both aspirin and clopidogrel in order to evaluate the CV safety profile of omeprazole, the COGENT study (Bhatt et al., 2010). The results of this trial, enrolling 3761 patients who had acute coronary syndrome or underwent coronary stent placement, did not found any different CV outcome (myocardial infarction, stroke, coronary artery bypass graft or CV death) in patients receiving omeprazole when compared to those receiving placebo (Hazard Risk: 0.99), while confirming a reduced risk of GI adverse events (Hazard risk: 0.34). However, this strong evidence is limited by the premature closure of this trial (both enrollment and follow-up) due to bankrupt of the sponsorship, significantly limiting the power of the conclusion.

Keypoint I - Difference between PPIs in clopidogrel-receiving patients:

Retrospective studies showed, in some cases, an overall increased CV toxicity (Rassen et al., 2009; Ho et al., 2009; Laine and Hennekens, 2010; Ray, 2010) while others identified specific molecule-related effects (i.e. an increased risk for pantoprazole in nested case-control retrospective study of Stockl et al., 2010). On the opposite, a population-based study (Juurlink et al., 2009) identified an increased CV risk for all patients receiving PPIs other than pantoprazole. Finally, the only prospective evidence available did not identify an increased risk for omeprazole (Bhatt et al., 2010). However, no prospective trial (either published or ongoing) compared the clinical events related to different PPIs in patients receiving dual antiplatelet therapy. Therefore, guidelines do not suggest any recommendation for a specific molecule (Abraham et al., 2010).

Keypoint II – Timing and dosing:

Pharmacokinetic and pharmacodynamic properties of both these drug classes suggest a reduced interaction if the two administrations were separated from at least 12 hours (both PPI and clopidogrel present a plasma half-life of less than 2 hours). However, only a prospective trial tested this hypothesis, using a surrogate end-point (platelet aggregation). Further studies, evaluating the clinical outcome, are necessary to corroborate this result. Until now, there is no clinical study evaluating different PPI doses.

In conclusion, even if some observational retrospective studies suggested a small increase (relative risk <2) in CV adverse events, large, prospective, controlled trial are necessary to validate this finding. Finally, although interrupted before the designed conclusion of enrollment and follow-up, the only prospective RCT available suggest a non-increased CV risk in patients receiving omeprazole plus dual antiplatelet therapy (Bhatt et al., 2010).

In all patients, especially in those with both CV and GI risk factors, prescription of NSAIDs, antiplatelet agents and gastroprotection must be based on an accurate risk/benefit analysis. Antiplatelet agents are necessary in patients with CV co-morbidities, specially in those with prior acute coronary syndrome or with a recent stent placement; however, prescription of aspirin, clopidogrel or both is associated with an increased risk of GI bleeding.

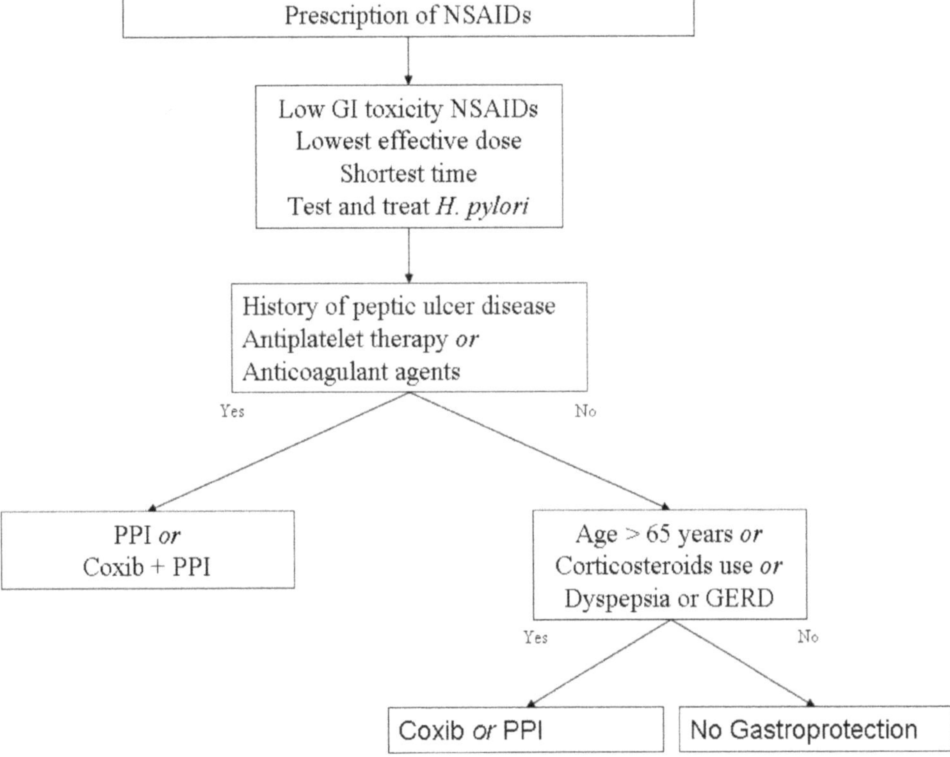

Fig. 1. Suggested management strategy in order to minimize upper GI adverse events in patients receiving chronic NSAIDs therapy.

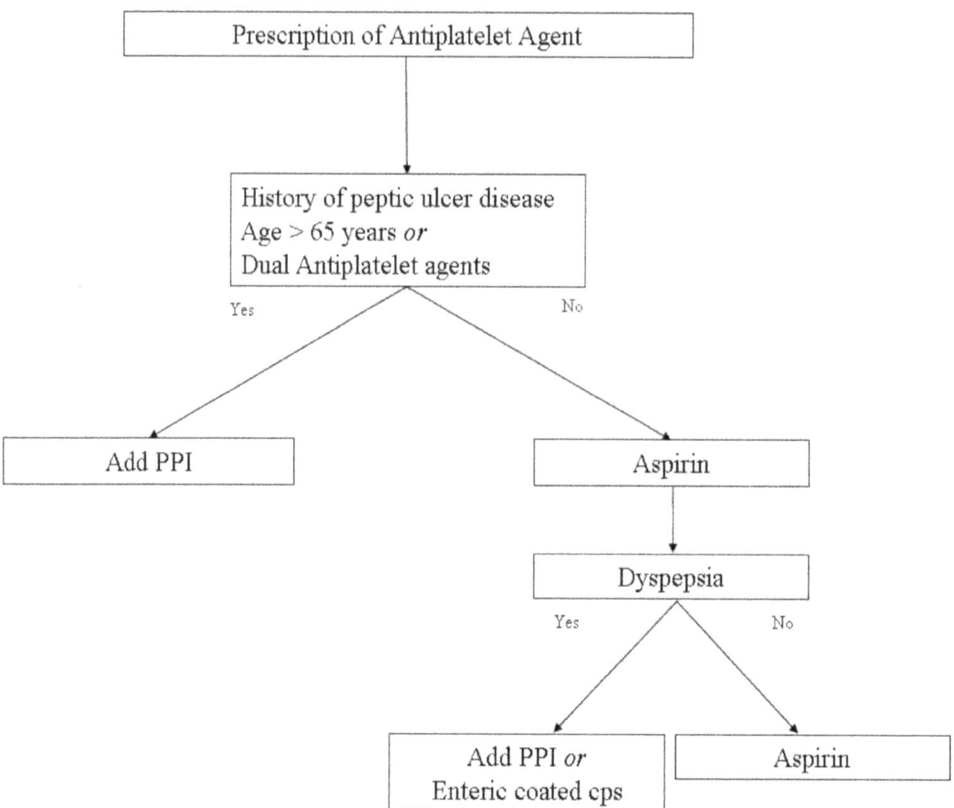

Fig. 2. Suggested management strategy in order to minimize upper GI adverse events in patients receiving antiplatelet agents.

The need of a gastroprotection must be evaluated on the basis of GI risk factors. High risk patients require gastroprotection with PPIs, while low risk population receives only a small benefit from PPIs prescription; in this setting, the increased risk of CV adverse events, related to the possible interaction between PPI and clopidogrel, suggest the use of antiplatelet therapy without gastroprotection.

PPIs are demonstrated to be more effective than H2RAs (Ng et al., 2010); however, although to a minor extent, H2RAs (other than cimetidine, because of its hepatic metabolism through CYP2C19) appear to be an alternative option in decreasing risk of gastric and duodenal ulcers (also among antiplatelet-receiving patients) (Lin et al., 2011). H2RAs, because of the low cost and low interaction, could be a good choice in patients with low risk for GI bleeding presenting peptic symptoms or NSAID-related dyspepsia.

6. List of abbreviations

NSAIDs, Non-Steroidal Anti-Inflammatory Drugs; COX, Cyclooxygenase; GI, GastroIntestinal; CV, CardioVascular; Coxib, selective COX2 inhibitor; *Hp, Helicobacter Pylori*; H2RA, histamine-2 receptor antagonist; PPI, proton pump inhibitor; HCl,

Hydrochloric Acid; PG, Prostaglandin; nsNSAID, non-selective NSAID; NO, Nitric Oxide;
TxA2, Thrombooxane A2; CINOD, COX-inhibiting NO-donating drug; ASA, Acetylsalicylic
Acid.

7. References

Aalykke C, Lauritsen JM, Hallas J, et al. *Helicobacter pylori* and risk of ulcer bleeding among
    users of nonsteroidal anti-inflammatory drugs: a case-control study.
    Gastroenterology. 1999;116:1305–1309.

Abraham NS, El-Serag HB, Johnson ML, Hartman C, Richardson P, Ray WA, Smalley
    W.National adherence to evidence-based guidelines for the prescription of
    nonsteroidal anti-inflammatory drugs. Gastroenterology. 2005 Oct;129(4):1171-8.

Abraham NS, El-Serag HB, Hartman C, Richardson P, Deswal A. Cyclooxygenase-2
    selectivity of non-steroidal anti-inflammatory drugs and the risk of myocardial
    infarction and cerebrovascular accident. Aliment Pharmacol Ther. 2007;25:913–24.

Abraham NS, Hlatky MA, Antman EM, Bhatt DL, Bjorkman DJ, Clark CB, Furberg CD,
    Johnson DA, Kahi CJ, Laine L, Mahaffey KW, Quigley EM, Scheiman J, Sperling LS,
    Tomaselli GF; ACCF/ACG/AHA. ACCF/ACG/AHA 2010 Expert Consensus
    Document on the concomitant use of proton pump inhibitors and thienopyridines:
    a focused update of the ACCF/ACG/AHA 2008 expert consensus document on
    reducing the gastrointestinal risks of antiplatelet therapy and NSAID use: a report
    of the American College of Cardiology Foundation Task Force on Expert
    Consensus Documents. Circulation. 2010 Dec 14;122(24):2619-33.

Agrawal NM, Campbell DR, Safdi MA, *et al.* Superiority of lansoprazole vs ranitidine in
    healing nonsteroidal anti-inflammatory drug-associated gastric ulcers: results of a
    double-blind, randomized, multicenter study. NSAID-Associated Gastric Ulcer
    Study Group. *Arch Intern Med* 2000;160:1455–61

Andreotti F, Testa L, Biondi-Zoccai GG, Crea F. Aspirin plus warfarin compared to aspirin
    alone after acute coronary syndromes: an updated and comprehensive meta-
    analysis of 25,307 patients. Eur Heart J. 2006;27:519 –26

Anon. Recommendations for the medical management of osteoarthritis of the hip and knee:
    2000 update. American College of Rheumatology Subcommittee on Osteoarthritis
    Guidelines. Arthritis Rheum 2000;43:1905-15.

Antman EM, DeMets D, Loscalzo J. Cyclooxygenase inhibition and cardiovascular risk.
    Circulation. 2005 Aug 2;112(5):759-70.

Barkin J. The relation between *Helicobacter pylori* and nonsteroidal anti-inflammatory drugs.
    Am J Med. 1998;105(suppl):22S–27S.

Bhatt DL, Scheiman J, Abraham NS, Antman EM, Chan FK, Furberg CD, Johnson DA,
    Mahaffey KW, Quigley EM; American College of Cardiology Foundation Task
    Force on Clinical Expert Consensus Documents. ACCF/ACG/AHA 2008 expert
    consensus document on reducing the gastrointestinal risks of antiplatelet therapy
    and NSAID use: a report of the American College of Cardiology Foundation Task
    Force on Clinical Expert Consensus Documents. Circulation. 2008 Oct
    28;118(18):1894-909.

Bhatt DL, Cryer BL, Contant CF, Cohen M, Lanas A, Schnitzer TJ, Shook TL, Lapuerta P, Goldsmith MA, Laine L, Scirica BM, Murphy SA, Cannon CP; COGENT Investigators. Clopidogrel with or without omeprazole in coronary artery disease. N Engl J Med. 2010 Nov 11;363(20):1909-17.

Bombardier C, Laine L, Reicin A, Shapiro D, Burgos-Vargas R, Davis B, Day R, Ferraz MB, Hawkey CJ, Hochberg MC, Kvien TK, Schnitzer TJ; VIGOR Study Group. Comparison of upper gastrointestinal toxicity of rofecoxib and naproxen in patients with rheumatoid arthritis. VIGOR Study Group. N Engl J Med. 2000 Nov 23;343(21):1520-8.

Brzozowski T, Konturek PC, Pajdo R, Ptak-Belowska A, Kwiecien S, Pawlik M, Drozdowicz D, Sliwowski Z, Brzozowski B, Konturek SJ, Pawlik WW. Physiological mediators in nonsteroidal anti-inflammatory drugs (NSAIDs)-induced impairment of gastric mucosal defense and adaptation. Focus on nitric oxide and lipoxins. J Physiol Pharmacol. 2008 Aug;59 Suppl 2:89-102.

Chan FKL, Sung JJY, Chung SCS, et al. Randomised trial of eradication of Helicobacter pylori before non-steroidal antiinflammatory drug therapy to prevent peptic ulcers. Lancet 1997; 350: 975–79.

Chan FK, Chung SC, Suen BY, et al. Preventing recurrent upper gastrointestinal bleeding in patients with *Helicobacter pylori* infection who are taking low-dose aspirin or naproxen. *N Engl J Med* 2001; 344: 967–73

Chan FKL, To KF, Wu JCY, et al. Eradication of *Helicobacter pylori* and risk of peptic ulcers in patients starting long-term treatment with non-steroidal anti-inflammatory drugs: a randomised trial. Lancet 2002; 359: 9–13.

Chan FK. *Helicobacter pylori*, NSAIDs and gastrointestinal haemorrhage. *Eur J Gastroenterol Hepatol.* 2002;14:1–3.

Chan FK, Ching JY, Hung LC, et al. Clopidogrel versus aspirin and esomeprazole to prevent recurrent ulcer bleeding. N Engl J Med. 2005;352:238–44.

Chan FK, Lanas A, Scheiman J, Berger MF, Nguyen H, Goldstein JL. Celecoxib versus omeprazole and diclofenac in patients with osteoarthritis and rheumatoid arthritis (CONDOR): a randomised trial. Lancet. 2010 Jul 17;376(9736):173-9

Clinard F, Bardou M, Sgro C, Lefevre N, Raphael F, Paille F, et al. Non-steroidal antiinflammatory and cytoprotective drug co-prescription in general practice. Eur J Clin Pharmacol. 2001;57:737–43.

Connolly SJ, Pogue J, Hart RG, Hohnloser SH, Pfeffer M, Chrolavicius S, Yusuf S, ACTIVE Investigators. Effect of clopidogrel added to aspirin in patients with atrial fibrillation. N Engl J Med. 2009 May 14;360(20):2066-78.

Covacci A, Censini S, Bugnoli M, et al. Molecular characterization of the 128-kDa immunodominant antigen of *Helicobacter pylori* associated with cytotoxicity and duodenal ulcer. *Proc Natl Acad Sci USA.* 1993;90:5791–5795.

Cuisset T, Frere C, Quilici J, Poyet R, Gaborit B, Bali L, Brissy O, Morange PE, Alessi MC, Bonnet JL. Comparison of omeprazole and pantoprazole influence on a high 150-mg clopidogrel maintenance dose the PACA (Proton Pump Inhibitors And Clopidogrel Association) prospective randomized study. J Am Coll Cardiol. 2009 Sep 22;54(13):1149-53.

Cullen DJ, HawkeyGM,Greenwood DC, et al. Peptic ulcer bleeding in the elderly: relative roles of *Helicobacter pylori* and non-steroidal anti-inflammatory drugs. *Gut.* 1997;41:459–462.

Cullen D, Bardhan KD, Eisner M, *et al.* Primary gastroduodenal prophylaxis with omeprazole for non-steroidal anti-inflammatory drug users. *Aliment Pharmacol Ther* 1998;12:135–40

Delaney JA, Opatrny L, Brophy JM, et al. Drug-drug interactions between antithrombotic medications and the risk of gastrointestinal bleeding. CMAJ 2007;177:347–351.

Derry S, Loke YK. Risk of gastrointestinal haemorrhage with long term use of aspirin: meta-analysis. BMJ. 2000;321:1183–7.

Din FV, Theodoratou E, Farrington SM, Tenesa A, Barnetson RA, Cetnarskyj R, Stark L, Porteous ME, Campbell H, Dunlop MG. Effect of aspirin and NSAIDs on risk and survival from colorectal cancer. Gut. 2010 Dec;59(12):1670-9

Donnelly MT, Goddard AF, Filipowicz B, Morant SV, Shield MJ, Hawkey CJ. Low-dose misoprostol for the prevention of low-dose aspirin-induced gastroduodenal injury. Aliment Pharmacol Ther. 2000; 14:529 –34.

Elwood PC, Gallagher AM, Duthie GG, Mur LA, Morgan G. Aspirin, salicylates, and cancer. Lancet. 2009 Apr 11;373(9671):1301-9

Farkouh ME, Kirshner H, Harrington RA, Ruland S, Verheugt FW, Schnitzer TJ, Burmester GR, Mysler E, Hochberg MC, Doherty M, Ehrsam E, Gitton X, Krammer G, Mellein B, Gimona A, Matchaba P, Hawkey CJ, Chesebro JH; TARGET Study Group. Comparison of lumiracoxib with naproxen and ibuprofen in the Therapeutic Arthritis Research and Gastrointestinal Event Trial (TARGET), cardiovascular outcomes: randomised controlled trial. Lancet. 2004 Aug 21-27;364(9435):675-84

FitzGerald GA, Patrono C. The coxibs, selective inhibitors of cyclooxygenase-2. N Engl J Med 2001;345:433–42.

Gabriel SE, Jaakkimainen L, Bombardier C. Risk for serious gastrointestinal complications related to use of nonsteroidal anti-inflammatory drugs: a meta-analysis. *Ann Intern Med.* 1991;115:787–796.

Garcia Rodriguez LA, Jick H. Risk of upper gastrointestinal bleeding and perforation associated with individual non-steroidal anti inflammatory drugs. Lancet 1994; 343: 769–72.

Gilard M, Arnaud B, Cornily JC, Le Gal G, Lacut K, Le Calvez G, Mansourati J, Mottier D, Abgrall JF, Boschat J. Influence of omeprazole on the antiplatelet action of clopidogrel associated with aspirin: the randomized, double-blind OCLA (Omeprazole CLopidogrel Aspirin) study. J Am Coll Cardiol. 2008 Jan 22;51(3):256-60.

Hallas J, Dall M, Andries A, et al. Use of single and combined antithrombotic therapy and risk of serious upper gastrointestinal bleeding: population based case-control study. BMJ. 2006;333:726.

Hawkey CJ, Karrasch JA, Szczepanski L, *et al.* Omeprazole compared with misoprostol for ulcers associated with nonsteroidal antiinflammatory drugs. Omeprazole versus Misoprostol for NSAID-induced Ulcer Management (OMNIUM) Study Group. *N Engl J Med* 1998;338:727–34

Hawkey CJ, Tulassay Z, Szczepanski L, et al. Randomised controlled trial of *Helicobacter pylori* eradication in patients on nonsteroidal anti-inflammatory drugs: HELP NSAIDs study. Helicobacter Eradication for Lesion Prevention. *Lancet.* 1998;352:1016–1021.

Hawkey C, Talley NJ, Yeomans ND, Jones R, Sung JJ, Langstrom G, et al. Improvements with esomeprazole in patients with upper gastrointestinal symptoms taking non-steroidal antiinflammatory drugs, including selective COX-2 inhibitors. Am J Gastroenterol. 2005;100:1028–36.

Henry D, Lim L-Y, Garcia Rodriguez LA, *et al.* Variability in risk of gastrointestinal complications with individual non-steroidal anti-inflammatory drugs: Results of a collaborative meta-analysis. *BMJ* 1996;312:1563–6.

Ho PM, Maddox TM, Wang L, et al. Risk of adverse outcomes associated with concomitant use of clopidogrel and proton pump inhibitors following acute coronary syndrome. JAMA 2009;301:937-44.

Hochain P, Berkelmans I, Czernichow P, *et al.* Which patients taking non-aspirin non-steroidal anti-inflammatory drugs bleed? A case-control study. *Eur J Gastroenterol Hepatol* 1995;7:419–26.

Holvoet J, Terriere L, Van Hee W, *et al.* Relation of upper gastrointestinal bleeding to non-steroidal anti-inflammatory drugs and aspirin: A case-control study. *Gut* 1991;32:730–4.

Hooper L, Brown TJ, Elliott R, Payne K, Roberts C, Symmons D. The effectiveness of five strategies for the prevention of gastrointestinal toxicity induced by non-steroidal anti-inflammatory drugs: systematic review. BMJ. 2004;329:948.

Huang JQ, Sridhar S, Hunt RH. Role of Helicobacter pylori infection and non-steroidal anti-inflammatory drugs in peptic-ulcer disease: a meta-analysis. Lancet 2002; 359: 14–22.

Ibanez L, Vidal X, Vendrell L, et al. Upper gastrointestinal bleeding associated with antiplatelet drugs. Aliment Pharmacol Ther 2006;23:235–242.

Ishizaki T, Horai Y. Review article: cytochrome P450 and the metabolism of proton pump inhibitors--emphasis on rabeprazole. Aliment Pharmacol Ther. 1999 Aug;13 Suppl 3:27-36.

Jawad AS. EULAR recommendations for the management of knee osteoarthritis. *Ann Rheum Dis* 2001;60:540.

Juni P, Nartey L, Reichenbach S, Sterchi R, Dieppe PA, Egger M. Risk of cardiovascular events and rofecoxib; cumulative meta-analysis. Lancet 2004;364;2021-9.

Juurlink DN, Gomes T, Ko DT, et al. A population-based study of the drug interaction between proton pump inhibitors and clopidogrel. CMAJ 2009;180:713-8.

Kitchingman GK, Prichard PJ, Daneshmend TK, Walt RP, Hawkey CJ. Enhanced gastric mucosal bleeding with doses of aspirin used for prophylaxis and its reduction by ranitidine. Br J Clin Pharmacol. 1989;28:581–5.

Lai KC, Lam SK, Chu KM, et al. Lansoprazole for the prevention of recurrences of ulcer complications from long-term low-dose aspirin use. N Engl J Med. 2002;346:2033–8.

Laine L, Marin-Sorenson M, Weistein WM. Nonsteroidal anti-inflammatory drug associated gastric ulcers do not require *Helicobacter pylori* for their development. *Am J Gastroenterol.* 1992;87:1398–1402.

Laine L, Harper S, Simon T, Bath R, Johanson J, Schwartz H, Stern S, Quan H, Bolognese J. A randomized trial comparing the effect of rofecoxib, a cyclooxygenase 2-specific inhibitor, with that of ibuprofen on the gastroduodenal mucosa of patients with osteoarthritis. Rofecoxib Osteoarthritis Endoscopy Study Group. Gastroenterology. 1999 Oct;117(4):776-83

Laine L. Stratifying the risk of clinical upper GI events in NSAID users: results from a double-blind outcomes study. Gastroenterology 2001;120:A552.

Laine L. Review article: the effect of *Helicobacter pylori* infection on nonsteroidal anti-inflammatory drug-induced upper gastrointestinal tract injury. *Aliment Pharmacol Ther.* 2002;16(suppl 1):34–39.

Laine L, Takeuchi K, Tarnawski A. Gastric mucosal defense and cytoprotection: bench to bedside. Gastroenterology. 2008 Jul;135(1):41-60.

Laine L, Curtis SP, Cryer B, Kaur A, Cannon CP. Risk factors for NSAID-associated upper GI clinical events in a long-term prospective study of 34701 arthritis patients. Aliment Pharmacol Ther. 2010 Nov;32(10):1240-8.

Laine L, Hennekens C. Proton pump inhibitor and clopidogrel interaction: fact or fiction? Am J Gastroenterol. 2010 Jan;105(1):34-41.

Lanas A, Bajador E, Serrano P, *et al.* Nitrovasodilators, low-dose aspirin, other nonsteroidal antiinflammatory drugs, and the risk of upper gastrointestinal bleeding. *N Engl J Med* 2000;343:834–9.

Lanas A. Review article: recommendations for the clinical management of patients taking non-steroidal anti-inflammatory drugs – a gastroenterologist's perspective. Aliment Pharmacol Ther 2005;1:16-19

Lanas A, García-Rodríguez LA, Arroyo MT, Bujanda L, Gomollón F, Forné M, Aleman S, Nicolas D, Feu F, González-Pérez A, Borda A, Castro M, Poveda MJ, Arenas J; Investigators of the Asociación Española de Gastroenterología (AEG). Effect of antisecretory drugs and nitrates on the risk of ulcer bleeding associated with nonsteroidal anti-inflammatory drugs, antiplatelet agents, and anticoagulants. Am J Gastroenterol. 2007 Mar;102(3):507-15.

Lanas A, Baron JA, Sandler RS, Horgan K, Bolognese J, Oxenius B, Quan H, Watson D, Cook TJ, Schoen R, Burke C, Loftus S, Niv Y, Ridell R, Morton D, Bresalier R. Peptic ulcer and bleeding events associated with rofecoxib in a 3-year colorectal adenoma chemoprevention trial. Gastroenterology. 2007 Feb;132(2):490-7.

Langman MJS, Weil J, Wainwright P, et al. Risks of bleeding peptic ulcer associated with individual non-steroidal anti-infl ammatory drugs. Lancet 1994; 343: 1075–78.

Lanza FL, Fakouhi D, Rubin A, Davis RE, Rack MF, Nissen C, et al. A double-blind placebo-controlled comparison of the efficacy and safety of 50, 100, and 200 micrograms of misoprostol q.i.d. in the prevention of ibuprofen-induced gastric and duodenal mucosal lesions and symptoms. Am J Gastroenterol. 1989;84:633–6.

Lanza FL, Chan FK, Quigley EM. Guidelines for prevention of NSAID-related ulcer events. Am J Gastroenterol 2009;104:728-38.

Lauer MS. Aspirin for primary prevention of coronary events. *N Engl J Med.* 2002;346:1468–1474.

Lawrence RC, Helmick CG, Arnett FC, et al. Estimates of the prevalence of arthritis and selected musculoskeletal disorders in the United States. Arthritis Rheum. 1998;41:778 –99.

Lewis SC, Langman MJS, Laporte JR, *et al.* Dose-response relationships between individual non-aspirin non-steroidal anti-inflammatory drugs (NANSAIDs) and serious upper gastrointestinal bleeding: a meta-analysis based on individual patient data. *Br J Clin Pharmacol* 2002;54:320–6.

Li L, Kelly LK, Ayub K, et al. Genotypes of *Helicobacter pylori* obtained from gastric ulcer patients taking or not taking NSAIDs. *Am J Gastroenterol.* 1999;94:1502–1507.

Li WQ, Andersson TB, Ahlstrom M, et al. Comparison of inhibitory effects of the proton pump-inhibiting drugs omeprazole, esomeprazole, lansoprazole and rabeprazole on human cytochrome P450 activities. Drug Metab Dispos 2004;32:821-7

Lin KJ, Hernández-Díaz S, García Rodríguez LA. Acid suppressants reduce risk of gastrointestinal bleeding in patients on antithrombotic or anti-inflammatory therapy. Gastroenterology. 2011 Jul;141(1):71-9.

Loeb DS, Talley NJ, Ahlquist DA, et al. Long-term nonsteroidal anti-inflammatory drug use and gastroduodenal injury: the role of *Helicobacter pylori* infection. *Gastroenterology.* 1992;102:1899–1905.

Ma L, Elliott SN, Cirino G, Buret A, Ignarro LJ, Wallace JL. Platelets modulate gastric ulcer healing: role of endostatin and vascular endothelial growth factor release. Proc Natl Acad Sci U S A. 2001 May 22;98(11):6470-5.

Ma TK, Lam YY, Tan VP, Kiernan TJ, Yan BP. Impact of genetic and acquired alteration in cytochrome P450 system on pharmacologic and clinical response to clopidogrel. Pharmacol Ther. 2010 Feb;125(2):249-59.

MacDonald TM, Morant SV, Robinson GC, et al. Association of upper gastrointestinal toxicity of non-steroidal anti-inflammatory drugs with continued exposure: cohort study. BMJ 1997;315:1333-7.

MacLean CH. Quality indicators for the management of osteoarthritis in vulnerable elders. Ann Intern Med. 2001;135:711–21

Malfertheiner P, Megraud F, O'Morain C, et al. Current concepts in the management of *Helicobacter pylori* infection: the Maastricht III Consensus Report. *Gut* 2007; 56:772–81.

Malfertheiner P, Chan FK, McColl KE. Peptic ulcer disease. Lancet. 2009 Oct 24;374(9699):1449-61.

McQuaid KR, Laine L. Systematic review and meta-analysis of adverse events of low-dose aspirin and clopidogrel in randomized controlled trials. Am J Med. 2006;119:624 –38.

Mega JL, Close SL, Wiviott SD, Shen L, Hockett RD, Brandt JT, Walker JR, Antman EM, Macias W, Braunwald E, Sabatine MS. Cytochrome p-450 polymorphisms and response to clopidogrel. N Engl J Med. 2009 Jan 22;360(4):354-62.

Moens HJ, van Croonenborg JJ, Al MJ, et al. Guideline 'NSAID use and the prevention of gastric damage'. Ned Tijdschr Geneeskd 2004;148:604-8.

Ng FH, Lam KF, Wong SY, Chang CM, Lau YK, Yuen WC, Chu WM, Wong BC. Upper gastrointestinal bleeding in patients with aspirin and clopidogrel co-therapy. Digestion. 2008;77(3-4):173-7.

Ng FH, Wong SY, Lam KF, Chu WM, Chan P, Ling YH, Kng C, Yuen WC, Lau YK, Kwan A, Wong BC. Famotidine is inferior to pantoprazole in preventing recurrence of aspirin-related peptic ulcers or erosions. Gastroenterology. 2010 Jan;138(1):82-8.

O'Donoghue ML, Braunwald E, Antman EM, Murphy SA, Bates ER, Rozenman Y, Michelson AD, Hautvast RW, Ver Lee PN, Close SL, Shen L, Mega JL, Sabatine MS, Wiviott SD. Pharmacodynamic effect and clinical efficacy of clopidogrel and prasugrel with or without a proton-pump inhibitor: an analysis of two randomised trials. Lancet. 2009 Sep 19;374(9694):989-97.

Ofman JJ, MacLean CH, Straus WL, et al. A meta-analysis of severe upper gastrointestinal complications of nonsteroidal antiinflammatory drugs. J Rheumatol. 2002;29:804 – 12.

Papatheodoridis GV, Sougioultzis S, Archimandritis AJ. Effects of *Helicobacter pylori* and nonsteroidal anti-inflammatory drugs on peptic ulcer disease: a systematic review. Clin Gastroenterol Hepatol 2006; 4: 130–42.

Pearson TA, Blair SN, Daniels SR, et al. AHA guidelines for primary prevention of cardiovascular disease and stroke: 2002 update: Consensus Panel Guide to Comprehensive Risk Reduction for Adult Patients Without Coronary or Other Atherosclerotic Vascular Diseases. American Heart Association Science Advisory and Coordinating Committee. Circulation. 2002;106:388 –91.

Perini RF, Ma L, Wallace JL. Mucosal repair and COX-2 inhibition. Curr Pharm Des 2003: 9: 2207

Peters RJ, Mehta SR, Fox KA, et al. Effects of aspirin dose when used alone or in combination with clopidogrel in patients with acute coronary syndromes: observations from the Clopidogrel in Unstable angina to prevent Recurrent Events (CURE) study. Circulation. 2003;108:1682–7.

Pilotto A, Leandro G, Di Mario F, et al. Role of *Helicobacter pylori* infection on upper gastrointestinal bleeding in the elderly: a case control study. *Dig Dis Sci.* 1997;42:586–591.

Ramey DR, Watson DJ, Yu C, et al. The incidence of upper gastrointestinal adverse events in clinical trials of etoricoxib vs. non-selective NSAIDs: an updated combined analysis. Curr Med Res Opin 2005;21:715-22.

Rassen JA, Choudhry NK, Avorn J, Schneeweiss S. Cardiovascular outcomes and mortality in patients using clopidogrel with proton pump inhibitors after percutaneous coronary intervention or acute coronary syndrome. Circulation. 2009 Dec 8;120(23):2322-9.

Ray WA, Murray KT, Griffin MR, Chung CP, Smalley WE, Hall K, Daugherty JR, Kaltenbach LA, Stein CM. Outcomes with concurrent use of clopidogrel and proton-pump inhibitors: a cohort study. Ann Intern Med. 2010 Mar 16;152(6):337-45.

Rockall TA, Logan RF, Devlin HB, et al. Incidence of and mortality from acute upper gastrointestinal haemorrhage in the United Kingdom. Steering Committee and members of the National Audit of Acute Upper Gastrointestinal Haemorrhage. BMJ 1995;311:222–6.

Roden DM, Stein CM. Clopidogrel and the concept of high-risk pharmacokinetics. Circulation. 2009 Apr 28;119(16):2127-30.

Rostom A, Dube C, Wells G, Tugwell P, Welch V, Jolicoeur E, et al. Prevention of NSAID-induced gastroduodenal ulcers. Cochrane Database Syst Rev. 2002;(4):CD002296.

Rothwell PM, Wilson M, Elwin CE, Norrving B, Algra A, Warlow CP, Meade TW. Long-term effect of aspirin on colorectal cancer incidence and mortality: 20-year follow-up of five randomised trials. Lancet. 2010 Nov 20;376(9754):1741-50.

Scheiman JM, Yeomans ND, Talley NJ, Vakil N, Chan FK, Tulassay Z, et al. Prevention of ulcers by esomeprazole in at-risk patients using non-selective NSAIDs and COX-2 inhibitors. Am J Gastroenterol. 2006;101(4):701–10.

Schnitzer TJ, Burmester GR, Mysler E, Hochberg MC, Doherty M, Ehrsam E, Gitton X, Krammer G, Mellein B, Matchaba P, Gimona A, Hawkey CJ; TARGET Study Group. Comparison of lumiracoxib with naproxen and ibuprofen in the Therapeutic Arthritis Research and Gastrointestinal Event Trial (TARGET), reduction in ulcer complications: randomised controlled trial. Lancet. 2004 Aug 21-27;364(9435):665-74.

Shaheen NJ, Hansen RA, Morgan DR, et al. The burden of gastrointestinal and liver diseases, 2006. Am J Gastroenterol. 2006;101:2128 –38.

Siller-Matula JM, Spiel AO, Lang IM, Kreiner G, Christ G, Jilma B. Effects of pantoprazole and esomeprazole on platelet inhibition by clopidogrel. Am Heart J. 2009 Jan;157(1):148.e1-5.

Silverstein FE, Graham DY, Senior JR, et al. Misoprostol reduces serious gastrointestinal complications in patients with rheumatoid arthritis receiving nonsteroidal anti-inflammatory drugs: a randomized, double-blind, placebo-controlled trial. Ann Intern Med. 1995;123:241–9.

Silverstein FE, Faich G, Goldstein JL, Simon LS, Pincus T, Whelton A, Makuch R, Eisen G, Agrawal NM, Stenson WF, Burr AM, Zhao WW, Kent JD, Lefkowith JB, Verburg KM, Geis GS. Gastrointestinal toxicity with celecoxib vs nonsteroidal anti-inflammatory drugs for osteoarthritis and rheumatoid arthritis: the CLASS study: A randomized controlled trial. Celecoxib Long-term Arthritis Safety Study. JAMA. 2000 Sep 13;284(10):1247-55

Singh G, Rosen Ramey D. NSAID induced gastrointestinal complications: the ARAMIS perspective--1997. Arthritis, Rheumatism, and Aging Medical Information System. J Rheumatol Suppl 1998;51:8–16

Singh M, Thapa B, Arora R. Clopidogrel pharmacogenetics and its clinical implications. Am J Ther. 2010 May-Jun;17(3):e66-73.

Skelly MM, Hawkey CJ. Potential alternatives to COX 2 inhibitors. BMJ. 2002 Jun 1;324(7349):1289-90

Somerville K, Faulkner G and Langman M. Non-Steroidal anti-inflammatory drugs and bleeding peptic ulcer. Lancet 1986; 327: 462-4

Sostres C, Gargallo CJ, Arroyo MT, Lanas A. Adverse effects of non-steroidal anti-inflammatory drugs (NSAIDs, aspirin and coxibs) on upper gastrointestinal tract. Best Pract Res Clin Gastroenterol. 2010 Apr;24(2):121-32.

Stockl KM, Le L, Zakharyan A, Harada AS, Solow BK, Addiego JE, Ramsey S. Risk of rehospitalization for patients using clopidogrel with a proton pump inhibitor. Arch Intern Med. 2010 Apr 26;170(8):704-10.

Suerbaum S, Michetti P. *Helicobacter pylori* infection. *N Engl J Med.* 2002;347:1175–1186.

Taha AS, Hudson N, Hawkey CJ, Swannell AJ, Trye PN, Cottrell J, et al. Famotidine for the prevention of gastric and duodenal ulcers caused by nonsteroidal anti-inflammatory drugs. N Engl J Med. 1996;334:1435–9.

Targownik LE, Nabalamba A. Trends in management and outcomes of acute nonvariceal upper gastrointestinal bleeding: 1993e2003. Clin Gastroenterol Hepatol 2006;4:1459-66.

Targownik LE, Metge CJ, Leung S, Chateau DG. The relative efficacies of gastroprotective strategies in chronic users of nonsteroidal anti-inflammatory drugs. Gastroenterology. 2008;134: 937–44.

Tiroch KA, Sibbing D, Koch W, Roosen-Runge T, Mehilli J, Schömig A, Kastrati A. Protective effect of the CYP2C19 *17 polymorphism with increased activation of clopidogrel on cardiovascular events. Am Heart J. 2010 Sep;160(3):506-12.

van Doorn LJ, Figueiredo C, Sanna R, et al. Clinical relevance of the cagA, vacA, and iceA status of *Helicobacter pylori*. *Gastroenterology*.1998;115:58–66.

van Hecken A, Depre M, Wynants K, et al. Effect of clopidogrel on naproxen-induced gastrointestinal blood loss in healthy volunteers. Drug Metabol Drug Interact 1998;14:193–205.

Vergara M, Catalan M, Gisbert JP, Calvet X. Meta-analysis: role of Helicobacter pylori eradication in the prevention of peptic ulcer in NSAID users. Aliment Pharmacol Ther 2005; 21: 1411–18.

Wallace JL, McKnight W, Reuter BK, Vergnolle N. NSAID-induced gastric damage in rats: requirement for inhibition of both cyclooxygenase 1 and 2. Gastroenterology. 2000;119:706 –14.

Weil J, Langman MJ, Wainwright P, *et al.* Peptic ulcer bleeding: accessory risk factors and interactions with non-steroidal anti-inflammatory drugs. *Gut* 2000;46:27–31.

Wolfe M, Lichtestein D, Singh G. Gastrointestinal toxicity of nonsteroidal anti-inflammatory drugs. *N Engl J Med.* 1999;340:1888–1899.

Yeomans ND, Tulassay Z, Juhasz L, *et al.* A comparison of omeprazole with ranitidine for ulcers associated with nonsteroidal antiinflammatory drugs. Acid Suppression Trial: Ranitidine versus Omeprazole for NSAID-associated Ulcer Treatment (ASTRONAUT) Study Group. *N Engl J Med* 1998;338:719–26.

Yusuf S, Zhao F, Mehta SR, Chrolavicius S, Tognoni G, Fox KK; Clopidogrel in Unstable Angina to Prevent Recurrent Events Trial Investigators. Effects of clopidogrel in addition to aspirin in patients with acute coronary syndromes without ST-segment elevation. N Engl J Med. 2001 Aug 16;345(7):494-502. Erratum in: N Engl J Med 2001 Nov 15;345(20):1506. N Engl J Med 2001 Dec 6;345(23):1716.

Khurram Z, Chou E, Minutello R, et al. Combination therapy with aspirin, clopidogrel and warfarin following coronary stenting is associated with a significant risk of bleeding. J Invasive Cardiol. 2006;18:162– 4.

8

Swallowing Disorders
Related to Vertebrogenic Dysfunctions

Eva Vanaskova, Jiri Dolina and Ales Hep
Department of Rehabilitation,
University Hospital, Hradec Kralove
Clinic of Internal Medicine, Gastroenterology,
University Hospital, Brno
Czech Republic

1. Introduction

In recent years, a growing interest in functional gastrointestinal problems can be noticed. In Western Europe, there is prevalence of functional disorders of the gastrointestinal tract in nearly 40% of the population. In Great Britain, 8 to 10% of patients visiting general practitioners have gastrointestinal problems, and approximately 50% of these are functional disorders (Becker & Aroldo, 1990). In the United States, 14% of the population are treated annually for functional gastrointestinal disorders, and in 50 to 70% of patients sent to a gastroenterologist, no significant pathology is detected (Mathias & Clench, 1995).

One of the seldom explored disability symptoms related to functional gastrointestinal problems are swallowing dysfunctions that are difficult to verify and quantify. Swallowing problems are often underestimated and attributed to psychological problems or negative mechanical effects of spinal morphological changes. The aim of our overview is to describe in detail the relationship between clinical disability of locomotor system and functional dysphagia.

2. Functional disorders of the gastrointestinal tract

The digestive tube is one of the systems most affected in terms of functional disorders. Rich gastrointestinal tract innervation of mainly vegetative nerve fibers is closely connected with and thereby influences function and activity of the central nervous system.

Gastrointestinal tract disturbances can be divided into esophageal (chest pain, functional heartburn, functional dysphagia), gastroduodenal (functional dyspepsia, etc.), intestinal disorders (irritable bowel syndrome, functional constipation or diarrhea), functional abdominal pain, biliary disorders, and anorectal disorders. In terms of pathogenesis, functional gastrointestinal motility disorders, visceral hypersensitivity, and intolerance to certain food components have been cited as principal contributing factors. Although musculoskeletal changes occur in approximately 60% of patients with functional bowel disorders, relatively little research has examined vertebrovisceral functional relationships.

3. Anatomy and function of the esophagus

The esophagus is a muscular tube that can be divided into three anatomic areas: The pars cervicalis, pars thoracica, and pars abdominalis. It has two layers of muscles - the inner circular and outer longitudinal. The proximal portion of the esophagus consists of striated muscle, distal smooth muscle, and a middle part consisting of smooth and striated muscles.

In terms of nerves, the esophagus is innervated from the plexus esophageus that consists of a large number of nerves of different diameters covering the area from the nn. vagi via nn. laryngei recurrentes. Branches provide connections with four or five cranial ganglia of the upper section of truncus sympathicus. These are autonomous fibers with a smaller component of sensory fibers. Plexus esophageus is located on the surface of the esophagus and continues caudally to truncus vagalis anterior and posterior. Both front and rear truncus vagalis contain left and right vagus nerve fibers.

Afferent signals apparent during the swallowing reflex are directed from sensitive fibers of the trigeminal nerve, n. glossopharyngeus and n. vagus. Efferent arm is successively comprised of the nerve hypoglossal motor fibers, n. trigeminus, n. facialis, n. glossopharyngeus and the n. vagus.

In terms of functions, the esophagus can be divided into the upper esophageal sphincter, the muscle's own tube (body), and the lower esophageal sphincter. All these parts play an important role with the following functions: Transport and swallowing, removal of gastric contents, and prevention of tracheobronchial aspiration.

Swallowing is divided into three phases:

An oral phase, which is a voluntary act that proceeds as the food or liquid is shifted towards the larynx.

A pharyngeal phase in which the muscles of the larynx and pharynx close all openings except the Killian sphincter where the food is passed.

An esophageal phase. Shortly after the contraction of the pharynx, the upper sphincter of the esophagus flags at about 0.5 seconds and at this time it creates a primary peristaltic wave. In about two seconds, the lower esophageal sphincter is extended and then relaxed for 5 to 10 seconds. Relaxation is terminated with a contraction lasting about a tenth of a second. In addition to the primary peristaltic wave, there is a secondary peristaltic contraction that forces regurgitated food or liquid. During swallowing, the upper sphincter closes periodically.

In the first phase of the voluntary swallowing act, food is transported from the mouth into the pharynx by the tongue's pressure against the palate with lips and teeth together. The tongue and soft palate shape the food during this process. Cranial hyoid bone muscles raise the hyoid bone with pharynx. The bite of food then inches behind the isthmus faucium and the second phase begins.

The second phase is involuntary reflex and begins as the soft palate makes contact with food or liquid. The soft palate rises and stretches along the upper pharyngeal constrictors closing the nasopharynx from the oral cavity. Mm. constrictores pharyngis (medius et inferior) shift the food, mm levatores rise up the pharynx with the larynx, the epiglottis is bending, and closes before the food passes the aditus laryngis.

In the next phase, which is a continuation of the swallowing reflex and is not considered a separate phase, the lower pharyngeal sphincter activity shifts the bite to the beginning of the esophagus, followed by transport due to esophageal muscle activity. Elevated pharynx and larynx return caudally. At the same time, swallowing ventilates the middle-ear cavity. Transport of food from the mouth into the upper esophagus is related to the coordinated relaxation of the upper esophageal sphincter, which is a consequence of inhibitory signals from the masticatory center through n. vagus. Sphincter tone can be influenced by local factors such as pH in the esophagus.

In the third phase, food is propelled by the coordinated peristaltic wave of esophagus muscles that move aborally at the rate of 3 cm/s when the lower esophageal sphincter is relaxed. Peristaltic wave speed is affected by many factors, especially by the temperature and volume of the swallowed food. If the interval between swallowing two mouthfuls is less than 10 seconds, swallowing is often not followed by a peristaltic wave.

The lower esophageal sphincter is a smooth muscle area with a length of 3 cm that separates the esophagus from the stomach. It prevents reflux of gastric contents back into the esophagus during swallowing and performs coordinated relaxation allowing the passage of food from the esophagus to the stomach. Its activity can be influenced by myogenic, neural, and humoral factors. The pressure increase is caused by gastrin, motilin, prostaglandin, and histamine. By contrast, a reduction occurs under the influence of cholecystokinine, secretine, glucagone, progesterone, neurotensin. The physiological significance of some of these substances is questionable.

The function of the esophagus is affected by autonomic innervation activity. The enteric system is relatively independent and regulates many functions of the digestive tube. Enteric system (myenteric and submucous) is under the influence of signals from CNS and receptors in the tube wall (mechanoreceptors, chemoreceptors, and thermoreceptors) (Bharucha & Camilleri, 2003, Bielefeldt & Gebhart, 2004).

The autonomic nervous system does not work separately from cortical and subcortical structures. The peripheral autonomic nervous system function is subject - to a large extent - to the regulations of the central nervous system (except the voluntary control), which provides a comprehensive and targeted response. Another function of the digestive tube modulation is the relationship between the enteric nervous system, central nervous system, and the immune system in the gastrointestinal tract. This can explain the influence of stress on the occurence or worsening of symptoms in the digestive tract.

4. Differential diagnosis of swallowing disorders

Dysphagia is a symptom of numerous organic and functional disorders. Impaired swallowing can be high (oropharyngeal) or low (esophageal). Organic dysphagia is characterized by permanent dysphagia (stricture, tumor). Functional dysphagia is that one caused by motility disorders (usually spasms) and has the character of intermittent problems. With these distinct characteristics, patient's history is important in terms of a major or single base diagnosis. The causes of dysphagia are varied and numerous.

Obstructive swallowing disorders: Esophageal tumor, extramural compression, congenital abnormalities (stenosis, atresia), inflammation, trauma (burns, scars, foreign bodies).

Non-obstructive swallowing disorders: Neuromuscular diseases (pseudobulbar syndrome, bulbar syndrome, lower motor neuron dysfunction, neuromuscular disorders, muscle disease), autoimmune disease, achalasia, idiopathic spastic dysphagia, psychogenic and functional disorders.

The most common types of non-obstructive swallowing disorders are:

- Motility disorders in diabetic neuropathy, alcoholism, psychiatric illness.
- Scleroderma – an autoimmune disease that causes weakening of the esophagus tissues.
- Achalasia – with the loss of ganglion cells in the wall, increases the tone of the lower sphincter at first (loss of inhibitory stimuli), followed by the loss of peristalsis in the proximal parts of the esophagus with subsequent accumulation of food and dilation of the esophagus.
- Primary esophageal spasm with unclearly identified pathophysiology – diffuse spasms that block the transport of food and fluids through the esophagus, leading to an increase in lower esophageal sphincter tone and nonspecific motility disorders.
- Functional and psychogenic dysphagia – no signs of organic impairment, it may be associated with stress.
- Age-related changes in motor function of the esophagus.
- Inflammation associated with the use of drugs (pill esophagitis).
- Inflammation associated with gastroesophageal reflux.

Sometimes, globus pharyngicus (hystericus) is classified as a functional swallowing disorders. Patients describe sensation of a lump in the throat with a characteristic absence of dysphagia. The food does not stick in the throat and fluids pass freely when swallowing, this condition can alleviate symptoms. Some studies suggest an increase in upper esophageal sphincter pressure or abnormal mobility of the hypopharynx. The occurence of these problems is usually associated with psychosocial factors, especially depression and anxiety. Medical treatment usually does not bring relief, although patients may benefit from psychotherapy.

5. Vertebral dysfunction in relation to internal organ disease

Vertebral dysfunction is caused by a combination of morphological and functional disorders. The musculoskeletal system has passive components (bones, joints, ligaments) and active components (muscles, fascia). These components create static and dynamic spinal function. Vertebral disorders should not be considered as only morphological disturbances. Functional disorders of the intervertebral joints, movement problems, altered muscle tone status and abnormalities may also be classified as vertebral disorders. Morphological and functional disorders should therefore be considered simultaneously, as symptoms for both dysfunctions frequently appear together (Lewit, 2010)

Vertebrovisceral relations are determined by segmental somatic and autonomic innervation. Myotome, dermatome, viscerotome, and sclerotome are innervated in each spinal segment. Failure in one of the reflex arc sectors often causes dysfunction in parts or the entire segment. In terms of etiopathogenesis, two types of functional disorders are generated. If there is a primary spinal defect which reflexively induces changes in viscerotom, we can simply, although not precisely, refer to vertebrovisceral syndromes. Reflective changes in the spine lead to a number of significant clinical manifestations-primarily pain along with other symptoms (Nansel & Szalazak, 1995). The musculoskeletal system can cause problems that mimic symptoms of visceral organ disorder.

We refer to viscerovertebral syndromes when there are primary defects in the visceral organ which can cause segment changes and changes in the functional state of the axial organ. The internal organ problems may cause changes, such as changes in muscle tone, tendons, fascia, subcutaneous tissue, and skin. Often it is difficult to establish a differential diagnosis that distinguishes the primary cause, and inaccurate or erroneous treatment could be the consequence.

In very broad terms, the four possibilities should be envisaged:

1. The spinal column (motion segment) is causing symptoms that are mistaken for visceral disease.
2. Visceral disease is causing symptoms that are interpreted as a lesion in some part of the locomotor system.
3. Visceral disease is producing changes in the locomotor system, such as movement restriction, etc.
4. A disturbance in the motion segment is triggering visceral disease or (more likely) is activating already latent visceral symptoms (hypothetical).

The first two points highlight the necessity for precise differential diagnosis and the problems associated with this. The spinal column with its motion segments can in fact produce symptoms that may mimic symptoms arising in the viscera. If such symptoms stem from the motor system, it is not surprising that drug treatment aimed at organic visceral disease fails. This causes frustration in many patients as the true cause of symptoms is not recognized (Nansel & Szalazak, 1995; Hülse, 1991).

If the mechanism causing visceral dysfunction is disturbed function of the motor system, better understanding of this would be of great practical interest, as more effective treatment by the technique of musculoskeletal (manual) medicine would be more widely applied.

Point 2 is the warning that pain perceived in the locomotor system may be a deceptive sign masking serious underlying visceral disease. This suspicion is strengthened if the symptoms of spinal segmental disturbance tend to relapse repeatedly without obvious cause. While the error in point 1 is more common, that in point 2 is all the more fraught with danger.

Point 3 is of major theoretical significance and demonstrates that visceral disease is actually one of the possible causes of dysfunction in the motion segment. Clinical experience teaches that certain visceral diseases are associated with characteristic patterns in the locomotor system. They are so specific that their recurrence is in all probability predictive of a recurrence of the visceral disease.

Point 4 it would seem justifiable to assume that lesion in a motion segment of the spinal column may impair function in the corresponding internal organs. This is borne out by the vasomotor response in the whole segment to which pain is referred. In such cases we can see the disorder clearing up as soon as we treat the motion segment. Reactions of this kind have been noted particularly in connection with the cervicocranial syndrome, especially at the craniocervical junction, including disturbances of equilibrium. Similar phenomena have been observed in connection with certain cardiac arrhythmias. A motion segment dysfunction may activate latent disease in an internal organ. Multiple pathogenic factors may also need to be considered in terms of their cumulative impact. As well as those that affect the locomotor system, other factors may be important in terms of their influence on the organism as a whole, for example infections, metabolic disturbances, diet, etc. None of these individual factors on its own would be sufficient to provoke disease but it is legitimate to refer to them as risk factors (Lewit 2010).

Motor system statics and dynamics are dependent on the physiological state of central regulatory mechanisms. Pain and stress play important roles. Chronic state pattern and disability severity are not represented with an individual musculoskeletal disorder, and the clinical picture is affected by the patient psychological condition. Vertebrovisceral relations are very complex. In many cases pathogenesis is due to more than one factor, and it is better to speak of disease with vertebrogenic factor (Lewit 2010).

In the medical literature the spinal column is mainly mentioned as a cause of dysphagia in the form of a possible mechanical obstacle causing compression of the esophagus by anterior osteophytes: they are believed to produce both dysphagia and dysphonia and even difficulty in breathing (Kodama et al, 1995; Krause & Castro, 1994, Richter et al., 1995; Valadka et al., 1995). Hughes (Hughes et al., 1994) even described patients in whom osteophytes caused dysphagia combined with apnea during sleep. Fuhrmann (Fuhrmann & Neufang, 1994) described similar cases due to disk protrusion. In such cases even surgical treatment was considered. Retropharyngeal hematoma, too, has been described, causing dysphagia and hoarseness (Shaw, 1995). Therefore it is mandatory to have the patient thoroughly examined clinically and by X-ray, ultrasound and esophageal endoscopy, etc.

6. Vertebral dysfunction and functional disorders of the esophagus

Vertebrovisceral relations are seldom explored as possible etiological factors of gastrointestinal tract functional disorders. Musculoskeletal changes occur in approximately 60% of patients with functional bowel disorders. Pain of the cervical and upper thoracic spine is often referred to as a focal point in terms of vertebrovisceral relationships. Functional dysphagia represents intermittent problem caused by motility disorders (usually spasm). In a patient group with evidence of spinal and thoracic, cervical dysfunctions and swallowing problems, functional dysphagia was quantified by measuring the dynamic esophageal scintigraphy detected with prolonged passage of marked fluid (Hep et al., 1999).

Disorders of the upper cervical spine are sometimes associated with the emergence of the swallowing difficulty termed globus pharyngicus, which is considered one of the functional disorders. In the past, the relationship between cervical spine disability, dysphonia, and globus formation was described. This relationship is a vertebrovisceral-induced impairment of the spine in the C 1- 4 segments. Globus is a typical syndrome for hyperfunctional dysphonia. Therefore, it is not accurate to designate or consider globus hystericus as a symptom of hysteria (Becker & Aroldo, 1990).

Functional dysphonia is associated with dysfunction of the upper cervical spine. Innervation of the vocal cords through n. laryngeus superior and n. laryngeus recurrens has no relationship with the disability of the spine but cervical spine changes have influence on a number of other muscles and thus affect the relative position of laryngeal cartilage and the tonus of vocal ligaments. They are innervating m. geniohyoideus of segments C1 and C2 (n. hypoglossus), followed by m. omohyoideus, m. sternohyoideus, m. thyreohyoideus, and m.

sternothyreoideus, that are innervated mainly from segments C2 and C3. M. cricothyreoideus and m. laryngopharyngeus are also innervated by n. laryngicus cranialis of cervical segments C 1-4. The treatment using musculoskeletal (manual) medicine techniques lead to an improvement of laryngeal difficulties (Hulse, 1991).

Inclusion of functional dysphagia as a vertebrovisceral disorder is generally recognized, but this conditon has not been studied extensively. This is because functional dysphagia borders with four fairly distant branches of medicine—gastroenterology, neurology, otorhinolaryngology, and musculoskeletal medicine. And an objective assessment of this disease is a complicated issue as well.

7. Diagnosis of functional swalloving disorders

Conventional radiology, computed tomography, ultrasound scans, and magnetic resonance imaging facilitate visualization of gastrointestinal tract organ morphology, but these scans cannot precisely quantify their function. In the diagnosis of esophagus disease, fluoroscopy has been used with non-physiological contrast materials, and this is not a quantitative evaluation either. The use of endoscopy or manometry is an invasive way of investigating the organ condition. The use of nuclear medicine can quantify gastrointestinal organ function assessment by measuring the passage of isotope-labeled material (Russel et al., 1981). At the investigation of patients with dysphagia and normal manometric and endoscopic findings, 50% of them presented dysmotility when dynamic scintigraphy was used (Kjellen et al., 1984). A positive diagnoses of functional gastrointestinal disorders are a result of an expert gastroenterologist's work. Usually, this diagnosis is determined after exclusion of all other potential causes of dysfunction.

However, it is necessary to take into account the importance of psychological factors that may be the cause of motility disorders of the esophagus. Studies using sophisticated psychometric instruments, dealing with the importance of psychological factors in patients with painful esophageal motility disorders, identified a number of mutual relations. Groups of patients with esophageal spasm, with irritable colon, with benign abnormalities of the impaired esophagus were compared with a control set of healthy persons. Patients with esophageal motility and irritable colon had significantly higher scores than other groups with somatic anxiety and gastrointestinal susceptibility. This shows that certain patients tend to have a significant interest in the somatic function and have more frequent and severe gastrointestinal symptoms due to stress (Waterman et al., 1989).

When 50 referred patients with pathogenic esophageal manometry underwent a psychiatric examination, abnormalities were detected in 21 out of 25 patients with motility disorders of the distal esophagus. On the contrary, abnormalities were found in only 4 out of 13 patients with normal manometric findings. The most common findings were somatization disorders, anxiety, and depression. (Clouse & Lustman, 1983).

8. Treatment of esophagus functional disorders caused by vertebral dysfunction

In addition to patients with clearly defined pathomorphological esophageal changes, a group of patients without obvious morphological variations had functional spinal disorders. The positive effect of manipulation therapy to relieve pain of the spine and affected organs has been known since the beginning of the twentieth century — originally cited in the works of Palmer and Still, and later referred to by Pikalov. (Pikalov & Kharin, 1994). In the past, it was found that somatic changes in the body caused by irritation are accompanied by an autonomic nervous system reaction that affects gastrointestinal system organs (Sato & Tera, 1976). The Beal study demonstrated a close relationship between changes in soft tissues and corresponding changes in the segmental innervation area (Beal, 1983, 1984).

Musculoskeletal (manual) medicine techniques can reduce pain and normalize the dysphagia. Using scintigraphy, this can be objectively measured. A significant relationship between dynamic scintigraphy and nonobstructive dysphagia/swallowing and spinal axis problems has been observed. Dynamic scintigraphy allowed for an objective treatment assessment (Vanaskova et al., 2001).

The effect of functional disorder treatment significantly influences psychological and emotional status of the patients. It is necessary to positively motivate the patient and then provide relaxation for both the body and the mind. From clinical practice and sports medicine we know that the use of methods of rehabilitation medicine can affect pain perception threshold, release tension and provide a feeling of well being by achieving stimulation of attention. Changes after therapy affect the function of the locomotor system, reflex actions, and internal organs. The effect of manipulative (manual) therapy in reducing anxiety and improving ability to solve numerical tasks were documented in the EEG records by Field and colleagues (Field et al, 1996).

9. Conclusions

In functional swallowing disorders related to spinal dysfunctions, pharmacologic treatment often fails. Many patients become disappointed with the treatment failure and seeming inability of physicians to identify the cause of their discomfort. On the other hand, rehabilitation therapy focused on the musculoskeletal system can sometimes suprisingly and quickly treat patient ailments. The vertebrogenic mechanism of functional dysphagia is therefore not only of academic significance but of clinical importance as well. Swallowing disorders can be due not only to structural changes, but frequently to dysfunction of the spinal column and its musculature.

10. References

Beal, M. & Dvorak, J. (1984). Palpatory examination of the spine: a comparison of the results of two methods and their relationship to visceral disease. *Manual Medicine*, Vol. 1, (1984), pp. 25-32, ISSN 0254-9522

Beal, M. (1983). Palpatory testing for somatic dysfunction in patients with cardiovascular disease. *Journal of the American Osteopathic Association*, Vol. 82, No. 11, (July 1983), pp. 822-831, ISSN 0098-6151

Becker, D. & Arold, A. (1990). Übungsschema zur Behandlung von Globusbeschwerden. *Sprache-Stimme-Gehör*, Vol.14, No.1, (1990), pp. 38-40, ISSN1439-1260

Bharucha, A. E. & Camilleri, M. (2003). Gastrointestinal dysmotility and sphincter dysfunction, In: *Neurological Therapeutics : Principles and practice, 2 Volume Set (Addendum included)*, Noseworthy, J. H. , pp. 3060-3064, Taylor & Francis, ISBN 1–85317-623-0, London

Bielefeldt, K. & Gebhart, G. F. (2004). Gut – to – Brain Signaling: Sensory Mechanisms, In: *Pathophysiology of the Enteric Nervous System : A Basis for Understanding Functional Diseases*, Spiller, R. & Grundy, D., pp. 24-43, Blackwell Publishing, ISBN 1-4051-2361-3, Oxford

Clouse, R. E. & Lustman, P. J. (1983). Psychiatric illness and contraction abnormalities of the esophagus. *New England Journal of Medicine*, Vol. 309, No. 22, (December 1983), pp. 337-1342, ISSN 0028-4793

Field, T., Ironson, G., Scafidi, F., Nawrocki, T., Goncalves, A., Burman, I., Pickens, J., Fox, N., Schanberg, S. & Kun, C. (1996). Massage therapy reduces anxiety and enhances EEG pattern of alertness and math computations. *International Journal of Neuroscience*, Vol. 86, No. 3-4, (September 1996), pp. 197-205, ISSN 0020-7454

Fuhrmann, R. & Neufang, K. F. (1994). Dysphagie als Symptom eines ventralen zervikalen Bandscheibenvorfalls. *Aktuelle Probleme in Chirurgie und Orthopädie*, Vol. 43, (1994), pp. 134-138, ISSN 0378-8504

Hep, A., Vanaskova, E., Tosnerova, V., Prasek, J., Vizda, J., Dite,P., Ondroušek, L. & Dolina, J. (1999). Radionuclide oesophageal transit scintigraphy - a useful method for verification of oesophageal dysmotility by cervical vertebropathy. *Disease of the Esophagus*, Vol. 12, No. 1, (1999), pp. 47-50, ISSN 1120-8694

Hughes, T. A., Wiles, C. M., Lawrie, B. W. & Smith, A. P. (1994). Case report: dysphagia and sleep apnoea associated with cervical osteophytes due to diffuse idiopathic skeletal hyperostosis (DISH). *Journal of Neurology, Neurosurgery, and Psychiatry*, Vol. 57, No. 3, (March 1994), pp. 384, ISSN 0022-3050

Hülse, M. (1991). Zervikale Dysfonie. *Folia Phoniatrica*, Vol. 43, No. 4, (1991), pp. 181-196, ISSN 0015-5705

Kjellén, G., Svedberg, J. B. & Tibbling, L. (1984). Solid bolus transit by esophageal scintigraphy in patients with dysphagia and normal manometry and radiography. *Digestive Diseases and Sciences*, Vol. 29, No. 1, (January 1984), pp. 1-5, ISSN 0163-2116

Kodama, M., Sawada, H., Udaka, F., Kameyama, M. & Koyama T. (1995). Dysphagia caused by an anterior cervical osteophyte: case report. *Neuroradiology*, Vol. 37, No. 1, (1995), pp. 58-59, ISSN 0028-3940

Krause, P. & Castro, W. H. (1994). Cervical hyperostosis: a rare cause of dysphagia. Case description and bibliographical survey. *European Spine Journal*, Vol. 3, No. 1, (1994), pp. 56-58, ISSN 0940-6719

Lewit, K. (2010). Theoretical considerations, In: *Manipulative Therapy Musculoskeletal Medicine*, pp. 9-38, Churchill Livingstone Elsevier, ISBN 9-780-7020-3056-7, Oxford

Mathias, J. R., & Clench, M. H. (1995). Neuromuscular diseases of the gastrointestinal tract. Specific disorders that often get a nonspecific diagnosis. *Postgraduate Medicine*, Vol. 97, No. 3, (1995), pp. 95-108, ISSN 0032-5481 .

Nansel, D. & Szlazak, M. (1995). Somatic dysfunction and the phenomenon of visceral disease simulation: a probable explanation for the apparent effectiveness of somatic therapy in patients presumed to be suffering from true visceral disease. *Journal of Manipulative and Physiological Therapeutics*, Vol. 18, No. 6, (July-August 1995), pp. 379-397, ISSN 0161-4754

Pikalov, A. A. & Kharin, V. V. (1994). Use of spinal manipulative therapy in the treatment of duodenal ulcer: a pilot study. *Journal of Manipulative and Physiological Therapeutics*, Vol. 17, No. 5, (June 1994), pp. 310-313, ISSN 0161-4754

Richter, D., Ostermann, P. A., Schumann, C., David, A. & Muhr, G. (1995). Die ventrale Hyperostose der Halswirbelsäule - eine seltene Differentialdiagnose der Dysphagie. *Chirurg*, Vol. 66, No. 4, (April 1995), pp. 431-433, ISSN 0009-4722

Russell, C. O., Hill, L. D., Holmes, E. R. 3rd, Hull, D. A., Gannon, R. & Pope, C. E. 2nd (1981). Radionuclide transit: a sensitive screening test for esophageal dysfunction. *Gastroenterology*, Vol. 80, No. 5 Pt 1, (May 1981), pp. 887-892, ISSN 0016-5085

Sato, Y. & Terui, N. (1976). Changes in duodenal motility produced by noxious mechanical stimulation of the skin in rats. *Neuroscience Letters*, Vol. 2, No. 4, (June 1976), pp. 189-193, ISSN 0304-3940

Shaw, C. B., Bawa, R., Snider, G. & Wax, M. K. (1995). Traumatic retropharyngeal hematoma: a case report. *Otolaryngology – Head and Neck Surgery*, Vol. 113, No. 4, (October 1995), pp. 485-488, ISSN 0194-5998

Valadka, A. B., Kubal, W. S. & Smith, M. M. (1995). Updated management strategy for patients with cervical osteophytic dysphagia. *Dysphagia*, Vol. 10, No. 3, (Summer 1995), pp. 167-171, ISSN 0179-051X

Vanaskova, E., Hep, A., Lewit, K., Tosnerova, V., Prasek, J., Vizda, J., Dite, P. & Dolina, J. (2001). Cervical dysfunction with disturbed oesophageal motility - scintigraphic assessment. *Journal of Orthopaedic Medicine*, Vol. 23, No. 1, (2001), pp. 9-11, ISSN 1753-6146

Waterman, D. C., Dalton, C. B., Ott, D. J., Castell, J. A., Bradley, L. A., Castell, D. O. & Richter, J. E. (1989). Hypertensive lower esophageal sphincter: what does it mean? *Journal of Clinical Gastroenterology*, Vol. 11, No. 2, (April 1989), pp. 139-146, ISSN 0192-0790

9

Enhanced Ulcer Recognition from Capsule Endoscopic Images Using Texture Analysis

Vasileios Charisis, Leontios Hadjileontiadis and George Sergiadis
Aristotle University of Thessaloniki
Greece

1. Introduction

The five senses constitute some of the most substantial elements of the human nature. Beyond their importance in daily life and perception of the world, they play crucial role in knowledge acquisition as well. For instance, medicine was one of the first domains where the conceptual tools of rationality and empiricism were combined with techniques of investigation to make the human body an object of knowledge (Foucault, 1973). In this context, the techniques mentioned above are based on the application of senses in order to acquire medical knowledge. More precisely, vision and hearing became specific objects of knowledge over the course of the 19th century, supplemented through technique and technology. Thus, seeing and hearing are to be understood as fundamentally and absolutely different modes of not only knowing the world, but also reaching a medical diagnosis.

A branch of medicine closely associated with one of these techniques, namely visual inspection, is gastroenterology. In the field of gastroenterology, vision is widely understood as the fundamental mode of knowing the state of the gastrointestinal (GI) tract. The advent of medical imaging technologies, such as radiography (in the wider sense), tomography and especially endoscopy, promoted this thesis (Lorenz *et al.*, 1993; Rutgeerts *et al.*, 1980) by enabling the visual examination without demanding to gain physical access. In case of visual inspection, as in case of auscultation, there are specific properties observed in order to assess the image content, no matter how simple or sophisticated the imaging technology is. During a stethoscope examination, for instance, the clinician attempts to identify frequency, pitch and duration deviations from the normal lung sounds. Similarly, during the observation of a medical image, there are image properties, corresponding to the acoustic ones of the pulmonary system, which may reveal the existence of illness. In the case of endoscopic GI tract images, these features essentially include texture, color and shape. The procedure that a clinician subconsciously follows in order to examine the images and reach a diagnosis is to seek for distortions. Distortions mainly in texture and color of the examined tissue, as compared to the features considered empirically or conceptually healthy. While color and shape are quite tangible approaches, the concept of texture is more abstract and subjectively defined and interpreted; however, embodies valuable information that can be used to identify or describe an image (Haralick *et al.*, 1973). The vagueness of this concept is evidenced by the fact that there is no universally agreed-upon definition of what image texture is and, in general, different researchers use different definitions depending upon the particular area of application (Tuceryan & Jain, 1998). The most widely used and accepted definition of texture in the field of medical image analysis, which is also adopted in this chapter, is the one that defines texture as the spatial variation of pixel intensities. In other words, texture describes the relationship between the intensities of neighbouring pixels (not necessarily adjacent). Texture is a fundamental characteristic that entails substantial information about the structural arrangement of surfaces and their relationship to the surrounding environment. This information may be applied to estimate shape, surface orientation, depth changes and construction materials. Texture is an innate property of virtually all surfaces; the grain of the wood, the weave of a fabric, the pattern of crops in a field, rugae on the mucous membrane of the stomach, the mucosa of colon and small intestine. An example of various texture patterns is given in Fig. 1. This structural information has been proven crucial for medical image analysis and interpretation (Miller & Astley, 1992; Xie *et al.*, 2005). This is the case especially for gastroenterology where the internal mucous membranes of the digestive tract exhibit strong textural features and distinctive patterns. For instance, an eroded ulcerous region or a protruded cancerous tissue is visually distinguished, mainly, by its alternated texture. Another image property also important for abnormal tissue evaluation is color. Ulcers, for instance, exhibit greenish-yellow hues while an active bleeding spot is characterized by deep red tones. On the contrary, the normal intestinal mucous membrane is reddish-pink in color. Nevertheless, color cannot be utilized as a standalone objective modality for abnormal tissue detection, since it is not perceptually uniform. The perceived color is highly conditioned by the nature and the amount of ambient luminosity (Berlin & Kay, 1969). Despite the color constancy effect (Foster *et al.*, 1997) of the human color perception system, whereby the color perception of objects remains relatively constant under varying environmental and visual conditions, serious color variations and color casts exist because of the intervention of an endoscope or a camera between the intestinal tissue and the physician's eye. For these reasons, gastroenterologists use color and texture information together, as the visual clues, along with other complementary examinations (i.e., blood tests, urine tests etc.), in order to reach a diagnosis.

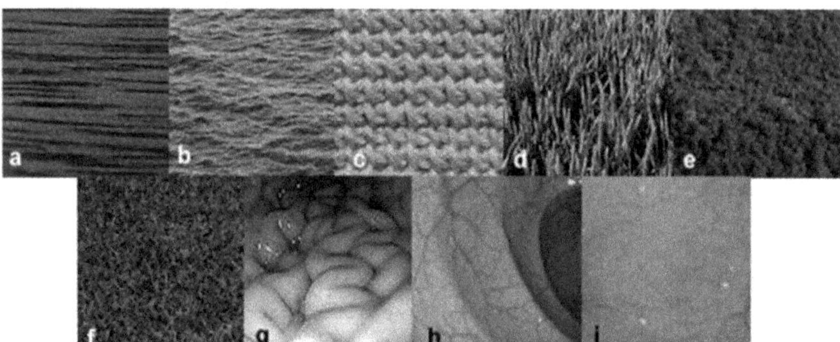

Fig. 1. Digital images with visibly different texture regions: a) grain of wood, b) water, c) cloth, d) corn crops, e) forest, f) grass, g) stomach, h) colon, i) esophagus.

The advent of Wireless Capsule Endoscopy (WCE) and the gastroenterologists' requirement for faster and more secure diagnoses necessitated the development of effective intestinal-disorder recognition systems and automated WCE image analysis/inspection techniques.

The aim of WCE image processing techniques is to help the physician draw more reliable conclusions by generating enhanced and more informative images. During an examination with a stethoscope the physician instructs the patient how to breathe in order to get the best possible auscultation. In a similar way, a gastroenterologist who reviews an endoscopic video would desire the images to be as much informative as possible, but, without the opportunity to either give instructions to the patient or guide the capsule. The automated intestinal-disorder recognition systems target to detect potential regions of abnormal tissue in order to help the physician reach a diagnosis more quickly. This is particularly essential in WCE due to the vast amount of images produced (over 55.000) and the highly time-consuming task of reviewing them (more than two hours) (Maieron *et al.*, 2004). The fact that abnormal findings might not be clearly apparent to the naked eye further renders computer-aided image analysis imperative. It is not rare that abnormal findings are visible in only one or two WCE frames and easily missed by the physician. Additionally, contrast between malignant and normal tissue may be present but below the threshold of human perception. The human visual system fails to detect certain textured patterns. Julesz, an experimental psychologist, was an early pioneer in the visual perception of texture. He verified that human eye can discriminate textures that differ up to second order statistics (Julesz, 1975). In other words, a deliberate amount of effort is required to discriminate between two textures with identical second order statistics. Last but not least, the young age of WCE implies that most clinicians are inexperienced in this examination and automatic diagnostic systems could be great tools for those who wish to become experts in WCE. In this context, automatic inspection and analysis of WCE images is of immediate need.

From the aforementioned perspectives, it becomes clear that the auxiliary automatic diagnostic systems should exploit the texture and color features of the endoscopic images. Many efforts and computational approaches towards WCE image analysis have been reported in the literature. More specifically, researchers are concerned with malicious tissue detection which refers to detection of abnormal regions, such as tumors, polyps, bleeding and ulcer. To cope with this matter, traditional pattern recognition methods are applied, utilizing both chromatic and achromatic image domains. In particular, detection of abnormal patterns is achieved by employing local color features (Li & Meng, 2007), texture unit number (NTU) transformation and texture spectrum (Kodogiannis *et al.*, 2007a, 2007b) and synergistic methodologies, such as L-G graphs and image registration (Bourbakis, 2005). Local binary patterns (Iakovidis *et al.*, 2006) with the aid of G-statistic (Wang *et al.*, 2006), co-occurrence matrices (Ameling *et al.*, 2009), and discrete wavelet transform in conjunction with second-order statistics (Karkanis *et al.*, 2007; Magoulas, 2006) contributed to polyp and tumor detection. Regarding ulcer recognition, the related research is quite limited, no matter how common and important this disease is. The techniques proposed include feature extraction from a curvelet-based uniform local binary pattern (Iakovidis *et al.*, 2006; Li & Meng, 2009b), chromaticity moments calculated with the aid of Chebychev polynomials (Li & Meng, 2009a), texture spectrum (Kodogiannis *et al.*, 2007b), MPEG-7 descriptors (Coimbra & Cunha, 2006) and Red-Green-Blue (RGB) pixel values evaluation (Gan *et al.*, 2008). However, their success rate is limited.

This chapter sheds light upon one of the main issues of the WCE image analysis field, i.e., the overall detection enhancement of one of the most common diseases in the GI tract, namely ulcer; hence, enriching the inadequate existing literature. This goal is achieved by emphasizing on efficient elicitation of the structure characteristics of ulcerations and by introducing new feature vectors (FVs). In particular, this chapter describes the use of innovative computer vision approaches towards the evaluation of ulcer-related content of WCE images. These approaches are similar to those employed by physicians in clinical practice to reach a diagnosis, i.e., the concept of color-texture characteristics. More specifically, they include sophisticated image processing tools with robust mathematical background, drawn from the field of Multi-Resolution Analysis, resulting in discrimination between ulcer and healthy regions. Additionally, innovative feature extraction algorithms, structured in both space and space-frequency domains, are presented, along with their application to real WCE data, collected from patients with ulcerous diseases. The chapter concludes by pointing out the potential of the proposed approaches towards efficient automated ulcer detection systems that will moderate the labour of the gastroenterologist and, consequently, the cost of the WCE examination.

2. Wireless Capsule Endoscopy (WCE)

In gastroenterology, the most common and established technique to visually inspect the GI tract and diagnose its diseases is endoscopy. The traditional endoscopic examinations applied for diagnosis in the upper and lower part of the GI tract, including esophagus, stomach, duodenum, terminal ileum and colon, are highly invasive causing discomfort to the patients. The visual inspection of the entire small intestine, in particular, has posed a challenge to gastroenterologists due to the strain of physically reaching it. Its important length and numerous windings make the examination extremely difficult, painful and not always possible, since usually there is a dead space in the middle part. Some imaging techniques used for the small intestine inspection include enteroclisis, small bowel follow through, push, sonde, and double balloon enteroscopy. Nevertheless, they are deeply inconvenient for the patients and require highly experienced gastroenterologists.

In 2000, advances in high integration and miniaturization allowed the researchers of Given Imaging to draw the attention of the GI community by unveiling what is now called endoscopic capsule. Wireless capsule endoscopy (WCE) (Iddan *et al.*, 2000) is a novel medical procedure, which has revolutionized endoscopy, as it has enabled, for the first time, a painless and effective diagnosis inside the GI tract. A WCE system consists of the capsule endoscope, a data recorder system and computer software for WCE data processing. The capsule endoscope is a disposable, pill-shaped device which consists of a CMOS camera, four light sources, two batteries and a radio transmitter. The patient shallows the capsule which captures images of the GI tract at a speed of two frames per second (fps). These images are compressed with JPEG algorithm and transmitted wirelessly to a special recorder attached to the patient's waist. The entire process lasts approximately 8 hours until the batteries exhaust. Finally, the images stored in the recorder are downloaded to a computer and the physicians, with the aid of the special software, can review the images and analyse potential sources of various GI diseases. The capsule travels along the digestive tract with the physiological peristalsis, without the need for air insufflation and sedation. Thus, the examination of the entire small intestine has become the most comfortable endoscopic examination for the patient to undergo. In this way WCE is suitable even for children and elderly.

WCE has proven invaluable in evaluating various diseases of the small bowel (Friedman, 2004; Pennazio, 2005), such as obscure bleeding (Mylonaki *et al.*, *2003*), polyps and neoplasm, Crohn's disease, celiac disease and mucosal ulcers (Aronott & Lo, 2004). Ulcer is one of the most common lesions of the GI tract that affects approximately 10% of the people. The most usual causes are Helicobacter pylori bacteria and use of nonsteroidal anti-inflammatory drugs (NSAID). Ulcer is a chronic inflammatory sore or erosion on the internal mucous membranes that arises in small intestine, especially in duodenum (the upper part of the small intestine) and in stomach. Some serious diseases are associated with ulcer, like Crohn's disease and ulcerative colitis. Although ulcer by itself is not lethal, complications are capable of causing death. That is the reason why early diagnosis and treatment is extremely essential.

2.1 Side effects

WCE is a well-tolerated and safe procedure with very few and rare complications. The main risk of WCE is capsule retention. Despite the small diameter of the capsule, a narrowing of the small bowel may cause it to become retained at a site of stricture. However, retention is estimated to occur in less than 1% of cases (Liao et al., 2010). The 2005 International Conference on Capsule Endoscopy reached a consensus stating that a capsule would be deemed to have been retained if it could be shown to be remaining in the GI tract more than two weeks, without symptoms, after it had been ingested. The causes of capsule retention are bowel obstructions narrower than the size of the capsule (11mm diameter). Small bowel strictures are a frequent complication of Crohn's disease (Cheifetz et al., 2006) and prolonged use of NSAID (Meredith et al., 2009). The risk of capsule retention is also high for patients with a history of bowel obstruction or a previous gastrointestinal surgery. In case of retention, the removal of the capsule is most commonly performed by surgery (Barkin & Friedman, 2002), often resecting the obstructing lesion at the same time. However, there are cases where the removal is possible with traditional endoscopic techniques.

In order to reduce the risk of retaining the capsule, a barium small bowel examination should be performed or a biodegradable patency capsule (Fig. 2) (Riccioni et al., 2003) should be digested prior to WCE. However, two studies (Meredith et al., 2009) indicated that small bowel follow through radiography (SBFT) investigations were not effective at excluding patients at risk of retention. Additionally, patients with abnormal SBFT can have successful WCE. The patency capsule is exactly the same size as the capsule endoscope but it is made from lactose, with 10% barium sulphate to make it radiopaque, and surrounded by

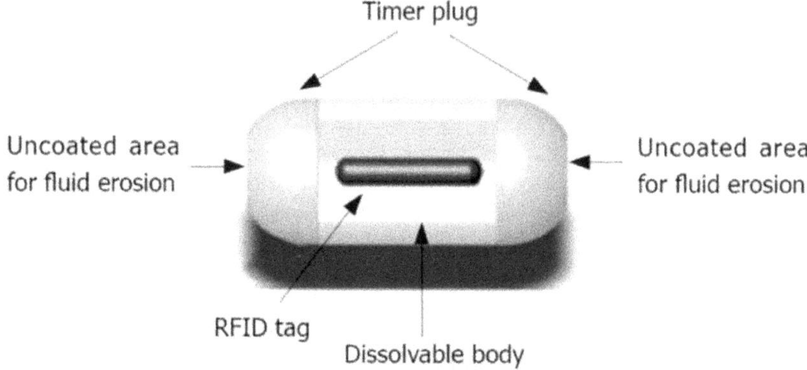

Fig. 2. Schematic drawing of a biodegradable patency capsule.

a cellophane coating. It has a timer plug which is slowly dissolved by gastric fluids, giving a disintegration time of 40-100 hours post ingestion, and contains a very small radiofrequency identification tag (RFID) which can be used to tract its location in the small bowel without the use of ionizing radiation. The patency capsule remaining in one area for a large period of time can suggest retention. Early experience with this biodegradable capsule indicates that it allows accurate and objective evaluation of potentially obstructing small bowel lesions prior to WCE (Belvin *et al.*, 2003; Cauendo *et al.*, 2003). Although the patency capsule is mostly soluble, there needs to be further research to determine whether its use will reduce the risk of the patient, requiring surgery to remove there is a pathological stricture present. Successful passing of this patency capsule intact and without pain can provide evidence that a capsule endoscope will have a similar successful journey.

To conclude, the retention of a capsule endoscope can be a significant complication procedure, requiring corrective surgery. Whilst the overall risk of retention is low, factors that increase this risk include known or suspected Crohn's disease, a history of NSAID use and previous small bowel surgery. Taking a careful medical history can identify those patients at higher risk of retention, and for those identified, the administration of a patency capsule allows the assessment of the patient's risks from swallowing a small bowel WCE.

2.2 Advances in wireless capsule endoscopy

WCE is still an under development technology, which may change endoscopy forever. However, there are technical limitations that raise some serious questions. Will capsule endoscopy replace traditional upper gastrointestinal endoscopy and colonoscopy? Will capsule endoscopy be able to deliver therapy? The answer is probably yes, but, there are major challenges that the capsule technology needs to overcome, to compete with probe gastroscopy and colonoscopy. As mentioned before, WCE is especially recommended for exploration of the small bowel, while it exhibits poorer diagnostic efficacy for the examination of esophagus, stomach and colon (Van Gossum *et al.*, 2009). The limitations/challenges include: power management, camera speed and image quality, controllable manoeuvring, and interventional capabilities (Swain, 2008).

The first endoscopic capsule, due to limited power supply, ceased image capturing before crossing the entire GI tract. It was even possible that transmission stopped before the end of ileum, in case of extended residence in stomach. Consequently, visualization of colon was impossible. In this context, researches were directed towards a more energy efficient capsule, capable of exploring the entire digestive tract. Technological advances allowed researchers to make radical changes in WCE design and energy supply (Moglia *et al.*, 2009). In particular, two breakthroughs took place. Firstly, the advent of more efficient battery materials (i.e., carbon nanotubes and buckytubes) led to batteries smaller in size with better electrical conductivity leaving room for a third battery in the capsule with a slight increase in size. Secondly, an intelligent power management system was introduced in the data recorder that saves energy by regulating the image transmission rate and applying a sleep mode to the capsule. The recorder recognizes the location of the capsule inside the GI tract and adjusts the transmission rate accordingly. The capturing of images starts half an hour after ingestion to allow travelling to the target area (sleep mode). When the capsule arrives in stomach, the recorder recognizes it and maintains a slow transmission rate of six images per minute. The recorder is also able to detect when the capsule enters small intestine and raises the transmission rate. Additionally, the recorder identifies if the capsule is in motion or stationary. If the capsule is moving the camera captures up to 35 images per second. Last but not least, the recorder has the intelligence to notify the patient with a sound signal and a vibration to ingest a prokinetic agent if the capsule resides in stomach for over an hour. This new design and technical achievements are very impressive. Yet the critical question to be addressed is whether this new capsule endoscope leads to improved diagnostic performance compared to traditional colonoscopy. Studies (Adler & Metzger, 2011) indicate that the diagnostic yield of WCE in colon has increased but still cannot surpass colonoscopy.

Currently, researchers intensely strive to unravel the issue of limited energy store inside the capsule by developing external wireless power transmission systems (Carta *et al.*, 2010). These approaches are based on magnetic fields and three-dimensional (3D) coils through a process that is known as inductive coupling. According to this phenomenon, an alternating magnetic field induces electrical voltage and electrical current to a coil that resides inside the field. Thus, the concept is to create a magnetic field around the human body that will transmit power to the capsule. To accomplish this, the capsule is equipped with windings of very thin copper wires (Fig. 3) around a ferrite core towards all three directions (3D coil). Ferrite is a lightweight material with efficient electromagnetic characteristics that support the formation of magnetic field. The existence of a ferrite core inside a coil has the effect of locally intensifying the magnetic field; hence, increasing the amount of collected power. On the contrary, the absence of the ferrite core would necessitate a larger coil for the same amount of received power. External power transmission systems seem promising and safe. Over 300mW usable power can be delivered while the maximum specific adsorption rate (SAR) does not exceed 0,329 W/Kg (Xin *et al.*, 2010), under the basic restrictions of the International Commission on Non-ionizing Radiation Protection (ICNIRP). However, there are major issues to deal with. The orientation of the capsule inside the body highly affects the stability of the received power. The amount of received power may drop over 55% for specific orientations which affects the proper operation of the capsule. Moreover, there is extensive power loss (over 70mW) in the electronic circuit that accompanies the coil inside the capsule. Another, equally important, problem is the stability of the external magnetic field which is altered by the human body. Despite the aforementioned issues, great steps forward have been made and it is likely, in the near future, an externally powered capsule endoscope to be realized.

The development of imaging technology and miniaturization resulted in size reduction of the image sensors and expansion of the camera angle of view. A wider viewing angle means

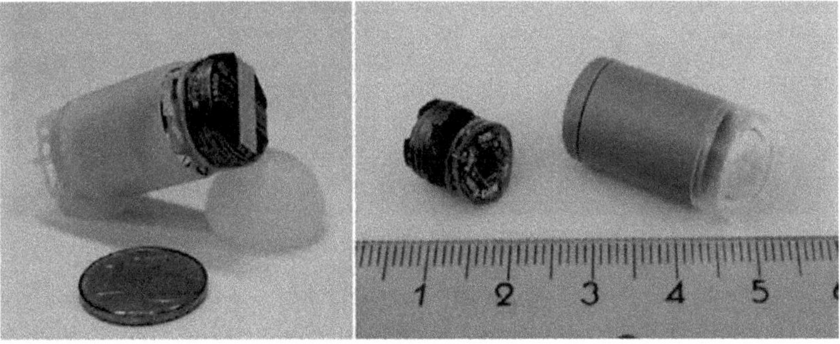

Fig. 3. 3D coil inside capsule endoscope for wireless power transmission (Carta *et al.*,2010).

more panoramic images. Smaller cameras contributed to increased free space inside the capsule, and as a result, the inclusion of a second camera. The twin camera capsule with a wider angle of view combined with the increased transmission frame rate enabled esophageal WCE (Waterman & Granlnek, 2009) with promising diagnostic efficiency. The size reduction of image sensors is, also, expected to result in increasing number of pixels and solve the problem of low resolution WCE images. New and more efficient image compression algorithms will, additionally, assist towards quality and color enhancement. Image compression is essential in WCE in order to significantly reduce the size of the image and, consequently, the storage space and transmission time required. However, the compression procedure lowers image quality by smoothing the razor-sharp details.

Gastroenterologists eagerly look forward the day that they will be able to control and steer the capsule endoscope as they do in standard endoscopy. This would give them control in maintaining the capsule steady in selected areas and hold the view in order to examine carefully the opposite wall of the bowel. To solve this problem, magnetic manoeuvring has recently become a thrust research area. The proposed approaches rely on a magnetic field applied to the capsule from the exterior of the patient, exploiting the principle that a magnet inside a magnetic field aligns with the direction of the field. The magnetic field can be used to control the movement trajectory, the position and the orientation of the endoscopic capsule. By changing the direction of the magnetic field, the direction of the capsule also changes. For this purpose, various techniques have been proposed in order to make an endoscopic capsule responsive to an external magnetic field. These include either magnetic parts and induction coils to be arranged inside the capsule, or magnetic shells to be reversibly applied to the capsule externally (Capri *et al.*, 2007) (Fig. 4). Capsule motions can readily be induced with hand-held/hand-guided magnets, as demonstrated even in the esophagus and stomach of a volunteer (Swain, 2010). This system is only available for research purposes. Nevertheless, the main issue related to the development of a clinically applicable technique is the generation and precise control of a stable magnetic field, really capable of guaranteeing accurate and reliable manoeuvrings of an endoscopic capsule. Such techniques start to emerge (Capri *et al.*, 2011; Gao *et al.*, 2010) and the realization of a self-propelled capsule is close.

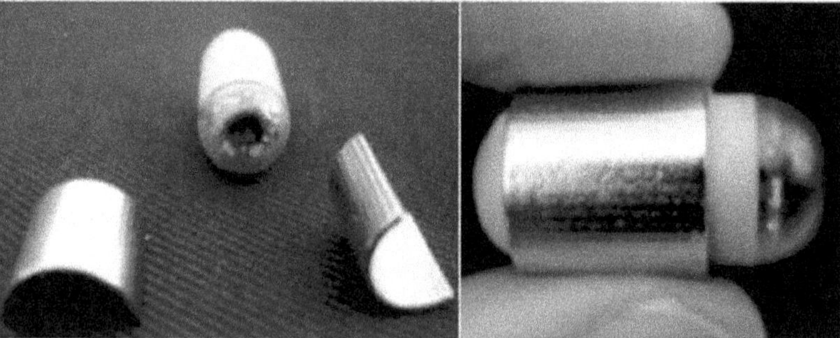

Fig. 4. Capsule with magnetic shield for controllable maneuvering (Capri *et al.*, 2011).

At present, WCE remains just a diagnostic tool that has yet to prove its potential. The endoscopic capsule is passive and cannot obtain biopsies, aspirate fluid, deliver drugs or brush lesions for cytology. The main pressure is to reduce the capsule size, which will release space that could be used for other interactive functions, and maximize power supply. New engineering methods for constructing tiny moving parts, miniature actuators and even motors into capsule endoscopes are being developed. However, these moving components require considerable amounts of power. Another limitation to therapeutic capsule endoscopy is the low mass of the capsule endoscope (approximately 4 grams). A force exerted on tissue, for example, by biopsy forceps may push the capsule away from the tissue. Opening small biopsy forceps to grasp tissue and pull it free will require different solutions to those used at conventional endoscopy. All these interventional capabilities seem to be something of a pipe dream at present but the huge technological leaps pave the way for an active therapeutic capsule.

The ideal WCE of the gastroenterologist's imagination should be remote controlled and capable of performing an ordinary biopsy as well as stop bleeding using adrenaline injection or a heat probe. The ultimate capsule would include special detectors for white blood cells and be able to measure various cytokines, pH, temperature and pressure, in addition to delivering drugs. Finally, the optimal WCE needs to contain a computerized system for automatic detection of pathologies, such as ulcer and polyps, in order to overcome the drawback of time-consuming viewing the video (Fireman, 2010). Technology for improving the capability of the future generation capsule is almost within grasp and it would not be surprising to witness the realization of these giant steps within the coming decade.

3. The concept of image decomposition

Automated knowledge extraction from medical images is a fast growing field of interest for the researchers. The attainment of this objective requires image decomposition to its components that will disclose the inherent structural characteristics of the image. In this context, this section presents Bidimensional Ensemble Empirical Mode Decomposition, a novel tool for image analysis.

3.1 Empirical Mode Decomposition (EMD)

In 1998, Huang *et al.* introduced a novel, intuitive and alternative signal decomposition technique for time-frequency analysis, namely Empirical Mode Decomposition (EMD) (Huang *et al.*, 1998). The major characteristic of EMD that renders it superior to traditional analysis methods, such as Fourier and Wavelets, is its adaptive nature. The decomposition does not require the use of *a priori* basis function. On the contrary, it is totally data driven. The concept that lies behind EMD is the existence of oscillations in every signal, at a very local level. Therefore, its target is to seek and reveal these inherent oscillatory modes, called Intrinsic Mode Functions (IMFs). EMD is designed to estimate IMFs of a signal so that, no matter how complicated the signal is, it embeds. A given signal $x(t)$ can be decomposed into n IMFs as:

$$x(t) = \sum_{i=1}^{n} c_i(t) + r_n(t), \tag{1}$$

where $c_i(t)$ is i^{th} IMF (IMF i) and $r_n(t)$ is the low frequency trend of $x(t)$ (residue). The highest frequency component of $x(t)$ corresponds to the lowest value of index i, i.e., $c_1(t)$ (IMF 1).

While the value of i increases, lower frequency components are obtained. An example is given in Fig. 5a, where the signal is decomposed into five IMFs plus residue. The process to calculate each $c_i(t)$ is called sifting process. The local extrema are defined and interpolated, resulting in two fitting curves, one for the maxima and one for the minima. Then, the mean curve is calculated and subtracted from the signal. This procedure continues until a stopping criterion is satisfied. The signal that remains after the last subtraction is $c_1(t)$. Next, $c_1(t)$ is subtracted from the initial signal and the remainder constitutes the new initial signal on which the above procedure is applied in order to extract the following IMFs until the desired number is obtained.

3.2 Ensemble EMD (EEMD)

Despite the great advantage of EMD, deficiency arises when the extrema of the original signal are unevenly distributed. In such a case, the IMFs are incorrectly calculated, since either a single IMF contains signals of widely disparate scales or a single mode of oscillations resides in two or more IMFs. This phenomenon is called *mode mixing* and an example is depicted in Fig. 5b. It is clear that the first two IMFs, apart from the high frequency component of the signal, incorrectly include a low frequency oscillation. To overcome this issue, Huang *et al.* proposed a noise-assisted version of EMD, namely ensemble EMD (EEMD) (Wu & Huang, 2009). EEMD requires the generation of an ensemble that contains multiple copies of the original signal that are distorted by white Gaussian noise, different for each copy, of finite amplitude. EMD is applied on every member of the ensemble and the final IMFs of the initial signal are derived by averaging the corresponding IMFs of each member of the ensemble. The concept of EEMD is grounded on the intuitive characteristics of white noise. White noise populates the whole time-frequency space uniformly and, as a result, establishes proper reference scales for the IMFs. The inherent modes of the signal are triggered by the noise and are projected accurately on the correct

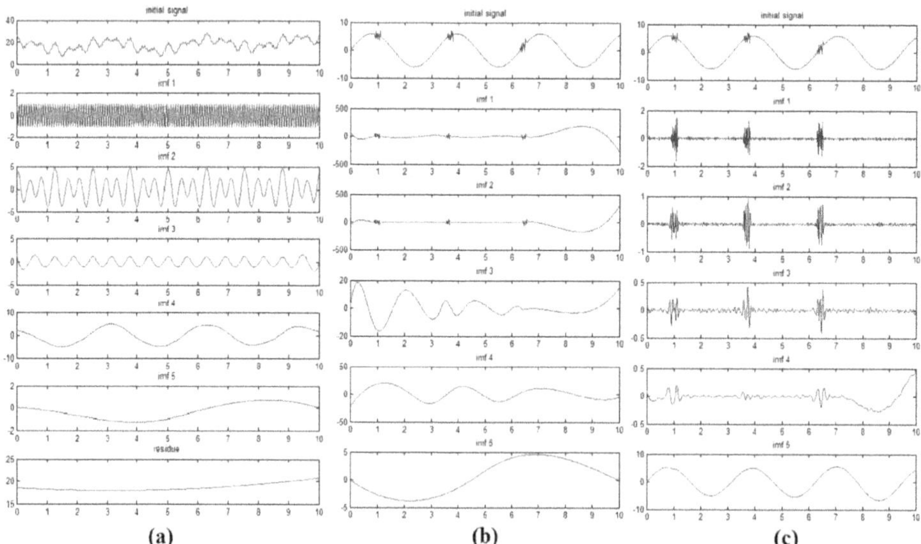

Fig. 5. (a) EMD analysis, (b) mode mixing phenomenon, (c) ensemble EMD analysis.

scales. The IMFs of each ensemble member are noisy but the final average IMFs are noise-free, since white noise cancels itself for a large number of ensemble members. Figure 5c presents the correct decomposition (using EEMD) of the signal in Fig. 5b. IMFs 1-3 include only the high frequency components while IMF5 contains the sinusoidal oscillation of the initial signal.

3.3 Bidimensional EEMD (BEEMD)

A multidimensional approach of EMD is required in case of a multidimensional signal. The extension of EMD in two dimensions (2D), namely Bidimensional EMD (BEMD), is an alternative multi-resolution analysis technique for image analysis and pattern discrimination. BEMD decomposes a 2D signal in 2D IMFs in the same way as eq. (1) demonstrates. However, there are two approaches for the realization of 2D extension. The first approach treats 2D data (images) as a collection of 1D slices (rows/columns) and applies 1D EMD on each row/column of the image (pseudo-BEMD). The second approach directly transplants the idea of 1D EMD algorithm in 2D data (genuine BEMD) after applying the appropriate changes (for example, fitting surfaces replace fitting curves). The first approach has the advantage of higher speed, while the latter exhibits improved performance, since the correlation among rows/columns of the image is taken into account. Bidimensional EEMD is the extension of EEMD in 2D (Wu *et al.*, 2009).

4. Texture extraction

Texture is a major property of any image that is useful in machine vision applications, especially for medical purpose. There are many approaches for texture analysis proposed in the literature. This paragraph describes the concept of Differential Lacunarity, an efficient tool for texture features extraction and identification.

4.1 Lacunarity Analysis (Lac)

Lacunarity (Lac) was introduced by Mandelbrot (Mandelbrot, 1993) as a fractal property, counterpart to fractal dimension (Mandelbrot, 1982), that describes the texture of a fractal. *Fractal dimension* is a measure of how much space is filled without consideration about the space-filling characteristics of data. In other words, two datasets with identical fractal dimensions can have distinct patterns with great differences in appearance. The introduction of Lac addressed this issue. Lac analyzes *how space is filled and consequently, can discriminate textures and natural surfaces that share the same fractal dimension.* In this direction, Lac has been used as a general technique to analyze patterns of spatial dispersion (Plotnick *et al.*, 1996). The term "lacunarity" has been used to evaluate and describe the distribution of gap sizes along datasets. A set with gaps of widely disparate sizes is considered heterogeneous and is characterized by high Lac, while a homogeneous set, with uniform gap sizes, exhibits lower Lac. It should be highlighted that homogeneous sets at large scales can be quite heterogeneous when examined at smaller scales and vice versa. From this perspective, Lac can be considered as a scale dependent tool to measure the heterogeneity or texture of an object (Gefen *et al.*, 1983).

Various algorithms have been proposed to calculate and quantify Lac, but the most popular are based on the "gliding box algorithm" (GBA) (Allain & Coitre, 1991) that is straightforward and computationally simple. GBA is applicable on binary datasets, although it can be extended to real datasets by converting the numerical data to dyadic by thresholding (Plotnick *et al.*, 1996).

4.2 Differential Lacunarity Analysis (DLac)

Most real life, image analysis applications need to extract texture information from either grayscale or color images without the option of thresholding. To this end, Dong (Dong, 2000) introduced a new version of Lac, namely Differential Lacunarity (DLac), suitable for grayscale image analysis. DLac is calculated by a differential box counting method. This algorithm employs a gliding box r of size r x r pixels and a gliding window w of size w x w pixels with $r<w$. Window w is initially positioned at the up left corner of the image and, by moving one by one columns to the left, scans the whole image. For every position of the window w, box r is placed inside the window at the up left corner and scans the image pixels bounded by the window (Fig. 6a) in order to calculate a value called "box mass". In other words, window w designates a region of the image (different each time until the entire image is covered) on which box mass is calculated with the aid of box r. According to the pixel values included in the box (r x r neighborhood) a column of more than one cubes of size (r x r x r) may be needed to cover the image intensity surface (Fig 6b). Numbers 1, 2, ... are assigned to the cubes from bottom to top and the differential height of the column $n(i,j)$ is calculated (i, j is the position of the box). Let the minimum and maximum pixel values reside in the cubes u and v, respectively. The differential height of the column is defined as

$$n(i,j) = v - u - 1. \tag{2}$$

As the box glides inside the window, the sum

$$M = \sum_{i,j} n(i,j), \tag{3}$$

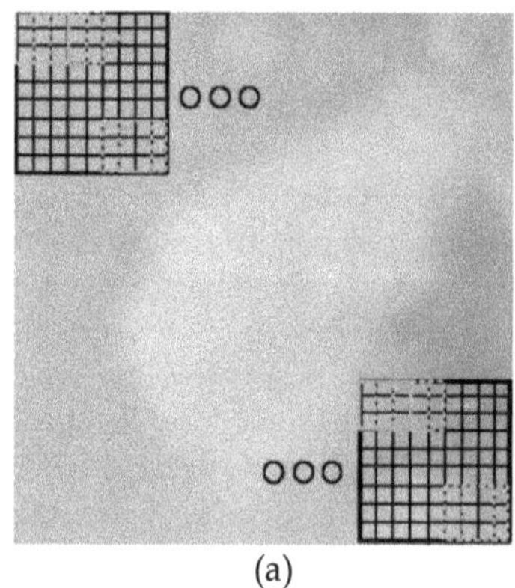

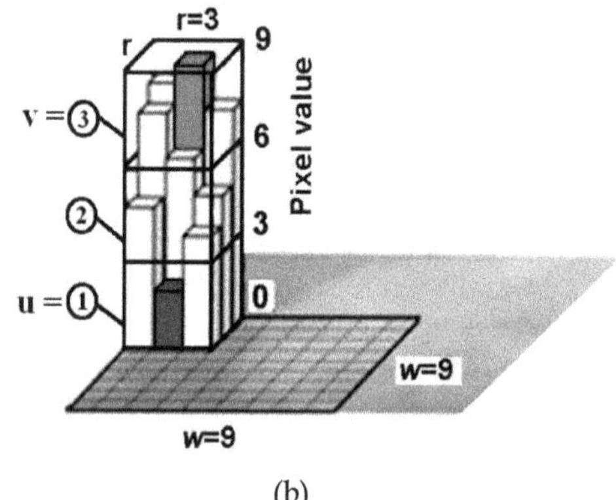

(a)   (b)

Fig. 6. (a) gliding box (green) and gliding window (black) movement throughout the image, (b) differential box counting method for box mass calculation (box size r=3, window size w=9, differential height of the column n=3-1-1=1).

is the box mass of the window w at a specific place. Let n(M,r) be the number of windows w with box mass M calculated by a box r. The probability function Q(M,r) is obtained by dividing n(M,r) by the total number of windows. The DLac of the image at scale r given a window w is defined as

$$\Lambda(r) = \frac{\sum_M M^2 Q(M,r)}{\left[\sum_M MQ(M,r)\right]^2}. \qquad (4)$$

5. The proposed automated ulcer tissue identification scheme

This section presents our proposed approach for color-texture-based automatic discrimination between ulcer and healthy tissue from WCE images. The color-texture concept was motivated by gastroenterologists' clinical practice, where the colour and texture properties of WCE images are utilized for reaching a diagnosis. More specifically, our scheme, named AR-DLac, combines BEEMD analysis to achieve adaptive image refinement (AR) with DLac analysis for efficient extraction of ulcer texture information. BEEMD-DLac combination for WCE image analysis was firstly introduced in (Charisis *et al.*, 2010b). The overall structure of the propose scheme is depicted in Fig. 7.

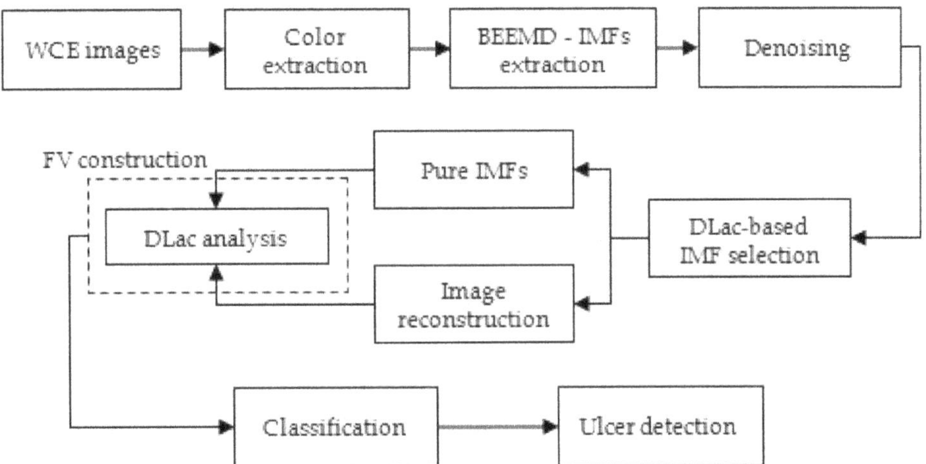

Fig. 7. The proposed AR-DLac scheme.

5.1 Color information

Each pixel in an image is characterized by a 3D color vector, i.e. three values that determine the color of the pixel. Various colour spaces exist to represent colour information. One of the most common color spaces is the hardware-oriented RGB (Red-Green-Blue). The majority of digital cameras, including the camera of a WCE system, utilize image sensors that capture colour images on the basis of the RGB model. In RGB, each colour is determined by the amount of red (R), green (G) and blue (B) present in the colour. In this context, a coloured WCE image comprises from three monochromatic components, one for each colour (R, G and B), whose combination provides the final colourful image.

Previous studies (Charisis *et al.*, 2010a, 2011) have shown that RGB is the most efficient space for WCE image analysis (compared to other colour spaces, i.e., HSV and CIE Lab). More specifically, the majority of ulcer texture information resides in green component of the RGB space. This conclusion coincides with the yellow-greenish appearance of ulcer regions. Thus, the proposed AR-DLac scheme is applied on the green channel extracted from each image.

5.2 Image denoising

The next step of our approach includes image purification by applying a denoising procedure. In order to facilitate texture-pattern extraction, the images need to be refined and smoothed by eliminating any distorting information. Endoscopic images from a WCE examination are prone to misleading content. Hardware limitations (quality of the image sensor and lens, non-adjustable light source) and adverse filming conditions (non-uniform lighting, reflections of the light on intestinal juices and lens cover, peptic content) are likely to cause high levels of noise to reside in total or part of the image (e.g., underexposed). To address this issue, we apply BEEMD analysis and each image is decomposed in eight 2D IMFs and residue. The first two IMFs contain the high frequency components of the image, i.e., the noise that may exist. Therefore, they are discarded and not utilized in the subsequent analysis and for image reconstruction. Figure 8 presents a worst case scenario, where artificial high level noise was added to an ulcer image. The distorted image is decomposed with BEEMD into eight IMFs and residue. The result (reconstructed image) proves that BEEMD is capable of dealing successfully with extreme cases of noise. Sheer

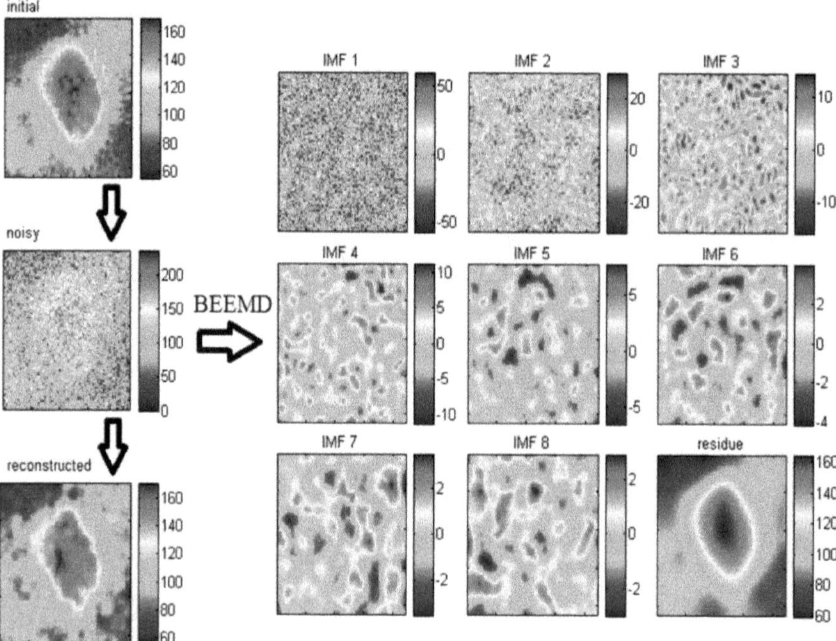

Fig. 8. Ulcer image with high-level, artificial noise decomposed in 8 IMFs plus residue and purified by BEEMD analysis.

noise reduction would be achieved by extracting three or four IMFs only. However, we opted for eight, since our target is to decompose the image to its components towards examining how intestinal information is distributed on a broad range of frequency scales and create a new, reconstructed image that reveals more efficiently ulcer texture information.

The motive for using BEEMD instead of other denoising techniques, such as Gaussian filter or wavelets, lies on the characteristics of the WCE images and the properties of BEEMD. The spatial characteristics of noise in WCE images and the spatial-frequency information representation of BEEMD, combined with its adaptive-to-the-data nature, provides a great advantage over a simple Gaussian filter. Moreover, ulcer regions are characterized by many and varying appearances and irregular shapes and sizes and do not have strong directional elements. Consequently, a tool, free from directional limitations, that permits multi-scale analysis is essential. Wavelet analysis has poor orientation selectivity (horizontal, vertical, diagonal) rendering BEEMD as a more efficient option.

5.3 AR-DLac scheme

In order to follow the WCE image characteristics and focus upon the ones that mostly relate to ulcer, an AR approach was developed. The aforementioned capabilities of EMD were exploited by developing a new DLac-based approach for the optimized selection of IMFs that correspond to ulcer characteristics of a WCE image. Towards this direction, DLac analysis is applied to every IMF of a decomposed image. The selected IMFs are used either to reconstruct a new image (R-case), or provide separate images (NR-case) that represent specific modes of oscillations coexisting in the initial WCE image. Apart from the optimal IMF selection, we are able to investigate how ulcer texture information are distributed across the frequency scales of WCE images.

5.3.1 Proposed DLac analysis

The great advantage of DLac is the ability to perform texture analysis in various scales. The coarseness of the scale is primarily determined by the size of window w, which designates the size of the neighbourhood for box mass calculation; the greater the window, the coarser the analysis scale. In the case of ulcer tissue recognition, a multi-scale texture analysis is required considering the great variability in size and appearance of ulcer regions. In this context, DLac is calculated for a variety of window sizes, given a constant, relative small box size r, in order to achieve pattern analysis at different scales, while identifying slight variations in neighbouring pixels (due to small value of r). An example of DLac-w (r=3, w=4-30) curves that correspond to images b, d, e and f from Fig. 1 is given in Fig. 9a. The curves are distinct, however, obvious discrimination is not achieved. To deliver greater differentiation between the curves an identical reference level has to be secured (Hadjileontiadis, 2009). Thus, DLac-w curves are normalized to the DLac value that corresponds to the smallest w. The resulting curves (Fig. 9b) provide quite clear discrimination between the four patterns. From now on, any reference to DLac-w curves implies normalized curves.

5.3.2 Optimized IMF selection

The selection of optimum IMFs is based on the characteristics of DLac-w curve of each IMF. The motive for such an approach lies in the concept that IMFs with possible useful texture

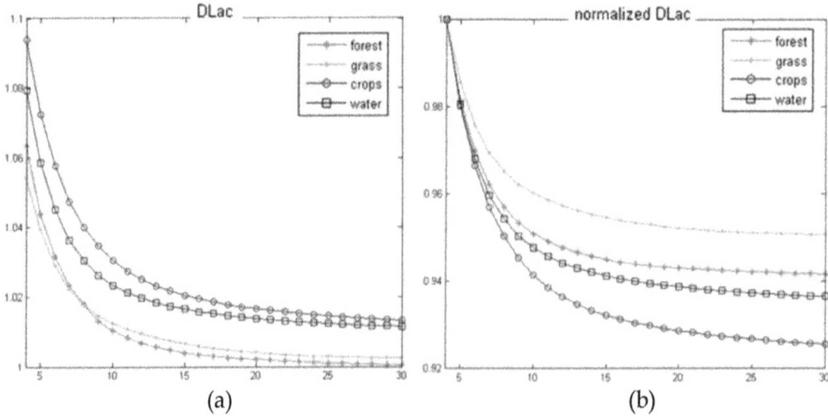

Fig. 9. DLac (a) and normalized DLac (b) curves for various window sizes (4 to 30 pixels) for images b, d, e and f from Fig. 1.

information should provide DLac-w curves that bear resemblance to the curves estimated on ulcer images. In this context, it has been observed that the slope of DLac-w curves of ulcer images lies within specific limits for the majority of ulcer cases. This observation led us to a slope-based criterion for IMF selection. The IMFs that provide DLac curves with slopes within the limits, specified by DLac curves of ulcer images, were selected. Figure 10 shows the selection probability of each IMF. According to the diagram, IMF5, IMF6 and IMF8 were selected for the majority of images implying that the information included in these IMFs should be taken under consideration.

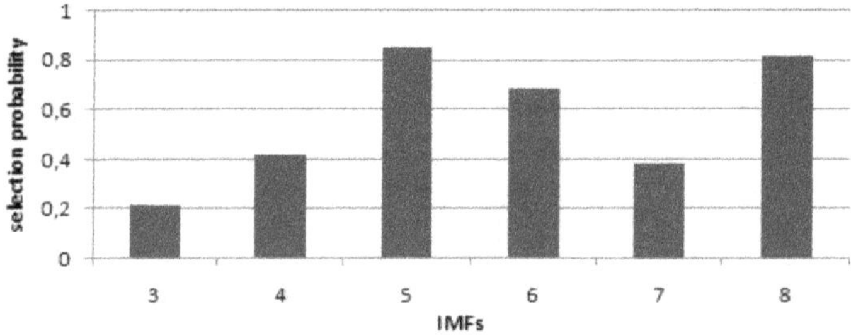

Fig. 10. Selection probability for each IMF.

5.3.3 DLac-based feature vector

In image pattern detection applications, feature vector (FV) is the set of features that characterize and represent an image and are utilized for the discrimination between various patterns. The DLac-based FV extraction was implemented in two different approaches, following the R-case and NR-case scenario. From a general perspective, the previously described DLac-w curve is used to form the FV. In our approach DLac-w curve is calculated for w=5-30 pixels. These 26 DLac values consist an extensive FV, subject to the "curse of dimensionality". The essence of reducing the feature space dimension without omitting any crucial information introduces the concept of modelling DLac-w curves with another function L(w). The normalized DLac-w curves in Fig. 9b expose an attitude that bears resemblance to the one of hyperbola. On this ground, the function

$$L(w) = \frac{a}{w^b} + c, \quad w=[5\text{-}30], \tag{5}$$

was chosen to model the normalized DLac-w curves (Hadjileontiadis, 2009). Parameter a represents the concavity of hyperbola, b portrays the convergence of L(w), and c is the translational term. The best interpretation of DLac-w by the model L(w) is computed as the solution of a least squares problem where parameters a, b, c are the independent variables. Parameters a, b, c embody the global behaviour of the DLac curve, i.e., all the substantial information. However, preliminary studies have shown that local behaviour of DLac curve is also important in ulcer tissue classification. Consequently, FV consists of parameters a, b, c plus five DLac values that correspond to the five smallest values of w (i.e., L(6) - L(10); L(5) is discarded as it always equals to one due to normalization). The values L(6) – L(10) were selected empirically after exhausting experiments. In this manner, FV embodies both local and global trend of DLac curve achieving a significant size reduction (eight rather than 26 values).

More specifically, in R-case scenario the selected IMFs and the residue recompose a new image on which the DLac-w curve is calculated and FV is extracted (FV^R) as described above. In NR-case scenario, the final FV (FV^{NR}) contains the FV from each selected IMF (FV_i, i=3 to 8). However, different number of IMFs is selected for every image with the subsequent problem of changing FV size. To address this issue, FV is designed to include the FVs from IMFs 5, 6 and 8 (i.e., $FV^{NR} = \{FV_5, FV_6, FV_8\}$) which are the most frequently chosen IMFs (Fig. 10) for all images in the dataset, implying that they contain the majority of beneficial information. Last but not least, the ability of texture information of each individual IMF to discriminate ulcer from normal images is investigated. In this case, the final FV (FV^{indiv}) consists of the FV from an individual IMF, different each time, i.e. $FV^{indiv} = FV_i$ for i=1 to 8. IMFs 1 and 2 are included, despite their noise contamination, for an overall assessment.

5.4 Classification

The last step of ulcer detection scheme is the classification procedure. This procedure involves the classification of extracted FVs into healthy/ulcerous and is accomplished by algorithms called "classifiers". The target of a classifier is to identify the population (e.g., healthy or abnormal) to which a FV belongs on the basis of a training set of FVs whose population is already known. It is usual that 90% of the sample dataset is used for training the classifier and 10% for testing. This procedure is repeated ten times (10-fold cross validation) with random training and test sets in order to acquire more accurate results. The classification performance is measured with the aid of accuracy (acc.), sensitivity (sens.) and specificity (spec.) indexes. The average acc., sens. and spec. are obtained in case of 10-fold cross validation technique. Various classification algorithms have been proposed in the literature. For an extensive evaluation of the classification performance of the proposed AR-DLac scheme, the widely used classification algorithms, i.e., LDA (Linear Discriminant Analysis), QDA (Quadratic Discriminant Analysis), MD (Mahalanobis Distance) (Krzanowski, 2000), and SVM (Support Vector Machine) (Cristiani & Shawe-Taylor, 2000), were adopted.

6. Experimental phase

The WCE images used in this study for the development and assessment of the proposed approach were drawn from six patients with ulcerous diseases, such as unexplained ulceration, ulceration from NSAID, ulcerative colitis and Crohn's diseases, who have undertaken a WCE examination in NIMTS Gastroenterology Clinic in Athens, Greece. The examinations were conducted with Pillcam SB (Given Imaging) WCE system. Rapid Reader 6.0 software (Given Imaging) was employed to export the images from the video sequence.

The dataset collected consists of 87 ulcer and 87 normal images. An example of the two categories is given in Fig. 11. The images were obtained by manual segmentation of the initial, complete WCE images. Two gastroenterologists reviewed the endoscopic video and manually isolated regions of interest (ROI), as the ones shown in Fig. 11, according to their expertise and upon agreement. It must be highlighted that the 87 ulcer images were obtained from 87 different events (ulcer regions) to achieve the lowest possible similarity. Furthermore, the normal images include both simple and confusing healthy tissue (folds, villus, bubbles etc.) in order to hamper the discrimination process. The ROI for the normal images varies from 110x110 to 220x220 pixels whereas the crop area of the ulcer images depends on the size, shape and position of the ulcer. The variety in ROI sizes does not affect the tissue discrimination procedure, since the feature vectors extracted from the images are utilized as the basis for comparison instead of the images themselves.

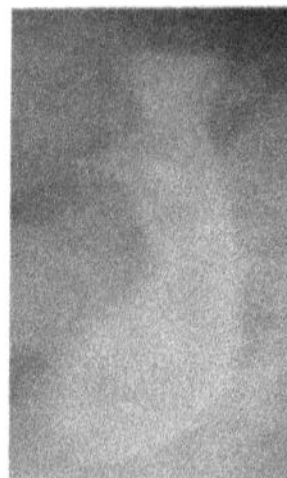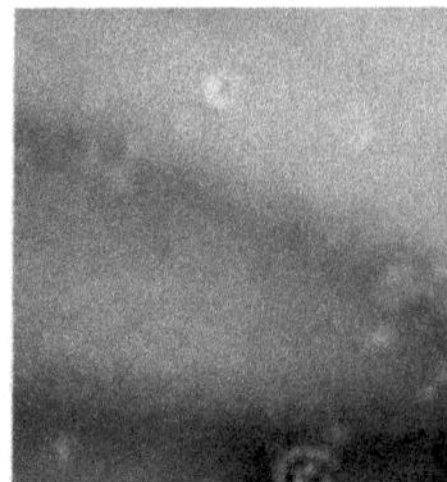

Fig. 11. An example of ulcerous (left) and normal (right) region of interest.

7. Results and discussion

The performance of the proposed AR-DLac scheme is evaluated through the experimental results derived from the application of the introduced approach to the dataset described in §6. To this end, results from every individual IMF analysis as well as results from both AR-DLac implementation scenarios (i.e., R-case and NR-case) are presented in this section.

7.1 Individual IMFs

Table 1 tabulates the classification performance achieved by the texture information extracted from each individual IMF ($FV^{indiv}=FV_i$, where FV_i is the feature vector constructed from IMFi as described in §5.3.3) for all classifiers. The highest classification rates obtained for each IMF are noted in bold. The format %±% corresponds to mean acc., sens. and spec. ± standard deviation.

The low classification rates for IMFs 1-2 denote their inefficiency in discriminating between ulcer and normal tissue. The performance of IMF1, in terms of classification accuracy, ranges from 51.9% to 61.3%, while the one of IMF2 varies from 53.3% to 62.0%. The sensitivity index is even lower (up to 29.1 percentage points) for the majority of classifiers (i.e., LDA, QDA and SVM). This performance implies that the texture information that lies in IMFs 1 and 2 is not eligible for ulcer detection. This behaviour is consistent with the concept of noise "contamination" of IMF1-2 and validates the noise reduction procedure described in §5.2 and illustrated in Fig 8. IMFs 1-2 contain the high frequency components of the image (i.e., the noise) and, therefore, should be discarded. On the contrary, the classification accuracy of IMF3-8 is 24.8% to 35.5% improved. IMF3 and IMF5 exhibit the lowest (77.4%) and highest (84%) performance (in terms of accuracy), respectively. Despite the superior classification rates, the performance of individual IMFs indicates that texture information that resides in a single image component is inadequate for efficient ulcer detection. Additionally, low classification sensitivity (<76%) suggests extensive misidentification of ulcer regions as healthy. It should be highlighted that IMFs 5, 6 and 8, that are the most commonly selected IMFs (Fig. 10) in IMF selection procedure, deliver the three highest classification accuracy rates among the IMFs. The convergence of these results testifies the optimal IMF selection procedure.

As far as the classification algorithms are concerned, the results in Table 1 imply that the most efficient classifiers include SVM and QDA. SVM achieves the best performance for the majority of IMFs (1-4, 8) due to its more advanced nature. However, the capabilities of QDA should not be underestimated since it exhibits 4.6, 5.7 and 4.8 percentage points higher classification accuracy than SVM for IMF5-7. LDA also proves competent, delivering slightly inferior performance. At last, MD is the most inappropriate classifier for our approach. The extremely high classification sensitivity (up to 99.2% for IMF6) in conjunction with the extremely low classification specificity (down to 15.6% for IMF6) denote over fitting to ulcer texture information.

Classifier		IMF							
		1	2	3	4	5	6	7	8.
LDA	Acc.	55.1±1.7	58.7±1.7	76.9±0.9	78.9±0.7	81.6±0.6	**80.0±1.1**	78.7±1.0	82.3±0.8
	Sens.	35.9±2.4	51.8±2.4	71.1±1.4	71.3±1.4	70.4±0.9	**72.2±1.7**	73.4±1.5	82.1±1.4
	Spec.	74.4±2.1	65.5±2.4	82.8±1.4	86.5±0.7	92.7±1.1	**87.7±1.6**	83.9±1.4	82.5±0.7
QDA	Acc.	59.5±0.8	59.9±1.4	77.1±0.9	79.7±0.7	**84.0±0.9**	78.2±0.8	**79.5±1.3**	80.5±0.9
	Sens.	30.4±1.4	42.3±2.2	66.2±1.4	64.9±1.1	**72.0±1.3**	67.1±1.6	**74.0±1.9**	65.7±1.5
	Spec.	88.6±1.1	77.5±1.7	88.1±1.5	94.4±0.9	**96.0±1.2**	89.2±0.6	**85.1±1.9**	95.3±1.1
MD	Acc.	51.9±0.7	53.3±1.4	61.2±1.1	66.3±1.0	61.3±1.0	57.4±1.4	62.4±1.1	68.5±1.1
	Sens.	98.3±0.8	96.6±1.2	93.8±1.0	93.8±1.0	97.1±0.9	99.2±0.9	98.3±0.9	96.5±1.0
	Spec.	5.6±1.3	10.0±2.7	28.5±1.9	34.6±1.9	25.5±1.8	15.6±2.5	26.5±2.1	40.5±1.9
SVM	Acc.	**61.3±1.6**	**62.0±1.5**	**77.4±1.1**	**79.8±1.0**	79.4±0.8	72.5±1.1	72.7±1.1	**82.5±0.5**
	Sens.	**42.9±2.0**	**59.8±1.8**	**74.2±1.2**	**75.9±1.3**	74.3±1.0	64.1±1.6	62.4±1.3	**67.7±0.9**
	Spec.	**79.8±2.2**	**64.2±2.6**	**80.5±1.6**	**83.5±1.6**	84.5±1.3	80.9±1.3	83.1±1.7	**93.3±1.0**

Table 1. Mean classification accuracy, sensitivity and specificity (%) for each individual IMF (FV_i, i=1 to 8), for all classifiers (LDA, QDA, MD, SVM).

7.2 Reconstruction (R-case) – Non Reconstruction (NR-case) scenarios

The proposed AR-DLac scheme, thoroughly described in §5.3, selects the optimum IMFs. In the reconstruction scenario (R-case) the selected IMFs and the residue reconstruct a new image from which the FV is extracted, while in non reconstruction scenario (NR-case) the FVs from the selected IMFs are concatenated in order to form the final FV. The results of both scenarios are tabulated in Table 2, for all classifiers. The best classification rates for each implementation scenario are notated in bold. The format %±% corresponds to mean acc., sens. and spec. ± standard deviation.

Classifier	Implementation scenario					
	R-case			NR-case		
	Acc.	Sens.	Spec.	Acc.	Sens.	Spec.
LDA	95.5±0.5	94.8±0.8	96.2±0.4	89.2±0.9	84.3±1.7	94.1±0.4
QDA	95.8±0.6	93.9±1.1	97.7±0.3	**91.2±0.9**	**86.2±1.3**	**95.9±1.1**
MD	96.3±0.2	96.0±0.1	96.6±0.6	78.7±1.4	98.3±0.9	58.3±2.7
SVM	**96.7±0.6**	**96.5±0.3**	**96.9±0.9**	89.7±0.8	87.5±1.0	91.9±0.9

Table 2. Mean classification rates (%) for both R-case and NR-case scenarios, for all classifiers (LDA, QDA, MD, SVM).

The most efficient performance of the proposed AR-DLac scheme is delivered in R-case scenario where the classification accuracy reaches 96.7% by exploiting SVM classifier. However, the difference between the most (SVM) and the least (LDA) efficient classifier is only 1.2 percentage points, in terms of accuracy, implying that the features extracted by the proposed analysis are quite robust, exhibiting advanced overall performance regardless of the classification algorithm engaged. It is also remarkable the fact that the high accuracy rate is accompanied by high and relatively consistent rates for both sensitivity (96.5%) and specificity (96.9%). These results indicate that AR-DLac scheme is capable of equally recognising ulcer and normal data without exhibiting bias towards a specific pattern. This behaviour applies to all examined classifiers since the difference between sensitivity and specificity does not exceed 2.6 percentage points.

The classification results of the NR-case, suggest inferior performance of the AR-DLac scheme during the non reconstruction scenario. The most effective classifier for NR-case is QDA delivering 91.2% accuracy, 86.2% sensitivity and 95.9% specificity. These rates, compared to those of R-case, are 5.5, 10.3 and 1.0 percentage points lower, respectively. Even the worst scenario for R-case (LDA classifier) achieves 4.3 percentage points higher accuracy than QDA in NR-case. Moreover, the balance between sensitivity and specificity rates deteriorated ranging from 4.4 (for SVM) to 40 (for MD) percentage points. MD, as in the individual IMF case, fails to recognize correctly the normal images since the specificity rate is 58.3%. The divergence in performance between R-case and NR-case indicates that the recomposed image by the optimal IMFs and the residue represents more efficiently the intestinal texture information than the individual components of the image. This may be explained by the fact that in NR-case the trend of the image (residue) is ignored. Moreover, the fact that FV^{NR} includes 3 IMFs x 8 features = 24 features in total (33% larger than FV^{R}) may also affect the classification performance.

The comparison of the results in Tables 1 and 2 denotes the inability of a single IMF to separate ulcer from normal images. R-case and NR-case deliver 12.7 and 7.2 percentage points improved classification accuracy compared to the most effective IMF (i.e., IMF5), respectively. The superiority of NR-case suggests that the utilization of a group of individual IMFs is more fruitful than standalone IMF exploitation.

8. Overall perspective and future work

The aforementioned experimental results highlight the potential of the proposed scheme towards ulcer and healthy intestinal tissue discrimination. The optimum image components (IMFs) that contain the majority of texture information include IMFs 5, 6 and 8. Individual IMFs score up to 84% classification accuracy, while their exploitation as a group enhances the detection rate up to 91.2%. On the contrary, the refined image reconstruction process achieves 96.7% successful tissue identification. When compared with other approaches, the proposed scheme seems to be more effective exhibiting increased classification ability by using a smaller feature vector. One of the most efficient ulcer detection approaches (Kodogiannis *et al.*, 2007b), used as a comparison baseline, employs 54 features (instead of 8) and results in 94.5% accuracy when applied to our dataset (Charisis *et al.*, 2011).

In spite of the promising performance of the proposed scheme, there are still some issues for improvements that should be taken under consideration for its use in a future computer aided diagnosis system. Firstly, the number of ulcer and normal images should be increased in order to secure maximum diversity between the ulcer cases, develop more robust algorithms and obtain more accurate conclusions. Secondly, automatic segmentation of the regions of interest (ROI) is mandatory. In our approach, WCE images are manually cropped to the ROI. A potential solution is to divide each WCE image (576x576) into small patches (64x64) and choose the patches that depict mucosa. These patches contain almost all possible ROI by covering the most valid area of the original WCE image. At last, the computational cost of the proposed techniques should be revised. In this work, the introduction of a real time application was not our objective. In this context, the computational cost of the current unoptimized MATLAB code is 9.3 seconds per ROI, considering an average size of 145x145 pixels. BEEMD analysis consumes 83.4% of this time while DLac analysis and classification absorb 16.2% and 0.4%, respectively. When focusing on real time application, dedicated hardware and programming languages, more efficient implementation algorithms (for BEEMD and DLac) and multithreading programming should be considered.

9. Conclusion

Wireless capsule endoscopy (WCE) is a novel, non-invasive form of endoscopy that has started a new era for the visual inspection of the entire small bowel. A WCE system consists of a pill-shaped, wireless capsule that the patient swallows. The capsule, propelled by the natural bowel movements, captures and transmits images from the internal mucous membranes, along its journey through the digestive tract. Despite the revolution WCE has introduced, there are several limitations that pose serious questions about the competency of WCE compared to probe gastroscopy and colonoscopy. Some of the major challenges include camera speed/quality, power supply, controllable manoeuvring and interventional capabilities. Significant research is conducted towards this direction, various approaches have been proposed and the first achievements have emerged. A new capsule equipped with two cameras and increased battery life has been developed for colon and esophagus examination. Magnetically remote controlling and wireless power transmission concepts are in experimental phase. Apart from the hardware-oriented limitations and approaches there is a major issue concerning the vast amount of data produced by a WCE examination. The optimal WCE needs to contain a computerized system for automatic detection of pathologies such as ulcer and polyps in order to overcome the drawback of time-consuming reviewing of the video (Fireman, 2010). In this context, researchers aim to develop automatic diagnosis systems. The main contribution of this work is the presentation of a novel tool for WCE image analysis and classification by exploiting color-texture features. This color-texture perspective was inspired by the one the gastroenterologist usually adopts in clinical practice for successful diagnosis of pathologies and, especially, ulcer. The proposed AR-DLac scheme is based on the ingenious combination of BEEMD and DLac, applied on the green component of WCE images in order to identify ulcerations. BEEMD, apart from an adaptive image denoising tool, was exploited to reveal the intrinsic components (IMFs) of the images in order to achieve data driven, adaptive image refinement (AR), boost the distinctness between normal and ulcer regions and facilitate DLac analysis to extract efficient texture characteristics. AR entailed optimum IMF selection, based on the structure patterns of IMFs disclosed by DLac. The optimum IMFs were used either to reconstruct a new, refined image, or provide separate images. The proposed AR-DLac approach was evaluated on selected WCE images, captured from patients, depicting ulcer and healthy tissue. Experimental results have shown that AR-DLac scheme exhibits quite satisfactory overall classification performance. Intestinal texture information is distributed along IMFs 3 to 8; thus, the utilization of a single IMF for the detection procedure is not recommended. The classification performance of individual IMFs does not exceed 84% (classification accuracy), with IMF5 being the most efficient. When individual images (i.e., optimum IMFs) are employed (non reconstruction case) the performance improves and accuracy reaches 91.2%. However, the best results are delivered in the reconstruction case, where accuracy, sensitivity and specificity exceed 96.5%. The advanced overall classification performance of AR-DLac approach paves the way for its use in a provisional automatic diagnosis system.

10. References

Adler, S.N. & Metzger, Y.C. (2011). PillCam COLON capsule endoscopy: recent advances and new insights, *Therapeutic Advances in Gastroenterology*, Vol.4, No.4, pp. 265-268

Allain, C. & Coitre, M. (1991). Characterizing the lacunarity of random and deterministic fractal sets, *Physical Review A*, Vol.44, No.6, pp. 3552-3558

Ameling, S.; Wirth, S.; Paulus, D.; Lacey, G. & Vilarino, F. (2009). Texture-based polyp detection in colonoscopy, *Proc. of Bildverarbeitung fur die Medizin 2009*, pp. 364-350, Berlin, Germany, March 22-25, 2009

Aronott, I.D.R. & Lo, S.K. (2004). The clinical utility of wireless capsule endoscopy, *Digestive Diseases and Sciences*, Vol.49, No.6, pp. 893–901

Barkin, J.S. & Friedman, S. (2002). Wireless capsule endoscopy requiring surgical intervention: the world's experience, *The American Journal of Gastroenterology*, Vol.97, No.9, pp. S298

Belvin, ML.; Voderholzer, WA. & Loch, S. (2003). Diagnosing small intestinal strictures: first experience with the M2A patency capsule, *Endoscopy*, Vol.35, Suppl. II, pp. A184

Berlin, B. & Kay, P. (1969). *Basic Color Terms: Their Universality and Evolution*, University of California Press, ISBN 1-57586-162-3, Berkeley, California

Bourbakis, N. (2005). Detecting abnormal patterns in WCE images, *Proc. of 5th IEEE Symposium on Bioinformatics and Bioengineering*, pp. 232-238, Minneapolis, U.S.A., October 19-21, 2005

Capri, F.; Galbiati, S. & Capri, A. (2007). Controlled navigation of endoscopic capsules: Concept and preliminary experimental investigations, *IEEE Trans. on Biomedical Engineering*, Vol.54, No.11, pp. 2028–2036

Capri, F.; Kastelein, N.; Talcott, M. & Pappone, C. (2011). Magnetically Controllable Gastrointestinal Steering of Video Capsules, *IEEE Trans. on Biomedical Engineering*, Vol.58, No.2, pp. 231-234

Carta, R.; Thone, J. & Puers, R., Wireless power and data transmission for robotic endoscopic capsules, *Proc. of 12th Mediterranean Conference on Medical and Biological Engineering and Computing*, pp. 232-235, Chalkidiki, Greece, May 27-30

Cauendo, A.; Rodriquez- Teilez, M.; Hernandez- Duran, M. *et al.* (2003). Evaluation of M2A patency capsule in the gastrointestinal tract: one-capsule preliminary data from a multicentre prospective trial, *Endoscopy*, Vol.35, Suppl.II, pp. A182

[a]Charisis, V. *et al.* (2010). Abnormal Pattern Detection in Wireless Capsule Endoscopy Images Using Nonlinear Analysis in RGB Color Space, *Proc. of 32nd International Conference of IEEE Engineering in Medicine and Biology Society*, pp. 3674-3677, Buenos Aires, Argentina, August 31- September 4

[b]Charisis, V. *et al.* (2010). Ulcer Detection in Wireless Capsule Endoscopy Images Using Bidimensional Nonlinear Analysis, *Proc. of 12th Mediterranean Conference on Medical and Biological Engineering and Computing*, pp. 236-239, Chalkidiki, Greece, May 27-30

Charisis, V.; Hadjileontiadis, L.J.; Liatsos, C.N.; Mavrogiannis, C.C. & Sergiadis, G.D. (2011). Capsule Endoscopy Image Analysis Using Texture Information from Various Color Models, *Computer Methods and Programs in Biomedicine*, under revision.

Cheifetz, A.S. *et al.* (2006). The risk of retention of the capsule endoscope in patients with known or suspected Crohn's disease, *The American Journal of Gastroenterology*, Vol.101, No.10, pp. 2218-2222

Coimbra, M. & Silva Cunha, J.P. (2006). MPEG-7 visual descriptors-contributions for automated feature extraction in capsule endoscopy, *IEEE Trans. on Circuits and Systems for Video Technology*, Vol.16, No.5, pp. 628-637

Cristianini, N. & Shawe-Taylor, J. (2000). *An Introduction to Support Vector Machines and Other Kernel-based Learning Methods*, Cambridge University Press, ISBN 0-52-178019-5, Cambridge, UK

Dong, P. (2000). Test of a new lacunarity estimation method for image texture analysis, *International Journal of Remote Sensing*, Vol.21, No.17, pp. 3369-3373

Fireman, Z. (2010). Capsule endoscopy: Future horizons, *World Journal of Gastrointestinal Endoscopy*, Vol.2, No.9, pp. 305-307

Foster, D.H. *et al.* (1997). Four issues concerning colour constancy and relational colour constancy, *Vision Research*, Vol.37, No.10, pp. 1341-1345

Foucault, M. (1973). *The Birth of the Clinic: An Archaeology of Medical Perception*, ISBN 0-415-30772-4, Pantheon Books, New York, USA

Friedman, S. (2004). Comparison of capsule endoscopy to other modalities in small bowel, *Gastrointestinal Endoscopy Clinics of North America*, Vol.14, No.1, pp. 51–60

Gan, T.; Wu, J.-C.; Rao, N.-N.; Chen, T. & Liu, B. (2008). A feasibility trial of computer-aided diagnosis for enteric lesions in capsule endoscopy, *World Journal of Gastroenterology*, Vol.14, No.45, pp. 6929-6935

Gao, M.; Hu, C.; Chen, Z.; Zhang, H. & Liu, S. (2010). Design and Fabrication of a Magnetic Propulsion System for Self-Propelled Capsule Endoscope, *IEEE Trans. on Biomedical Engineering*, Vol.57, No.12, pp. 2891–2902

Gefen, Y.; Meir, Y.; Mandelbrot, B.B. & Aharony,A. (1983). Geometric implementation of hypercubic lattices with noninteger dimensionality by use of low lacunarity fractal lattices, *Physical Review Letters*, Vol.50, No.3, pp. 145–148

Hadjileontiadis, L.J. (2009). A texture-based classification of crackles and squawks using lacunarity, IEEE Trans. on Biomedical Engineering, Vol.56, No.3, pp. 718-732

Haralick, R.M.; Shanmugam, K. & Dinstein, I. (1973). Textural features for image classification, *IEEE Trans. on Systems, Man and Cybernetics*, Vol.3, No.6, pp. 610-621

Huang, N.E. *et al.* (1998). The empirical mode decomposition and the Hilbert spectrum for nonlinear and non-stationary time series analysis, *Proc. of Royal Society of London A*, Vol.454, No.1971, pp. 903–995

Iakovidis, D.K.; Maroulis, D.E.& Karkanis, S.A. (2006). An intelligent system for automatic detection of gastrointestinal adenomas in video endoscopy, *Computers in Biology and Medicine*, Vol.26, No.10, pp. 1084-1103

Iddan, G.; Meron, G.; Glukhovsky, A. & Swain, P. (2000). Wireless capsule endoscopy, *Nature*, Vol.405, No.6785, pp. 417-417

Julesz, B. (1975). Experiments in the visual perception of texture, *Scientific American*, Vol. 232, No.4, pp 34-43

Karkanis, S.A.; Iakovidis, D.K.; Maroulis, D.E.; Karras, D.A. & Tsivras, M. (2007). Computer-aided tumor detection in endoscopic video using color wavelet features, *IEEE Trans. on Information Technology in Biomedicine*, Vol.7, No.3, pp. 142-151

[a]Kodogiannis, V.S.; Boulougoura, M.; Lygouras, J.N. & Petrounias, I. (2007). A neuro-fuzzy-based system for detecting abnormal patterns in wireless-capsule endoscopic images, *Neurocomputing*, Vol. 70, No.4-6, pp. 704-717

[b]Kodogiannis, V.S.; Boulougoura, M.; Wadge, E. & Lygouras, J.N. (2007). The usage of soft-computing methodologies in interpreting capsule endoscopy, *Engineering Applications of Artificial Intelligence*, Vol.20, No.4, pp. 539-553

Krzanowski, W.J. (2000). *Principles of multivariate analysis: A user's perspective*, Oxford University Press, ISBN 0-19-850708-9, New York, USA

Li, B. & Meng, M.Q.-H. (2007). Analysis of the gastrointestinal status from wireless capsule endoscopy images using local color feature, *Proc. of 2007 International Conference on Information Acquisition*, pp. 553-557, Jeju, Korea, July 8-11, 2007

[a]Li, B. & Meng, M. Q.-H. (2009). Computer-based detection of bleeding and ulcer in wireless capsule endoscopic images by chromaticity moments, *Computers in Biology and Medicine*, Vol.39, No.2, pp. 141-147

[b]Li, B. & Meng, M. Q.-H. (2009). Texture analysis for ulcer detection in capsule endoscopy images, *Image and Vision Computing*, Vol.27, No.3, pp. 1336-1342

Liao, Z.; Gao, R.; Xu, C. & Li, ZS. (2010). Indications and detection, completion, and retention rates of small-bowel capsule endoscopy: a systematic review, *Gastrointestinal Endoscopy*, Vol.71, No.2, pp. 280-286

Lorenz, R.; Jorysz, G. & Classen, M. (1993). The value of endoscopy and endosonography in the diagnosis of the dysphagic patient, *Dysphagia*, Vol.8, No. 2, pp. 91-97

Magoulas, G. (2006). Neuronal networks and textural descriptors for automated tissue classification in endoscopy, *Oncology Repots*, Vol.15, pp. 997–1000

Maieron, A. *et al.* (2004). Multicenter retrospective evaluation of capsule endoscopy in clinical routine, *Endoscopy*, Vol.36, No.10, pp. 864-868

Mandelbrot, B.B. (1982). *The Fractal geometry of nature*, W. H. Freeman, ISBN 0-7167-1186-9, New York, USA

Mandelbrot, B.B. (1993). A fractal's lacunarity, and how it can be tuned and measured, In: *Fractals in Biology and Medicine*, T.F. Nonnenmacher, G.A. Losa, and E.R. Weibel (eds.), pp. 8-21, Birkhauser, ISBN 978-3-7643-2989-1, Basel, Switzerland.

Meredith, A.; Nightngale, J. & Eden, J.K. (2009). Capsule endoscopy: The risk of retention, *Synergy*, July 2009

Miller, P. & Astley, S. (1992). Classification of breast tissue by texture analysis, *Image Vision Computing*, Vol.10, No.5, pp. 277–282

Moglia, A.; Menciassi, A.; Dario, P. & Cuschieri, A. (2009). Capsule endoscopy: Progress update and challenges ahead, *Nature Reviews Gastroenterology & Hepatology*, Vol.6, pp. 353–362

Mylonaki, M.; Fritscher- Ravens, A. & Swain, P. (2003). Wireless capsule endoscopy: A comparison with push enteroscopy in patients with gastroscopy and colonoscopy negative gastrointestinal bleeding, *Gut*, Vol.52, No.8, pp. 1122–1126

Pennazio, M. (2005). Diagnosis of small-bowel diseases in the era of capsule endoscopy, *Expert Review of Medical Devices*, Vol.2, No.5, pp. 587–598

Plotnick, R.E.; Gardner, R.H.; Hargrove, W.W.; Prestegaard, K. & Perlmutter, M. (1996). Lacunarity analysis: A general technique for the analysis of spatial patterns, *Physical Review E*, Vol.53, No.5, pp. 5461-5468

Riccioni, M.E. *et al.* (2003). M2A patency capsule in the evaluation of patients with intestinal stricture: preliminary results, *Endoscopy*, Vol.35, Suppl.II, pp. A6

Rutgeerts, P. *et al.* (1980). Crohn's Disease of the Stomach and Duodenum: A Clinical Study with Emphasis on the Value of Endoscopy and Endoscopic Biopsies, *Endoscopy*, Vol.12, No.6, pp. 288-294

Swain, P. (2008). The future of wireless capsule endoscopy, *World Journal of Gastroenterology*, Vol.14, No.26, pp. 4142–4145

Swain, P. *et al.* (2010). Remote magnetic manipulation of a wireless capsule endoscope in the esophagus and stomach of humans, *Gastrointestinal Endoscopy*, Vol.71, No.7, pp. 1290–1293

Tuceryan, M. & Jain, A.K. (1998). Texture Analysis, In: *The handbook of pattern recognition and computer vision*, C.H. Chen; L.F. Pau, & P.S.P. Wang, (Eds), 207-248, World Scientific Publishing Co., ISBN 9-810-23071-0, Singapore

Van Gossum, A. *et al.* (2009). Capsule endoscopy versus colonoscopy for the detection of polyps and cancer, *The New England Journal of Medicine*, Vol.361, No.3, pp. 264–270

Wang, P.; Krishnan, S.M.; Kugean,C.& Tjoa, M.P. (2001). Classification of endoscopic images based on texture and neural network, *Proc. of 23rd International Conference of the IEEE Engineering in Medicine and Biology Society*, Vol. 4, pp. 3691-3695, Istanbul, Turkey, October 25-28, 2001

Waterman, M. & Gralnek, I.M. (2009). Capsule endoscopy of the esophagus, *Journal of Clinical Gastroenterology*, Vol.43, No.7, pp. 605-612

Wu, Z. & Huang, N.E.(2009). Ensemble empirical mode decomposition: A noise-assisted data analysis method, *Advances in Adaptive Data Analysis*, Vol.1, No.1, pp. 1-41

Wu, Z.; Huang, N.E. & Chen, X. (2009). The multi-dimensional ensemble empirical mode decomposition method, *Advances in Adaptive Data Analysis*, Vol.1, No.3, pp. 339-372

Xie, J.; Jiang, Y. & Tsui, HT. (2005). Segmentation of kidney from ultrasound images based on texture and shape priors, *IEEE Trans. on Medical Imaging*, Vol.24, No.1, pp. 45–57

Xin, W.; Yan, G. & Wang, W. (2010). Study of a wireless power transmission system for an active capsule endoscope, *International Journal of Medical Robotics and Computer Assisted Surgery*, Vol.6, No.1, pp. 113-122

10

Methods of Protein Digestive Stability Assay – State of the Art

Mikhail Akimov and Vladimir Bezuglov
Shemyakin-Ovchinnikov Institute of Bioorganic Chemistry, Russian Academy of Science
Russian Federation

1. Introduction

The evaluation of protein stability in digestive tract is an important topic in various fields of biomedical sciences. The most straightforward task within it is the evaluation of food quality, as during the food processing the digestibility of a protein could fall dramatically. Another task, tightly connected with the previous one, is the evaluation of protein allergenicity. This parameter is shown to be dependent on protein's digestibility, the less digestible ones having the highest probability to induce immune response. Finally, the task of development of new peptide drugs also requires digestive stability check for *per os* drug forms that are the most convenient for a patient.

Current knowledge on protein digestion suggests it to be a multistage process, starting from pepsin cleavage in stomach and proceeding through trypsin and chymotrypsin digestion in intestinal lumen, and finally involving cleavage by intestinal surface and intracellular proteases. The latter two protease groups accomplish the most deep protein degradation. An intriguing point is that in spite of this knowledge the models, which include all stages of protein digestion, are used primarily in food quality control.

Protein digestion, specific enzymes, involved in this process, as well as research area specific methodology for protein digestibility evaluation is regularly reviewed. However, as a common rule, the authors of latter group of reviews ignore the existence of methods with similar goals in other research areas, as well as the question of a degree to which any given method represents a living organism. The aim of this review is to describe existing models for evaluation of protein digestibility with a special emphasis on biological relevance provided by distinct model as well as on productivity of each methodology.

2. Protein and peptide digestion

Before a discussion of protein digestibility evaluation methods, it seems worthwhile to introduce a reader to the current understanding of protein and peptide digestion process in order to provide him with a holistic picture of what could happen to an ingested protein. That is why this section will give a short description of digestive tract and an evaluation of enzymes involved in protein digestion in stomach and intestine. A special emphasis will be laid on characterization of intestinal wall peptidases (surface as well as intracellular) with description of their specificities and their role in overall protein digestion.

2.1 An overview of the protein digestion in the digestive tract

First of all, is should be noted, that excellent reviews and textbooks are readily available on the topic of digestive tract physiology and biochemistry (Freeman & Kim 1978; Widmaier et al. 2011), and we refer a curious reader them for more details; here only a short overview of this process is presented.

The digestive tract consists of several interconnected compartments: mouth (grinding and moisturizing of food), esophagus (connection and separation), stomach, small intestine (food digestion and absorption), and large intestine (food remnants digestion by symbiotic microbiota and undigested material excretion). Protein digestion is initiated in lumen of stomach, then proceeds in the intestinal lumen and is finalized at the surface and in the cytoplasm of intestinal mucosa cells. Additional digestion events occur in large intestine, where symbiotic microorganisms either digest protein remnants to amino acids, or convert them to other compounds of nutritional value.

Stomach is the first compartment, which is chemically active towards proteins. Its acidic pH serves three major functions: it sterilizes the ingested material, denatures food protein and activates local proteolytic enzymes. Only one protease, pepsin, is secreted in stomach. Pepsin does not destruct proteins to amino acids, rather it splits them to smaller parts to increase its accessibility for successive digestion steps (Widmaier et al. 2011).

The core function of stomach is the control of graduated food delivery into small intestine, and so it is rather dispensable for the overall protein assimilation. The experimental data on animals and patients with total gastrectomy show that the organism even under this condition retains the ability to assimilate dietary protein adequately and remains in positive nitrogen balance (Freeman & Kim 1978).

The next digestion phase, pancreatic, occurs in small intestine. It is thought to be more critical than the gastric phase. Here the pH changes to more basic and several different sources of proteases come into play. The most abundant ones: trypsin, chymotrypsin, elastase and several carboxypeptidases, are secreted by pancreatic acinar cells in a form of precursors, which are activated by proteolytic cleavage (Widmaier et al. 2011). The first three enzymes are endopeptidases; they cleave protein or polypeptide substrates at different specific peptide linkages within their secondary structures. Carboxypeptidases are exopeptidases and act on terminal peptide bonds at the carboxyl terminus of protein. The products of the combined action of the aforementioned enzymes are small peptides and amino acids. These small peptides consist of 2-6 amino acid residues and account for over 60% of luminal amino nitrogen; the remaining 40% is associated with amino acids (Freeman & Kim 1978).

The results of Savoie *et al.* indicate that the amount and size of the resultant peptides and their stability and resistance to exhaustive hydrolysis is strongly influenced by the nature of the source protein. For example, while casein and gluten have the highest proportion of the 1-10 kDa peptide fraction in the first 2 h of digestion, the peptides from gluten are evidently less degraded in the subsequent 4 h. The folding and spatial orientation of the protein chains could explain this observation; the high number of Pro and Glu residues is expected to have contributed heavily in the low accessibility and efficacy of the hydrolytic action of pancreatic enzymes on Pro- and Glu-reach proteins (Savoie et al. 2005).

The core properties of the luminal proteases are summarized in table 1, to give the reader an understanding of the processes, which take place at different stages of digestion. It should be noted that most digestive enzymes are present not as a single entity, but rather as a group of slightly different molecules with quite similar substrate specificity and kinetic properties. Some authors suggest it to be a sign of evolutionary importance of these enzymes (Silk et al. 1976). A detailed discussion of these enzymes is, however, beyond the scope of this chapter, and we refer a curious reader to the excellent reviews available (Freeman & Kim 1978; Turner 1968; Whitcomb & Lowe 2007).

Besides the common luminal enzymes, which are secreted by specialized organ – pancreas, a significant amount of intestinal wall proteases is also present in the lumen. The sources of these enzymes are desquamated mucosal cells resulting from active replacement of the lining epithelium. An approximate quantity of these enzymes is about 30 g per day (Freeman & Kim 1978; Gropper et al. 2009).

Chemical assay data, thermostability studies, and examination of electrophoretic mobilities of luminal peptide hydrolases indicate that aforementioned jejunal enzymes originate predominantly from the cytoplasm of intestinal mucosal cells, whereas the brush border of mucosal cells is a major source of the enzymes in the ileum. All of these enzymes recognize primarily short peptides and are aminopeptidases; they are discussed in more detail in the next section.

The products of luminal proteolysis are free amino acids and small peptides having a chain length of two to six amino acid residues. Analysis of post-prandial intestinal contents aspirated from human jejunum reveals that approximately only one-third of the total amino acid content exists in the free form (Silk et al. 1985). Some of the short peptides are directly absorbed by specific transport systems. However, to increase the overall efficiency of the assimilation process the mucosal cells of intestinal wall provide an additional source of proteolytic enzymes. As these cells line the intestinal wall and are intensively shed into lumen, they contribute both to luminal and parietal digestion. A profound characteristic of mucosal cells is high aminopeptidase activity. This peptidase activity is located in two main subcellular fractions: the cytoplasm and the brush border membrane. The brush border membrane fraction is associated with less than 10% of the total hydrolytic cellular activity for dipeptides but as much as 60% for tripeptides (Freeman & Kim 1978; Sterchi & Woodley 1980a).

The whole digestion process is quite rapid in man, as well as in rat. So, according to the data of Curtis *et al.*, 44.9 % of the meal had left the stomach of a rat in 30 min, and 84.7 % of the meal had left the stomach in 60 min. At 30 min and thereafter, negligible amounts of ^{14}C-labeled protein, which was included in the meal, were detected in intestinal contents of proximal third of small intestine. At 30 min and 1 hr, ^{14}C accumulated in medial and distal thirds of small intestine. At 2, 3 and 4 hr small quantities of ^{14}C were detected in intestinal contents of distal third of small intestine and the colon. The absorption of ingested protein was virtually complete 2 hr after administration of the meal (Curtis et al. 1978). In human, the situation is quite the same: digestion and absorption of dietary protein are completed in the jejunum, the whole process of digestion and absorption reaches its maximum at about 45 min or possibly earlier, and absorption may be largely complete within 75 to 90 min. However, the data of some studies show that the remnants of dietary protein can be recovered from the ileum as late as 4 hr after a meal (Adibi 1976). Nevertheless, it appears

Enzymes	Compartment and localization	Properties	References
Stomach proteases			
Pepsins: Pepsin, pepsin B, gastricsin, chymosin A, renin	Stomach lumen	Endopeptidase, cleaves at Phe, Tyr, Leu, and Val	(Freeman & Kim 1978; Szecsi 1992; Turner 1968; Whitecross et al. 1973)
Pancreatic proteases			
Trypsins: Cationic trypsin, anionic trypsin, mesotrypsin, pancreasin	Ileum lumen	Endopeptidase; cleaves peptide bond at Lys and Arg	(Feinstein et al. 1974; Freeman & Kim 1978; Savoie et al. 2005; Whitcomb & Lowe 2007)
Chimotrypsins: Two isoforms + chymotrypsin-like protease	Ileum lumen	Endopeptidase, cleaves bonds at aliphatic amino acid residues	(Bender & Killheffer 1973; Savoie et al. 2005; Whitcomb & Lowe 2007)
Elastases: Two isoforms	Ileum lumen	Endopeptidase, cleaves at Ala, Gly, Ser	(Whitcomb & Lowe 2007)
Carboxypeptidases A: A1, A2, A3	Ileum lumen	Exopeptidase, cleaves aromatic amino acids from carboxyl terminus of substrate	(Whitcomb & Lowe 2007)
Carboxypeptidases B: B1, B2, N, M, E, AEBP1	Ileum lumen	Exopeptidase, cleaves Arg or Lys from C-terminus of substrate	(Whitcomb & Lowe 2007)
Intestinal wall proteases			
Brush border aminopeptidases (distinct enzymes): aminopeptidase 1, aminopeptidase 2, dipeptidylpeptidase IV, gamma-glutamyltranspeptidase, aminopeptidase A, aminopeptidase M	Small intestine epithelium brush border	Hydrolyze amino acid residue at the N-terminus of hexa- to tripeptides	(Kim et al. 1972; Sterchi & Woodley 1980b)
Cytoplasmic aminopeptidases: four distinct enzymes	Small intestine epithelium cytoplasm	Hydrolyze amino acid residue at the N-terminus of tri- and dipeptides	(Kim et al. 1972; Schiller et al. 1977)

Table 1. Principal properties of protein hydrolases

reasonable to assume that under normal conditions the greatest portion of dietary proteins is digested and absorbed in the upper small intestine (Adibi 1976; Silk 1980; Silk et al. 1985).

2.2 Enzymes of the intestinal wall

In addition to the luminal proteases, the mucosal cells that line the intestinal wall also possess two kinds of proteolytic enzymes: membrane-bound, which are primarily localized in the brush border area, and cytoplasmic. The core difference of these enzymes from the luminal ones is that they are oligopeptidases, that is, recognize only short peptides of 2-6 amino acids in length. The profound characteristics of these enzymes are that they are aminopeptidases, so the N-terminal amino acid residue of peptides is the determinant of their rate and substrate specificity, and all have pH optima in alkaline (7.5-8.5) range (Adibi 1976).

To date, in brush border membranes in human and rat were identified at least 6 aminopeptidases (aminopeptidase 1, aminopeptidase 2, dipeptidylpeptidase IV, gamma-glutamyltranspeptidase, aminopeptidase A and aminopeptidase M) (Kim et al. 1972; Sterchi & Woodley 1980b), and in the cytosol of the mucosal epithelial cells at least 4 enzymes were detected (Kim et al. 1972; Schiller et al. 1977). The specificity towards peptide length is distributed unequally between the subcellular fractions: the majority of dipetides (80 to 95%) are hydrolyzed by cytoplasmic enzymes (Adibi 1976; Krzysik & Adibi 1977), 10-60% of the tripeptidase activity is also in the brush border membrane (Sterchi & Woodley 1980a), and activity against tetrapeptides is located exclusively in the brush border membrane (Sterchi & Woodley 1980a). The ability of brush border enzymes to hydrolyze penta- and hexapeptides has been reported (Adibi 1976), however, little details are still known about this activity.

Some, but not all, cytosolic and brush border membrane peptidases also display some preference to the amino acid composition of substrate. Thus, aminopeptidase 1 from brush border is most active towards aliphatic tripeptides (Sterchi & Woodley 1980b), although most activity against aliphatic peptides is located in cytosol; dipeptidases of brush border prefer substrates with aromatic amino acid at the N-terminus (Sterchi & Woodley 1980a). An interesting exception are proline-containing peptides, which are hydrolyzed by a special hydrolase in the cytosolic fraction (Freeman & Kim 1978; Smith & Bergmann 1944). In normal conditions, 80-90% of hydrolase activity in rat and human is localized within the cytosolic fraction (Kim et al. 1972), starvation increases the peptide hydrolase activity of the cytosol fraction, while that of the brush border fraction is decreased (Adibi 1976).

The distribution of peptide hydrolase activity between brush border membrane and cytosol varies considerably with species (Sterchi & Woodley 1980a), the enzymes from different species have different electrophoretic mobility, but, at the same time, by the activity and substrate preference they often could be grouped in a strikingly similar manner (Kim et al. 1972).

2.3 Peptide and protein transport across the intestinal wall

The absorption is the last and the most controversial phase of protein digestion. Theoretically, an organism requires only amino acids to produce energy and rebuild lost proteins. The foreign proteins and peptides should be avoided, as they could transmit unwanted signals or even be toxic or mutagenic. The reality, however, is much more complicated. Although amino nitrogen in postprandial blood is almost entirely in the form of free amino acids, few small peptides do appear in portal blood. These include short proline- and hydroxyproline-containing peptides after gelatin ingestion, and both carnosine and anserine after ingestion of certain meats, specifically chicken breast. Significant amounts of whole protein and other large macromolecules are absorbed intact by fetal and neonatal small intestine (Freeman & Kim 1978).

The transport of amino acids is active and depends on a gradient of sodium ions across the brush border membrane of intestinal epithelial cell. Three major group-specific active transport systems exist for: a) monoamino monocarboxylic (neutral) amino acids, b) dibasic amino acids and cysteine, and c) dicarboxylic (acidic) amino acids (Silk et al. 1985). Methionine and the branched chain amino acids (leucine, isoleucine, and valine) are absorbed most rapidly from amino acid mixture. Among the 18 common dietary amino acids, aspartate and glutamate are most slowly absorbed, as are tryptophan and threonine among the eight essential amino acids. As a group, essential amino acids are better absorbed than nonessential amino acids (Adibi 1976).

Small peptides are also actively absorbed, but their transporters are different from those for amino acids. As such, dipeptides and tripeptides are actively transported against a concentration gradient, and they share a common transport mechanism. There are at least two general strategies for transport of small peptides. First, small peptides resistant to brush border membrane peptidases appear to be transported intact across the brush border membrane and are later hydrolyzed by the cytoplasmic peptidases. Second, small peptides, having a higher affinity for brush border membrane peptidases are likely hydrolyzed primarily at the brush border membrane. The hydrolysis products, including free amino acids and dipeptides or tripeptides, are then absorbed by their respective transport systems (Freeman & Kim 1978; Sterchi & Woodley 1980a). There are little data on the active transport of tetrapeptides, and these data do not support the hypothesis on existence of such process (Silk et al. 1985).

One of important differences between amino acid and small peptide transport is that the capacity of free amino acid absorption is far greater in the jejunum than in the ileum, while that for peptide transport is evenly distributed. High-affinity amino acids competitively inhibit the absorption of low-affinity amino acids. However, absorption rates of amino acids by the intestinal epithelial cells are significantly greater in the form of low molecular weight peptides than the corresponding free amino acids, with the competition between amino acids being abolished. These spatio-temporal events directly influence amino acid concentration in blood flow, which in turn affects many physiological and metabolic phenomena as well as influencing the overall rate of protein synthesis (Savoie et al. 2005).

As to the peptide and protein molecules that are larger than 6 amino acids, so they pass through the intestinal wall differently. There are several routes, which allow the more or less non-specific passage of molecules: specialized microfold cells of Peyer's patches, isolated lymphoid follicles, through the epithelial cells (transcellular pathway) and between these cells (paracellular pathway) (Perrier & Corthésy 2011). The mucosa-associated lymphoid tissue, comprising Peyer's patches and isolated lymphoid follicles, is covered by the follicle-associated epithelium containing microfold cells. These cells have the capacity to engulf particulate antigens, and transport them to underlying dendritic cells thus contribute towards possible immune response. Paracellular transport across the epithelial barrier is highly regulated and is able to leave access to small molecules (44 angstroms), but also allows the passage of larger molecules including small peptides and bacterial lipopolysaccharides (500-1500 Da). A particular subset of dendritic cells (CX3CR11) is known to extend their dendrites in the lumen to collect bacteria under steady-state conditions, a process further accentuated upon inflammation. It is not yet clear whether this process can also take place for food antigens and whether this could contribute to the selective passage of antigens across the intestinal barrier and further presentation to the mucosal immune system (Perrier & Corthésy 2011).

Normally, large molecules are restricted from access to the intestinal wall by the mucus layer, which blocks passage of molecules of over 17 kDa (Jin et al. 2006). The intestinal cell layer permeability towards peptides and large molecules, on the other hand, is tightly bound to the external conditions. Thus, during fasting the efficiency of small peptide absorption increases (Silk et al. 1985). Then, a specific consequence of allergic reactions is the increased permeability towards large molecules via paracellular pathway, which can persist for a significant time after acute immune response is over (Perrier & Corthésy 2011). *In vitro* studies on confluent cultures of the enterocyte-like cell line Caco-2 have shown, that a model protein beta-lactoglobulin is taken by endocytosis, and whilst the majority of the protein was degraded intracellularly, around a third was transported across the cells (Wickham et al. 2009).

2.4 Comparison of relative roles of protein digestion stages

The functional importance of different stages of protein digestion process is unequal, albeit the exact significance of each of them varies depending on whether food toxicity/allergenicity or nutritive value is considered. As one could expect, the nutritive value of a protein is the most stable characteristic in context of the involvement of different digestive tract compartments. Thus, stomach and mucosal peptidases are dispensable for this function, and individual amino acid transport is also not very important if peptide transport is alive. The core functionality appears to be the one of pancreatic endopeptidases, which should split food protein into peptides of 3-2 amino acids; this activity is logically protected by the existence of multiple enzyme isoforms.

In addition to this, it should be noted, that peptide transport role is more impotant than the amino acid one. In evaluations involving both highly digestible proteins such as egg and less digestible protein sources such as corn as well as free amino acid mixtures, the food source of protein routinely gave better nitrogen balance test results than did the counterpart amino acid diets. Explanations for these results included the following: (a) that the immediate availability of purified amino acids might lead to overall overtaxing of absorption mechanism systems or competition among particular amino acids might lead to selected competitive inhibition of absorption of particular amino acids and hence to reduced efficiency of their utilization; (b) that rapid absorption of amino acids over a short period of time rather than over a longer period of time might overtax the body's ability to efficiently use amino acids for protein synthesis purposes, thus leading to increased deamination of amino acids and utilization for energy purposes; (c) that experimental diets containing purified amino acids were not truly matched to those containing food proteins in contents of all trace nutrients and results reflected these deficits (Kies 1981).

The situation changes significantly, as one tries to evaluate food protein toxicity and allergenicity. In this case stomach phase value greatly increases, as the low pH in this compartment often provides denaturation and thus inactivation and detoxification of ingested proteins. The oligopeptidases of the intestinal mucosa are not very important for the toxicity prevention, albeit they play a role as protectors against exogenous signals, as many proteins could possess hormonal properties (Widmaier et al. 2011). The pancreatic enzymes are still important for the defensive function, as they split large proteins into small chunks, thus destroying potential immunological epitopes.

3. The evaluation of protein and peptide digestibility

There are several approaches to the evaluation of protein digestibility. The most common of these include single-enzyme systems, based on pepsin and/or trypsin; whole-organ systems; cannula incision; and immobilized multiple digestive enzymes system. The latter model provides the most relevant data, while pepsin hydrolysis is the simplest. Several more rare models will be also described (for example, the use of cell fractions of small intestine, culture of Caco-2 cells, yeast surface enzymes, tissue fragments).

3.1 Isolated enzymes

One of the simplest models of protein digestion is the use of the purified major enzymes of stomach (pepsin) and pancreas (trypsin and chymotrypsin) (Horii et al. 2009; Huang et al. 2010; Kamata et al. 1982; Nielsen et al. 1988; Stanic et al. 2010; Yagami et al. 2000), implemented either separately of subsequently. The products of the digestion are usually analyzed using SDS-PAGE with the separation range from 3 to 20-30 kDa (Stanic et al. 2010; Yu et al. 2011) or reverse-phase HPLC (Bublin et al. 2008). In rare cases, mass spectrometry is also employed to characterize the digestion products (Dupont et al. 2010).

The procedure of pepsin and trypsin/chymotrypsin digestion is defined in the US and EU Pharmacopoeias (Council of Europe 2004; United States Pharmacopeial Convention 2006), and prescribes the exact composition of the incubation medium, enzyme to protein ratio and incubation time.

Several optimizations of enzyme digestion assay exist. First of all, the inclusion of non-protein components of gastric and intestinal juice, such as phosphatidyl choline and bile, and some potential food components (pectin) could significantly change the analysis result (Bublin et al. 2008; Dupont et al. 2010; Mandalari et al. 2009; Polovic et al. 2010). Not all proteins respond to such changes, but sometimes partially unfolded form of the protein is able to penetrate into the phosphatidyl choline vesicles. These interactions are probably responsible for slowing of gastric digestion by reducing the accessibility of the protein to pepsin (Moreno et al. 2005). Another option is the use not only of the major luminal proteases, but also of other enzymes: aminopeptidase M, leucine aminopeptidase, carboxypeptidase A and carboxypeptidase Y (Dizdaroglu et al. 1984; Tonglet et al. 2001), or modeling of the subsequent interaction of food protein with saliva, gastric juice and duodenal juice (Versantvoort et al. 2005), and heating during food processing (Nielsen et al. 1988), a group of approaches which should be definitively considered if some protein seems to be stable. Horii *et al.* implemented another interesting modification of enzyme digestion procedure. They introduced test protein into the incubation medium not as a solution of individual molecules, but as a component, expressed on the surface of a whole yeast cell. The aim of this study was to check the stability of expressed oral vaccine, and it has shown that indeed, a protein displayed on the yeast cell surface had an increased resistance to pepsin, possibly due to pepsin underwent steric hindrance and only digested the outermost side of the yeast cell wall protein (Horii et al. 2009).

An unquestionable advantage of individual enzyme digestion method is its simplicity and speed, as the whole analysis takes only about 2 to 3 hours to complete (including the products separation) and does not require any specific instrumentation or animal procedures. Wickham *et al.*, however, notices, that such models «are particularly useful where there is limited digestion, e.g. stomach, but are less applicable for total digestion studies. These types of models are predominately used for digestion studies on simple foods and isolated or purified nutrients, and are therefore ideal for assessments of the digestibility of isolated allergenic proteins» (Wickham et al. 2009).

3.2 Isolated digestive tract compartments

An intermediate between *in vivo* and *in vitro* protein digestibility assays is the utilization of isolated digestive tract compartments (Polovic et al. 2010; Wickham et al. 2009). The experimental procedure requires an animal to be sacrificed immediately before the measurement. After that, the required compartment is surgically removed and either placed into a vial with a simulated fluid of this compartment, or sealed both sides with the salt mixture with substrate within. A variation of this technique implies the inversion of a digestive tract compartment inside out before sealing, so the resultant bag is put into a beaker with the substrate-containing solution, and the digestion products diffuse to the internal volume of such bag. Some researchers add glucose to the incubation medium to provide the tissue with energy.

The strong point of this approach is that the digestion and absorption systems of the intestine remain intact, and so the biological significance of the obtained results is very high, and the question on whether the digestion products really pass through the intestinal wall is immediately answered. The isolation of reaction products is also rather simple, as they are automatically separated from the source protein and mucosal proteins (if a sealed compartment bag is employed). The downsides of this method are, of course, high animal requirements and low suitability for high-throughput screening.

3.3 *In vivo* methods

In vivo methods, albeit the most complex ones, are at the same time the most informative ones. The two possible strategies within this group are based on the evaluation of either the remnants of the substrate within or at the end of digestive tract, or of the assimilation of the digestion products by the organism.

The methods based on protein nitrogen utilization by an organism are subject of several great reviews, and we refer a curious reader to them for more details (Bender 1958; Darragh & Hodgkinson 2000; von der Decken 1983). Below, a short description of method families will be given.

The first group of methods (protein efficiency ratio, net protein retention, rat-repletion method) use direct determination of the weight of animals, fed with a test protein. The variations of this method lie in the employment of non-protein diet fed rats as a control group or starvation of animals before the introduction of a test meal (Bender 1958; Henry 1965). A variation of these methods suggests the determination not of the animal weight, but rather of amount of a specific tissue (liver, muscle, *etc.*), laid down while feeding on a test protein (Bender 1958; Mokady et al. 1969). These include protein retention efficiency and liver protein utilization. It should be noted, that the original growth determination methods are very animal-sparing, while the more advanced assays usually implicate animal death in order for some parameter to be determined.

Another group of methods, developed with the aim to overcome the not-so-obvious relationship between protein in diet and growth rate, introduces direct determination of nitrogen either in food before and after passage through digestive tract, or in animal carcass; a variant of latter analysis implicates the division of animal group in several parts with subsequent determination of carcass nitrogen at different time points (Bender 1958). The methods in this group are Thomas-Mitchell method, N-balance index method, carcass-nitrogen method and growth and nitrogen balance method. In some variations of nitrogen retention methods protein isotope labeling is required.

The further development of nitrogen analysis concept led researchers to the development of some biochemical methods for protein nutritive value determination. These methods are based on several parameters, which strongly correlate with tissue growth: polyribosomal profiles or ribosome activity and content; the activity of enzymes involved in urea metabolism or transamination reactions; 3-methylhistidine (an excreted-only myosin component) production and creatinine excretion (Bender 1958; von der Decken 1983). Ribosome activity is quite informative, as it is sensitive enough to detect small differences in protein quality. The latter two parameters, on the other hand, are measured in urine and thus are suitable for humans.

The current recommendation, when calculating a protein digestibility, is to determine the digestibility of a dietary protein across the entire digestive tract, using the rat as a model animal for humans. This fecal digestibility value is subsequently corrected for endogenous contributions of protein using a metabolic nitrogen value determined by feeding rats a protein-free diet, a task for which the protein digestibility-corrected amino acid score (PDCAAS) was introduced. To calculate a PDCAAS, the availability of the amino acids in a dietary protein is assessed based on the digestibility of total nitrogen (N) in that dietary protein. Digestibility is defined as the difference between the amount of N ingested and excreted, expressed as a proportion of N ingested. Although accepted as the recommended procedure, the use of fecal digestibility coefficients to evaluate amino acid availability is thought to be inherently inaccurate due to the metabolism of both dietary and endogenous proteins by the hindgut microbial population (Darragh & Hodgkinson 2000; Kies 1981).

In fact, the aforementioned techniques are not precisely suitable for protein digestibility evaluation. The problem is that they measure protein assimilation and do not provide any data on how exactly a particular protein was or was not digested and transported. This hindrance is circumvented in the second group of *in vivo* approaches, which include swallowed probe utilization, anastomosis and cannula incision (Darragh & Hodgkinson 2000; Faber et al. 2010).

Anastomosis involves transecting the ileum anterior to the ileocecal junction and attaching this to the descending colon. This allows a quantitative collection of ileal digesta, but many studies have shown that anastomosed animals have an altered physiology compared with intact animals. It should be noted that human ileostomates may also have an altered physiology compared with intact humans, which could also call into question the validity of using human ileostomates for the collecttion of ileal digesta (Darragh & Hodgkinson 2000).

The insertion of a re-entrant cannula involves transecting the terminal ileum and sealing the two ends. A cannula is inserted into each end of the sealed ileum and the two cannulae are joined. This allows a quantitative collection of digesta. The surgery to insert a re-entrant cannula is complex, however, and involves total transection of the ileum. Blockage of the cannula is a common complication. Simple T-piece cannulation and postvalve T-cecum cannulation have the distinct advantage of maintaining the ileocecal valve intact and avoiding ileal transection; in this case there is also no surgical interference with the small intestine. In addition to that, most of the digesta should pass through such cannula during sampling, as the ileocecal value protrudes directly into it (Darragh & Hodgkinson 2000).

The *in vivo* methods of protein bioaccessibility determination, such as retained nitrogen analysis, cannula incision and swallowed probe sampling, undoubtedly provide the most relevant data. However, their major drawback is experimental complexity and practical impossibility of any reasonable screening.

3.4 Digestive tract simulators

Most of the aforementioned models, excluding the animal ones, lack two important characteristics of digestive tract – the mechanical forces, exerted by stomach and intestinal walls, and the fact that food arrives into stomach and upper intestine not as a solution or an emulsion, but rather as a bolus with different accessibility of its internal and external contents for the enzymatic machinery. The digestive tract simulators try to overcome this situation. Usually they represent complex devices, consisting of several mixing chambers with programmatically controlled pH, mixing speed, temperature and valves between them, which provide a definite transition time from one compartment to another. The compartments that imitate intestine contain immobilized enzymes, either trypsin and chymotrypsin, or more complex mixtures including proteases of intestinal wall. The system is filled with simulated gastric and intestinal fluid plus phospholipids and/or bile, and the test substances are delivered into the system either in form of solution or within agarose beads (a way to mimic food bolus). The result of protein digestion in such system could be analyzed at any stage; the commonly employed analytical methods are SDS-PAGE (mass range 2-15 or 14-60 kDa) and reverse phase HPLC.

The most representative example of such device is the Dynamic Gastric Model, described by Vardakou et al. (Vardakou et al. 2011). It is composed of three parts, the main body (fundus), the antrum and the valve assembly. In the main body of the model the inhomogeneous mixing of the stomach is reproduced by gentle contractions induced by computer-controlled changes in the applied pressure of water in the thermostated water bath surrounding the main body. Gastric acid and enzymes are added from a dispenser that is floating on the top of the main body contents. The dispenser is designed in such a way as to deliver the enzyme and acid evenly from the sides of the main body, replicating the human gastric secretions originating from the walls of the stomach. The rate of addition of both enzymatic and acid secretions is also computer-controlled. The food material is allowed to move from the main body into the antrum, and *vice versa*. The artificial antrum simulates the strong shear forces of the human antrum to reproduce the breakdown of the food particles and the preferential sieving observed *in vivo*. The mechanical processing of the food within the antrum is achieved by the sliding of a piston within a barrel, which forces the material through an elastic annulus where selective sieving takes place. Once ready, the processed bolus is ejected through the valve assembly and can be collected for further analysis.

Another widely used system is the Immobilized Digestive Enzyme Assay (IDEA), developed by Schasteen et al. (Schasteen et al. 2002). This system is somewhat more simple, and concentrates not on the grinding forces, but rather on the mixing of the «ingested» components and the food transition times through various digestive tract compartments. The overall digestion procedure consists of a stepwise acid solubilization, pepsin digestion, neutralization, trypsin, chymotrypsin and intestinal peptidase digestion followed by analysis of hydrolysis products. As follows from the model name, it relies on the glass beads-immobilized enzymes, and this allows for substantial costs reduction. The downside of this particular model is very long analysis time — up to 2.5 days.

The digestive tract simulators possess several advantages. They are more efficient at predicting of the fate of tablets within the gastrointestinal tract and more accurate at the simulation of the interaction of investigated protein or peptide with other meal and chyme components. The use of immobilized enzymes allows the reduction of experiment costs. However, the pay-off of these systems lies within their design: the complete analysis procedure usually takes a day or even two, and the complexity of the system dramatically reduces the throughput, as usually only one protein could be analyzed by one device at once. Finally, such machines are usually too complex to build by a research team, and thus require a substantial capital investment at the initial stage of a research project.

3.5 Other approaches

Beyond aforementioned widely used approaches to study of protein digestibility, several less common or hybrid ones also exist.

First of all, when it comes to the evaluation of protein nutritive value, the simplest way to determine it is to calculate relative quantity of essential amino acids in the test protein relative to some well-known food protein. Hansen et al. (Hansen 1975) describes two such indices: Essential Amino Acid Index (EAAI) and Arnoulds index. The reference protein in both cases is egg protein; the latter index differs by including of the sum of the non-essential amino acids (NEAA) as part of equation. An unquestionable advantage of the amino acid scores is very low requirement of experimental work for production of preliminary estimates about a protein. However, this method does not take into account any properties of a protein, thus making impossible to draw any conclusions on its real bioaccessibility.

Then, von der Decken et al. point out to the fact, that the protozoan *Tetrahymena pyriformis W* has a proteolytic enzyme to digest proteins and similar to human needs for essential amino acids, and thus could be a model for protein digestion (von der Decken 1983). Time consumption of such model is, however, rather high (48 to 66 hours), and the details of animal digestion process are missed as well.

Our group has recently suggested an assay, that tries to replicate the conditions of parietal digestion in small intestine, at the same time maintaining capability for high-throughput sample analysis (Akimov et al. 2010). The active component of this system is a fragment of rat stomach or intestinal wall, immersed in simulated gastric or intestinal fluid. The products are analyzed by HPLC. The utilization of tissue fragments allows for reduction of animal consumption, while still maintaining the whole set of intestinal peptidases and providing some phosphatidyl choline in the medium. The assay design is suitable for the processing of 40 samples per day.

To simultaneously determine protein digestibility in small intestine and transport through epithelial cells, a hybrid model is often employed (Dhuique-Mayer et al. 2007; Jin et al. 2006; Versantvoort et al. 2005). The intestinal epithelium is represented by the Caco-2 cell culture, which is grown to the monolayer state on a membrane that separates two chambers. A test protein solution with digestive enzyme or after *in vitro* digestion is applied in one chamber and, if transport is possible, the products are collected from the second chamber. Two optimizations of this experimental design have been proposed: first, a mucin layer could be applied on the surface of the cell culture, thus mimicking the real mucus layer, which exists in intestine. Mucin protects cells from damage by luminal digestive enzymes and limits the passage of large (over 1500 Da) molecules to the cell surface (Jin et al. 2006). Second, Caco-2 cells could be co-cultured with HT29-MTX cells, which imitate mucus-producing cells of small intestine; this approach could be considered a more natural variant of previous modification (Yao et al. 2010). The core complication of such methods is the requirement for the facilities for operations with animal cell cultures. On the other hand, the model could be used for medium-sized screening, has a decent degree of intestinal wall imitation and thus the obtained results are quite relevant.

The final and most promising approach is the molecular modeling. In a work by Foltz et al. (Foltz et al. 2009) a special database was constructed to study the relationship between peptide structure and activity, permeability, and digestive stability. For this purpose, a total of 228 dipeptides were synthesized and their intestinal stability was evaluated by *in vitro* digestion. Then, a quantitative structure-activity relationship (QSAR) modeling was performed using partial least squares regression based on 400 molecular descriptors. The correlation coefficient for the best fit model was 0.76, and proteolytic stability for 12 new peptides was successfully predicted. As it is seen from the description above, molecular modeling has one major drawback: it requires a huge amount of preliminary data to build an efficient model. After that, it offers great speed and low experimental costs, but the aforementioned initial stage makes this approach suitable only for large screening experiments.

4. Current view of protein stability evaluation in different fields

The common approaches to the determination of the protein and peptide digestibility in different areas of research varies significantly:

- Allergenicity studies are usually the simplest ones and rely on direct hydrolysis of test substrate by pepsin and a combination of trypsin with chymotrypsin in simulated gastric and intestinal fluids.
- Biological value is most commonly determined using animal assays.

- The studies on the properties of digestive enzymes rely on the purified enzymes or on fractionated homogenates of the parts of gastrointestinal tract.
- Pharmacological studies tend to use complicated devices for the evaluation of the ability of a particular pharmacological form to degrade in specific compartment of digestive tract.

In fact, the stability towards protease degradation is not considered to be a basic method for the evaluation of potential protein allergenicity, albeit the resistant proteins are usually allergenic (Fu 2002). To better understand the data on the digestibility of any potential immunogenic peptide, a basic picture of the underlying mechanisms is necessary (for more details reader is referred to an excellent review by Huby et al. (Huby et al. 2000)).

Allergic sensitization to proteins involves the induction of IgE type antibodies production of sufficient magnitude by differentiated B-lymphocytes to facilitate the elicitation of an inflammatory reaction following subsequent exposure to the same (or a cross-reactive) allergen. For a B cell to differentiate into a plasma cell and produce antibodies, the B-cell receptor expressed on its surface must bind to specific B epitopes on the surface of the protein antigen. The antibodies subsequently produced by the plasma cell, into which the B cell differentiates, have the same specificity as the B-cell receptor, and are therefore able to bind specifically to the same B epitopes on the surface of the protein antigen. Efficient secretion of antibodies normally requires that the B cells receive help from T-helper cells that specifically recognize separate epitopes on the same protein antigen. Such recognition is mediated by the T-cell antigen receptor, which delivers stimulatory intracellular signals to the T cell. Allergenic proteins *per se* cannot be recognized by T cells; the proteins must first be processed and then presented by specialized antigen-presenting cells (APCs) (Gorovits 2010; Huby et al. 2000).

After the first contact with an antigen the T-helper-stimulated B-cells differentiate and become ready to produce antibodies. Thus, if such antigen is encountered for the second time, there will be some antibodies against it present in the blood flow, and the production of their large quantities will start immediately. The IgE antibodies, however, serve mainly as information transducers during allergic response. After antigen recognition they bind to the Fc receptors for IgE (FceR) on the surface of basophils and mast cells; for these cells to become activated and secrete histamine and other inflammatory mediators their receptors need to dimerize. Thus, the peptide is to be large enough to bind at least two antibodies, which will bring two FceR together. The minimal length of peptide chain, which could be recognized by IgE antibody (epitope), is 15 amino acids, and thus the minimum size of an immunogenic peptide should be around 30 amino acids or 5-6 kDa (Van Beresteijn et al. 1994). At the same time, the sensitization stage, when an antigen is recognized by T-cells and undifferentiated B-cells, requires only one epitope and thus a peptide size of around 3 kDa (Moreno 2007; Van Beresteijn et al. 1994).

The discussion above clearly indicates the valid conditions of digest products analysis: HPLC and MALDI are always informative enough, but SDS-PAGE is appropriate only if it includes molecular masses of 2-3 kDa, which unfortunately is not always the case (Huang et al. 2010; Yagami et al. 2000; Yu et al. 2011).

Even after all the requirements for the stability assay of a potential allergen are met, the results should be interpreted with caution, as some stable proteins are not allergens at all, and some other, which are completely degraded in the experimental conditions, still induce immune response *in vivo* (Faeste et al. 2007; Fu 2002; Jensen-Jarolim & Untersmayr 2006).

One of the complicated moments during the immune response is that depending on the type of T-cell, the type of antibodies produced by the B-cell could be changed: Th2 cells produce a cocktail of cytokines that, among other actions, encourage plasma cells to switch to synthesis of IgE, while Th1 cells typically produce interleukin 2, interferon gamma, and tumor necrosis factor (TNF)-alpha/beta, that together downregulate IgE synthesis. Only one type of stimulation could be active for a given antigen, as Th1 cytokines suppress Th2 cell development, and *vice versa*. Structural investigations of several allergens have identified T epitopes implicated in the selective development of Th2-type lymphocytes. Some allergens, such as ovalbumin, have only a few epitopes that preferentially induce a Th2 response, whereas others, such as beta-lactoglobulin, have many. The potential to induce a polarized (Th1 or Th2) response is not exclusively an intrinsic property of particular epitopes; the quality of the T-cell response to any given epitope depends upon many factors, including the dose of protein or peptide given, the affinity of the peptide for MHC class II receptor, and the longevity of the class II/peptide complex. Together, these parameters act to influence the dynamic epitope density on the surface of APCs. It is generally agreed that parameters that serve to increase ligand density, including greater affinity to MHC class II, higher levels of ligand loading, or longer-lived complexes favor Th1-type responses (Huby et al. 2000).

In addition to the possible anti-allergic action of Th1 epitopes, a significant variety into experimental results is introduced due to the experimental conditions differences. Several investigators term protein as «stable» after incubation times ranging from 8 to 60 min (Bannon et al. 2003; Fu 2002; Herman et al. 2006). As far as the unstable proteins usually survive less than 15 sec in the similar assay conditions, such conclusion seems to be quite correct. However, the 8-min survival could potentially be an indication of the protein instability, as the simplified conditions of simulated gastric and intestinal fluid do not take into account intestinal mucosa peptidases or minor luminal endopeptidases. Then, albeit standardized in the last period, the enzyme to substrate ratios vary between different research groups (Herman et al. 2006), and thus obtained stability or instability may not adequately reflect the reality.

Finally, the conditions inside the digestive tract during the potential allergen ingestion are of crucial importance. For example, during inflammation the permeability of digestive tract is increased (Perrier & Corthésy 2011); then, any elevation of the pH should result in hindrance of peptic degradation. Numerous situations with elevated stomach pH are known, e.g. in early childhood, in elderly, or in chronic atrophic gastritis. Moreover, there is a number of pathologies, like gastritis or ulcer, where acid neutralization or inhibition is an important therapeutic goal. Acid neutralization is state of the art during surgical care, corticosteroid or analgesic treatment. Moreover, anti-acids, H2-receptor blockers and proton pump inhibitors are increasingly consumed without prescriptions due to liberalization of the market by over-the-counter sale (Jensen-Jarolim & Untersmayr 2006).

As a logical consequence of the aforementioned complications, immunogenicity assessment is typically done using a multistage strategy, generally including an digestive stability and antibody affinity screening assay, a specificity confirmation step, and in some cases a characterization step. Samples are first evaluated in a screening assay, for which an assay threshold has been set based on the variability of samples from a drug naïve target patient population. Screen positive samples are further evaluated in a confirmatory assay to verify whether the signal observed in the screening assay is a result of a specific response to the protein therapeutic treatment. Confirmed positive samples are then put into downstream methods for sequential characterization based on the comprehensive consideration of immunogenicity risk assessment and mechanism of action for the protein therapeutic (Gorovits 2010; Peng et al. 2011).

The studies of protein nutritive value usually rely on the *in vivo* experiments or on the data on protein amino acid composition. The point is that the most important aim of such studies is to tell, whether a given protein (perhaps after some processing) is suitable for supplying body needs for energy and essential amino acids. The question on how does an organism manage to consume that protein is often ignored, albeit it is tempting to speculate that the exact metabolic route from the whole protein to the amino acids and energy inside body cells could be important as well. One should note that as it was shown in section 2, there are several conceptually different steps in protein digestion (denaturation and splicing in large chunks in stomach, splicing in tetra- to dipeptides and individual amino acids in small intestine and various processing by the large intestine microbiota), whose efficiency could be independently affected by the protein structure and modifications, and thus during some pathological conditions a protein of a high nutritive value could suddenly lose it.

The *in vivo* evaluation of nutritive value consists of animal feeding with test protein with subsequent analysis of either the amount of absorbed or unabsorbed protein fractions, or the degree to which such meal is able to sustain animal growth. The experiments are usually quite long, expensive and involve complex manipulations with animals. The direct determination of protein amino acid composition is much simpler. The only complication of such approach is that the degree to which the constituent amino acids of a food protein are actually available to the body is determined by such factors as protein configuration, amino acid bonding, other constituents of the diet, and the physiological condition of the gastrointestinal tract of the individual person or animal involved. However, the correlation between prediction and performance is quite good: prediction for poor performance of proteins devoid or nearly devoid of an essential amino acid as well as of good performance for proteins containing all essential amino acids according to idealized patterns is excellent. However, fine-line predictions of intermediate quality are less accurate, and surprises are not uncommon (Kies 1981). Thus the *in vivo* models are still a preferred way for nutritive value analysis.

Enzymatic studies are usually concerned not with the stability of a some protein, but rather with the distribution, specificity and kinetics of a particular enzyme, and thus they usually implement some procedures of purification from animal tissues (Krzysik & Adibi 1977; Smith & Bergmann 1944; Sterchi & Woodley 1980a) or of expression of a recombinant enzyme in some prokaryotic or eukaryotic cells (Hauri et al. 1985; Lentze 1995). The applicability of such procedures is usually quite legitimate, albeit the biological significance and theoretical value of the obtained results could vary. The enzyme-to-substrate ratios in such studies usually do not resemble the *in vivo* situation, and thus the real significance of a given enzyme for the digestive process could not always be predicted. The differences of purification procedures complicate the integration of data from various research groups into

Name	Reproduced conditions	Time to complete and special conditions	Reference
In vitro methods			
Simulated gastric fluid	Stomach lumen without mechanical forces after individual ingestion	Hours	(Thomas et al. 2004)
Simulated intestinal fluid	Intestinal lumen without shed mucosal cells and mechanical forces after individual ingestion	Hours	(Tonglet et al. 2001)
Amino acid score	Ability of protein to be a source of essential amino acids	Hours	(Hansen 1975)
Organ fragments	Mucosal and intracellular digestion	Hours; HPLC or MALDI analysis	(Akimov et al. 2010)
A device with immobilized enzymes	Luminal digestion with mechanical forces ant transitional times without mucosal enzymes	Hours (single compartment) to days (whole digestive tract); requires a special device	(Vardakou et al. 2011)
Ex vivo methods			
Caco-2 cell culture	Luminal and intracellular intestinal digestion, transport	Hours + cell culture preparation; requires animal cell culture facilities	(Dhuique-Mayer et al. 2007)
Isolated organs	Luminal, mucosal and intracellular digestion of a given organ, transport	Hours	(Curtis et al. 1978)
Bacterial culture	Microbial digestion in large intestine; ability to provide essential amino acids	Hours; requires microbiological facilities	(Bender 1958)
In vivo methods			
Nitrogen balance	Whole digestion process in a given health condition	Days-weeks; may require isotope labeling	(Mokady et al. 1969)
Cannula/probe	Digestive process up to the point of probing without data on digestion products	Days(cannula); hours(probe); applicable for human	(Darragh & Hodgkinson 2000; Faber et al. 2010)
In silico methods			
QSAR	Predicts degradation in any conditions depending on model	Minutes (computation), weeks to months (database and model development); requires large experimental body (data on 100-200 proteins)	(Foltz et al. 2009)

Table 2. A comparison of different method classes for protein digestibility evaluation

one picture (*cf.,* for example, the discussion in the work by Sterchi et al. (Sterchi & Woodley 1980a)).

The aim of a substantial part of pharmacological studies of peptide- and protein-based therapeutics is often the evaluation of the disintegration, dissolution and drug release profiles of oral drug formulations (Vardakou et al. 2011). Thus another aspect of food digestion becomes important – the mechanical grinding and mixing forces, exerted on a pharmaceutical formulation by various digestive tract compartments. To simulate such conditions devices of various complexity are employed (Schasteen et al. 2002; Vardakou et al. 2011). The applicability of such devices for the drug form disintegration testing is unquestionable, however, usually they reproduce only the luminal phase of food digestion. Thus the evaluation of the ability of released protein or peptide to get to the blood flow intact requires additional methods.

A short reference of available method types is provided in table 2. It should be noted, that some *in vitro* methods could be combined and expanded to provide more relevant data. For example, single-enzyme digestions by stomach and small intestine could be performed sequentially, the Caco-2 cell culture is often overlaid by a simulated gastric fluid and possibly mucin (to protect cells and imitate the similar layer present *in vivo*). The computational methods are the most adaptive and powerful ones, however, to date their usability is limited to large screening studies due to huge preparatory experimental work.

5. Conclusion

Significant progress has been made in the modeling of protein digestion and absorption in gastrointestinal tract since the first works on this topic in the beginning of the XX century. A multitude of methods of various complexity, biological significance, animal requirements and human applicability now exist to answer the question on digestibility of proteins and peptides. The degree of biological processes imitation ranges from single luminal enzymes in simulated gastric or intestinal fluid model to sophisticated devices, which take in account grinding, mixing and turbulence forces and transition times, as well as isolated animal organs.

There is, however, no single method, which will suit every possible research goal. The problem is, that as the biological significance increases, time and labor requirements also rise tremendously, and methods became progressively less suitable for high throughput screening, which is often required. In addition to this, there is no experimental model, which could imitate every last component of the digestion process. The enzyme-only models and organ fragments ignore mechanical forces, digestive devices lack intracellular hydrolases and transport steps, isolated organs usually represent only one compartment of the whole system, and they fail to exert mechanical forces as well. As there is no efficient methodology of sampling of the digested products after they are absorbed, but before they enter blood or lymph, whole animal models are also limited – they can only answer questions, whether a protein was absorbed and if it was suitable for the sustaining normal growth of an organism. A very promising approach has appeared with the development of the high-performance computation methods, that is, molecular modeling. Theoretically, mathematical modeling is able to join data on the digestion patterns of various proteins from *in vitro* experiments with the results of *in vivo* tests of the ability of an organism to utilize these proteins. However, a vast array of preliminary data is required for optimization and validation of such models, and so they are relatively rare.

Thus, when considering various methods of protein digestibility assay, one should first of all define the limitations of the research at hand. If a high throughput screening is required? If there is a need for any data on digestion products? If absorption efficiency could vary and is essential? If a protein should serve as food or not? A possible decision tree for method optimization is presented on figure 1, albeit it should be considered more as a reference than a rule.

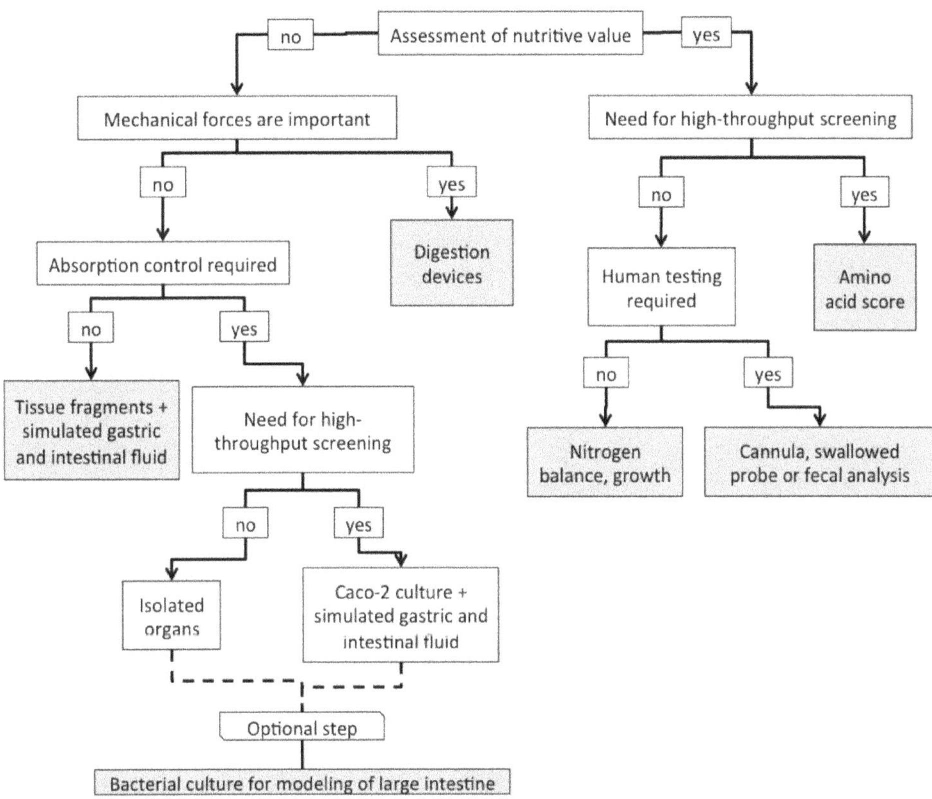

Fig. 1. A decision tree for protein or peptide digestibility assay choice

6. References

Adibi, S.A., (1976). Intestinal phase of protein assimilation in man. *American Journal of Clinical Nutrition*, Vol. 29, No. 2, (February 1976), pp. 205-215, ISSN 0002-9165

Akimov, M.G., Nazimov, I.V., Gretskaya, N.M., Deigin, V.I. & Bezuglov, V.V. (2010). Investigation of peptide stability upon hydrolysis by of fragments of the organs of the gastrointestinal tract of rats. *Russian Journal of Bioorganic Chemistry*, Vol. 36, No. 6, (November 2010), p. 690, ISSN 0132-3423

Bannon, G., Fu, T.J., Kimber, I. & Hinton, D.M. (2003). Protein digestibility and relevance to allergenicity. *Environmental Health Perspectives*, Vol. 111, No. 8, (June 2003), pp. 1122-1124, ISSN 1552-9924

Bender, A.E., (1958). Biological methods of evaluating protein quality. *Proceedings of the Nutrition Society*, Vol. 17, No. 01, pp. 85-91

Bender, M.L. & Killheffer, J.V. (1973). Chymotrypsins. *CRC Critical Reviews in Biochemistry*, Vol. 1, No. 2, (April 1973), pp. 149-199, ISSN 0045-6411

Bublin, M., Radauer, C., Knulst, A., Wagner, S., Scheiner, O., Mackie, A.R., Mills, E.N. & Breiteneder, H. (2008). Effects of gastrointestinal digestion and heating on the allergenicity of the kiwi allergens Act d 1, actinidin, and Act d 2, a thaumatin-like protein. *Molecular Nutrition and Food Research*, Vol. 52, No. 10, (October 2008), pp. 1130-1139, ISSN 1613-4133

Council of Europe (2004). *European pharmacopoeia: 2005*, Council of Europe, ISBN 9287152810, Strasbourg

Curtis, K.J., Kim, Y.S., Perdomo, J.M., Silk, D.B. & Whitehead, J.S. (1978). Protein digestion and absorption in the rat. *The Journal of Physiology*, Vol. 274, No. 1, (January 1978), p. 409, ISSN 1469-7793

Darragh, A.J. & Hodgkinson, S.M. (2000). Quantifying the digestibility of dietary protein. *Journal of Nutrition*, Vol. 130, No. 7, (July 2000), pp. 1850S-1856S, ISSN 0022-3166

Dhuique-Mayer, C., Borel, P., Reboul, E., Caporiccio, B., Besancon, P. & Amiot, M.J. (2007). Beta-cryptoxanthin from citrus juices: assessment of bioaccessibility using an in vitro digestion/Caco-2 cell culture model. *British Journal of Nutrition*, Vol. 97, No. 5, (May 2007), pp. 883-890, ISSN 0007-1145

Dizdaroglu, M., Gajewski, E. & Simic, M.G. (1984). Enzymatic digestibility of peptides cross-linked by ionizing radiation. *International Journal of Radiation Biology and Related Studies in Physics, Chemistry and Medicine*, Vol. 45, No. 3, (March 1984), pp. 283-295, ISSN 0020-7616

Dupont, D., Mandalari, G., Molle, D., Jardin, J., Léonil, J., Faulks, R.M., Wickham, M.S., Mills, E.N. & Mackie, A.R. (2010). Comparative resistance of food proteins to adult and infant in vitro digestion models. *Molecular Nutrition and Food Research*, Vol. 54, No. 6, (June 2010), pp. 767-780, ISSN 1613-4133

Faber, T.A., Bechtel, P.J., Hernot, D.C., Parsons, C.M., Swanson, K.S., Smiley, S. & Fahey, G.C. (2010). Protein digestibility evaluations of meat and fish substrates using laboratory, avian, and ileally cannulated dog assays. *Journal of Animal Science*, Vol. 88, No. 4, (April 2010), pp. 1421-1432, ISSN 1525-3163

Faeste, C.K., Løvberg, K.E., Lindvik, H. & Egaas, E. (2007). Extractability, stability, and allergenicity of egg white proteins in differently heat-processed foods. *Journal of AOAC International*, Vol. 90, No. 2, (March-April 2007), pp. 427-436, ISSN 1060-3271

Feinstein, G., Hofstein, R., Koifmann, J. & Sokolovsky, M. (1974). Human pancreatic proteolytic enzymes and protein inhibitors. *European Journal of Biochemistry*, Vol. 43, No. 3, (April 1974), pp. 569-581, ISSN 1742-4658

Foltz, M., van Buren, L., Klaffke, W. & Duchateau, G.S. (2009). Modeling of the relationship between dipeptide structure and dipeptide stability, permeability, and ACE inhibitory activity. *Journal of Food Science*, Vol. 74, No. 7, (September 2009), pp. H243-H251, ISSN 1750-3841

Freeman, H.J. & Kim, Y.S. (1978). Digestion and absorption of protein. *Annual Reviews in Medicine*, Vol. 29, (February 1978), pp. 99-116, ISSN 0066-4219

Fu, T.J., (2002). Digestion stability as a criterion for protein allergenicity assessment. *Annals of the New York Academy of Sciences*, Vol. 964, (May 2002), pp. 99-110, ISSN 0077-8923

Gorovits, B., (2010). Immunogenicity: prediction, detection and effective assay development. *Bioanalysis*, Vol. 2, No. 9, (September 2010), pp. 1539-1545, ISSN 1757-6199

Gropper, S.A.S., Smith, J.L. & Groff, J.L. (2009). *Advanced nutrition and human metabolism*, Wadsworth/Cengage Learning, ISBN 9780495116578, Australia; United States

Hansen, N.G., (1975). Comparison of chemical methods of protein evaluation with biological value determined on rats. *Zeitschrift fuer Tierphysiologie, Tierernahrung und Futtermittelkund*, Vol. 35, No. 6, (October 1975), pp. 302-310, ISSN 0044-3565

Hauri, H.P., Sterchi, E.E., Bienz, D., Fransen, J.A. & Marxer, A. (1985). Expression and intracellular transport of microvillus membrane hydrolases in human intestinal epithelial cells. *Journal of Cell Biology*, Vol. 101, No. 3, (September 1985), pp. 838-851, ISSN 0021-9525

Henry, K.M., (1965). A comparison of biological methods with rats for determining the nutritive value of proteins. *British Journal of Nutrition*, Vol. 19, pp. 125-135, ISSN 0007-1145

Herman, R.A., Storer, N.P. & Gao, Y. (2006). Digestion assays in allergenicity assessment of transgenic proteins. *Environmental Health Perspectives*, Vol. 114, No. 8, (August 2006), pp. 1154-1157, ISSN 0091-6765

Horii, K., Adachi, T., Tanino, T., Tanaka, T., Sahara, H., Shibasaki, S., Ogino, C., Hata, Y., Ueda, M. & Kondo, A. (2009). Evaluation of cell surface-displayed protein stability against simulated gastric fluid. *Biotechnology Letters*, Vol. 31, No. 8, (August 2009), pp. 1259-1264, ISSN 1573-6776

Huang, Y.Y., Liu, G.M., Cai, Q.F., Weng, W.Y., Maleki, S.J., Su, W.J. & Cao, M.J. (2010). Stability of major allergen tropomyosin and other food proteins of mud crab (Scylla serrata) by in vitro gastrointestinal digestion. *Food Chemistry and Toxicology*, Vol. 48, No. 5, (May 2010), pp. 1196-1201, ISSN 1873-6351

Huby, R.D.J., Dearman, R.J. & Kimber, I. (2000). Why are some proteins allergens? *Toxicological Sciences*, Vol. 55, No. 2, (June 2000), pp. 235-246, ISSN 1096-6080

Jensen-Jarolim, E. & Untersmayr, E. (2006). Food Safety: In Vitro Digestion Tests Are Non-Predictive for Allergenic Potential of Food in Stomach Insufficiency. *Immunology Letters*, Vol. 102, No. 1, (January 2006), pp. 118-119, ISSN 0165-2478

Jin, F., Welch, R. & Glahn, R. (2006). Moving toward a more physiological model: application of mucin to refine the in vitro digestion/Caco-2 cell culture system. *Journal of Agricultural and Food Chemistry*, Vol. 54, No. 23, (November 2006), pp. 8962-8967, ISSN 1520-5118

Kamata, Y., Otsuka, S., Sato, M. & Shibasaki, K. (1982). Limited proteolysis of soybean beta-conglycinin. *Agricultural and Biological Chemistry (Japan)*, Vol. 46, (November 1982), pp. 2829–2834, ISSN 0002-1369

Kies, C., (1981). Bioavailability: a factor in protein quality. *Journal of Agricultural and Food Chemistry*, Vol. 29, No. 3, (May-June 1981), pp. 435-440, ISSN 0021-8561

Kim, Y.S., Birtwhistle, W. & Kim, Y.W. (1972). Peptide hydrolases in the bruch border and soluble fractions of small intestinal mucosa of rat and man. *Journal of Clinical Investigation*, Vol. 51, No. 6, (June 1972), pp. 1419-1430, ISSN 0021-9738

Krzysik, B.A. & Adibi, S.A. (1977). Cytoplasmic dipeptidase activities of kidney, ileum, jejunum, liver, muscle, and blood. *The American Journal of Physiology*, Vol. 233, No. 6, (December 1977), pp. E450-E456, ISSN 0002-9513

Lentze, M.J., (1995). Molecular and cellular aspects of hydrolysis and absorption. *American Journal of Clinical Nutrition*, Vol. 61, No. 4 Suppl, (April 1995), pp. 946S-951S, ISSN 0002-9165

Mandalari, G., Adel-Patient, K., Barkholt, V., Baro, C., Bennett, L., Bublin, M., Gaier, S., Graser, G., Ladics, G.S., Mierzejewska, D., Vassilopoulou, E., Vissers, Y.M., Zuidmeer, L., Rigby, N.M., Salt, L.J., Defernez, M., Mulholland, F., Mackie, A.R., Wickham, M.S. & Mills, E.N. (2009). In vitro digestibility of beta-casein and beta-lactoglobulin under simulated human gastric and duodenal conditions: a multi-laboratory evaluation. *Regulatory Toxicology and Pharmacology*, Vol. 55, No. 3, (December 2009), pp. 372-381, ISSN 1096-0295

Mokady, S., Viola, S. & Zimmermann, G. (1969). A new biological method for estimating of protein nutritive value. *British Journal of Nutrition*, Vol. 23, No. 3, (August 1969), pp. 491-495, ISSN 0007-1145

Moreno, F.J., (2007). Gastrointestinal digestion of food allergens: effect on their allergenicity. *Biomed Pharmacother*, Vol. 61, No. 1, (January 2007), pp. 50-60, ISSN 0753-3322

Moreno, F.J., Mackie, A.R. & Mills, E.N. (2005). Phospholipid interactions protect the milk allergen alpha-lactalbumin from proteolysis during in vitro digestion. *Journal of Agricultural and Food Chemistry*, Vol. 53, No. 25, (December 2005), pp. 9810-9816, ISSN 1520-5118

Nielsen, S.S., Deshpande, S.S., Hermodson, M.A. & Scott, M.P. (1988). Comparative digestibility of legume storage proteins. *Journal of Agricultural and Food Chemistry*, Vol. 36, No. 5, (September 1988), pp. 896-902, ISSN 1520-5118

Peng, K., Siradze, K., Quarmby, V. & Fischer, S.K. (2011). Clinical immunogenicity specificity assessments: a platform evaluation. *Journal of Pharmaceutical and Biomedical Analysis*, Vol. 54, No. 3, (February 2011), pp. 629-635, ISSN 1873-264X

Perrier, C. & Corthésy, B. (2011). Gut permeability and food allergies. *Clinical and Experimental Allergy*, Vol. 41, No. 1, (January 2011), pp. 20-28, ISSN 1365-2222

Polovic, N., Obradovic, A., Spasic, M., Plecas-Solarovic, B., Gavrovic-Jankulovic, M. & Cirkovic Velickovic, T. (2010). In Vivo Digestion of a Thaumatin-Like Kiwifruit Protein in Rats. *Food Digestion*, Vol. 1, No 1-2, (December 2010), pp. 5-13, ISSN 1869-1978

Savoie, L., Agudelo, R.A., Gauthier, S.F., Marin, J. & Pouliot, Y. (2005). In vitro determination of the release kinetics of peptides and free amino acids during the digestion of food proteins. *Journal of AOAC International*, Vol. 88, No. 3, (May 2005), pp. 935-948

Schasteen, C., Wu, J., Schulz, M. & Parsons, C. (2002). An enzyme-based digestibility assay for poultry diets., *Proceedings of Multi-State Poultry Meeting*, May 14-16 2002

Schiller, C.M., Huang, T.I. & Heizer, W.D. (1977). Isolation and characterization of four peptide hydrolases from the cytosol of rat intestinal mucosa. *Gastroenterology*, Vol. 72, No. 1, (January 1977), pp. 93-100, ISSN 0016-5085

Silk, D.B., (1980). Digestion and absorption of dietary protein in man. *Proceedings of the Nutritional Society*, Vol. 39, No. 1, (February 1980), pp. 61-70, ISSN 0029-6651

Silk, D.B., Grimble, G.K. & Rees, R.G. (1985). Protein digestion and amino acid and peptide absorption. *Proceedings of the Nutritional Society*, Vol. 44, No. 1, (February 1985), pp. 63-72, ISSN 0029-6651

Silk, D.B., Nicholson, A. & Kim, Y.S. (1976). Hydrolysis of peptides within lumen of small intestine. *The American Journal of Physiology*, Vol. 231, No. 5 Pt. 1, (November 1976), pp. 1322-1329, ISSN 0002-9513

Smith, E.L. & Bergmann, M. (1944). The peptidases of intestinal mucosa. *Journal of Biological Chemistry*, Vol. 153, No. 2, (May 1944), pp. 627-651, ISSN 0021-9258

Stanic, D., Monogioudi, E., Dilek, E., Radosavljevic, J., Atanaskovic-Markovic, M., Vuckovic, O., Raija, L., Mattinen, M., Buchert, J. & Cirkovic Velickovic, T. (2010). Digestibility and allergenicity assessment of enzymatically crosslinked beta-casein. *Molecular Nutrition and Food Research*, Vol. 54, No. 9, (September 2010), pp. 1273-1284, ISSN 1613-4133

Sterchi, E.E. & Woodley, J.F. (1980a). Peptide hydrolases of the human small intestinal mucosa: distribution of activities between brush border membranes and cytosol. *Clinica Chimica Acta*, Vol. 102, No. 1, (March 1980), pp. 49-56, ISSN 0009-8981

Sterchi, E.E. & Woodley, J.F. (1980b). Peptide hydrolases of the human small intestinal mucosa: identification of six distinct enzymes in the brush border membrane. *Clinica Chimica Acta*, Vol. 102, No. 1, (March 1980), pp. 57-65, ISSN 0009-8981

Szecsi, P.B., (1992). The aspartic proteases. *Scandinavian Journal of Clinical and Laboratory Investigation. Supplementum*, Vol. 210, (1992), p. 5, ISSN 0085-591X

Thomas, K., Aalbers, M., Bannon, G.A., Bartels, M., Dearman, R.J., Esdaile, D.J., Fu, T.J., Glatt, C.M., Hadfield, N., Hatzos, C., Hefle, S.L., Heylings, J.R., Goodman, R.E., Henry, B., Herouet, C., Holsapple, M., Ladics, G.S., Landry, T.D., MacIntosh, S.C., Rice, E.A., Privalle, L.S., Steiner, H.Y., Teshima, R., Van Ree, R., Woolhiser, M. & Zawodny, J. (2004). A multi-laboratory evaluation of a common in vitro pepsin digestion assay protocol used in assessing the safety of novel proteins. *Regulatory Toxicology and Pharmacology*, Vol. 39, No. 2, (April 2004), pp. 87-98, ISSN 0273-2300

Tonglet, C., Jeusette, I., Istasse, L. & Diez, M. (2001). Prediction of protein digestibility in dog food by a multi-enzymatic method: a useful technique to develop. *Journal of Animal Physiology and Animal Nutrition (Berlin)*, Vol. 85, No. 7-8, (August 2001), pp. 189-194, ISSN 0931-2439

Turner, M.D., (1968). Pepsinogens and pepsins. *Gut*, Vol. 9, No. 2, p. 134, ISSN 0017-5749

United States Pharmacopeial Convention (2006). *The United States pharmacopeia*, United States Pharmacopeial Convention, ISBN 1889788473, Rockville, MD

Van Beresteijn, E.C.H., Peeters, R.A., Kaper, J., Meijer, R.J.G.M., Robben, A.J.P.M. & Schmidt, D.G. (1994). Molecular mass distribution, immunological properties and nutritive value of whey protein hydrolysates. *Journal of Food Protection*, Vol. 57, No. 7, (July 1994), pp. 619-625, ISSN 0362-028X

Vardakou, M., Mercuri, A., Barker, S.A., Craig, D.Q., Faulks, R.M. & Wickham, M.S. (2011). Achieving antral grinding forces in biorelevant in vitro models: comparing the USP Dissolution Apparatus II and the Dynamic Gastric Model with human in vivo data. *AAPS Pharmscitech*, Vol. 12, No. 2, (June 2011), pp. 620-626, ISSN 1530-9932

Versantvoort, C.H., Oomen, A.G., Van de Kamp, E., Rompelberg, C.J. & Sips, A.J. (2005). Applicability of an in vitro digestion model in assessing the bioaccessibility of mycotoxins from food. *Food Chemistry and Toxicology*, Vol. 43, No. 1, (January 2005), pp. 31-40, ISSN 0278-6915

von der Decken, A., (1983). Experimental studies on the quality of food proteins. *Comparative Biochemistry and Physiology, Part B*, Vol. 74, No. 2, pp. 213-220, ISSN 0305-0491

Whitcomb, D.C. & Lowe, M.E. (2007). Human pancreatic digestive enzymes. *Digestive Diseases and Sciences*, Vol. 52, No. 1, (January 2007), pp. 1-17, ISSN 0163-2116

Whitecross, D.P., Armstrong, C., Clarke, A.D. & Piper, D.W. (1973). The pepsinogens of human gastric mucosa. *Gut*, Vol. 14, No. 11, (1973), p. 850, ISSN 0017-5749

Wickham, M., Faulks, R. & Mills, C. (2009). In vitro digestion methods for assessing the effect of food structure on allergen breakdown. *Molecular Nutrition and Food Research*, Vol. 53, No. 8, (August 2009), pp. 952-958, ISSN 1613-4133

Widmaier, E.P., Raff, H., Strang, K.T. & Vander, A.J. (2011). *Vander's human physiology: the mechanisms of body function*, McGraw-Hill, ISBN 9780077350017, New York

Yagami, T., Haishima, Y., Nakamura, A., Osuna, H. & Ikezawa, Z. (2000). Digestibility of allergens extracted from natural rubber latex and vegetable foods. *Journal of Allergy and Clinical Immunology*, Vol. 106, No. 4, (October 2000), pp. 752-762, ISSN 0091-6749

Yao, L., Friel, J.K., Suh, M. & Diehl-Jones, W.L. (2010). Antioxidant properties of breast milk in a novel in vitro digestion/enterocyte model. *Journal of Pediatric Gastroenterology and Nutrition*, Vol. 50, No. 6, (June 2010), pp. 670-676, ISSN 1536-4801

Yu, H.L., Cao, M.J., Cai, Q.F., Weng, W.Y., Su, W.J. & Liu, G.M. (2011). Effects of different processing methods on digestibility of Scylla paramamosain allergen (tropomyosin). *Food Chemistry and Toxicology*, Vol. 49, No. 4, (April 2011), pp. 791-798, ISSN 1873-6351

11

Mesenteric Vascular Disease

Amer Jomha and Markus Schmidt
Klinikum Bad Hersfeld,
Academic Teaching Hospital of the Justus-Liebig-University, Giessen
Germany

1. Introduction

Mesenteric ischemia occurs when perfusion of the visceral organs fails to meet normal metabolic requirements. This disorder is categorized as either acute and chronic, based on the duration of symptoms. Acute mesenteric ischemia (AMI) occurs rapidly over hours to days and frequently leads to acute intestinal infarction requiring resection.

2. Anatomy of the visceral arteries

The celiac artery arises from the abdominal aorta just caudal to the diaphragm at the level of L1 and is bordered by the median arcuate ligament at the aortic hiatus superiorly and the superior border of the pancreas inferiorly.Traditionally, the three branches from this common trunk include the left gastric, splenic, and common hepatic arteries. However, multiple variations of the true "trifurcation" can exist. Most frequently, the common hepatic artery and its branches arise from the SMA or directly from the abdominal aorta (1).

The SMA arises a few centimeters caudal to the celiac trunk, and its origin is crossed by the neck of the pancreas and the splenic vein.

The IMA is usually located 3 to 4 cm cephalic to the aortic bifurcation, just to the left of midline, and usually arises at the level of the third lumbar vertebra.

2.1 Acute mesenteric ischemia

2.1.1 Embolism

The most common cause of AMI is embolization to the SMA. Arterial emboli are responsible for 40% to 50% of cases of AMI (2, 3, 4).The proximal source of the embolus is frequently intracardiac mural thrombus. Mural thrombus in proximal aneurysms in the thoracic or proximal abdominal aorta can also serve as embolic sources. Because the SMA arises at a less acute angle from the abdominal aorta compared with the other mesenteric vessels, it appears to be the most common final destination for mesenteric emboli. Additionally, such emboli tend to lodge several centimeters from the vessel's origin, usually distal to the middle colic artery.

2.1.2 Arterial thrombosis

Arterial thrombosis constitutes the next most common cause of AMI and occurs in 20% to 35% of cases (4, 5). Preexisting atherosclerotic plaque affecting all visceral vessels is the

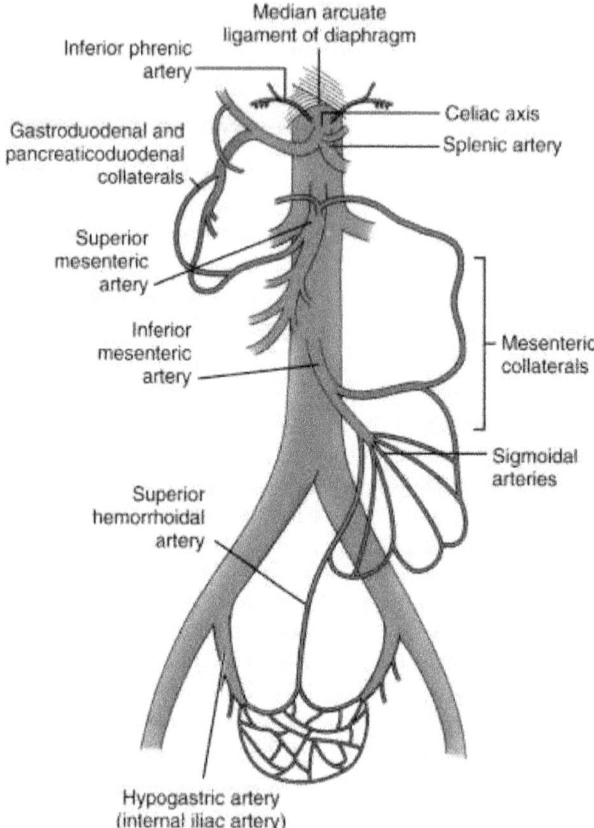

Fig. 1. Anatomy of the visceral arteries

most common finding. The affected segment of artery is usually its origin at the level of the aorta. Patients with acute arterial thrombosis frequently have preexisting symptoms of CMI. Acute extension of an aortic dissection can also serve as a mechanism for abrupt mesenteric vessel occlusion and thrombosis. The degree of intestinal infarction was significantly greater in patients with SMA thrombosis compared with embolus.

2.1.3 Nonocclusive mesenteric ischemia

Impaired intestinal perfusion in the absence of thromboembolic occlusion is termed nonocclusive mesenteric ischemia (NOMI). Symptomatic patients are frequently found to have extensive atherosclerosis, with involvement of all three visceral arteries. However, NOMI can also occur in patients without mesenteric arterial occlusive disease (6, 7, 8). Visceral ischemia can occur due to low-flow states, especially in conjunction with intestinal atherosclerotic disease. NOMI most commonly occurs secondary to cardiac disease, particularly severe congestive heart failure (9).

2.1.4 Mesenteric venous thrombosis

MVT constitutes 5% to 15% of all cases of mesenteric ischemia (10). Involvement is usually limited to the superior mesenteric vein but can also involve the inferior mesenteric vein and portal vein. The extent of bowel ischemia depends largely on the degree of venous involvement. Inherited or acquired hypercoagulable diseases, including protein-C and -S deficiency, polycythemia vera, antithrombin III deficiency, antiphospholipid antibody syndrome, and factor V Leiden mutation, are frequent causes.

3. Clinical presentation

3.1 Acute mesenteric ischemia

The most common symptom of AMI associated with arterial thromboembolic disease is the sudden onset of abdominal pain. Lack of collateral flow to the visceral organs leads to a more dramatic presentation in AMI, with severe, rapid clinical deterioration. Nausea, vomiting, diarrhea, emptying symptoms, and abdominal distention can also occur. Patients with NOMI or MVT typically present with a slower clinical course. Frequently, patients with NOMI are critically ill, hospitalized, intubated patients who experience a sudden deterioration in their clinical condition.

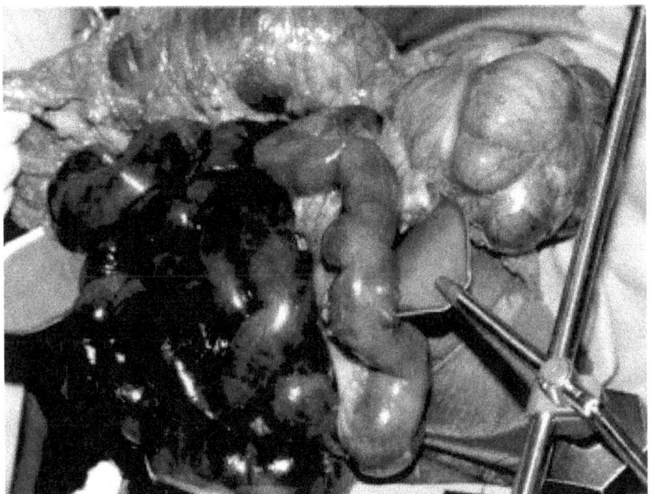

Fig. 2. Acute Mesenteric Ischemia (intraoperative photograph)

3.2 Chronic mesenteric ischemia

Postprandial abdominal pain and progressive weight loss are the most common symptoms in patients with CMI. Pain is often described as dull and crampy and located in the midepigastric region. The course of symptoms can be equated with intestinal claudication. Lack of energy leads to failure of the intestinal smooth muscle to relax, which intensifies the cramping pain. Pain often occurs 15 to 45 minutes after a meal, and the severity varies according to the size and type of meal. Patients typically develop "food fear" and decrease their oral intake in anticipation of severe pain after meals. Changes in bowel habits, nausea, and vomiting are less common findings. CMI is believed to be more prevalent in elderly women (11). The variable nature of symptoms often makes the diagnosis confusing and can result in delayed treatment. The traditional risk factors for atherosclerosis are usually present. A heavy smoking history is frequently obtained. The majority of patients also have a history of symptomatic manifestations in other vascular beds, most commonly cerebrovascular, coronary, and peripheral arteries.

Physical examination findings are usually nonspecific. Patients are commonly undernourished and cachectic.An abdominal bruit can sometimes be auscultated but is not always present. Bowel sounds are frequently hyperactive. Guarding and rebound tenderness are usually absent. Low prealbumin and albumin levels are often seen, owing to the patient's chronic malnourished state.

4. Diagnostic evaluation

4.1 Noninvasive evaluation

Duplex ultrasonography is a useful tool for the early, noninvasive diagnosis of visceral ischemic syndromes. Color Doppler scanning can be used to assess the flow velocities and resistance index in the splanchnic arteries and their arterial beds, as well to evaluate end-organ vascularity (12).

Computed tomography (CT) is an accurate, noninvasive imaging modality for diagnosing mesenteric ischemia, CTA diagnosed AMI with a sensitivity of 96% and a specificity of 94%.

Magnetic resonance angiography (MRA) is useful for diagnosing mesenteric occlusive disease. Because MRA takes significantly longer to perform than CTA, its role in evaluating patients with AMI is limited.

4.2 Invasive evaluation

Conventional angiography remains the "gold standard" in the diagnosis of mesenteric ischemia. Anteroposterior and lateral views of the visceral aorta as well as selective catheterization of the celiac trunk, SMA, and IMA, provide the most accurate and specific localization of stenotic and occlusive lesions. Therapeutic alternatives such as balloon angioplasty, stenting, and thrombolysis and percutaneous thrombus extraction can all be used to restore luminal visceral blood flow.

5. Treatment of acute and chronic mesenteric ischemia

Medical treatment alone is not effective in these patients. Preventive risk factor modification helps control the progression of atherosclerosis in the mesenteric circulation as well as other vascular beds. Patients with known risks for inheritable hypercoagulable disorders should undergo screening and should be treated with systemic anticoagulation if indicated.

5.1 Endovascular treatment

Advances in endovascular techniques have greatly expanded the role of percutaneous interventions for patients with mesenteric ischemia in recent years. However, endovascular management remains largely limited to patients with CMI. Balloon angioplasty and stenting are the most common interventions, and recent reports have documented excellent technical results with low patient morbidity.Endovascular therapy should be the treatment of choice in high-risk patients with CMI (13, 14, 15, 16). High technical success rates and decreased patient morbidity and mortality rates have been reasonably well established in such individuals.

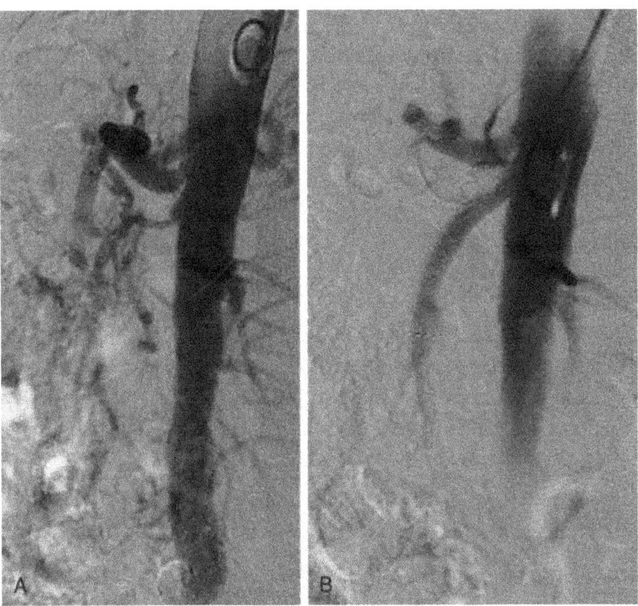

Fig. 3. A, Lateral arteriogram of the celiac axis and superior mesenteric artery. Note the mild orificial stenosis in the celiac axis and the severe stenosis in the proximal superior mesenteric artery. B, Completion study after angioplasty and stenting of the superior mesenteric artery stenosis. Note the widely patent superior mesenteric artery, with no evidence of stenosis

5.2 Surgical treatment

Laparotomy with visceral revascularization can be used to treat patients with both AMI and CMI. Patients presenting with signs and symptoms of AMI require urgent abdominal exploration, assessment of bowel viability, and revascularization. Several techniques for the restoration of intestinal perfusion are available to the vascular surgeon, and familiarity with a variety of options is crucial. Before revascularization, large segments of both small and large intestine may appear dusky, ischemic, or necrotic.

5.3 Acute mesenteric ischemia

5.3.1 SMA embolectomy

Perfusion of the mesenteric arteries is assessed by palpation and Doppler evaluation. In cases in which the obstruction is caused by an embolus, a proximal SMA pulse is often appreciated. Systemic heparinization is established. If the artery feels relatively soft and free of atherosclerotic disease, a transverse arteriotomy is performed distal to the area of obstruction, and the arterial lumen is assessed for thrombus. Balloon-tipped embolectomy catheters are gently passed proximally and distally until no more clot can be removed. Care must be taken not to overinflate the balloons and dissect the arterial intima. Distally, mesenteric vessels are very thin, and overinflation can result in rupture and intramesenteric extravasation. The transverse arteriotomy is then closed primarily with simple interrupted Prolene sutures if no endarterectomy is necessary. In cases in which a flow-limiting plaque is present, the arteriotomy is converted to a longitudinal one, and a local thromboendarterectomy is performed. Patch angioplasty with autogenous vein is the preferred method of revascularization owing to potential contamination from concomitant bowel resection. The arteriotomy site can also be used for distal anastomosis of an antegrade or retrograde bypass if necessary.

5.4 Chronic mesenteric ischemia

5.4.1 Transaortic endarterectomy

Advantages of this operation include removal of atheroma from the aorta and both visceral arteries simultaneously. Limitations include the need for extended exposure of the upper abdominal aorta via medial visceral rotation and incomplete plaque removal if the atheroma extends to the distal artery or if transmural calcification is present. It is suitable for selected patients with CMI undergoing elective revascularizaion (17).

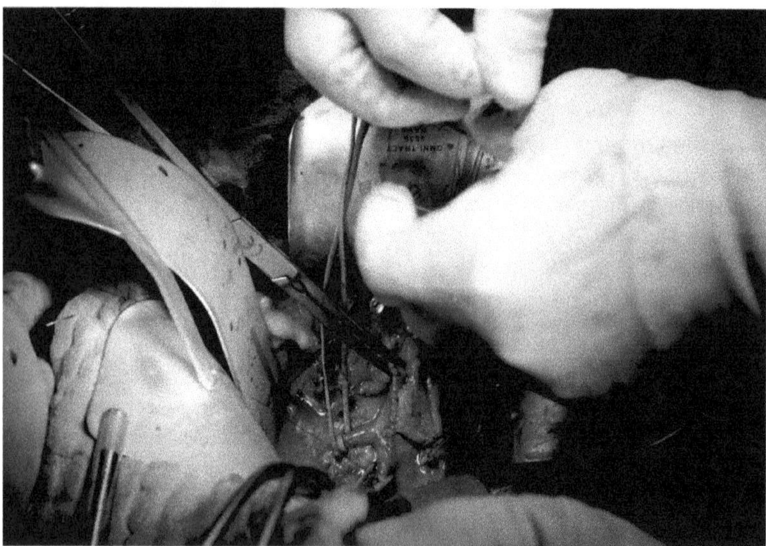

Fig. 4. Endarteriektomie of the SMA

5.5 Antegrade mesenteric bypass

Reconstruction of the celiac artery and the SMA with a bifurcated prosthetic graft originating from the supraceliac aorta. The operation is done through an upper midline or bilateral subcostal incision, depending on the patient's body habitus and costal cartilage flare. Supraceliac-origin grafts are a poor choice in patients with compromised cardiac or pulmonary function or those with extensive atherosclerosis or circumferential calcification of the supraceliac aorta. In these cases, infrarenal sources of inflow are preferred (18, 19, 21).

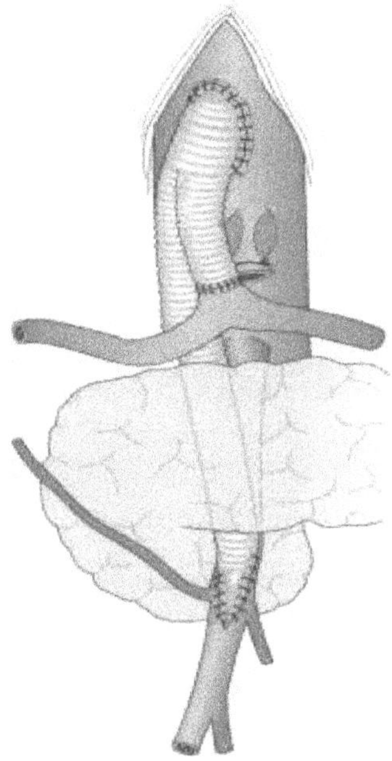

Fig. 5. Antegrade aortoceliac–superior mesenteric artery bypass

5.6 Retrograde mesenteric bypass

The infrarenal aorta, a prior infrarenal aortic graft, or the iliac artery are excellent inflow sources, Two-vessel reconstructions can be performed with retrograde grafts by doing a side-to-side anastomosis to the SMA and an end-to-side anastomosis to the common hepatic artery. These grafts may be passed on top of or beneath the pancreas and curved in a C shape toward the hepatic artery.

6. Treatment of nonocclusive mesenteric ischemia

The primary treatment for NOMI is medical, with extensive critical care support and prompt arteriography. Operative exploration is reserved for signs of peritonitis that suggest the presence of gangrenous bowel that requires excision. Interventional therapies can be initiated at the time of the diagnostic arteriogram and are targeted at relieving vasospasm using intra-arterial infusions of vasodilator medications. The most common intra-arterial agent is phosphodiesterase inhibitor papaverine and prostaglandin (22). Surgical exploration is required for all patients who have evidence of any threatened bowel, regardless of the underlying cause. The prognosis is poor, despite the absence of organic obstruction in the principal arteries.

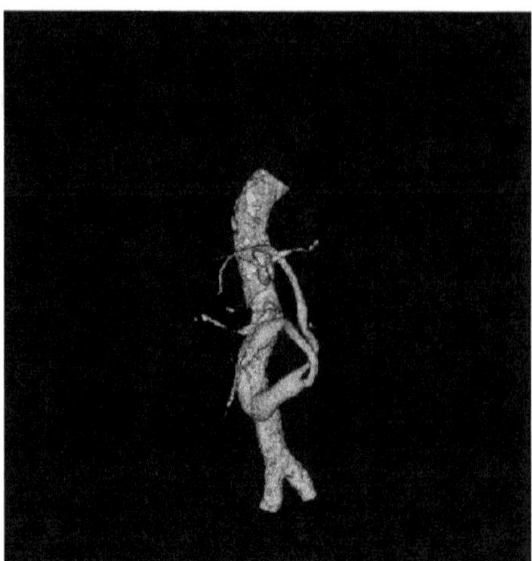

Fig. 6. Retrograde aortoceliac–superior mesenteric artery bypass

7. Treatment of mesenteric venous thrombosis

Initial anticoagulation with heparin is the treatment of choice in patients without peritonitis. After initial anticoagulation, continued treatment with low-molecular-weight heparin (LMWH) or VKA is advocated. Uncertainties about bowel viability are assessed through laparotomy or laparoscopy; it is safer to perform a laparotomy to check for bowel viability in patients with signs of peritonitis and rebound tenderness. Endovascular treatment in combination with heparin infusion, with or without bowel resection, is an additional treatment tool (23, 24, 25, 26, 27). The indications for surgery are peritonitis, severe gastrointestinal bleeding, late small bowel perforation, and intestinal stricture; the last is often associated with chronic diarrhea.

7.1 Splanchnic artery aneurysms

True aneurysms of splanchnic arteries are less common than visceral artery pseudoaneurysms, but they remain an important vascular disease. Nearly 22% of these present as clinical emergencies, including 8.5% that result in death (28). The pathogenesis and natural history of these aneurysms have been reassessed, and in most instances redefined, within the past three decades as advances in imaging technology and endovascular treatments have begun to influence diagnostic and management strategies. Recognition of splanchnic artery aneurysms has increased because of the greater availability and widespread use of advanced imaging capabilities such as high-resolution computed tomography (CT) scanning, magnetic resonance angiography (MRA), sophisticated ultrasonography, and angiography. Selective arteriography remains the most valuable examination in planning therapy but noninvasive imaging techniques for diagnosis and operative planning are becoming increasingly important.

Although surgery remains the mainstay of therapy for most splanchnic aneurysms, especially in the setting of rupture, many aneurysms (particularly those involving solid organs) are now treated with catheter-based interventions. Endovascular approaches are commonly used to control the bleeding that accompanies aneurysm rupture (29), and prophylactic treatment of incidentally discovered intact aneurysms has become common (particularly those well-collateralized aneurysms that are imbedded within the pancreatic or hepatic parenchyma). Embolization has become the preferred treatment in patients at high surgical risk or for aneurysms in locations that are difficult to approach surgically.

Arterial Location	Incidence of Aneurysms
Splenic	60.0%
Hepatic	20.0%
Superior mesenteric	5.5%
Celiac	4.0%
Gastric or gastroepiploic	4.0%
Jejunal, ileal, or colic	3.0%
Pancreaticoduodenal or pancreatic	2.0%
Gastroduodenal	1.5%
Inferior mesenteric	Rare

Table 1. Incidence of Aneurysms of the Splanchnic Arterial Circulation (30, 31)

7.2 Splenic artery aneurysm

The most common of the splanchnic artery aneurysms and account for as many as 60% of all reported splanchnic aneurysms (32). The most common clinical risk factors reported in association with Splenic Artery Aneurysm are female gender, a history of multiple pregnancies, and portal hypertension. A classic calcified ring may be noted in the left upper quadrant on a plain x-ray film of the abdomen.the patients may have an abdominal bruit, the majority of physical examinations are normal in patients with asymptomatic lesions. When rupture occurs, patients usually complain of acute left-sided abdominal pain. Shock, abdominal distention, and death can result from free intraperitoneal rupture of an Splenic Artery Aneurysm. The overall mortality of ruptured Splenic Artery Aneurysm is high (33).

Splenic aneurysms that have ruptured or are symptomatic require urgent treatment. Additionally, aneurysms in pregnant women or those of childbearing age also absolutely warrant treatment. Less stringent indications for treatment include aneurysms that are noted to be enlarging or those greater than 2 cm in diameter.

Endovascular exclusion of has been used more recently with general success. Treatment options include coil embolization of the splenic artery both proximal and distal to the aneurysm itself, thereby effectively "trapping" the lesion (34, 35).

7.3 Hepatic artery aneurysms

The hepatic artery is the second most common location for aneurysmal degeneration in the splanchnic circulation. The causes are degenerative ("atherosclerotic"), medial degeneration, fibrodysplasia, trauma, infection, biliary diseases and percutaneous or endoscopic procedures, polyarteritis nodosa, and congenital disorders.

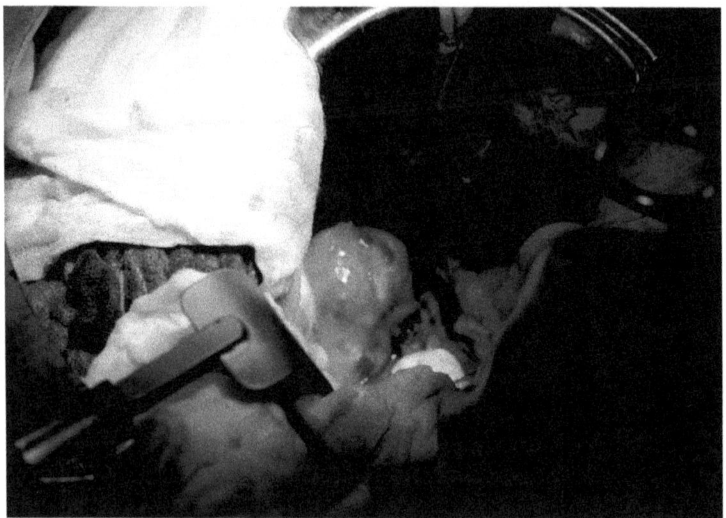

Fig. 7. Splenic Artery Aneurysm (intraoperative photograph)

Symptoms can include epigastric or right upper quadrant pain and subsequent gastrointestinal hemorrhage and jaundice. Treatment options depend to a large extent on the anatomic location and morphology of the Hepatic Artery Aneurysms, underlying etiology, and status of the end organ (36, 37, 38, 39).

7.4 Celiac artery aneurysms

In contrast to Splenic Artery Aneurysms are Celiac Artery Aneurysms more commonly found in men. The causes are medial degeneration or atherosclerotic disease. Less common causes include trauma, collagen vascular disease, arterial dissection, anomalous splanchnic circulation, and mycotic aneurysms. Open surgical options included aneurysmectomy, aneurysmorrhaphy, and ligation (40).

7.5 Superior mesenteric artery aneurysm

Most commonly found within the first 5 cm of the artery,, these aneurysms are particularly dangerous because complications such as aneurysm rupture, acute thrombosis, or distal embolization may jeopardize the entire small bowel.

Superior Mesenteric Artery Aneurysm associated with an infectious etiology in the majority of cases (Mycotic aneurysms). The majority of Superior Mesenteric Artery Aneurysms are symptomatic at initial evaluation. Treatment of Superior Mesenteric Artery Aneurysms should be considered regardless of size or symptomatology because of the high mortality risk associated with potential rupture. treatment must be individualized and based on the etiology, size, and anatomic location of the lesion; co-morbid conditions of the patient; and the potential morbidity of the proposed procedure (41, 42).

8. References

[1] Rosenblum JD, Boyle CM, Schwartz LB: The mesenteric circulation: anatomy and physiology. Surg Clin North Am 1997; 77:289-306.

[2] Foley MI, Moneta GL, Abou-Zamzam AM, et al: Revascularization of the superior mesenteric artery alone for treatment of intestinal ischemia. J Vasc Surg 2000; 32:37-47.

[3] Stoney RJ, Cunningham CG: Acute mesenteric ischemia. Surgery 1993; 114:489-490.

[4] McKinsey JF, Gewertz BL: Acute mesenteric ischemia. Surg Clin North Am 1997; 77:307-318.

[5] Park WM, Gloviczki P, Cherry Jr KJ, et al: Contemporary management of acute mesenteric ischemia: factors associated with survival. J Vasc Surg 2002; 35:445-452.

[6] Bradbury AW, Brittenden J, McBride K, et al: Mesenteric ischaemia: a multidisciplinary approach. Br J Surg 1995; 82:1446-1459.

[7] Mansour MA: Management of acute mesenteric ischemia. Arch Surg 1999; 134:328-330.

[8] Oldenburg WA, Lau LL, Rodenburg TJ: Acute mesenteric ischemia: a clinical review. Arch Intern Med 2004; 164:1054-1062.

[9] Thomas JH, Blake K, Pierce GE, et al: The clinical course of asymptomatic mesenteric arterial stenosis. J Vasc Surg 1998; 27:840-844.

[10] Kumar S, Sarr MG, Kamath PS: Mesenteric venous thrombosis. N Engl J Med 2001; 345:1683-1688.

[11] Schwartz LB, Gewertz BL: Mesenteric ischemia. Surg Clin North Am 1997; 77:275-507.

[12] Dietrich CF, Jedrzejczyk M, Ignee A: Sonographic assessment of splanchnic arteries and the bowel wall. Eur J Radiol 2007; 64:202-212.

[13] Sivamurthy N, Rhodes JM, Lee D, et al: Endovascular versus open mesenteric revascularization: immediate benefits do not equate with short-term functional outcomes. J Am Coll Surg 2006; 202:859-

[14] Sharafuddin MJ, Olson CH, Sun S, et al: Endovascular treatment of celiac and mesenteric arteries stenosis: applications and results. J Vasc Surg 2003; 38:692-698.

[15] Sarac TP, Altinel O, Kashyap V, et al: Endovascular treatment of stenotic and occluded visceral arteries for chronic mesenteric ischemia. J Vasc Surg 2008; 47:485-491.

[16] Brown DJ, Schermerhorn ML, Powell RJ, et al: Mesenteric stenting for chronic mesenteric ischemia. J Vasc Surg 2005; 42:268-274.

[17] Lau H, Chew DK, Whittemore AD, et al: Transaortic endarterectomy for primary mesenteric revascularization. Vasc Endovasc Surg 2002; 36:335-341.

[18] Jimenez JG, Huber TS, Ozaki K, et al: Durability of antegrade synthetic aortomesenteric bypass for chronic mesenteric ischemia. J Vasc Surg 2002; 35:1078-1084.

[19] Kansal N, LoGerfo FW, Belfield AK, et al: A comparison of antegrade and retrograde mesenteric bypass. Ann Vasc Surg 2002; 16:591-596.

[20] Kougias P, Lau D, El Sayed HF, et al: Determinants of mortality and treatment outcome following surgical interventions for acute mesenteric ischemia. J Vasc Surg 2007; 46:467-474.

[21] Mateo RB, O'Hara PJ, Hertzer NR, et al: Elective surgical treatment of symptomatic chronic mesenteric occlusive disease: early results and late outcomes. J Vasc Surg 1999.821-832.

[22] Mitsuyoshi A, Obama K, Shinkura N, et al: Survival in nonocclusive mesenteric ischemia: early diagnosis by multidetector row computed tomography and early

treatment with continuous intravenous high-dose prostaglandin E1. Ann Surg 2007; 246:229-235.

[23] Lopera JE, Correa G, Brazzini A, et al: Percutaneous transhepatic treatment of symptomatic mesenteric venous thrombosis. J Vasc Surg 2002; 36:1058-1061.

[24] Kim HS, Patra A, Khan J, et al: Transhepatic catheter-directed thrombectomy and thrombolysis of acute superior mesenteric venous thrombosis. J Vasc Interv Radiol 2005.1685-1691.

[25] Zhou W, Choi L, Lin PH, et al: Percutaneous transhepatic thrombectomy and pharmacologic thrombolysis of mesenteric venous thrombosis. Vascular 2007; 1:41-45.

[26] Grisham A, Lohr J, Guenther JM, et al: Deciphering mesenteric venous thrombosis: imaging and treatment. Vasc Endovasc Surg 2005; 39:473-479.

[27] Semiz-Oysu A, Keussen I, Cwikiel W: Interventional radiological management of prehepatic obstruction of [corrected] the splanchnic venous system. Cardiovasc Intervent Radiol 2007; 30:688-695.

[28] Pasha S.F., Gloviczki P., Stanson A.W., Kamath P.S.: Splanchnic artery aneurysms. Mayo Clinic Proc 2007; 82(4):472-479.

[29] Gabelmann A., Gorich J., Merkle E.M.: Endovascular treatment of visceral artery aneurysms. J Endovascular Therapie 2002; 9(1):38-47.

[30] Ruiz-Tovar J., Martinez-Molina E., Morales V., et al: Evolution of the therapeutic approach of visceral artery aneurysms. Scand J Surg 2007; 96(4):308-313.

[31] Huang Y.K., Hsieh H.C., Tsai F.C., et al: Visceral artery aneurysm: risk factor analysis and therapeutic opinion. Eur J Vasc Endovasc Surg 2007; 33(3):293-301.

[32] Miani S., Arpesani A., Giorgetti P.L., et al: Splanchnic artery aneurysms. J Cardiovasc Surg (Torino) 1993; 34(3):221-228.

[33] Carr S.C., Mahvi D.M., Hoch J.R., et al: Visceral artery aneurysm rupture. J Vasc Surg 2001; 33(4):806-811.

[34] Grego F.G., Lepidi S., Ragazzi R., et al: Visceral artery aneurysms: a single center experience. Cardiovasc Surg 2003; 11(1):19-25.

[35] Kanazawa S., Inada H., Murakami T., et al: The diagnosis and management of splanchnic artery aneurysms: report of 8 cases. J Cardiovasc Surg (Torino) 1997; 38(5):479-485.

[36] Lumsden A.B., Mattar S.G., Allen R.C., Bacha E.A.: Hepatic artery aneurysms: the management of 22 patients. J Surg Res 1996; 60(2):345-350.

[37] Abbas M.A., Fowl R.J., Stone W.M., et al: Hepatic artery aneurysm: factors that predict complications. J Vasc Surg 2003; 38(1):41-45.

[38] Parangi S., Oz M.C., Blume R.S., et al: Hepatobiliary complications of polyarteritis nodosa. Arch Surg 1991; 126(7):909-912.

[39] Erskine J.M.: Hepatic artery aneurysm. Vasc Surg 1973; 7(2):106-125.

[40] Bailey R.W., Riles T.S., Rosen R.J., Sullivan L.P.: Celiomesenteric anomaly and aneurysm: clinical and etiologic features. J Vasc Surg 1991; 14(2):229-234.

[41] Stone W.M., Abbas M., Cherry K.J., et al: Superior mesenteric artery aneurysms: is presence an indication for intervention?. J Vasc Surg 2002; 36(2):234-237.discussion, 7

[42] Geelkerken R.H., van Bockel J.H., de Roos W.K., Hermans J.: Surgical treatment of intestinal artery aneurysms. Eur J Vasc Surg 1990; 4(6):563-567.

12

A Case Based Approach to Severe Microcytic Anemia in Children

Andrew S. Freiberg
Pennsylvania State University
USA

1. Introduction

Clinicians are traditionally taught that the differential diagnosis of microcytic anemia is limited to a very few causes, with iron deficiency anemia on top of that list. While this may be true, the specific etiology of these causes and specifically the exact cause of the iron deficiency in each case is of clinical importance, as treatment of the anemia is very different for each cause. Just as the most common reason for severe microcytic anemia at any age is iron deficiency, the most common reasons for that deficiency at any age involve the gastrointestinal tract. The gastrointestinal tract is both the site of iron uptake and the most common site of blood loss. Thus, the gastrointestinal specialist plays a key role in diagnosing and managing microcytic anemia and must understand the various etiologies of microcytic anemia that are likely or possible in the population seen, including those cases that do not have a GI cause. In this chapter we will explain in a case based format the proper workup of the child and adolescent with microcytic anemia, emphasizing the role of the GI tract in the mechanism and of the GI specialist in the diagnosis and management.

2. Overview of anemia

Anemia refers to a hemoglobin (Hgb) or hematocrit (Hct) level lower than adult range or the age-adjusted range for healthy children. Normal values also vary depending on the gender and race of the patient. Since the main physiological role of red blood cells (RBCs) is to deliver oxygen to tissues, anemia is a condition where the body's metabolic demands for oxygen may not be adequately achieved. The condition is usually secondary to various pathologic processes and is not considered a disease in itself.

The causes for anemia can be broadly categorized into three pathological processes: decreased or ineffective erythropoiesis, increased hemolysis, and blood loss. However, cases where anemia is multifatorial in origin can exist. Anemia can also be further classified as microcytic, normocytic or macrocytic, referring to the mean corpuscular volume (MCV) which measures RBCs size, ranging from small, normal and large, respectively. This chapter will focus on microcytic anemia in children. The cases and information given are applicable to the general practitioner, but are aimed specifically at the pediatric gastroenterologist, focusing specifically on *severe* anemias that are *severely* microcytic, because these are the cases that impact the gastroenterologist most. An effort will be made to clarify much of the commonly thought but vague and misleading information about this condition.

There have been numerous reviews on the evaluation of anemia and microcytic anemia in children (Jain & Kamat 2009, Janus & Moerschel 2010). Although these reviews attempt to be comprehensive, they tend to be overly simplistic and misleading. Specifically with regard to microcytic anemia, the impression given is that nutritional deficiency is the most frequent cause of iron deficiency and hence microcytic anemia. Although this may be true for mild anemia, it is certainly not true for severe anemia, where blood loss is far more common. While a child with a hemoglobin of 11 g/dL and mild microcytosis may have a lack of sufficient iron in his or her diet, a hemoglobin of 5 g/dL and MCV of 55 fL cannot be due to nutrition alone. Anyone at any age with such values requires investigation for a serious condition and should not be treated with iron supplementation alone. To assume that most cases of microcytosis should be treated with supplemental iron alone is to miss the opportunity and the necessity of the proper workup for significant pathology.

2.1 Epidemiology of iron deficiency in children

Iron deficiency and iron deficiency anemia affect a large proportion of people worldwide (Beard & Stoltzfus, 2001; Benoit 2001; Stoltzfus, 2001). According to the Fourth National Health and Nutrition Examination Survey (NHANES IV), iron deficiency without anemia exists in 7% of toddlers aged 1 to 2 years, 9% of adolescent girls, and 16% of women of childbearing age, (Looker, 2002) a true public health concern. Unfortunately, studies of the prevalence of iron deficiency anemia use arbitrary definitions of anemia and iron deficiency, such as a hemoglobin less than 11 (Eden & Mir, 1997). There is often no attempt to separate iron deficiency based on severity, so that the true incidence of *severe* iron deficiency anemia is unknown.

It must be remembered that iron deficiency and iron deficiency anemia are somewhat distinct, but overlapping and related disorders. Although confirmatory studies are lacking, it is probably true that the greatest cause of iron deficiency worldwide and in the United States is nutrition, i.e. lack of sufficient iron in the diet, and the greatest cause of iron deficiency *anemia* worldwide and in the United States is slow gastrointestinal bleeding. Statistics stating the leading causes of these conditions can easily mislead the practitioner, since the epidemiology of iron deficiency and iron deficiency are different, and also varies by age, gender, socioeconomic status and geography. Worldwide, and especially in poor countries, infestation by hookworm (mostly Necator americanus and Ancylostoma duodenale) is the leading cause of gastrointestinal blood loss leading to iron deficiency and iron deficiency anemia. Infestation by Trichuris trichiura, the cause of trichuriasis (whipworm) infection is common throughout many parts of the world, and symptomatic infestations leading to iron deficiency or growth retardation preferentially affect children between 2 and 10 years of age. By contrast, in the United States, parasitic infestation has become distinctly rare due to improved sanitation and the fact that most children in the U.S. now wear shoes when outdoors. In the United States, cultural differences in feeding practices affect the incidence of iron deficiency anemia (Kwiatowski, 1999)

2.2 Health effects of iron deficiency

The association between iron deficiency anemia and impaired neurocognitive function is well established, and is independent of psychosocial and environmental factors. The association is especially strong in young children and infants (Oski, 1979). There is evidence that iron deficiency that has not progressed to anemia is also associated with poor neurocognitive function (Akman et al., 2004; Cook & Lynch 1986; Grantham-McGregor & Ani, 2001; Oski, 1983, 1985; Pollitt et al., 1986). Many possible mechanisms for the association have been suggested and investigated, but the true etiology is unknown (Beard, 2001; Erikson et al., 2001; Ortiz et al., 2004). Whether and to what extent this poor neurocognitive function can be reversed by correcting the deficiency is debated (Akman et al, 2004; Lozoff et al., 1982, 1996, 2000; Oski, 1983; Walter et al., 1989)

Many types of anemia such as hemoglobinopathies, hemolytic anemias and iron deficiency lead to increased absorption of both iron and lead from the GI tract. Coupled with the increased incidence of pica in these anemias, one effect of anemia, including that due to iron deficiency, is the increased incidence of lead poisoning and its health effects.

3. Differential diagnosis of microcytic anemia

Students are traditional taught that the differential diagnosis of microcytic anemia includes five possible conditions:

1. Iron deficiency anemia
2. Thalassemia trait
3. Lead poisoning
4. Chronic disease
5. Sideroblastic anemia

Figure 1 shows a general schema for distinguishing these disorder based on RBC size (MCV) and hemoglobin level. The figure is not meant to show the exact values for these disorders, but to emphasize the relative values and emphasizes their overlap. After considering some of the disorders that overlap with iron deficiency, this chapter will focus on the severe anemias that are severely microcytic, i.e. those that are most likely due to iron deficiency. Note that lead poisoning is not included in the figure because as explained below it is now considered more of a consequence than a cause of iron deficiency; sideroblastic anemia is also not seen because it is not a distinct condition and thus shows considerable heterogeneity in hemoglobin and MCV. Likewise, bone marrow failure syndromes such as Diamond-Blackfan anemia, the erythropoietin deficiency of end stage renal failure, transient erythroblastopenia of childhood, and leukemia encompass a wide variety of separate disorders with different combinations of MCV and hemoglobin, but none of these are microcytic.

It is important to keep in mind that the presence of one disorder does not exclude others. For example, iron deficiency may occur in patients with thalassemia, and patients may have concomitant acute and chronic bleeding. Also, the relationship is altered by therapy; hence patients who have been partially or inadequately treated may have values that do not fit the expected relationships.

From a practical sense, when considering the above five disorders, the severely microcytic anemias limit this differential for the most part to the top two, and further considering only those that are severely anemic to a large extent eliminates all but the first. As we shall see, a large part of microcytic anemia in children, as in adults, and certainly the severe clinically important cases, is due to iron deficiency anemia. As will be discussed, once iron deficiency

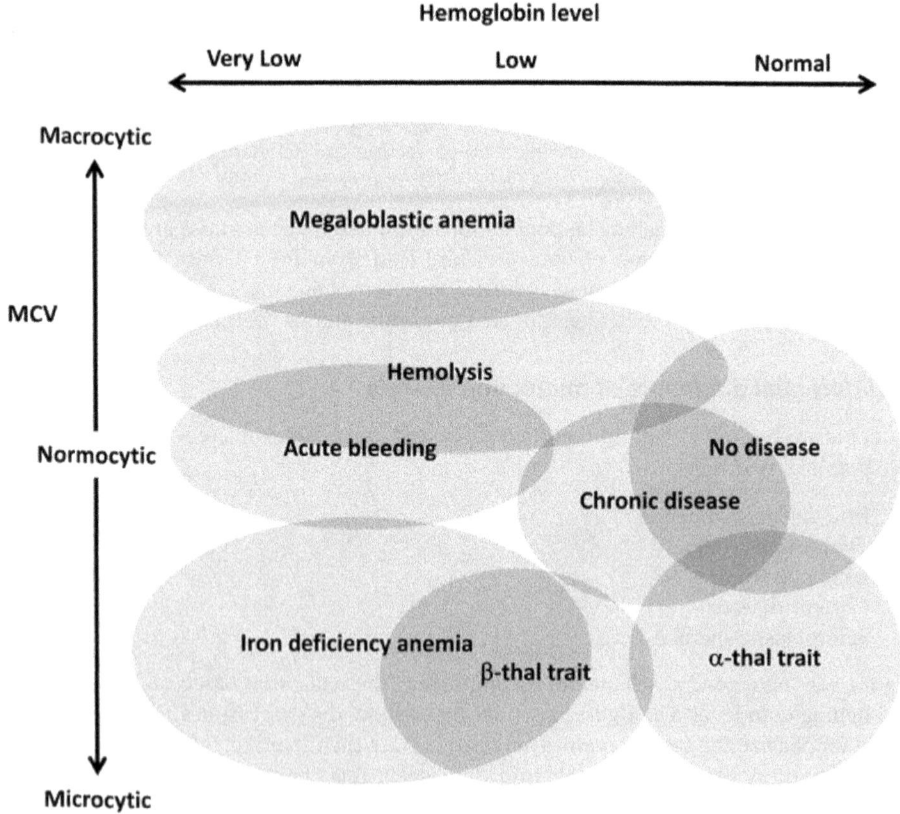

Fig. 1. Approximate relationship of anemias according to hemoglobin and red cell size (MCV)

is determined to be likely, the cause of the deficiency must be determined, and it is important for the clinician to distinguish blood loss from other causes. This list of causes varies depending on the age of the patient, the severity of the anemia and the severity of microcytosis. The chapter will outline a more thorough differential for all causes, leading towards a proper diagnosis before initiating treatment. We will emphasize that iron therapy alone is not adequate therapy; as such treatment alone will leave the cause of the anemia undiagnosed and untreated.

3.1 Acute blood loss

Since iron deficiency anemia is almost always due to chronic blood loss, the distinction between acute and chronic blood loss must be made. While both lead to anemia, the causes as well as the signs and symptoms are profoundly different between the two. As to the cause, acute blood loss can occur externally by any route or internally into practically any space, including intracranial, intrathoracic, retroperitoneal and abdominal. Isolated acute blood loss is normocytic, with a reticulocyte count that is not elevated until several days after the event, providing the patient survives and has adequate iron stores, i.e. there is not coexistent chronic blood loss. Therefore the anemia of acute blood loss is due to blood loss, while the anemia of iron deficiency is due to iron loss, and is in fact a bone marrow failure syndrome limited to red cells due to lack of substrate (iron).

Signs and symptoms of acute blood loss are very different from those of chronic blood loss. Acute blood loss leads to volume depletion and can rapidly progress to tissue hypoperfusion and shock, while the slow onset of anemia that occurs with chronic blood loss allows hemodynamic compensation. Children especially can tolerate extremely low hemoglobins if gradual in onset, without cardiac decompensation and no end organ effects. These children will appear pale, and have compensatory tachycardia, and may have dyspnea and headache on exertion, but very small children may have no signs other than pallor and mild fussiness. Some children will appear "yellow" due to underlying skin pigmentation, especially if the diet includes yellow vegetables, but actual jaundice is easy to exclude due to the lack of scleral icterus.

We will now discuss in some detail the five traditional causes of microcytic anemia, using some specific cases to illustrate.

3.2 Sideroblastic anemia

The sideroblastic anemias are a heterogeneous group of congenital and acquired bone marrow disorders defined by the presence of pathologic iron deposits within the mitochondria of erythroid precursors. The anemia may be mild, moderate or severe and may be normocytic, microcytic, or macrocytic and is typically characterized by a relative reticulocytopenia (Flemming, 2009). There are several known and incompletely characterized congenital causes, but all are rare including atransferrinemia, hypotranferrinemia (Shamsian et al., 2009), and others (Iolascon et al., 2009). Acquired causes include a variety of toxic exposures, drugs, and myelodysplastic syndromes, as well as copper deficiency. Many of these, although included in a full discussion of anemia and microcytic anemia, do not need to be considered in this chapter because they only rarely present as a severe anemia that is severely microcytic. Copper deficiency, for example is extremely rare, is usually normocytic, and the major manifestations are neurologic rather than hematologic.

3.3 The anemia of "chronic disease" (Case 1)

A 10 year old boy was referred to pediatric hematology clinic for anemia occurring on a previous blood test. Two months earlier he had been hospitalized briefly for a high fever and rash. While in the hospital, a CBC showed a mild microcytic anemia (hgb 10.0 g/dL (normal 11.9-15.4 g/dL), MCV 75 fL (normal 80-95 fL). He recovered well and was subsequently discharged. He had since been well, with no subsequent fevers, and no weight loss or night sweats. He had had no increased fatigue or exercise intolerance. His family history was negative for any hematologic disorders or malignancies. He had no chronic medical conditions, took no medications, and had no known drug allergies.

In clinic, he appeared healthy, cooperative and in no distress. His skin showed no rash, bruises, jaundice, or pallor. He had no lymphadenopathy, scleral icterus, or conjunctival pallor. His lungs were clear with no wheezes, and his heart sounds were normal with no murmur. His abdomen was soft and nontender with no organomegaly, although his liver was palpable and slightly tender to palpation, but his spleen was not palpable. His extremities were well perfused with no edema. Two months after his original CBC his hemoglobin had risen to 11 g/dL (normal 12-15 g/dL), and MCV was 72.9 fL (normal 74-82). His ferritin was 38 ng/mL (normal 10-200 ng/mL). Iron studies were normal as was his hemoglobin electrophoresis and blood smear.

3.3.1 Discussion

Typically the anemia of chronic disease, also called the anemia of inflammation, is a mild normocytic or mildly microcytic anemia. Usually it is associated with chronic conditions such as IBD, and the anemia resolves with effective treatment of the underlying condition. As this case illustrates however, the anemia of "chronic" disease can be associated with inflammatory conditions of shorter duration such as chronic strep infections, recurrent otitis media, or viral infections. The RDW is often slightly elevated as a result of slight anisocytosis, reflecting ineffective iron recycling. The anemia itself is mild and asymptomatic and will not respond to iron unless there is concomitant iron deficiency. Since ferritin is an acute phase reactant, an elevated level does not imply the patient has adequate iron stores, but a low level indicates inadequate stores. Again, this type of anemia is included in a full discussion of microcytic anemia in children, but will not be discussed further in this chapter because the anemia by itself does not have the features that would or should bring it to the attention of a gastroenterologist, i.e. by the severity of the anemia or the microcytosis, although the underlying inflammatory condition itself may involve the GI tract. Distinguishing iron deficiency from the anemia of inflammation is usually not difficult from the history and CBC, but serum transferrin receptor (sTfR) levels, if available, have been shown to help distinguish them (Oliveras et al., 2000; Skikne, 1998, Vazquez et al., 2006).

3.4 Lead poisoning

The association between lead poisoning and microcytic anemia has long been assumed to be a direct inhibition of lead on heme synthesis, leading to a sideroblastic effect. This mechanism is supported by the basophilic stippling present and the markedly elevated free erythrocyte protoporphyrin values in these patients. More likely, however, the lead poisoning is a secondary effect of severe iron deficiency. The mechanism is twofold, in that severe iron deficiency increases the incidence of pica (Buchanan, 1999, 2003; Eden, 1999), and increases the absorption of lead from the gut. The incidence of Pica may be higher than generally assumed (Corbett et al., 2003). The precise pathophysiology of Pica is unknown, but is probably related to CNS iron deficiency. Patients often consume laundry starch, ice, soil, or clay. Both clay and starch can bind iron in the gastrointestinal tract and exacerbate iron deficiency (Crosby, 1982; Gonzalez et al., 1982; Thomas et al., 1976). At any concentration of lead, inhibition of ferrochelatase is most marked when the iron concentration is lower (Piomelli et al., 1987), but the neurologic effects of lead may be severe in the absence of anemia in children. Thus, it is important to address both the lead poisoning and the anemia and to find and treat the cause of the bleeding rather than solely addressing the lead poisoning. There is evidence that replacing iron in patients with concomitant iron deficiency and lead poisoning helps the body eliminate lead (McGeehan, 2003; Rondó et al., 2006; Wright et al., 2003).

3.5 Thalassemia trait (Case 2)

A 23 month old girl was referred to Pediatric Hematology for investigation of anemia. Thalassemia was suspected due to a family history of "Mediterranean anemia." Her father and some of his family members were known to be a carrier for thalassemia. He had been treated with high dose iron, but said that it did not help and made him ill. His family was originally from Sicily, where he lived for 8 years. She had no siblings.

The patient had generally been healthy, with normal growth and development, except for a brief febrile seizure a few months earlier. Her diet included fruits, vegetables, pasta, and lentils. She took no medications. On exam, she appeared healthy and alert. She was engaging and playful. She was slightly pale but showed no signs of icterus, petechiae, or ecchymoses. She had no adenopathy or splenomegaly. Her heart rate was regular, and her lungs were clear.

Screening lab work was remarkable for a mild anemia that was severely microcytic with a hemoglobin of 11 g/dL (normal 10.5-14 g/dL), MCV 60.2 fL (normal 70-90 fL) a year earlier and more recently 9.6 g/dL and 54.9 fL. A hemoglobin electrophoresis was remarkable for an elevated hgb A2 of 5.5 percent. Molecular studies had been done and showed that she was a carrier of two separate thalassemia mutations.

3.5.1 Discussion

This patient is a carrier of beta thalassemia, as is clear from the history as well as lab results. The clue is the relatively mild anemia with severe microcytosis. The blood smear in thalassemia trait typically has significant target cells present, and usually a hemoglobin electrophoresis shows an elevated hemoglobin A2 or F percentage. More quantitative ways to distinguish thalassemia trait from iron deficiency include the Mentzer index (Mentzer, 1973), as well as a variety of other methods of varying degrees of sensitivity and specificity (Demir et al. ,2002; Piomelli et al., 1976). The Mentzer index is calculated as the MCV divided by the RBC; a value over 13 is somewhat predictive of iron deficiency, while a value below 13 is more typical of beta thalassemia trait. Unfortunately in a practical sense, many cases fall near the line, especially those that are not clinically obvious one way or the other. The RDW is of limited use since it is increased in iron deficiency as well as a variety of hemoglobinopathies including thalassemia.

The presence of thalassemia trait does not exclude iron deficiency, which usually can be ruled out with a ferritin level and iron studies. Without iron deficiency, regular iron supplementation should not be given; not only will iron not improve the mild anemia, but over time could lead to iron overload, particularly because the mild anemia causes increased iron absorption form the gut. Thalassemia trait itself requires no therapy or follow-up, but genetic counseling should be considered because of the risk of having children with thalassemia major. To avoid unnecessary lab evaluations and therapy, the patient and family need to have a clear understanding of these points. Iron or folic acid deficiency, pregnancy or intercurrent illness may exacerbate the anemia in patients with thalassemia trait. The specific clinical phenotype depends on the precise genetic defect in heterozygous and especially homozygous individuals. In patients with microcytosis, hypochromia and erythrocytosis but without evidence of iron deficiency or elevated hgb A2 and Hgb F levels, one of the alpha thalassemia carrier states is likely. These too are benign conditions where proper genetic and medical counseling of the patient and family is imperative.

4. Iron deficiency

As is evident above, cases of microcytic anemia that are NOT due to iron deficiency are usually easy to distinguish. The remaining cases in this chapter are all due to iron deficiency. With two notable exceptions, severely microcytic severe anemias in children are due to chronic gastrointestinal blood loss. Figure 2 shows the relative frequencies of the major causes of iron deficiency anemia to be explained in the following sections, illustrating the 2 major sites of blood loss (gastrointestinal and vaginal) and the two major gastrointestinal etiologies (blood loss and iron malabsorption).

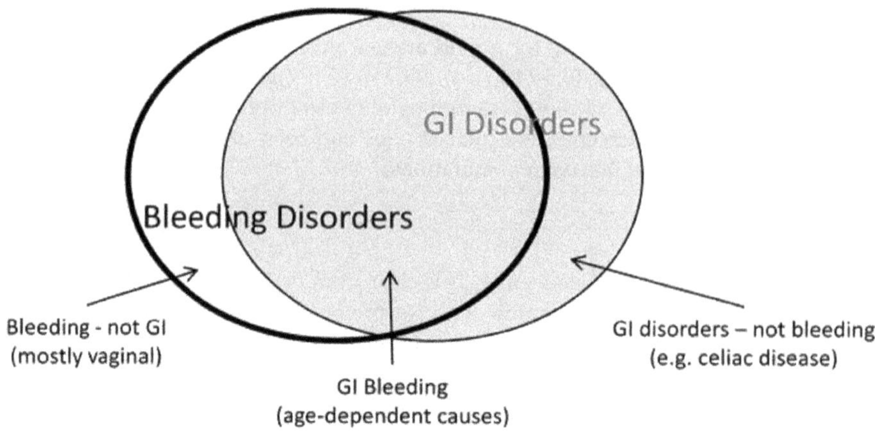

Fig. 2. Relative frequencies of causes of iron deficiency anemia (not to scale)

Because so much of the body's iron resides in hemoglobin, anemia is one of the first signs of iron deficiency, but anemia is actually a late stage of iron depletion. Iron deficiency leading to anemia is a continuum, but there are three recognized phases:

1. *Prelatent iron deficiency* occurs when tissue stores are depleted, without a change in hemoglobin level. The serum ferritin level will be low.
2. *Latent iron deficiency* occurs with depletion of iron from the reticuloendothelial system. TIBC increases and the serum iron level will fall as newly produced erythrocytes will be iron deficient, but the overall hemoglobin level and MCV remain normal.
3. *Iron deficiency anemia* occurs when a substantial portion of the erythrocyte population is affected, resulting in anemia, microcytosis and hypochromia.

With adequate treatment, these stages occur in reverse, i.e. the anemia resolves before adequate iron stores are replenished.

Several pediatric cases will be presented and discussed to illustrate the importance of the gastrointestinal tract in severe iron deficiency anemia. However, the initial case is of severe microcytic anemia occurring in an adult to make the connection between microcytic anemias and gastrointestinal blood loss clear.

4.1 Severe microcytic anemia in an adult (Case 3)

A 63 year old male presented to his physician with complaints of fatigue and shortness of breath, progressive over several weeks. The physician noted that the patient looked pale and ordered a complete blood count. The CBC revealed a hemoglobin of 5.9 g/dL and an MCV of 59 fL. The physician correctly interpreted this as a severe microcytic anemia, and that this anemia was of relatively recent onset. The physician considered transfusions and a prescription for oral iron as therapy for the anemia. However, upon considering the etiology of the anemia with the above history, he knows that the microcytosis is not consistent with a lesion leading to acute blood loss. Chronic blood loss is the only possibility, and that blood loss MUST be gastrointestinal. He referred the man to a gastroenterologist for a thorough investigation.

4.1.1 Discussion

For this patent, while several more benign lesions leading to chronic blood loss can be responsible, the lesion must be found, as colon cancer must be considered highly likely until proven otherwise. The sequence of events is therefore clear: The patient has developed a lesion in his GI tract that has been losing blood slowly over at least several months. Since the blood loss is relatively slow, the patient's bone marrow easily makes up for the anemia at first, but eventually stores of iron are depleted from his liver and other sites. At that point his anemia becomes more severe and begins to be microcytic, until the anemia itself becomes severe enough to cause the complaints that lead him to seek help from his physician. In retrospect the patient may or may not have noticed the typically black or tarry stools, depending on the rate of bleeding, and in fact the stool may not even consistently test positive for blood since the bleeding is often intermittent. In fact, testing the stool for blood in such a case is not necessary, as there can be no other cause of this type of anemia in this man but gastrointestinal bleeding. A negative stool test is in no way reassuring; this man must be referred to find the specific lesion. Transfusion and iron therapy do not treat the bleeding. It should even be stated that in such a case of anemia the hematologist plays no role. At any age the more severe the anemia and the microcytosis, the more likely that blood loss rather than a nutritional cause is the responsible mechanism.

The following pediatric cases will use the same concepts illustrated in the above case to emphasize the role of the gastroenterologic system in the etiology and therapy of severe microcytic anemias.

4.2 Milk enteropathy (Case 4)

A 14 month old boy presented to his pediatrician for a one year well child checkup. At the visit however his parents explained to the pediatrician that he had been pale for about the last month or so, not feeding well, and had some pica like behaviors. He had recently been more fussy and was sleeping poorly. They denied any jaundice, change in bowel or urinary habits or breathing difficulties. They denied bloody or black stools. They reported poor feeding when offered a variety of foods, and until very recently his diet relied heavily on milk, and he would typically go through a gallon every other day. The family lived in an older apartment with chipping paint that the parents admitted the child sometimes peeled from the walls. His growth and development had otherwise been normal. He took no medications and had no known allergies. He had three healthy half siblings. His mother was of German ancestry and had been anemic herself in the past. The father also denied any significant family history.

In clinic, the patient was alert and active but fussy during the exam. He was markedly pale, with no jaundice, bruising, petechiae, or rash. His tympanic membranes and oropharynx were clear. He had no adenopathy. His lungs were clear with no wheezes, and heart sounds were normal with no murmurs. His abdomen was soft and nontender with no hepatosplenomegaly. His extremities were well perfused with no edema.

Blood work was remarkable for a hemoglobin of 4.7 g/dL and MCV of 63 g/dL, a severe (and severely microcytic) anemia. His CBC was otherwise unremarkable except for red cell morphologic abnormalities consistent with severe iron deficiency. A serum lead level was only 4 mcg/dL.

The patient had a severe microcytic, hypochromic anemia, but was well compensated with no sign of heart failure. His parents were instructed to stop his milk entirely and he was started on therapeutic iron supplements. They were instructed that concomitant intake of orange juice would aid absorption of the iron. Follow-up labs were planned to assure his anemia was improving, but the plan was for him to continue taking the iron for several months after his anemia resolved, in order to replenish his iron stores. Milk could be added back to the diet, but only with meals, as soon as the anemia had begun to improve.

4.2.1 Discussion

This child presents with a common cause of iron deficiency anemia in the 1-2 year old. Just as in the adult male in the first case above, he has an *acquired, severe* anemia that is *severely* microcytic, and by far the most likely cause is chronic gastrointestinal blood loss. And like the adult, this child requires a GI workup. However, in this case an adequate workup consists mostly of the history of excess milk consumption along with the physical exam and some simple labs to classify the severity and type of anemia, so no referral to a pediatric gastroenterologist is required, and endoscopic procedures are not needed. If the history of excessive milk consumption were not present, then such a referral would be required, and procedures such as a Meckel's scan or endoscopy would be needed to find another cause, i.e. a specific gastrointestinal lesion.

Consumption of cow's milk may contribute to iron deficiency through several mechanisms. Whole milk given to young infants under a year of age, especially under 6 months of age, leads to iron deficiency anemia (American Academy of Pediatrics, 1992; Chessare, 1988; Fomon et al., 1981; Tunnessen & Oski, 1987; Wilson et al., 1964). Cow's milk and human milk both have low iron content, but the bioavailability of iron in human milk is greater. (Picciano & Deering, 1980) Cow's milk also replaces iron-rich foods in the diet. In addition, components in cow's milk such as calcium and caseinophosphopeptide can directly interfere with iron absorption (Ani-Kibangou et al., 2005; Hallberg et al., 1992). For severe anemia, these mechanisms can exacerbate the anemia, along with increased demand from the neonatal growth spurt, but the major mechanism is direct gastrointestinal bleeding.

Whole milk protein causes an enteropathy in the immature gut that leads to GI bleeding. What is not generally understood however is that these same effects continue into the second year of life for some children, so that *excessive* whole milk given to some toddlers causes an enteropathy with enough chronic blood loss to create severe iron deficiency anemia (Buchanan, 1999; Kwiatowski et al., 1999). For these severe anemias the cause is often misunderstood to be "nutritional" due to the above mechanisms of poor iron bioavailability and absorption. While inadequate iron in the diet might lead to a mild iron deficiency, the severe anemia in the case above can only be caused by chronic gastrointestinal bleeding. As for the adult, testing for occult blood is not needed. The etiology of the blood loss is exposure of the gut to the excessive milk protein. Treatment includes iron supplementation, but the enteropathy must be treated as well, by removing the excess milk from the diet. Transfusion therapy is usually not needed regardless of how low the hemoglobin, unless signs of decompensation such as heart failure are present, and in those cases must be done cautiously. A reasonable approach in these severe cases is to stop the milk entirely and provide therapeutic iron. After several weeks, when labs indicate improvement in the hemoglobin from the therapeutic iron, milk can be restarted, in moderate amounts with meals.

Compliance with iron therapy can be an issue, especially in this age group. Intravenous iron can be considered in these cases, or other forms of iron such as heme iron (Proferrin®, Colorado Biolabs, Inc.), (Nissenson et al. , 2003) that can be more palatable and well absorbed with fewer side effects, but efficacy studies in children are lacking.

4.3 Crohn's disease (Case 4)

A 14-year-old male was seen in pediatric hematology clinic in consultation for anemia. A month earlier he had had two episodes of pneumonia and bronchitis that were treated with antibiotics. He then started complaining of fatigue, prompting a CBC that revealed microcytic anemia that was subsequently shown to be due to iron deficiency.

The patient reported a long history of diarrhea once or twice a day, associated with bloating and cramping, especially after eating but could not relate it to any particular food. He denied any history of bloody stools, hematuria, or mucosal bleeding. There was no history of fevers, weight loss, cough, or difficulty breathing, and the rest of the review of systems was negative. His development had been normal. He had had no previous hospitalizations or surgeries. His immunizations were up-to-date. His only current medication was iron 325 mg PO daily started a week prior.

The patient had four healthy sisters. His mother had a history of iron deficiency with heavy periods but there was no other history of anemia in the family. His paternal grandfather has a history of diverticulitis and a cousin of his father had a history of Crohn's disease.

On exam his weight was 59.5 kg, between the 25th and 50th percentiles for age. His exam was mostly normal, with some voluntary guarding but no obvious abdominal tenderness, masses or organomegaly. Abdomen was nondistended, soft, nontender, with active bowel sounds. His extremities showed full range of motion of all joints, nontender, and well perfused, and his neurologic exam was grossly intact.

His CBC was normal except for a microcytic anemia (hgb 10.2 g/dL, MCV 67.1 fL), and a mild thrombocytopenia, all consistent with iron deficiency anemia. Hemoglobin electrophoresis was normal and his blood smear was normal.

The patient was referred to Pediatric Gastroenterology where endoscopic exam showed mild esophagitis, chronic gastritis, a normal duodenum, lymphoid aggregates and a focal granuloma in his colon, consistent with Crohn's disease. Medical treatment was successful in alleviating his symptoms and his anemia.

4.3.1 Discussion

This boy presented with an acquired moderate anemia that was severely microcytic. As with the previous two cases, chronic slow gastrointestinal bleeding is the likely cause, leading to iron loss, eventually leading to depletion of stores of iron and the characteristic anemia. A full discussion of the pathophysiology and therapy of Crohn's disease and inflammatory bowel disease is beyond the scope of this chapter but the hematologic manifestations are likely due to the slow blood loss, although the anemia of inflammation may play a role as well.

4.4 Iron deficiency from gastrointestinal bleeding – Summary

In all three of these cases, the microcytic anemia was due to slow gastrointestinal blood loss, although the specific cause of the blood loss was different, and to a large extent age dependent. The approach to the underlying cause is therefore age dependent:

Toddler	Excessive whole milk ingestion
	Other causes, e.g. Meckel's diverticulum
School age/Teen	Inflammatory bowel disease
	Menorrhagia
	Other causes, e.g. AV malformation, ulcer
Adult	Colon Cancer
	Other causes, e.g. ulcer

One common feature of the above cases is that although all presented with a severe microcytic anemia, none of the underlying causes were fundamentally hematologic in nature. Therefore in the overwhelming majority of cases of microcytic anemia, these patients have a gastrointestinal cause (slow gastrointestinal blood loss) and need to be referred to a gastroenterologist for diagnosis of the underlying cause. There are two exceptions to the above generalizations. One is a special case of non gastrointestinal blood loss, and the other is due to a defect in iron absorption, although even that cause is still gastrointestinal. These exceptions are illustrated in the two cases below:

5. Iron deficiency not due to gastrointestinal bleeding

5.1 Menorrhagia (Case 6)

A 12-year-old female was referred to pediatric hematology clinic for a possible bleeding disorder. She had had heavy menstrual periods since menarche 6 months previously. She had been admitted to a local community hospital 4 months earlier at which time she was found to be profoundly anemic with a hemoglobin of 5.9 g/dL, MCV 68.2 fL with symptoms of anemia requiring several blood transfusions. She was started on oral birth control pills with resolution of her menorrhagia. She was also started on daily iron sulfate tablets.

Apart from dysfunctional uterine bleeding, the patient did not have a past medical history of bleeding problems, nosebleeds, easy bruising, petechiae or mucosal bleeding. She denied any loose, bloody, tarry stools or abdominal pain. She had no food allergies. She was healthy before the onset of menarche except for daily headaches which had been evaluated by CT. Her father said he experienced similar headaches as an adolescent. Her father denied a family history of bleeding disorders or menorrhagia. She was doing well in 7th grade and enjoyed cheerleading.

In clinic the patient was alert and in no apparent distress. She was afebrile, with normal vital signs. Skin was unremarkable with no petechiae or bruising. Her conjunctivae were pink without pallor. Abdomen was soft, nontender, nondistended without hepatosplenomegaly. A comprehensive coagulation workup showed no evidence of a systemic bleeding disorder. At the time of her visit to pediatric hematology clinic her hemoglobin was 12.5 g/dL, MCV 82.4, fL, both normal. A ferritin level was normal.

5.1.1 Discussion

As demonstrated by the first three cases above, acquired severe microcytic anemias are almost always due to chronic gastrointestinal blood (i.e. iron) loss. One notable exception is demonstrated in this case, in which the route of bleeding is vaginal. There is a common misconception that menstruating females have lower average hemoglobin levels because of normal menstrual bleeding. While there is overlap between the normal ranges of males and female hemoglobins, the lower average values in females are due to lower testosterone levels, not vaginal bleeding. Hence adults have higher hemoglobins than children, and males have higher values than females. Normal menstruation can lead to iron deficiency but not anemia; therefore actual anemia implies abnormal bleeding. Abnormal bleeding can be an acute vaginal hemorrhage from a single or a few heavy periods, but it is chronic bleeding from many heavy periods that leads to iron deficiency anemia, as in this case.

As most cases of severe microcytic anemia have a GI cause, a gastroenterologist rather than a hematologist should be involved. Dysfunctional uterine bleeding requires a gynecologic workup, but a proportion of these cases have an underlying bleeding disorder, so it is these cases that should also be referred to a hematologist for an adequate workup for conditions such as von Willebrand's disease and platelet function disorders. Women with menorrhagia, especially if present since menarche, have an incidence of von Willebrand's disease of around 13%, considerably higher than the general population incidence of 1% to 2% (Kadir et al., 1998; Lukes et. al., 2005). For the most part however, the management involves oral contraceptive pills. It should be noted that if there is not a convincing history of several heavy periods, a gastrointestinal cause should still be sought.

Other causes of chronic bleeding and iron loss leading to iron deficiency anemia are rare and usually obvious from the history. Iron deficiency and iron deficiency anemia can result from pulmonary hemosiderosis and from renal bleeding in Berger's disease. These rare routes should be considered if the history is not consistent with the more common causes or if the patient does not respond adequately to therapy.

5.2 Celiac disease (Case 7)

A five year old boy presented to his primary care physician with pallor and was found to have a severe microcytic anemia. Stool was negative for occult blood. He was referred to a pediatric hematologist who diagnosed iron deficiency anemia. He had occasional complaints of abdominal pain but no vomiting, diarrhea or constipation. He had not lost any weight but had grown poorly over the past year, falling from the 60th to the 30th percentile for weight and the 50th to the 40th for height. He was referred to a pediatric gastroenterologist, where further studies were done, including an endoscopy showing villous atrophy with increased numbers of intraepithelial lymphocytes consistent with celiac disease. He was placed on a gluten free diet. Three months later his hemoglobin was normal and his weight had increased to the 50th percentile.

5.2.1 Discussion

Although chronic gastrointestinal bleeding is the major cause of severe iron deficiency anemia, there are notable exceptions that involve the GI tract, and lead to severe anemia due to poor iron absorption alone. The model disorders that fit into this category are celiac disease and tropical sprue (Lombardo, 2006). Celiac disease has been shown to be a relatively common cause of anemia in adults, and therefore may be underdiagnosed in children; it is increasingly recognized as presenting with a spectrum of severity (Van Heel, 2005). Genetics play a strong role in susceptibility but the full genetic pattern is incompletely understood.

Iron absorption may also be disrupted when substantial segments of bowel, particularly the proximal duodenum, are removed surgically. Intractable inflammatory bowel disease, traumatic abdominal injury, and structural defects such as intestinal volvulus or intussusception, as well as necrotizing enterocolitis and typhlitis may necessitate intestinal resection, leading to a defect in iron absorption that may take years to manifest clinically. There are also rare gastrointestinal disorders leading to either malabsorption of iron or chronic blood loss or both, such as collagenous gastritis (Suskind et al., 2009), epidermolysis bullosa (Fridge & Vichinsky, 1998) and short gut syndromes.

To the general practitioner however, it is enough to remember that unless dysfunctional uterine bleeding is elicited from the history, or for any male or prepubertal female, the cause of any *severe, acquired severely microcytic* anemia must be gastrointestinal, which should guide the appropriate referral.

6. Initial workup of suspected anemia in children

In a child with suspected anemia based on history and exam, a minimal workup should be obtained. The goal is to characterize the anemia, and to evaluate the other cell lines (platelets, granulocytes) that define bone marrow function. In most cases a CBC with differential, reticulocyte count, iron panel, ferritin level, and lead level give a strong indication as to the cause and define the therapy.

In general, the more cell lines that are depressed, and the lower the values, the more likely is an underlying marrow disease. Hence, pancytopenia (neutropenia, anemia, and thrombocytopenia) makes leukemia more likely while an isolated single cytopenia (neutropenia, anemia, *or* thrombocytopenia) makes a peripheral disorder outside the marrow more likely. If leukemia or a primary marrow failure is suspected, referral to a pediatric hematologist/oncologist should be made promptly for further testing, including a marrow evaluation. An isolated severe microcytic anemia is not consistent with leukemia and indicates slow blood (i.e. iron) loss (gastrointestinal or vaginal), or in the case of celiac disease, lack of iron absorption. The severe depletion of iron leads to marrow failure in a sense, in that the marrow is unable to complete heme synthesis. Despite the marrow "failure," further marrow evaluation of marrow function is not part of the evaluation, as the underlying cause is entirely outside the marrow.

In iron deficiency anemia a clue to otherwise normal marrow function is often provided by a "left shift" of the other cell lines; leukocytosis, elevated neutrophil count, increased bands and other immature forms, and an elevated platelet count with large platelets. The reticulocyte count is often only mildly elevated, reflecting the lack of iron substrate. Hemolytic anemias such as sickle cell disease, autoimmune hemolytic anemia and hereditary spherocytosis also shift cell lines to the left, but are not microcytic and present with a much higher reticulocyte count. A high reticulocyte count makes a hemolytic anemia likely, especially if the anemia is normocytic or mildly macrocytic. B12 and folate deficiency are not microcytic and are considerably rarer than iron deficiency. The iron panel is usually consistent with other studies, but serum iron may be misleading, as recent ingestion of iron may elevate the value. Ferritin, as an acute phase reactant, may also be elevated in a deficiency state, but low values always represent iron deficiency, and occur in no other condition. A lead level should be considered, not as a cause of microcytic anemia, but because of its association with iron deficiency due to pica and increased lead absorption, especially in small children.

Children, especially the very young tolerate chronic anemia extremely well. It is not unusual for a toddler with a hemoglobin well below five to act perfectly normal, with the very slow onset of pallor as the only manifestation of the anemia. Some fussiness and irritability might be noticed in retrospect. Often these children appear yellow due to underlying normal pigments. True jaundice can be ruled out if the sclerae are white, and lab evaluation of liver function is therefore not necessary. Hepatosplenomegaly is unusual, as is true decompensation e.g. heart failure, but shortness of breath on exertion and headache are common in older children and young adults.

7. Therapy of iron deficiency anemia

The therapy of iron deficiency anemia is strongly guided by the cause. Iron therapy is only part of the treatment. For mild anemias due to previous iron loss that has resolved, oral iron is all that is required. If bleeding is ongoing, iron may partially correct the anemia without affecting the underlying cause, leading to delay in diagnosis and therapy of the underlying cause. The most egregious example is the adult with colon cancer; Iron therapy alone would allow the cancer to progress without diagnosis.

Transfusions are usually not required, especially in children, but should be considered in cases of decompensation or heart failure. It is said that transfusions for chronic anemia in children are given because of the elevated heart rate of the doctor, rather than the patient. If used, packed red cells should be given slowly under the direction of a pediatric hematologist or other experienced clinician to avoid the risk of fluid overload due to the hyperdynamic state of chronic severe anemia.

Response to therapy depends on the disorder, the severity of the deficiency and compliance, not only with the prescribed iron, but in removing the bleeding source. Especially in children whose bleeding is due to excess whole milk, the response to oral iron will be slow or nonexistent if the milk intake is not severely cut back or eliminated from the diet. Intake of acid foods such as orange juice aid iron absorption, and hypochorhydric states, such as produced by proton pump inhibitors, has been reported to impair absorption (Sharma et al., 2004). The amount of iron in typical vitamin supplements (about 10 mg of elemental iron daily), while sufficient to prevent deficiency, is well below the 3-6 mg *per kg* required as treatment. If compliant with therapy, the hemoglobin should rise by 1 g/dL or more during the first week, along with an increased reticulocyte count, and the hemoglobin should be nearly normal by 4-6 weeks. Iron therapy should be continued for several weeks beyond normalization of the hemoglobin, as pointed out previously, in order to replenish iron stores in the body.

8. Conclusion

Iron deficiency anemia is the leading cause of microcytic anemia when both the anemia and the microcytosis are severe. Regardless of the age of the patient, gastrointestinal disorders are the most frequent causes, and most of these are due to chronic gastrointestinal bleeding. The frequency of the specific causes of the bleeding varies with age. In most cases of severe microcytic anemia in children, as in adults, referral to a gastroenterologist is appropriate or required.

9. Acknowledgment

I thank Eric Vargas for his help in initiating this project.

10. References

Akman, M.; Cebeci, D.; Okur, V.; Angun, H.; Abali, O. & Akmun, A. (2004). The Effects of Iron Deficiency on Infants' Developmental Test Performance. *Acta Pædiatr*, Vol.93, No.10, pp. 1391-6, ISSN 0803-5253

American Academy of Pediatrics Committee on Nutrition (1992). The Use of Whole Cow's Milk in Infancy. *Pediatrics*, Vol 89, No.6, pp. 1105-1109, ISSN 0031-4005

Ani-Kibangou, B.; Bouhallab, S.; Mollé, D.; Henry, G; Bureau, F.; Neuville, D.; Arhan, P. P & Bouglé, D. (2005). Improved Absorption of Caseinophosphopeptide-bound Iron: Role of Alkaline Phosphatase. *J Nutr Biochem*, Vol 16, No.7, pp. 398-401, ISSN 0955-2863

Beard, J. & Stoltzfus, R. (2001). Forward. *J. Nutr*, Vol.131, No.2, p563S, ISSN 0022-3166

Beard, J. (2001). Iron Biology in Immune Function, Muscle Metabolism and Neuronal Functioning. *J Nutr*, Vol.131, No.2, pp. 568S-80S, ISSN 0022-3166

Benoist, B. (2001) Introduction. *J. Nutr*, Vol.131, No.2, p564S, ISSN 0022-3166

Buchanan, G. (1999). The Tragedy of Iron Deficiency During Infancy and early Childhood. *J Pediatr*, Vol.135, No.4, pp 413-5, ISSN 0022-3476

Buchanan, G. (2003). Iron Deficiency and Blood Lead Levels. *J Pediatr*, Vol.143, No 2, p 281, ISSN 0022-3476

Chessare, J. (1988). Whole Cow Milk versus Iron–Fortified Formula. *J Pediatr.* Vol.112, No.6, pp 1049-50, ISSN 0022-3476

Cook, D. & Lynch, S. (1986). The Liabilities of Iron Deficiency. *Blood.* Vol.68, No.4, pp 803-9, ISSN 0006-4971

Corbett, R; Ryan, C. & Weinrich, S. (2003). Pica in Pregnancy; does it Affect Pregnancy Outcomes? *Am J Matern Child Nurs.* Vol.28, No.3, pp183-9, ISSN 0361-929X

Crosby, W. (1982). Clay Ingestion and Iron Deficiency Anemia. *Ann Intern Med.* Vol.97, No.3, p 456, ISSN 0003-4819

Demir, A.; Yarali, N.; Fisgin, T.; Duru, F. & Kara, A. (2002) Most Reliable Indices in Differentiation between Thalassemia Trait and Iron Deficiency Anemia. *Pediatr Int.* Vol.44, No.6, pp. 612-6, ISSN 1328-8067

Eden, A. & Mir, M. (1997). Iron Deficiency in 1- to 3-year-old Children A Pediatric Failure? *Arch Pediatr Adolesc Med.* Vol.151, No.10, pp 986-8, ISSN 1072-4710

Eden. A. (2003). Iron Deficiency and Blood Lead Levels. *J Pediatr.* Vol.143, No.2, p 281-2 ISSN 0022-3476

Erikson K.; Jones B.; Hess E.; Zhang, Q. & Beard, J. (2001). Iron Deficiency Decreases Dopamine D_1 and D_2 Receptors in Rat Brain. *Pharmacol Biochem Behav.* Vol.69, No.3-4, pp 409-18, ISSN 0091-3057

Flemming, M. (2009). Sideroblastic Anemias, In: *Hematology of Infancy and Childhood, 7th Edition.* Okin, S.; Nathan, D.; Ginsgurg, D.; Look, A.; Fisher, D. & Lux, S. pp 547-551, Saunders, ISBN 978-1-4160-3430-8, Philadelphia, PA

Fomon, S.; Ziegler, E.; Nelson, S. & Edwards, B. (1981). Cow Milk Feeding in Infancy: Gastrointestinal Blood Loss and Iron Nutritional Status. *J. Pediatr.* Vol.98, No.4, pp 540-5, ISSN 0022-3476

Fridge J. & Vichinsky, E. (1998). Correction of the Anemia of Epidermolysis Bullosa with Intravenous Iron and Erythropoietin. *J Pediatr.* Vol.132, No.5, pp 871-3, ISSN 0022-3476

Gonzalez, J.; Owens, W.; Ungaro, P.; Werk, E. & Wentz, P. (1982). Clay Ingestion: A Rare Cause of Hypokalemia. *Ann Intern Med.* Vol.97, No.1, pp 65-6, ISSN 0003-4819

Grantham-McGregor, S. & Ani, C. (2001). A Review of Studies on the Effect of Iron Deficiency on Cognitive Development in Children. *J Nutr.* Vol.131, No.2, pp 649S-68S, ISSN 0022-3166

Hallberg, L.; Rossander-Hultén, L.; Brune, M. & Gleerup, A. (1992). Bioavailability in Man of Iron in Human Milk and Cow's Milk in Relation to Their Calcium Contents. *Pediatr Res.* Vol.31, No.5, pp 524-7, ISSN 0031-3998

Iolascon, A.; De Falco, L. & Beaumont, C. (2009). Molecular Basis of Inherited Microcytic Anemia due to Defects in Iron Acquisition or Heme Synthesis. *Haematologica.* Vol.94, No.3, pp 395-408, ISSN 1592-8721

Jain, S. & Kamat, D. (2009). Evaluation of Microcytic Anemia. *Clinical Pediatrics.* Vol.48, No.1, pp 7-13, ISSN 0009-9228

Janus, J. & Moerschel, S. (2010). Evaluation of Anemia in Children. *American Family Physician.* Vol.81, No.12, pp 1462-71, ISSN 0002-838X

Kadir, R.; Economides, D.; Sabin, C.; Owens, D. &Lee, C. (1998). Frequency of Inherited Bleeding Disorders in Women with Menorrhagia. *Lancet.* Vol.351, No.9101, pp 485-9, ISSN 0140-6736

Kwiatowski, J.; West, T.; Heidary, N.; Smith-Whitney, K. & Cohen, A. (1999). Severe Iron Deficiency Anemia in Young Children. *J Pediatr.* Vol.135, No.4, pp 514-6, ISSN 0022-3476

Lombardo, T.; Ximenes, B.; & Ferro, G. (2006). Hypochromic Microcytic Anemia as a Clinical Presentation of Celiac Disease. *Clin Lab.* Vol.52, No.5-6, pp 231-6, ISSN 1433-6510

Looker, A. (2002). Iron deficiency — United States, 1999–2000. *MMWR Morb Mortal Wkly Rep.* Vol.51, No.40, pp 897-9, ISSN 0149-2195

Lozoff, B.; Brittenham, G.; Viteri F.; Wolf, A. & Urrutia, J. (1982). Developmental Deficits in Iron-Deficient Infants: Effects of Age and Severity of Iron Lack. *J Pediatr.* Vol.101, No.6, pp 948-52, ISSN 0022-3476

Lozoff, B.; Jimenez, E.; Hagen, J.; Mollen, E. & Wolf, A. (2000). Poorer Behavioral and Developmental Outcome More Than 10 Years after Treatment for Iron Deficiency in Infancy. *Pediatrics,* Vol.105, E51, ISSN 1098-4275

Lozoff, B.; Wolf, A. & Jimenez, E. (1996). Iron-Deficiency Anemia and Infant Development: Effects of Extended Oral Iron Therapy. *J Pediatr.* Vol.129, No.3, pp 382-9, ISSN 0022-3476

Lukes, A.; Kadir R.; Peyvandi F. & Kouides P. (2005). Disorders of Hemostasis and Excessive Menstrual Bleeding: Prevalence and Clinical Impact. *Fertil Steril.* Vol.84, No.5, pp 1338-44, ISSN 0015-0282

McGeehan, M. (2003). Getting the Lead Out: Can Iron Help? *J. Pediatr.* Vol.142, No.1, pp 3-4, ISSN 0022-3476

Mentzer, W. (1973). Differentiation of Iron Deficiency from Thalassemia Trait. *Lancet.* Vol.301, No.7808, p 882, ISSN 0140-6736

Nissenson, A.; Berns, J.; Sakiewicz, P.; Gheddar, S.; Moore, G.; Schleicher, R. & Seligman, P. (2003). Clinical Evaluation of Heme Iron Polypeptide: Sustaining a Response to rHuEPO in Hemodialysis Patients. *Am J Kidney Dis.* Vol.42, No.2, pp 325-30, ISSN 0272-6386

Olivares, M.; Walter, T.; Cook, J.; hertrampf, E. & Pizarro, F. (2000). Usefulness of Serum Transferrin Receptor and Serum Ferritin in Diagnosis of Iron Deficiency in Infancy. *Am J Clin Nutr.* Vol.72, No.5, pp 1191-5, ISSN 0002-9165

Ortiz E.; Pasquini, J.; Thompson, K.; Felt, B.; Butkus, G.; Beard, J. & Connor, J. (2004). Effect of Manipulation of Iron Storage, Transport, or Availability on Myelin Composition and Brain Iron Content in Three Different Animal Models. *J Neurosci Res.* Vol.77, No.5, pp 681-689, ISSN 0360-4012

Oski, F. (1979). The Nonhematologic Manifestations of Iron Deficiency. *Am J Dis Child.* Vol.133, No.3, pp 315-22, ISSN 0096-8994

Oski, F. (1985). Is Bovine Milk a Health Hazard? *Pediatrics.* Vol.75(suppl), pp 182-6, ISSN 0031-4005

Oski, F.; Honig, A.; Helu, B. & Howanitz, P. (1983). Effect of Iron Therapy on Behavior Performance in Nonanemic, Iron-Deficient Infants. *Pediatrics.* Vol.71, No.6, pp 877-80, ISSN 0031-4005

Picciano, M. & Deering, R. (1980). The Influence of Feeding Regimens on Iron Status During Infancy. *Am J Clin Nutr.* Vol.33, No.4, pp 746-53, ISSN 0002-9165

Piomelli, S.; Brickman, A. & Carlos, E. (1976). Rapid Diagnosis of iron Deficiency by Measurement of Free Erythrocyte Porphyrins and Hemoglobins: the FEP/Hemoglobin Ratio. *Pediatrics.* Vol.57, No.1, pp 136-41, ISSN 0031-4005

Piomelli, S.; Seaman, C. & Kapoor S. (1987). Lead-Induced Abnormalities of Porphyrin Metabolism. The Relationship with Iron Deficiency. *Ann NY Acad Sci.* Vol.514, p 278-88, ISSN 0077-8923

Pollitt, E.; Saco-Pollitt, C.; Leibel, R. & Viteri F. (1986). Iron Deficiency and Behavioral Development in Infants and Preschool Children. *Am J Clin Nutr.* Vol.43, No.4, pp 555-65, ISSN 0002-9165

Rondó, P.; Carvalho, F.; Souza, M. & Moraes, F. (2006). Lead, Hemoglobin, Zinc Protoporphyrin and Ferritin Concentrations in Children. *Rev Saude Publica.* Vol.40, No.1, pp 71-6, ISSN 0034-8910

Shamsian, B.; Rezaei, N.; Arzanian, M.; Alavi, S.; Khojasteh, O. & Eghbali, A. (2009). Severe Hypochromic Microcytic Anemia in a Patient with Congenital Atransferrinemia. *Pediatr Hematol Oncol.* Vol.26, No.5 pp 356-62, ISSN 0888-0018

Sharma, V.; Brannon, M. & Carloss, E. (2004). Effect of Omeprazole on Oral Iron Replacement in Patients with Iron Deficiency Anemia. *Southern Medical Journal.* Vol.97, No.9, pp 887-9, ISSN 0038-4348

Skikne, B. (1998). Circulating Transferrin Receptor Assay—Coming of Age. *Clin Chem.* Vol.44, No.1, pp 7-9, ISSN 0009-9147

Stoltzfus, R. (2001). Defining Iron-Deficiency Anemia in Public Health Terms: A Time for Reflection. *J Nutr.* Vol.131(suppl), pp 565S-7S, ISSN 0022-3166

Suskind, D.; Wahbeh, G.; Murray, K.; Christie, D. & Kapur, R. (2009). Collagenous Gastritis, a New Spectrum of Disease in Pediatric Patients: Two Case Reports. *Cases J.* Vol.2, No.7511, ISSN 1757-1626

Thomas, F.; Falko, J. & Zuckerman, K. (1976). Inhibition of Intestinal Iron Absorption by Laundry Starch. *Gastroenterology.* Vol.71, No.6, pp 1028-32, ISSN 0016-5085

Tunnessen, W. & Oski, F. (1987). Consequences of Starting Whole Cow Milk at 6 Months of Age. *J Pediatr.* Vol.111, No.6, pp 813-6, ISSN 0022-3476

Van Heel, D. & West, J. (2006). Recent Advances in Coeliac Disease. *Gut.* Vol.55, No.7, pp 1037-46, ISSN 0017-5749

Vazquez Lopez, M.; Carracedo, A.; Lendinez, F.; Muñoz, J.; Lopez, J. & Muñoz, A. (2006). The Usefulness of Serum Transferrin Receptor for Discriminating Iron Deficiency without Anemia in Children. *Haematologica.* Vol.91, No.2, pp 264-5, ISSN 1592-8721

Walter, T.; De Andraca, I.; Chadud, P. & Perales, C. (1989). Iron Deficiency Anemia: Adverse Effects on Infant Psychomotor Development. *Pediatrics.* Vol.84, No.1, pp 7-17, ISSN 0031-4005

Wilson, J.; Heiner, D. & Lahey, M. (1964). Milk-Induced Gastrointestinal Bleeding in infants
    with Hypochromic Microcytic Anemia. *JAMA*. Vol.189, No.7, pp 568-72, ISSN 0098-
    7484

Wright, R.; Tsaih, S.; Schwartz, J.; Wright, R. & Hu, H. (2003). Association Between Iron
    Deficiency and Blood Lead Level in a Longitudinal Analysis of Children
    Followed in an Urban Primary Care Clinic. *J Pediatr*. Vol.142, No.1, pp 9-14, ISSN
    0022-3476

Section 3

Pathophysiology and Treatment of Pancreatic and Intestinal Disorders

13

Emerging Approaches for the Treatment of Fat Malabsorption Due to Exocrine Pancreatic Insufficiency

Saoussen Turki and Héla Kallel
Unité de Biofermentation, Institut Pasteur de Tunis
Tunisia

1. Introduction

The main purpose of the gastrointestinal tract is to digest and absorb nutrients (fat, carbohydrates, and proteins), micronutrients (vitamins and trace minerals), water, and electrolytes. Digestion involves both mechanical and enzymatic breakdown of food. Mechanical processes include chewing, gastric churning, and the to-and-fro mixing in the small intestine. Enzymatic hydrolysis is initiated by intraluminal processes requiring gastric, pancreatic, and biliary secretions. The final products of digestion are absorbed through the intestinal epithelial cells.

Malabsorption is a state arising from abnormality in absorption of food nutrients across the gastrointestinal (GI) tract. Depending on the abnormality, impairment can be of single or multiple nutrients leading to malnutrition and a variety of anaemias. Symptoms of malabsorption are varied because the disorder affects so many systems. General symptoms may include loss of appetite (anorexia), weight loss, fatigue, shortness of breath, dehydration, low blood pressure, and swelling (edema). Nutritional disorders may cause anemia (lack of iron, folate and vitamin B12), bleeding tendency (lack of vitamin K), or bone disease (lack of vitamin D). Gastrointestinal symptoms include flatulence, stomach distention, borborygmi (rumbling in the bowels), discomfort, diarrhea, steatorrhea (excessive fat in stool) and frequent bowel movements (Bai, 1998). Intestinal malabsorption can be due to : mucosal damage (enteropathy), congenital or acquired reduction in absorptive surface, defects of specific hydrolysis, defects of ion transport, impaired enterohepatic circulation or pancreatic insufficiency (Walker-Smith & al.,2002). This chapter will particularly focus on fat malabsorption, the overriding problem caused by severe pancreatic insufficiency.

Pancreatic insufficiency is a condition commonly associated with diseases such as pancreatitis or cystic fibrosis. Patients suffering from these pathologies show a shortage of the digestive enzymes necessary to break down food. Hence, a common feature of these diseases is a severe dietary malabsorption due to the poor hydrolysis of lipid in the lumen of small intestine. Digestive lipases are the key enzymes of fat digestion. The most common example of these enzymes is human pancreatic lipase. Nevertheless, the human lipases include the pre-duodenal lingual and gastric lipase, the extra-duodenal pancreatic, hepatic, lipoprotein and the recently described endothelial lipase. In this chapter, a short basic overview of these fat-digesting enzymes and their physiological contribution to fat digestion is first presented. Thereafter, pathophysiology of fat malabsorption resulting from exocrine pancreatic insufficiency, clinical symptoms, incidence and diagnosis of the pathology are described as well.

Standard strategies for exocrine pancreatic insufficiency management are based on oral administration of porcine derived pancreatic extracts. Unfortunately, this approach is being unsatisfactory for many reasons. Greater attention has been paid over the last decade to optimize correction of fat malabsorption and essential fatty acid deficiency in order to improve the quality of life and extend the life span of patients with severe pancreatic insufficiency. Hence, we interestingly discuss herein drawbacks of therapeutic use of currently available lipase preparations before focusing mainly on research forces joined for the development of new oral enzyme substitution approaches and future promising opportunities to treat intestinal fat malabsorption caused by exocrine pancreatic insufficiency.

2. Human digestive lipases

Lipases are key enzymes responsible for digesting lipids in the digestive system. In humans, gastrointestinal lipases include pre-duodenal lipases (gastric lipase and lingual lipase) and the other members of the lipase gene family: pancreatic, hepatic, lipoprotein and endothelial lipases. The chromosomal localization of genes encoding these lipases and their tissue of origin has been described (Table 1).

Lipase	Chromosomal localization of gene	Tissue of origin	References
Lingual lipase	-*	Serous glands of the tongue	Hamosh, 1990
Gastric lipase	10q23.2	Fundic mucosa of the stomach	Bodmer & al., 1987
Pancreatic lipase	10q26.1	Pancreas	Sims & al., 1993
Hepatic lipase	15q21–q23	Liver	Ameis & al., 1990
Lipoprotein lipase	8p22	Adipose, heart, skeletal muscle	Wion et al., 1987
Endothelial lipase	18q21.1	Endothelial cells, liver, lung, kidney, placenta	Hirata et al., 1999

* Unknown data

Table 1. Human digestive lipases

2.1 Lingual lipase

The serous von Ebner glands of the tongue secrete lingual lipase in the saliva. Unlike rodents, lingual lipase is present in trace amounts in humans (Hamosh, 1990). Human lipase purified from lingual serous glands or gastric juice has a MW of 45 kDa to 51 kDa but tends to aggregate (MW 270-300 kDa and 500 kDa) and is highly hydrophobic (Hamosh, 1990). Lingual lipase has unique characteristics including an optimum activity at pH 4,5 – 5,4 and ability to catalyze reactions without bile salts (Hamosh & Scow, 1973). Lingual lipase breaks down short and medium chain saturated fatty acids and helps in their digestion. It has been stated that 10 to 30% of dietary fat is hydrolyzed in the stomach by lingual lipase. The enzyme uses a catalytic triad consisting of Aspartatic Acid-203 (Asp), Histidine-257 (His), and Serine-144 (Ser), to initiate the hydrolysis of a triglyceride into a diacyglyceride and a free fatty acid (Hamosh & Scow, 1973). Secreted in the buccal cavity, lingual lipase is one of the key components that make the digestion of milk fat in newborns possible. In humans lipolytic activity is present in gastric aspirates as early as 26 weeks of gestational age which is evidence enough for the fact that lingual lipase is present at birth (Hamosh, 1979). New born infants indeed secrete only low amounts of pancreatic lipase and bile salts and it has been demonstrated that pancreatic lipase alone does not readily hydrolyze a lipid emulsion as well as native milk fat globules (Miled & al., 2000).

2.2 Gastric lipase

Gastric lipase (EC 3.1.1.3) is the predominant pre-duodenal lipase in humans. The enzyme is secreted in the gastric juice by the chief cells of fundic mucosa in the stomach (Moreau & al., 1988). The pre-duodenal enzyme was purified from human gastric aspirates and its N-terminal amino-acid sequence was determined. The amino-acid sequence from the isolated protein and the DNA sequence obtained from the cloned gene indicated that human gastric lipase consists of a 379 amino acid unglycosylated polypeptide with a molecular weight of 43 162 Da (Bodmer & al., 1987). However, native human gastric lipase (HGL) (molecular weight 50 kDa) is a highly glycosylated protein with four potential glycosylation sites (Bodmer & al., 1987). Human gastric and rat lingual lipase share a high degree of sequence homology and have identical gene organizations (Lohse & al., 1997). Gastric lipase belongs to the α/β-hydrolase-fold family. It possesses a classical catalytic triad (Ser-153, His-353, Asp-324) and an oxyanion hole (backbone NH groups of Gln-154 and Leu-67) analogous to serine proteases (Roussel & al., 1999). It has an optimum pH activity around 5.4, hydrolyzes long-, medium- and short-chain triacylglycerols and do not require bile acid or colipase for optimum enzymatic activity (Denigris et al., 1985). For many years, the exact physiological contribution of gastric lipase to the overall process of lipolysis was unknown. Carrière et al. (1993a) established, for the first time, that most of the HGL secreted in the stomach was still active in the duodenum. They estimated that the gastric lipase contribution in the hydrolysis of triglycerides is about 25 %. The stereoselectivity of HGL toward triglycerides was also investigated. It was clearly demonstrated that HGL shows a stereopreference for the sn-3 position of the triglyceride (Rogalska & al., 1990).

Hence, gastric lipase, together with lingual lipase, make up 30% of lipid hydrolysis occurring during digestion in the human adult, with gastric lipase contributing the most of the two acidic lipases. In neonates, these acidic pre-duodenal lipases are much more important, they have the unique ability to initiate the degradation of maternal milk fat globules.

2.3 Pancreatic lipases

A limitation of acidic lipases is that they remove only one fatty acid from each triacylglycerol. The free fatty acid can readily cross the epithelial membrane lining the gastrointestinal tract, but the diacylglycerol cannot be transported across. Hence, hydrolysis of dietary triacylglycerols by both gastric and pancreatic lipase is essential for their absorption by enterocytes. Human pancreatic lipase (HPL) (EC 3.1.1.3) is produced by the pancreatic acinar cells. The lipase is located into the zymogen granules, together with many other enzymes and secreted into the intestinal lumen together with the bile (Miled & al., 2000). Contrary to most of the pancreatic enzymes which are secreted as proenzymes and further activated by proteolytic cleavage in the small intestines, HPL is directly secreted as an active enzyme. Purified from pancreatic juice, the protein showed to have a molecular weight of 48 kDa (De Caro & al., 1977) and has been characterized as a glycoprotein consisting of 449 amino acid polypeptide (Lowe & al., 1989). The resolution of the HPL 3D structure (Fig.1) revealed the presence of a catalytic triad (Ser[152]-Asp[176] –His[263]) similar to that found in other serine hydrolases, Ser [152] being part of the G-X-S-X-G consensus sequence (Lowe & al., 1989). Pancreatic lipase acts maximally around pH 8-9 (Winkler et al., 1990) and was found to be poorly stereoselective (Rogalska & al., 1990). Unlike pre-duodenal lipases, pancreatic lipase requires colipase—a pancreatic protein—as cofactor for its enzymatic activity (Fig.1). Colipase relieves phosphatidyl choline-mediated inhibition of the interfacial lipase–substrate complex, helps anchor the lipase to the surface and stabilizes it in the 'open', active conformation (Brockman, 2000; Lowe, 1997).

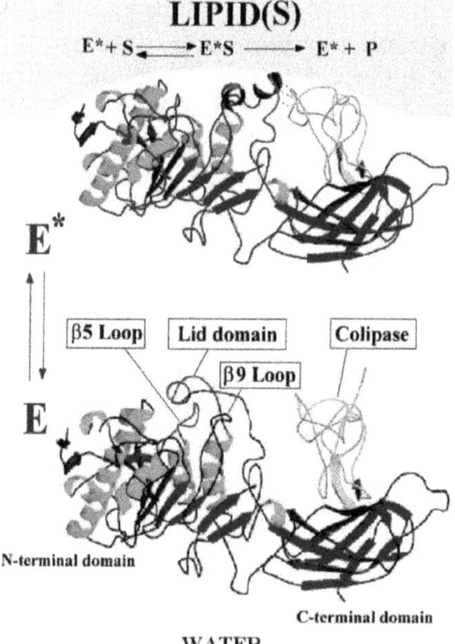

Fig. 1. 3-D Structure of the HPL-procolipase complex in the closed conformation (E) and in the open conformation (E*). These two diagrams show the conformational changes in the lid, the β-5 loop and the colipase during interfacial activation (Adapted from Miled et al., 2000 as cited in van Tilbeurgh et al., 1992; 1993).

The lipase gene family includes also two other pancreatic proteins: pancreatic lipase related proteins 1 and 2, with strong nucleotide and amino acid sequence homology to pancreatic triglyceride lipase. All three proteins have virtually identical three-dimensional structures (Lowe, 2000). Of the pancreatic triglyceride lipase homologues, only pancreatic lipase related protein 2 has lipase activity (Table 2).

Enzyme Name	Substrate specificity	References
Pancreatic lipase	Triglycerides (lipid-droplet)	Thirstrup & al., 1994
Pancreatic lipase related protein 1 (PLRP1)	Unknown Inhibitory effect of HPL (regulatory effect of TG digestion in the duodenum?)	Crenon & al., 1998 Berton & al., 2009
Pancreatic lipase related protein 2 (PLRP2)	Broad range of substrate specificity Triglycerides (milk lipid-droplet) Synergistic effect of HPL (regulatory effect of TG digestion in the duodenum?) Phospholipids Galactolipids Esters of vitamin A	Berton & al., 2009 Thirstrup & al., 1994 Sias & al., 2004 Reboul & al., 2006
Carboxyl ester lipase	Nonspecific enzyme Esters of lipid-soluble vitamins Esters of cholesterol Triglycerides, diglycerides, monoglycerides Phospholipids Ceramides	Hui & Howles , 2002
Phospholipase A2	Phospholipids	Verheij & al., 1983

Abbreviations: HPL, human pancreatic lipase; TG, triglycerides

Table 2. Human pancreatic enzymes involved in lipid digestion

It should be stressed that adult pancreas also produces an enzyme equivalent to the colipase-dependant pancreatic lipase (CDL) called bile-salt-stimulated lipase (BSSL) or carboxyl ester lipase (EC 3.1.1.1) (Hui & Howles, 2002). Originally discovered in milk of humans and various other primates (Swan & al., 1992), BSSL participates to the intestinal digestion of dietary lipids (Table 2). While colipase-dependent pancreatic lipase facilitates the uptake of fatty acids, bile-salt-stimulated lipase facilitates the uptake of free cholesterol from the intestinal lumen (Sahasrabudhe & al., 1998). A distinguishing feature of this 722 - amino acid native protein is that it requires primary bile salts for the hydrolysis of emulsified long chain triacylglycerols (Sahasrabudhe & al., 1998).

The exocrine pancreas secretes another group of phospholipid-hydrolyzing enzymes including phospholipase A1 (EC 3.1.1.32), and phospholipase A2 (EC 3.1.1.4). These enzymes are secreted in their zymogen form and activated by trypsin on entering the duodenum (Nouri-Sorkhabi & al., 2000).

PLA1 catalyzes the hydrolysis of fatty acids exclusively at the sn-1 position of phospholipids. A free fatty acid (FFA) and a lysophospholipid (lysoPL) are the products of this reaction. However, this class of phospholipase is not well understood, and no crystal structures exist. The assignment of a function for this pancreatic enzyme has yet to be firmly established (Richmond & Smith, 2011).

In intraluminal digestion, phospholipase A2 is primarily responsible for hydrolyzing phosphatidyl-choline to 2-lysophophatidyl-choline. This reaction is important in triglyceride digestion as the amphipathic phosphatidyl-choline, in a manner similar to bile salts, will adsorb to the surface of the lipid droplets, preventing contact between the lipase-colipase complex and its lipid substrate. Hydrolysis of phosphatidyl-choline by phospholipase 2 will allow desorption of lysophosphatidyl-choline, which is water soluble. The subsequent mucosal absorption of lysophosphatidyl-choline is important in the generation of enterocyte phospholipids and lipoproteins and, thus, chylomicron formation (Nouri-Sorkhabi & al., 2000).

2.4 Hepatic lipase

As the name suggests, hepatic lipase (EC 3.1.1.3) is synthesized mostly by hepatocytes in the liver and found localized at the surface of liver sinusoidal capillaries (Perret & al., 2002). The human hepatic lipase presents four glycosylation sites, which are localized at positions 20, 56, 340, and 375, and a molecular mass around 65 kDa (Ben-Zeev & al., 1994 ; Wolle & al., 1993). Together with lipoprotein lipase (LPL), hepatic lipase (HL) could be considered as a lipase of the vascular compartment (Perret & al., 2002). Unlike pancreatic lipase, hepatic lipase does not require a cofactor for its activity; is stable at high salt concentrations and is inactivated by sodium dodecyl sulfate (Mukherjee, 2003). HL exerts both triglyceride lipase and phospholipase A1 activities, and is involved at different steps of lipoprotein metabolism (Santamarina-Fojo & al., 2004). The preferred physiological substrate of hepatic lipase is triglyceride of intermediate density lipoprotein (IDL) particle, which it hydrolyses to form triglyceride-poor and cholesterol-rich low-density lipoprotein (LDL). Hepatic lipase also converts post-prandial triglyceride rich high-density lipoprotein (HDL) particle (i.e.HDL2) to post-absorptive triglyceride poor HDL (i.e. HDL3) (Mukherjee, 2003).

2.5 Lipoprotein lipase

Lipoprotein lipase (EC 3.1.1.34) (LPL) is a non-covalent homodimeric protein produced mainly by the adipose, heart and muscle tissue and to some extent by macrophages (Camp & al., 1990). LPL is secreted from parenchymal cells as a glycosylated homodimer, after which it is translocated through the extracellular matrix and across endothelial cells to the capillary lumen. After secretion, however, the mechanism by which LPL travels across endothelial cells is still unknown (Braun & Severeson 1992; Mead & al., 2002). The glycosylation sites of LPL are Asn-43, Asn-257, and Asn-359 (Mead & al., 2002). Lipoprotein lipase has multiple functional domains including lipid-binding, the dimer formation, heparin binding, cofactor interaction and fatty acid-binding domains (Santamarina-Fojo & Dugi, 1994). Interaction of the enzyme with the lipoprotein substrate takes place in the lipid-binding domain. This results in a conformational change that leads to the movement of a short helical segment or 'lid' to expose the active site containing the Ser-Asp-His catalytic triad, where hydrolysis of triacylglycerol takes place (Emmerich & al., 1992). As a homodimer, LPL has the dual function of triglyceride hydrolase and ligand/bridging factor for receptor-mediated lipoprotein uptake. Through catalysis, triacylglycerol present in very low-density lipoprotein (VLDL) and chylomicron particles is converted to triglyceride-poor intermediate-density lipoprotein (IDL) and chylomicron remnants, respectively (Mukherjee, 2003). Apolipoprotein CII (ApoCII) present on VLDL particles is the co-factor required for activating the enzyme (Mukherjee, 2003).

2.6 Endothelial lipase

Endothelial lipase (EC 3.1.1.3) which was firstly characterized in 1999 was also added to the lipase gene family (Jaye & al., 1999). Mature endothelial lipase is a 68 kDa glycoprotein with five potential N-linked glycosylation sites (Yasuda & al., 2010). It has 44% primary sequence homology with lipoprotein lipase, 41% with hepatic lipase and 27% with pancreatic lipase (Choi & al., 2002). The enzyme is secreted by endothelial cells from various tissues like lung, liver, kidney and placenta. However, heart and skeletal muscles do not express endothelial lipase (Jaye & al., 1999). Endothelial lipase differs from the other enzymes of the lipase gene family in the sequence of the 'lid' domain. Its 19-residue 'lid' region is 3 residues shorter and less amphipathic than 'lid' region of lipoprotein or hepatic lipase indicating a different enzymatic function (Jaye & al., 1999). Indeed, unlike lipoprotein or hepatic lipases that have triacylglycerol lipase activity, endothelial lipase has primarily a phospholipase A1 activity. It was suggested that endothelial lipase plays a physiologic role in HDL metabolism probably by catalyzing hydrolysis of HDL phospholipids thereby facilitating a direct HDL receptor-mediated uptake (Cohen, 2003). Endothelial lipase may also facilitate the uptake of apolipoprotein B-containing remnant lipoprotein. As the placental tissue abundantly expresses endothelial lipase, it may also have a role in the development of fetus (Choi & al., 2002).

3. Human dietary lipid digestion process and regulation of pancreatic fluid in healthy state

Protein digestion begins in the stomach with the concomitant action of hydrochloric acid and pepsin, continues with pancreatic proteases in the duodenum, and finishes with numerous brush border peptidases located all over the small intestine (Fieker & al., 2011 as cited in Alpers, 1994). Starch digestion begins in the mouth with salivary amylase, continues with pancreatic amylase, and ends with several intestinal brush border oligosaccharidases (Fieker & al., 2011 as cited in Alpers, 1994). In contrast, the majority of lipid digestion and absorption occurs between the pylorus and the ligament of Treitz. Prior to this step, 5% to 40% of the dietary triglyceride acyl chains are released in the stomach by gastric lipase (Armand & al., 1994, 1996, 1999; Carrière & al., 1993b ; Hamosh, 1990) which continues its action in the duodenum together with pancreatic lipase until these enzymes are degraded by pancreatic proteases. Although a pH of 8 to 9 appears to be optimal for pancreatic lipase activity *in vitro*, bile salts allow the enzyme to work efficiently at a pH of 6 to 6.5 *in vivo* (Borgstrom, 1964; Carrière & al., 2005). HPL is responsible for the hydrolysis of 40% to 70% of triglycerides (Fig.2).

The pancreatic lipase-related 2 protein (hPLRP2), with a broader substrate specificity, hydrolyzes milk triglycerides (Berton & al., 2009) phospholipids (Jayne & al., 2002; Lowe, 2002; Thirstrup & al., 1994) galactolipids (Sias & al., 2004) and esters of lipid-soluble vitamins (Reboul & al., 2006). Carboxyl ester lipase (also called bile salt-stimulated lipase,

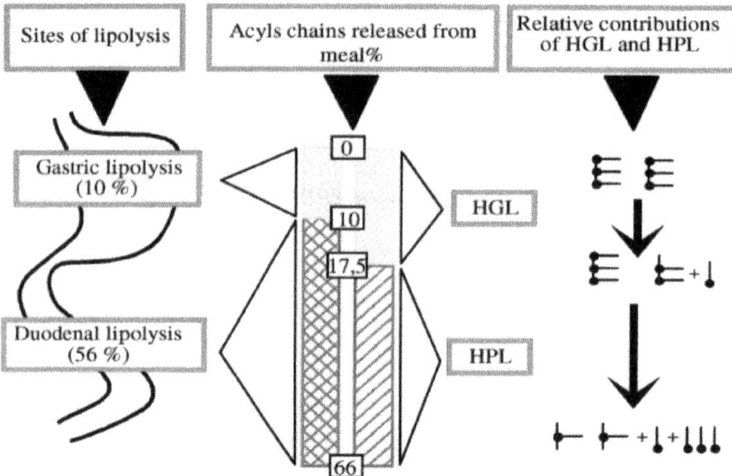

Fig. 2. Schematic representation of the relative contributions of HGL and HPL to the overall digestion of dietary triacylglycerides. On a weight basis, the ratio of pancreatic lipase to gastric lipase total secretory outputs was found to be around four after 3 hours of digestion. The level of gastric hydrolysis was calculated to be 10% of the acyl chains released from the meal triglycerides. Gastric lipase remained active in the duodenum where it might still hydrolyze 7.5% of the triglyceride acyl chains. Hence, globally, during the whole digestion period, gastric lipase hydrolyzes 17.5% of all the triglyceride acyl chains. (Reproduced from Carrière & al., 1993b).

(BSSL)) will hydrolyze triglycerides, diglycerides, phospholipids, and esters of lipid-soluble vitamins and of cholesterol (Hui & Howles, 2002). Phospholipase A2 hydrolyzes phospholipids to lysophospholipids20 which is essential for an optimal absorption of lipid nutrients (Fieker & al., 2011, as cited in Tso, 1994).

Products generated during lipolysis are solubilized in bile salts–mixed micelles and liposomes (vesicles) which allow absorption across the intestinal villi. Once absorbed, the digested lipids are converted back to triglycerides, phospholipids, and esters of cholesterol and of lipid-soluble vitamins, then packaged as chylomicrons and transported through the thoracic duct into the systemic circulation for delivery to various sites throughout the body (Fieker & al., 2011, as cited in Tso, 1994).

To execute this digestive function, postprandial pancreatic juice secretion can increase up to 1 to 2 L per day in response to physiologic stimuli, mainly secretin and vagal output (Lee & Muallem, 2009). Appropriate enzyme delivery in the duodenum is allowed through a specific orchestration of the pancreatic fluid secretion during the fed state. In fact, during the gastric phase, digestion of proteins by pepsin and of triglycerides by gastric lipase generates amino acids and free fatty acids, respectively (Fieker & al., 2011, as cited in Alpers, 1994). When delivered through the pylorus, they become powerful stimulants of the cholecystokinin hormone (CCK) produced by the duodenal endocrine cells which stimulates pancreatic enzymes secretion and controls the gastric emptying rate. The acidic pH of the chyme entering the duodenum stimulates the release of secretin, which increases the secretion of water and bicarbonate ions from the pancreas (Fieker & al., 2011 as cited in

Solomon, 1994). This gastric phase of digestion represents an important aspect in the overall postprandial regulation of pancreatic secretion. During the intestinal phase, enterohormones, such as CCK, together with neurotransmitters and neuropeptides further stimulate pancreatic secretion (Chey & Chang, 2001). Thus, digestive pancreatic enzyme response to a meal follows a specific pattern in which the degree and duration depend on nutrient composition, caloric content and physical properties of the meal. Enzyme secretion into the duodenum increases quickly reaching peak output within the first 20 to 60 minutes postprandially, then decreasing to a stable level before reaching an interdigestive level at the end of the digestive period, ie, about 4 hours after meal intake (Keller & Layer, 2005).

4. Exocrine pancreatic insufficiency & fat malabsorption

As previously described, the pancreas functions as the main factory for the digestive enzymes. The gland produces pancreatic juice that consists of a mixture of more than two dozen digestive enzymes in the pre-activated form, called zymogens. Zymogens are produced by acinar cells and mixed with a bicarbonate rich fluid that is produced by pancreatic ducts cells (Whitcomb & Lowe, 2007). Trypsin, chymotrypsin, amylase and lipase are responsible for the majority of the enzyme activity derived from the pancreas (Whitcomb & Lowe, 2007). Lipase is one of the most important enzymes because it plays a leading role in the digestion of fat, which is the highest dietary source of calories.

Pancreatic exocrine insufficiency, partial or complete loss of digestive enzyme synthesis, occurs primarily in disorders directly affecting pancreatic tissue integrity (Table 3).

Pancreatic parenchymal disease
Chronic pancreatitis Post-necrotizing acute pancreatitis Cystic fibrosis Pancreatic cancers/tumors Autoimmune pancreatitis
Extrapancreatic disease
Celiac disease Inflammatory bowel disease Diabetes mellitus Zollinger-Ellison syndrome
Postsurgical states
Gastric resection Whipple's pancreaticoduodenectomy Short bowel syndrome Bariatric surgeries (eg, gastric bypass)

Table 3. Conditions Causing EPI (adapted from Keller et al., 2009).

It is most frequently due to chronic pancreatitis (in adults) or cystic fibrosis (in children) (Keller & al., 2009). Other pancreatic causes include acute pancreatitis, pancreatic tumors and pancreatic surgery (Table 3).

While protein and starch digestion are usually maintained at a normal physiological level even in severe cases of pancreatic insufficiency, lipid malabsorption becomes the overriding problem and causes many of the clinical symptoms and nutritional deficiencies.

4.1 Pathophysiology

Clinically evident EPI occurs only when 90% of the function is lost and the secretion of pancreatic enzymes is less than 10% of normal (Lankisch & al., 1986; Layer & al., 1986). In chronic pancreatitis, an earlier decrease of lipase secretion is observed in comparison with amylase and protease. This is due to higher susceptibility of lipase to acidic pH caused by concomitant impairment of bicarbonate secretion, higher susceptibility of lipase to proteolytic destruction during small intestinal transit, additional acidic denaturation of bile acids and marked inhibition of bile acid secretion in malabsorptive states (Keller & Layer, 2005). Hence, in case of EPI, fat malabsorption precedes malabsorption of proteins and carbohydrates and is clinically more apparent. Additionally, due to the low bicarbonate secretion, the intraduodenal pH may drop below 4 late postprandially, bile salts may precipitate which leads to a decrease in post- prandial duodenal lipid solubilisation and contribute to impaired lipolysis (Zentler-Munro & al., 1984). The increased presence of lipids and other nutrients in the distal small bowel causes significant alterations in gut motility leading to accelerated gastric emptying and intestinal transit. This results in a marked decrease in the time available for digestion and absorption of nutrients, which also contributes to the malabsorption (Layer & al. 1997). However, more than 80% of carbohydrates can be digested and absorbed in the absence of pancreatic amylase activity and the colonic flora can further metabolizes malabsorbed carbohydrates (Layer & al., 1986). By contrast, gastric lipase, the only extrapancreatic source of lipolytic activity in humans, does not compensate efficiently for pancreatic lipase deficiency although it may be elevated in patients with chronic pancreatitis compared to healthy individuals (Carrière & al., 1993b). That's why fat malabsorption remains the first problem to be considered when treating EPI.

4.2 Clinical symptoms and complications

Maldigestion of fat results in steatorrhoea. In western countries steatorrhoea is diagnosed when daily stool fat content exceeds 7 g during ingestion of a diet containing 100 g fat per day. This corresponds to a decrease of the enteral absorption rate to less than 93% (Dimagno & al., 1973). Steatorrhoea causes symptoms such as foul-smelling, voluminous, greyish, fatty stools, abdominal cramps, bloating and chronic abdominal pain (Pasquali & al., 1996). It may also cause weight loss due to the loss of the highest dietary source of calories (fat contains 38 kJ/g, carbohydrates and protein contain 17 kJ/g) (Rosenlund & al., 1974). Steatorrhoea and weight loss are the overt clinical symptoms of EPI. They usually only occur if pancreatic enzyme secretion falls below 5–10% of normal levels (Keller & al., 2009).

Due to fat malabsorption fat-soluble vitamins (A, D, E and K), magnesium, calcium and essential fatty and amino–acids are insufficiently resorbed (Dutta & al., 1982; Keller & al., 2009) which results in a variety of associated complications. Deficiencies in these vitamins and nutrients may lead to tetany, glossitis, cheilosis, and in a more progressive stage, to peripheral neuropathy (Dimagno , 1993). Patients with PEI may exhibit low vitamin D levels and develop osteopathy, i.e. osteopenia, osteoporosis and osteomalacia. There are reports on vitamin A deficiency causing night-blindness, visual impairment and other ocular affections. As a consequence of vitamin E and K deficiencies neurologic symptoms or coagulopathy can occur (Keller & al., 2009). There seems also to be an increased risk for cardiovascular events in PEI, independent of life style factors (Gullo & al., 1996).

4.3 Incidence and diagnosis

The prevalence of EPI is increasing with the higher proportion of patients with cystic fibrosis who survive into adult life and the incidence of chronic pancreatitis, which rises in parallel with alcohol consumption. In fact, the incidence of cystic fibrosis is approximately 1 in 2500 live births. The lack of chloride secretion in the pancreatic duct is responsible for severe exocrine pancreatic insufficiency in approximately 85% of CF newborns (Levy, 2011). In case of chronic pancreatitis, an incidence of 8.2 per 100 000 population per year and a prevalence of 26.4 cases per 100 000 along with a 3.6-fold increase in mortality in patients with alcohol-induced chronic pancreatitis compared with a population without chronic pancreatitis has been signaled (Keller & al., 2009). Hence, to avoid malnutrition related morbidity and mortality, it is pivotal to start treatment as soon as EPI is diagnosed.

Several direct and indirect function tests are available for assessment of pancreatic function. Direct invasive function tests like the secretin-caerulein test are still the gold standard with highest sensitivity and specificity. However, their availability is limited to specialized centers, they are costly, time consuming and uncomfortable for the patient (Keller & al., 2009). Determination of fecal elastase is convenient and widely available but its sensitivity is low in mild to moderate cases. Moreover, due to low specificity, it is of limited value for differential diagnosis in patients with diarrhea (Dominguez-Munoz & al., 1995; Stein & al., 1996). Other non-invasive tests such as 13C-breath tests are becoming more important but are not widely established, yet (Dominguez-Munoz & al., 2007).

5. Standard approaches for the treatment of fat malabsorption due to exocrine pancreatic insufficiency

The main focus in the management of EPI is to prevent weight loss, EPI related symptoms, vitamin deficiencies, and to improve the patient's nutritional status. Whatever the aetiology, oral pancreatic enzyme supplements are widely used as the first-line approach to treat malabsorption secondary to exocrine pancreatic insufficiency (Breithaupt & al., 2007).

5.1 Formulations and galenic properties

Pancreatic enzyme preparations (PEPs) are typically a mixture of porcine-derived pancreatic enzymes. These preparations, also called pancreatin, contain a variable mixture of protease, lipase and amylase depending on the brand. Various preparations are commercially available. The main formulations are immediate-release, enteric-coated microspheres and minimicrospheres, enteric-coated microtablets and enteric-coated microspheres with a bicarbonate buffer (Table 4). A Comprehensive table of these preparations has been summarized in other reviews (Krishnamurty & al., 2009, Ferrone & al., 2007).

Formulation	Number of available products	Product example (manufacturer)
Immediate–release formulations	6	Pancrelipase tablets (various manufacturers) Vikokase powder (Axcan Scandipharm)
Enteric-coated microspheres	24	Lipram capsules (Global Pharmaceuticals) Pangestym (Ethex) Pancrelipase capsules (various manufacturers)
Enteric-coated microtablets	7	Pancrease (McNeil) Ultrase (Axcan Scandipharm)
Enteric-coated minimicrospheres	3	Creon capsules (Solvay Pharmaceuticals)
Enteric-coated microsphere with bicarbonate buffer	3	Pancrecarb (Digestive Care)

Table 4. Commercially available pancreatic enzyme formulations (adapted from Krishnamurty et al., 2009)

The uncoated formulations are susceptible to acidic inactivation in the stomach and are currently used largely in clinical practice to treat the pain of chronic pancreatitis and not malabsorption (Chauhan & Forsmark, 2010). The enteric-coated pancreatic enzyme formulations have been developed to solve problems associated with acid-mediated inactivation of pancreatic lipase, especially in patients with EPI who also show low pH values in the small intestine. First generation of these preparations was the enteric coated tablet with diameter of 11-20 mm. Due to their large size, these formulations did not empty into the duodenum as quickly as smaller food particles and did not show any additional benefits over conventional preparations (Meyer & al., 1988; Meyer & Lake, 1997). Next generation of enteric-coated preparations consist of capsules (over 2 mm in size) coated with acid resistant agents designed to release the enzyme between pH 5.0-5.5. No therapeutic benefit of these preparations was seen. Studies of labeled capsules suggest that even with varying sizes of microspheres, the ingested lipid may enter the duodenum in advance of the pancreatic enzyme (Meyer & Lake, 1997). Hence, newer formulations consisting of capsules containing mini-microspheres, pellets or micro-tablets of less than 2 mm in size were designed to promote an adequate intragastric mixture of exogenous enzymes with chyme. Whether the use of these enteric coated mini-microsphere preparations adds any special advantage over the existing treatment options remains, however, subject to great discussion (Halm & al., 1999; Stern & al, 2000).

The most recent innovation in the formulation of pancreatic enzymes supplements has been the development of enteric-coated "buffered" micro-sphere preparations which have 1.5-2.5 mEq of bicarbonate per capsule. Clinical trials conducted to compare these formulations to standard enteric coated microspheres showed controversy results (Brady & al., 2006; Kalnins & al., 2006).

In Europe, availability of preparations varies by country and they are regulated nationally and not by the European Medicines Agency. In products in which the enzyme content has been standardized, marked variability in particle size, enzyme release, and for some, acid stability has been noted and may result in differences in clinical effect (Walters & Littlewood, 1996; Aloulou & al., 2008; Löhr & al., 2009). In the United States, marked variation in the enzyme content of the various formulations especially with generic products has been attributed to a lack of stringent regulation (Fieker & al., 2011).

5.2 Dosage recommendation and schedule of administration

Some general guidelines are given in spite of the absence of an easy applicable and objective method to establish the adequate dose of oral pancreatic enzymes to treat exocrine pancreatic insufficiency.

In general, the recommended dosage of Pancreatic enzyme supplements (PES) for a main meal (breakfast, lunch, or dinner) ranges from 25,000 to 75,000 units of lipase and from 10,000 to 25,000 units of lipase for snacks, depending on the fat content of the meal (Sikkens et al., 2010). Initial dose must ensure supplementation of 60 UI/min of lipase activity in postparandial chyme throughout the digestive period; hence, dosing is adjusted considering this recommendation and the amount of lipase in the supplement (Krishnamurty et al., 2009) but it is not recommended to exceed 10,000 units of lipase per kg of body weight per meal (Fieker et al., 2011).

The timing of ingestion of the capsules is important to optimize therapeutic efficacy. A recent study compared three different administration schedules using enzyme replacement before, during or after meals. Better lipid digestion was found when giving enzymes during or after meals (Dominguez-Munoz & al., 2005).

5.3 Efficacy assessment of the treatment with pancreatic enzyme supplements

Numerous randomized placebo controlled trials have shown that treatment with pancreatic enzyme supplements improves steatorrhea, as measured by increased fat absorption, reduced fecal fat excretion, decreased stool weight and frequency, improved stool consistency and improved symptom scores (Guarner et al., 1993; O'keefe et al., 2001; Dominguez-Munoz et al., 2005; Safdi et al., 2006, Trapnell et al., 2009; Wooldridge et al., 2009; Whitcomb et al., 2010). Enzyme supplements have been found to improve lipid malabsorption in children even those who are younger than 7 years old (Graff et al., 2010a, 2010b). In yet other studies, increased cholesterol absorption and improved enterohepatic cycling of bile salts have been reported (Dutta et al., 1986; Vuoristo et al., 1992). Moreover, it has been demonstrated that improvement of lipid digestion contributes to effective correction of motility disorders (Mizushima et al., 2004). Altered levels of gastro-intestinal hormones were normalized (Nustede et al., 1991); accelerated gastric emptying and abnormal antroduodenal motility were corrected (Layer et al., 1997).

Even though, randomized controlled trials have suggested, years ago, that non-enteric coated pancreatic enzyme supplements reduce pain in chronic pancreatitis (Isaksson et al., 1983; Slaff et al., 1984), a more recent study did not support the use of these preparations for the relief of pain in all patients (Brown et al., 1997). Unfortunately, pancreatic enzyme supplements were reported to be not sufficient for correcting fat soluble vitamin deficiencies or B12 deficiency without simultaneous vitamin supplementation (Dutta et al., 1982; Bang et al., 1991).

The most surprising fact regarding efficacy assessment of this therapy is that few investigations are made considering nutritional status and quality of life improvements as well as weight gain (Czako et al., 2003; Trolli et al., 2001; Dominguez-Munoz, 2007). Reduction in stool fat achieved by pancreatic enzyme replacement therapy has not been proven by robust research to be correlated with a complete correction of nutritional deficiency in patients with pancreatic insufficiency. Accordingly, an overall assessment of this therapy efficacy is yet dependent on future demonstration of long-term interesting outcomes.

5.4 Safety concerns, side effect and treatment failure

Enzyme replacement therapy using pancrelipase (pancreatin) delayed-release capsules (i.e. Creon®, Solvay Pharmaceuticals, Inc., Marietta, GA, USA) have been available in the United States of America for more than 20 years with very few observed side effects (Krishnamurty et al., 2009). Meanwhile, allergic reactions to the porcine proteins and some others side effects may occur: Pancreatin extracts are prone to form insoluble complexes with folic acid resulting in folate deficiency (Russell & al., 1980). One serious adverse effect has been reported by Smyth et al. (1994, 1995). The authors described five children with cystic fibrosis in which a colonic obstruction developed due to fibrosing colonopathy (FC) after using very high doses of the enteric-coated micro- minisphere preparations (i.e. more than 20000 lipase units/capsule). Fortunately, the cases of reported FC have decreased considerably since the Medicine Control Agency (MCA) recommended in 1994 that the dose of pancreatic enzymes should not exceed 10,000 IU lipase/kg/day in patients with CF (Taylor , 2002 as cited in Medicine Control Agency, 1994).

Recently, Axcan Pharma Inc. and its subsidiaries received safety update reports describing a total of 46 adverse events observed in a clinical study carried out between 01 November 2008 and 31 May 2009 and involving three pancreatic enzyme preparations: ULTRASE®, VIOKASE® and PANZYTRAT® (Table 5). Fifty-three patients were enrolled, 40 of these patients completed the study.

In most cases, adverse effects were single occurrences. Drug ineffectiveness was the most frequently reported adverse effect for ULTRASE® (Table 5). A lack of therapeutic effect was also reported for some other preparations (Kraisinger et al., 1994). In fact, among marketed PEPs, great variability in the amount of enzymes included in each capsule has been noted (Case & al., 2005; US Food and Drug Administration, 2006; Wooldridge & al., 2009) due in part to the manufacturer practice of overfilling capsules to account for enzyme degradation that occurs over the course of the product's shelf life (US Food and Drug Administration, 2004). While instability of the enzymes results in delivery medications that contain less than the packaged amount of enzyme, the practice of "overfilling" in an effort to address enzyme degradation may result in excess enzyme content, resulting in formulations that deliver inadequate or excess amounts of enzyme.

The possible safety risk posed by high-dose enzyme therapy, particularly fibrosing colonopathy , in combination with the issue of enzyme overfill, recently prompted the FDA to require the manufacturers of PEPs to demonstrate drug efficacy and safety in randomized, placebo-controlled trials before approval (Trapnell & al., 2009). The FDA ruled that manufacturers of pancreatic enzyme supplements must file new drug applications

SOC / Preferred Term	ULTRASE®	VIOKASE®	PANZYTRAT®	Total
Cardiac disorders				
Cardio-respiratory arrest	0	1	0	1
Gastrointestinal disorders				
Abdominal pain	0	2	0	2
Abdominal pain upper	1	1	1	3
Abnormal faeces	0	1	0	1
Diarrhoea	1	3	1	5
Dyspepsia	0	1	0	1
Faecal volume increased	1	0	0	1
Frequent bowel movements	1	0	0	1
Gastritis	0	1	0	1
Glossodynia	0	1	0	1
Groin pain	0	1	0	1
Lip swelling	0	1	0	1
Nausea	0	1	1	2
Oral discomfort	0	1	0	1
Steatorrhoea	1	0	0	1
Swollen tongue	0	1	0	1
Tongue ulceration	0	1	0	1
Vomiting	0	0	1	1
General disorders and administration site conditions				
Asthenia	0	1	0	1
Drug effect decreased	1	0	0	1
Drug ineffective	4	0	0	4
Feeling abnormal	0	1	0	1
Product commingling	0	1	0	1
Therapeutic response decreased	0	1	0	1
Injury, poisoning and procedural complications				
Incorrect dose administered	0	1	0	1
Investigations				
Blood glucose increased	1	0	0	1
Blood sodium decreased	0	1	0	1
Blood sugar level fluctuation	0	1	0	1
Drug screen positive	0	1	0	1
Weight decreased	1	0	0	1
Metabolism and nutrition disorders				
Diabetes mellitus	1	0	0	1
Nervous system disorders				
Loss of consciousness	0	1	0	1
Respiratory, thoracic and mediastinal disorders				
Throat irritation	0	1	0	1
Skin and subcutaneous tissue disorders				
Rash macular	0	1	0	1
Urticaria	0	1	0	1

Coded with MedDRA dictionary

Table 5. Adverse Events (Preferred Term) Recorded for Pancreatic Enzyme Preparations in the Axcan Pharma Safety Database Classified by System Organ Class from November 1, 2008, to May 31, 2009 (Reproduced from Page 8 of the Safety Update for NDA 22-222 dated August 4, 2009).

(NDA) to ensure consistent efficacy, safety, and quality of these agents (US Food and Drug Administration, 2006). Therefore, in order to comply with the FDA 2004 mandate, several studies have been recently conducted to ensure safety and effectiveness of some new reformulated pancreatic enzyme supplements such as Creon® 24,000 and EUR-1008 (Zenpep™) (Wooldridge & al., 2009; Trapnell & al., 2009). Nevertheless, these products of animal origin present yet a risk of viral transmission. Accordingly, there remains a need for new alternatives to treat correctly exocrine pancreatic insufficiency.

6. Enzyme replacement therapy: What's in the pipeline?

6.1 Bovine enzymes

Even though bovine enzymes have been suggested as a potential alternative for individuals who refuse to consume porcine products for religious or other cultural reasons; there remain some safety concerns about transmittable pathogens such as Foot and mouth disease and Bovine spongiform encephalopathy from these preparations. Additionally, lipase activity is approximately 75% lower than the porcine preparations (Layer and Keller, 2003)

6.2 Recombinant mammalian/human lipases

Owing to rapid development of plant biotechnology in recent times, Merispase a recombinant mammalian gastric lipase was produced in transgenic corn by Meristem Therapeutics and proposed as new oral substitute for the treatment of pancreatic insufficiency. Dog gastric lipase was selected because it is naturally resistant to inactivation by stomach acids and maintains a high enzymatic activity after passage through the stomach. Enzyme expression was stable over 11 generations with an approximate level of 1,000 mg kg^{-1} kernel (Shama & Peterson, 2008). According to Fieker et al. (2011), this approach could be problematic for several reasons: gastric lipase specific activity is about 10 times lower than that of pancreatic lipase (measured on tributyrin), it is highly sensitive to trypsin proteolysis, and endogenous secretion of gastric lipase can be increased in patients with pancreatic insufficiency because of possible nutritional adaptation. Meanwhile, clinical trials showed that the recombinant gastric lipase is well tolerated and efficient when administered either alone or combined with porcine pancreatic extract to patients with cystic fibrosis (Fieker & al., 2011, as cited by Lenoir et al., 2006, 2008). The highest efficiency is obtained when 250 mg of recombinant gastric lipase is associated with low dose of pancreatic extract (Fieker & al., 2011, as cited by Lenoir et al., 2008). Despite these encouraging results, Mersitem therapeutics went out of business in September 2008 while the product was blocked in clinical phase II trial.

Expected to offer superior safety by decreasing the risk of allergic reactions, recombinant human bile salt- stimulated lipase was suggested as promising candidate for the treatment of lipid malabsorption in pancreatic insufficiency. Human bile salt-stimulated lipase is naturally acid resistant and able to: (i) hydrolyze triglycerides and phospholipids (Lindquist & Hernell, 2010) (ii) generate lysophospholipids necessary for an efficient lipid absorption rate by the small intestine (Fieker & al., as cited by Tso, 1994) (iii) participate in chylomicron assembly and secretion through its ceramidase activity (Hui and Howles, 2002). For these reasons, Swedish Orphan Biovitrum - a leading company focused on treatment of rare diseases developed two preparations of recombinant bile salt-stimulated lipase: Kiobrina for preterm infants and

Exinalda for cystic fibrosis patients. A phase I clinical trial showed that addition of recombinant bile salt-stimulated lipase to standard pancrelipase (Creon) enabled a dose reduction of pancrelipase. The treatment had the advantage of restoring a normal level and pattern of plasma chylomicron secretion (Fieker & al., 2011, as cited by Strandvik et al., 2004). The combined results from two Phase II studies evaluating Kiobrina in preterm infants demonstrated an increase in growth velocity and uptake of long chain polyunsaturated fatty acids such as docosahexanoic acid and arachidonic acid. The safety and tolerability profile of rhBSSL added to formula was similar compared to placebo (Maggio et al., 2010). Based on these encouraging results, Swedish Orphan Biovitrum enrolls in August 2011 the first patient in Kiorbina phase III clinical trial. An open-label exploratory phase II study on Exinalda (rhBSSL) in patients with cystic fibrosis and pancreatic insufficiency has been completed. The aim was to study the effect of Exinalda on fat absorption as well as safety in this patient population. The results showed that Exinalda is safe and tolerable at a dose level of 170 mg three times a day. In terms of efficacy (coefficient of fat absorption CFA) the primary endpoint was not met. Swedish Orphan Biovitrum is now assessing options to continue the development (Swedish Orphan Biovitrum website www. sobi.com).

6.3 Microbial and plant derived lipases

With the aim of developing porcine-free enzyme supplements and in order to avoid the short-life of lipolytic enzymes of pancreatic origin, microbial lipases of fungal or bacterial origin were suggested for replacement therapy. Therefore, potential efficacy of many fungal Lipases derived from *Aspergillus niger* (Griffin & al., 1989), *Rhizopus arrhizus* (Iliano & Lodewijk, 1990), *Rhizopus delemar* (Galle & al., 2004), *Candida cylindracea* (Schuler & Schuler, 2008) and *Yarrowia lipolytica* (Turki & al., 2010a) was investigated. The *Yarrowia lipolytica* lipase seemed to be of potential interest because of its acid and protease-stable properties and its resistance to the detergent action of bile salts as shown *in vitro* (Turki & al., 2010a). Supporting its use as a pharmaceutical, safety assessment of the enzyme in rats showed that there were no toxicologically severe changes in clinical signs, growth, hematology, clinical chemistry, organ weight and pathology related to oral administration of *Yarrowia lipolytica* lipase in animals (Turki & al., 2010b). Actually, a substitute for EPI treatment based on Lip2p is under investigation by Laboratoire Mayoly Spindler, a French pharmaceutical company specialized in gastroenterology therapeutics (Fickers & al., 2011, as cited in http://www.mayoly-spindler.com/). The process development in cGMP conditions for the production of the *Yarrowia lipolytica* MS1819 lipase was completed in 2009 with the Swiss biotech company DSM Nutritional Product Ltd (Fickers & al., 2011, as cited in http://www.dsm.com, press release, December 22th, 2009). In 2010, a drug development partnership was established with Protea Biosciences to initiate phase I/IIA clinical trials in France with the aim of demonstrating safety and proof-of-concept of the therapeutic use of this recombinant lipase (Fickers & al., 2011).

A pipeline preparation Liprotamase (formerly known as ALTU 135 and Trizytek) containing bacterial lipase, fungal protease and amylase was developed by Eli Lilly company (Eli Lilly, IN, USA, www. Lilly.com). An open-label Phase III safety study was carried out in order to evaluate 214 patients, of which 145 CF patients, ages 7 and above, completed 12 months of treatment with Liprotamase. Investigators found that 96 percent of all CF patients who received liprotamase for 12 months maintained or gained weight. Based on key nutritional parameters, the study showed that patients who completed 12 months of treatment with liprotamase demonstrated that they maintained their nutritional status; and survival in people living with cystic fibrosis was maintained too (Borowitz & al., 2011). Subsequent to the completion of the stage III clinical study on liprotamase, the drug's manufacturer submitted a New Drug Application to the U.S. Food and Drug Administration (FDA) for approval. However, on January 13th of this year, the FDA panel stated that he was not convinced that Liprotamase was any better than the current pancreatic enzyme products available now. The manufacturer disclosed that another clinical trial must be conducted before the FDA will consider the approval of this drug (Eli Lilly, IN, USA, www. Lilly.com).

In yet other approaches, plant acid-stable lipases were suggested as good alternatives to porcine preparations. Hence, considerable attention has focused in these enzymes and suitable techniques for isolating and purifying them have been well documented. A lipase sourced from *Carica papaya* latex has been recently proposed as suitable candidate for use as a therapeutic tool in patients with pancreatic exocrine insufficiency (Abdelkafi et al., 2009). The enzyme showed several biochemical properties enabling it to act in the gastro-intestinal tract like mammalian digestive lipases (Abdelkafi et al., 2009): (i) its activity on long-chain Triacylglycerols reaches an optimum at pH 6.0 in the presence of bile, (ii) it is only weakly inhibited by bile salts, (iii) it shows a similar pattern of regioselectivity to that of human pancreatic lipase, generating 2-Mono acylglycerol and free fatty acids (FFA), the lipolysis products absorbed at the intestinal level, and (iv) it shows significant levels of stability and activity at low pH values at a temperature of 37 °C. Therefore, *Carica papaya* lipase seems to be tailored to act optimally under the physiological conditions pertaining in the gastro-intestinal tract. However, its sensitivity to digestive proteases still needs to be tested.

6.4 Future therapies and new research areas

Development of non-porcine enzyme replacement therapies is currently extended to new research areas including design, by direct molecular evolution, of human pancreatic lipase variants that display lipolytic activity at acidic pH higher than that of the native enzyme. Colin et al. (2008) investigated, first, the feasibility of altering the pH optimum of pancreatic lipase to improve its performances in the intestinal conditions of cystic fibrosis by site-directed mutagenesis. Later, they demonstrated that directed molecular evolution approach combined to a sensitive screening strategy could be useful to improve pancreatic lipase activity at acidic pH. The authors showed that a single round of random mutagenesis was successful in identifying lipase variant with approximately 1.5-fold increased activity at low pH (Colin et al., 2010).

Future therapies may also include structuring food emulsions and creation of functional dietary lipids that are more effectively digested. This new area of research could substantially help patient suffering from pancreatic insufficiency with the design of specific more digestible or absorbable lipid sources. Hence, the addition of specific phospholipids able to enhance lipase activity in enzyme supplements or in formula would both increase lipase activity and, in parallel, enhance lipid nutrient absorption (Fieker et al., 2011).

7. Conclusion

Pancreatic exocrine insufficiency is a condition commonly associated with diseases such as pancreatitis or cystic fibrosis. When pancreatic insufficiency is severe, impaired absorption of nutrients by the intestines may result, leading to deficiencies of essential nutrients and the occurrence of loose stools containing unabsorbed fat (steatorrhea). A shortage of the digestive enzymes necessary to break down food is the main cause of this dietary malabsorption. Unlike protein and starch digestion, lipid malabsorption is the overriding problem and the main cause of clinical symptoms and nutritional deficiencies. Until recently, approaches used to address problem of fat malabsorption due to pancreatic insufficiency have been focusing primarily on oral administration of exogenous pancreatic enzymes extracted from porcine source. Standard clinical practices dictate administration of lipase 25,000-75,000 units/meal by using pH-sensitive pancrelipase microspheres, along with dosage increases, compliance checks, and differential diagnosis in cases of treatment failure. Various pancreatin preparations are available, however, differences in galenic properties and release kinetics and other factors such as early acid inactivation, under dosage and patient incompliance may decrease clinical efficacy of the treatment. The FDA decreed that all manufacturers of pancreatic enzyme supplements must file new drug applications (NDA) to ensure consistent efficacy, safety, and quality of these agents. Accordingly, improved approaches to treat efficiently problem of fat malabsorption secondary to pancreatic insufficiency are investigated. New alternatives of enzyme substitution therapy are being developed. Emerging therapeutic landscape includes use of porcine free - lipase preparations. Enzyme supplements either from human, mammalian, microbial or plant origins are wisely suggested. Interestingly, newest approaches state the design of acid -stable variants of human pancreatic lipase as well as creation of functional dietary food with specific more digestible/absorbable lipid sources. However, how these pipeline therapies may help meet the ongoing challenges in treating lipid malabsorption in patients with pancreatic insufficiency and improve the long-term outcomes of these patients remains yet to be assessed.

8. References

Abdelkafi, S.; Fouquet, B. ; Barouh, N. ; Durner, S. ; Pina, M. ; Scheirlinckx, F. ; Villeneuve, P. & Carrière F. (2009). In vitro comparisons between Carica papaya and pancreatic lipases during test meal lipolysis: Potential use of CPL in enzyme replacement therapy. *Food Chemistry*, Vol.115, No. 2, pp. 488–494

Aloulou, A. ; Puccinelli, D. ; Sarles, J. ; Laugier, R. ; Leblond, Y. & Carrière, F. (2008). In vitro comparative study of three pancreatic enzyme preparations: dissolution profiles, active enzyme release and acid stability. *Alimentary Pharmacology and Therapeutics.* Vol. 27, No. 3, pp. 283-392.

Ameis, D.; Stahnke, G.; Kobayashi, J.; McLean, J.; Lee, G.; Buscher, M.; Schotz, M.C. & Will, H. (1990). Isolation and characterization of the human hepatic lipase gene. *Journal of Biological Chemistry.* Vol. 265, pp. 6552–6555.

Armand, M.; Borel, P.; Dubois, C.; Senft, M.; Peyrot, J.; Salducci, J.; Lafont, H. & Lairon, D. (1994).Characterization of emulsions and lipolysis of dietary lipids in the human stomach. *American Journal of Physiology Gastrointestinal and Liver Physiology*, Vol., 266, No. 3, pp. 372-381.

Armand, M.; Hamosh, M.; Mehta, N.R.; Angelus, P.A.; Philpott, J.R.; Henderson, T.R.; Dwyer, N.K.; Lairon, D. & Hamosh, P. (1996). Effect of human milk or formula on gastric function and fat digestion in the premature infant. *Pediatric Research*. Vol. 40, No. 3, pp.429–437.

Armand, M. ; Pasquier, B.; Andre, M.; Borel, P. ; Senft, M.; Peyrot, J.; Salducci, J. ; Portugal, H. ; Jaussan, V. & Lauron, D. (1999). Digestion and absorption of 2 fat emulsions with different droplet sizes in the human digestive tract. *The American Journal of Clinical Nutrition*. Vol. 70, No. 6, pp.1096–1106.

Bai, J. (1998).Malabsorption syndromes. *Digestion*, Vol. 59, No.5, pp 530–546.

Bang Jørgensen, B.; Thorsgaard Pedersen, N. & Worning, H. (1991). Short report: lipid and vitamin B12 malassimilation in pancreatic insufficiency. *Alimentary Pharmacology & Therapeutics*, Vol. 5, No. 2, pp. 207-210.

Ben-Zeev, O.; Stahnke, G.; Liu, R.; Davis, C. & Doolittle, M. H. (1994). Lipoprotein lipase and hepatic lipase: the role of asparagine linked glycosylation in the expression of a functional enzyme. *Journal of Lipid Research*. Vol. 35, pp. 1511–1523.

Berton, A.; Sebban-Kreuzer, C.; Rouvellac, S.; Lopez, C. & Crenon, I. (2009) Individual and combined action of pancreatic lipase and pancreatic lipase-related proteins 1 and 2 on native versus homogenized milk fat globules. *Molecular Nutrition & Food Research*. Vol.53, No.12. pp.1592–1602.

Breithaupt, D. E.; Alpmann, A. & Carrière, F. (2007). Xanthophyll esters are hydrolysed in the presence of recombinant human pancreatic lipase. *Food Chemistry*, 103, 651–656.

Bodmer, M.W.; Angal, S.; Yarranton, G.T.; Harris, T.J.R.; Lyons, A.; King, D.J.; Pieroni, G.; Riviere, C.; Verger R. & Lowe P.A. (1987).Molecular cloning of human gastric lipase and expression of the enzyme in yeast, *Biochimica and Biophysica Acta*, Vol. 909, pp. 237–244.

Borgstrom, B. (1964). Influence of bile salt, pH, and time on the action of pancreatic lipase. *Journal of Lipid Research*. Vol. 5, pp.522–531.

Borowitz, D.; Stevens, C.; Brettman, L.R.; Campion, M.; Chatfield, B. & Cipolli, M. & for the Liprotamase 726 Study Group (2011).. International phase III trial of liprotamase efficacy and safety in pancreatic-insufficient cystic fibrosis patients. *Journal of Cystic Fibrosis*, In press doi:10.1016/j.jcf.2011.07.001 |

Brady, M.S.; Garson, J.L.; Krug, S.K.; Kaul, A.; Rickard, K.A.; Caffrey, H.H.; Fineberg, N., Balistreri, W.F.; Stevens, J.C. (2006). An enteric-coated high-buffered pancrelipase reduces steatorrhea in patients with cystic fibrosis: a prospective, randomized study. *Journal of American Dietetic Association*. Vol. 106, No. 8, pp. 1181-1186.

Braun, J.E. & Severson, D.L. (1992). Regulation of the synthesis, processing and translocation of lipoprotein lipase. *Biochemistry Journal*. Vol. 287, No 2, pp. 337–347.

Brockman, H.L. (2000). Kinetic behaviour of the pancreatic lipase– colipase–lipid system. *Biochimie*, Vol. 82, pp. 987–995.

Brown, A.; Hughes, M.; Tenner, S. & Banks, P.A. (1997). Does pancreatic enzyme supplementation reduce pain in patients with chronic pancreatitis: a meta-analysis. *American Journal of Gastroenterology*, Vol.92, pp. 2032–2035.

Case, C.L.; Henniges, F. & Barkin, J.S. (2005). Enzyme content and acid stability of enteric-coated pancreatic enzyme products in vitro. *Pancreas*, Vol. 30, No. 2, pp.180–183.

Carrière, F.; Barrowman, J.A. ; Verger, R. & Laugier, R. (1993a). Secretion and contribution to lipolysis of gastric and pancreatic lipases during a test meal in humans, *Gastroenterology*, Vol.105, pp. 876–888.

Carriere, F.; Laugier, R.; Barrowman, J.A.; Douchet, I.; Priymenko, N. & Verger, R. (1993b) Gastric and pancreatic lipase levels during a test meal in dogs. *Scandinave Journal of Gastroenterology.* Vol. 28, pp. 443–454.

Carrière, F.; Grandval, P.; Renou, C. ; Palomba, A. ; Priéri, F. ; Giallo, J. ; Henniges, F. ; Sander-Struckmeier, S. & Laugier, R. (2005). Quantitative study of digestive enzyme secretion and gastrointestinal lipolysis in chronic pancreatitis. *Clinical Gastroenterology & Hepatology.*Vol. 3, No 1, pp. 28–38.

Camp, L.; Reina, M.; Llobera, M.; Vilaro, S. & Olivecrona, T. (1990). Lipoprotein lipase: cellular origin and functional distribution, *American Journal of Physiology.* Vol. 258, pp. 673 – 681.

Chauhan, S. & Forsmark, C.E. (2010). Pain management in chronic pancreatitis: A treatment algorithm. *Best Practice Research in Clinical Gastroenterology.* Vol. 24, No. 3, pp. 323–335.

Chey, W.Y. & Chang, T. (2001). Neural hormonal regulation of exocrine pancreatic secretion. *Pancreatology.* Vol.1, No. 4, pp.320–335.

Choi, S.Y.; Hirata, K.; Ishida, T.; Quertermous, T. & Cooper, A.D. (2002). Endothelial lipase: a new lipase on the block. *Journal of Lipid Research.* Vol. 43, pp. 1763–1769.

Czakó, L.; Takács, T.; Hegyi, P., Prónai, L.; Tulassay, Z.; Lakner, L.; Döbrönte, Z.; Boda, K. & Lonovics, J. (2003). Quality of life assessment after pancreatic enzyme replacement therapy in chronic pancreatitis. *Canadian Journal of Gastroenterology*, Vol. 17, No. 10, pp. 597–560.

Crenon, I.; Foglizzo, E.; Kerfelec, B.; Vérine, A.; Pignol, D.; Hermoso, J.; Bonicel, J. & Chapus C. (1998). Pancreatic lipase-related protein type I: a specialized lipase or an inactive enzyme. *Protein Engineering.* Vol. 11, No. 2, pp.135–142.

Cohen, J.C. (2003). Endothelial lipase: direct evidence for a role in HDL metabolism. *Journal of Clinical Investigation.* Vol. 111, pp. 318–321

Colin,D.Y. ; Deprez-Beauclair,P. ; Allouche,M. ; Brasseur,R. & Kerfelec,B. (2008). Exploring the active site cavity of human pancreatic lipase. *Biochemical and Biophysical Research Communication*, Vol. 370, No. 3, pp. 394–398.

Colin,D.Y. ; Deprez-Beauclair,P.; Silva, N.; Infantes, L. & Kerfelec, B. (2010). Modification of pancreatic lipase properties by directed molecular evolution. *Protein Engineering, Design & Selection*, Vol. 23, No. 5, pp. 365–373.

De Caro, A.; Figarella, C.; Amic, J.; Michel, R. & Guy, O. (1977). Human pancreatic lipase: A glycoprotein. *Biochimica and Biophysica Acta (BBA)-Protein Structure*, Vol. 490, No 2, pp. 411-419.

DeNigris, S.J.; Hamosh, M.; Kasbekar, D.K.; Fink, C.S.; Lee, T.C. & Hamosh, P. (1985). Secretion of human gastric lipase from dispersed gastric glands. *Biochimica & Biophysica Acta (BBA) -Lipids and Lipid Metabolism.* Vol. 836, No 1, pp. 67-72.

DiMagno, EP. (1993). A short eclectic history of exocrine pancreatic insufficiency and chronic pancreatitis. *Gastroenterology*, Vol. 104, No. 5, pp. 1255 - 1262.

DiMagno, E.P.; Go, V.L. & Summerskill, W.H (1973). Relations between pancreatic enzyme outputs and malabsorption in severe pancreatic insufficiency. *New England Journal of Medecine,* Vol. 288, pp. 813–815.

Dominguez-Munoz, J.E., Hieronymus, C., Sauerbruch, T., & Malfertheiner, P. (1995). Fecal elastase test: evaluation of a new noninvasive pancreatic function test. *American Journal of Gastroenterology,* Vol. 90, No. 10, pp.1834–1837.

Domínguez-Muñoz, J.E.; Iglesias-García, J.; Iglesias-Rey, M.; Figueiras, A. & Vilariño-Insua, M. (2005). Effect of the administration schedule on the therapeutic efficacy of oral pancreatic enzyme supplements in patients with exocrine pancreatic insufficiency: a randomized, three-way crossover study. *Alimentary Pharmacology and Therapeutics.* Vol. 21, pp. 993-1000.

Dominguez-Munoz, J.E.; Iglesias-Garcia, J.; Vilarino-Insua, M. & Iglesias-Rey M. (2007). 13C-mixed triglyceride breath test to assess oral enzyme substitution therapy in patients with chronic pancreatitis. *Clinical Gastroenterology and Hepatology,* Vol. 5, pp. 484–488.

Dutta, S.K.; Bustin, M.P., Russell, R.M. & Costa, B.S. (1982). Deficiency of fat-soluble vitamins in treated patients with pancreatic insufficiency. *Annals of Internal Medcine,* Vol. 97, pp. 549–552.

Duttan, S.K.; Anand, K. & Gadacz, T.R. (1986). Bile salt malabsorption in pancreatic insufficiency secondary to alcoholic pancreatitis. *Gastroenterology,* Vol. 91, pp.1243–1249.

Eli Lilly, IN, USA, Liprotamase Liprotamase Regulatory Review Bus (Liprotamase) is a biologic entity that combines three biotechnology-produced enzymes. *http://www.lilly.com/SiteCollectionDocuments/FlashFiles/PipeLine/Clinical Development Pipeline/14.html.*

Emmerich, J.; Beg, O.U.; Peterson, J.; Previato, L.; Brunzell, J.D.; Brewer, J.r.H.B. & Santamarina-Fojo, S. (1992). Human lipoprotein lipase. Analysis of catalytic triad by site-directed mutagenesis of Ser-132, Asp-156 and His-241, *Journal of Biological Chemistry,* Vol. 267, pp. 4161–4165

Ferrone, M., Raimondo, M., Scolapio, J.S.(2007). Pancreatic enzyme pharmacotherapy. *Pharmacotherapy,* Vol. 27, No.6, pp. 910-920.

Fickers, P.; Marty, A. & Nicaud, J.M (2011). The lipases from *Yarrowia lipolytica:* Genetics, production, regulation, biochemical characterization and biotechnological applications, *Biotechnology Advances,* doi: 10.1016/j.biotechadv.2011.04.005

Fieker, A.; Philpott, J. & Armand, M. (2011). Enzyme replacement therapy for pancreatic insufficiency: present and future. *Clinical and Experimental Gastroenterology.* Vol. 4, pp. 55-73.

Galle, M.; Gregory, P.C.; Potthoff, A. & Henniges, F. (2004). Microbial enzyme mixtures useful to treat digestive disorders. US Patent 20040057944

Graff, G.R.; Maguiness, K.; McNamara, J.; Morton, R.; Boyd, D.; Beckmann, K. & Bennett, D. (2010a). Efficacy and tolerability of a new formulation of pancrelipase delayed-release capsules in children aged 7 to 11 years with exocrine pancreatic insufficiency and cystic fibrosis: a multicenter, randomized, double-blind, placebo-controlled, two-period crossover, superiority study. *Clinical Therapeutics*, Vol. 32, No. 1, pp. 89-103.

Graff, G.R.; McNamara, J.; Royall, J.; Caras, S.; Forssmann, K. (2010b). Safety and tolerability of a new formulation of pancrelipase delayed-release capsules (CREON) in children under seven years of age with exocrine pancreatic insufficiency due to cystic fibrosis: an open-label, multicentre, single-treatment-arm study. *Clinical Drug Investigation*, Vol.30, No. 6, pp. 351- 364.

Griffin, S. M.; Alderson, D.; Farndon, J.R. (1989). Acid resistant lipase as replacement therapy in chronic pancreatic exocrine insufficiency: a study in dogs. *Gut*, Vol. 30, pp. 1012-1015

Guarner, L. ; Rodriguez, R. ; Guarner, F. ; Malagelada, J. R. (1993). Fate of oral enzymes in pancreatic insufficiency. *Gut*, Vol. 34, pp. 708–712.

Gullo, L.; Tassoni, U.; Mazzoni, G. ; Stefanini F. (1996). Increased prevalence of aortic calcification in chronic pancreatitis. *American Journal of Gastroenterology*, Vol. 91, No. 4, pp. 759-761.

Halm, U.; Löser, C.; Löhr, M.; Katschinski, M. & Mössner, J. (1999). A double-blind, randomized, multicentre, crossover study to prove equivalence of pancreatin minimicrospheres versus microspheres in exocrine pancreatic insufficiency. *Alimentary Pharmacology and Therapeutics*. Vol. 13, No. 7, pp. 951-957.

Hamosh, M. (1979). The role of lingual lipase in neonatal fat digestion. *Ciba Foundation Symposium*, Vol. 16-18, No. 70, pp. 69-98.

Hamosh, M. (1990). Lingual and gastric lipase. *Nutrition*, Vol. 6, pp. 421–428.

Hamosh, M. & Scow, R.O. (1973). Lingual lipase and its role in the digestion of dietary lipid. *Journal of Clinical Investigation*. Vol. 52, No. 1, pp. 88–95.

Hirata, K.-I.; Dichek, H.L.; Cioffi, J.A.; Choi, S.Y.; Leeper, N.J.; Quintana, L.; Kronmal, G.S.; Cooper, A.D. & Quertermous, T. (1999). Cloning of a unique lipase from endothelial cells extends the lipase gene family. *Journal of Biological Chemistry*. Vol. 274, pp.14170 -14175.

Hui, D.Y. & Howles, P.N. (2002). Carboxyl ester lipase: structure-function relationship and physiological role in lipoprotein metabolism and artherosclerosis. *Journal of Lipid Research*. Vol. 43, No. 12, pp.2017-2030.

Iliano, L.O. & Lodewijk, J.S. (1990). A composition for the treatment of exocrine insufficiency of the pancreas, and the use of said composition. European Pat. ES 2059986 (T3).

Isaksson, G.; Ihse, I. (1983). Pain reduction by an oral pancreatic enzyme preparation in chronic pancreatitis. *Digestive Disease Science*, Vol. 28, pp. 97–102.

Jaye, M.; Lynch, K.J.; Krawiec, J.; Marchadier, D.; Maugeais, C.; Doan, K.; South, V.; Amin, D.; Perrone, M. & Rader, D.J. (1999). A novel endothelial-derived lipase that modulates HDL metabolism. *Nature Genetics*. Vol. 21, pp. 424–428.

Jayne, S.; Kerfelec, B.; Foglizzo, E.; Chapus, C. & Crenon, I. (2002). High expression in adult horse of PLRP2 displaying a low phospholipase activity. *Biochimica & Biophysica Acta*. Vol.1594, No. 4, pp. 255–265.

Kalnins, D., Ellis, L.; Corey, M.; Pencharz, P.B., Stewart, C., Tullis, E., Durie, P.R. (2006). Enteric-coated pancreatic enzyme with bicarbonate is equal to standard enteric-coated enzyme in treating malabsorption in cystic fibrosis. *Journal of Pediatric Gastroenterology and Nutrition.* Vol. 42, No. 3, pp. 256-261.

Keller, J. & Layer P. (2005). Human pancreatic exocrine response to nutrients in health and disease. *Gut.* Vol. 54, No. 6, pp.1-28.

Keller, J.; Aghdassi, A.A.; Lerch, M.M.; Mayerle, J.V. & Layer, P. (2009). Tests of pancreatic exocrine function – Clinical significance in pancreatic and non-pancreatic disorders. *Best Practice & Research Clinical Gastroenterology*, Vol. 23, pp. 425–439.

Krishnamurty, D. M.; Rabiee, A.; Jagannath, S. B. & Andersen, D.K. (2009) Delayed release pancrelipase for treatment of pancreatic exocrine insufficiency associated with chronic pancreatitis. *Therapeutics and clinical risk management*, Vol. 5, pp. 507-520.

Kraisinger, M.; Hochhaus, G.; Stecenko, A.; Bowser, E. & Hendeles, L. (1994). Clinical pharmacology of pancreatic enzymes in patients with cystic fibrosis and *in vitro* performance of microencapsulated formulations. *Journal of Clinical Pharmacology*, Vol. 34, No. 2, pp.158–166.

Lankisch, P.G.; Lembcke, B.; Wemken, G. & Creutzfeldt, W. (1986). Functional reserve capacity of the exocrine pancreas. *Digestion*, Vol. 35, No. 3, pp. 175 - 181.

Layer, P.; Go, V.L. & DiMagno, E.P. (1986) Fate of pancreatic enzymes during small intestinal aboral transit in humans.*American Journal of Physiology.* Vol. 251, No. 4, pp. 475- 480.

Layer, P.; vonderOhe, M.R.; Holst, J.J.; Jansen, J.B.; Grandt, D.; Holtmann, J. & Goebell, H. (1997). Altered postprandial motility in chronic pancreatitis: role of malabsorption .*Gastroenterology*, Vol. 112, No.5, pp. 1624- 1634.

Layer, P. & Keller J. (2003). Lipase Supplementation Therapy: Standards, Alternatives, and Perspectives. *Pancreas*, Vol. 26, No. 1, pp. 1-7.

Lee, M.G. & Muallem, S. (2009). Physiology of duct cell secretion, *In : The Pancreas: An Integrated Textbook of Basic Science, Medicine, and Surgery, Second Edition*, (eds H. G. Beger, A. L. Warshaw, M. W. Büchler, R. A. Kozarek, M. M. Lerch, J. P. Neoptolemos, K. Shiratori, D. C. Whitcomb and B. M. Rau), pp.78-90, Blackwell Publishing Ltd., 9781444300123, Oxford, UK.

Levy, E. (2011). Nutrition-related derangements and managements in patients with cystic fibrosis: Robust challenges for preventing the development of co-morbidities. *Clinical Biochemistry*, Vol. 44, pp. 489–490

Löhr, JM, Hummel FM, Pirilis KT, Steinkamp G, Körner A, Henniges F. (2009). Properties of different pancreatin preparations used in pancreatic exocrine insufficiency. *European Journal of Gastroenterology and Hepatology.* Vol. 21, No. 9, pp. 1024-1031.

Lohse, P.; Chahrokh-Zadeh, S. & Seidel, D. (1997). The acid lipase gene family: three enzymes, one highly conserved gene structure. *Journal of Lipid Research.* Vol. 38, pp. 880–891

Lowe, M.E. (1997). Molecular mechanisms of rat and human pancreatic triglyceride lipases. *Journal of Nutrition.* Vol. 127, pp.549–557.

Lowe, M.E. (2000). Properties and function of pancreatic lipase related protein 2. *Biochimie*, Vol. 82, No 11, pp. 997-1004.

Lowe, M.E. (2002). The triglyceride lipases of the pancreas. *Journal of Lipid Research*, Vol. 43, No. 12, pp. 2007–2016.

Lowe, M.E , Rosemblum, J.L. & Strauss, A.W. (1989). Cloning and characterization of human pancreatic lipase cDNA. *Journal of Biological Chemistry.* Vol. 264, pp. 20042-20048.

Lindquist, S. & Hernell, O. (2010). Lipid digestion and absorption in early life: an update. *Current Opinion of Clinical Nutrition Metabolism Care.* Vol. 13, No. 3, pp. 314-320.

Maggio, L.; Bellagamba, M.; Costa, S.; Romagnoli, C.; Rodriguez, M.; Timdahl, K.; Vågerö, M.; Carnielli, V.P. A prospective, randomized, double-blind crossover study comparing rhBSSL (recombinant human Bile Salt Stimulated Lipase) and placebo added to infant formula during one week of treatment in preterm infants born before 32 weeks of gestational age. Abstract EAPS meeting.

Mead, J.R.; Irvine, S.A. & Ramji, D.P. (2002). Lipoprotein lipase: structure, function, regulation, and role in disease. *Journal of Molecular Medecine.* Vol. 80, No. 12, pp. 753– 769.

Meyer, J.H.; Elashoff, J.; Porter-Fink, V., Dressman, J. & Amidon, G.L. (1988). Human postprandial gastric emptying of 1-3-millimeter spheres. *Gastroenterology*, Vol. 94, pp. 1315-1325.

Meyer, J.H. & Lake, R. (1997). Mismatch of duodenal deliveries of dietary fat and pancreatin from enterically coated microspheres. *Pancreas*, Vol. 15, pp. 226–235.

Miled, N.; Canaan, S.; Dupuis, L.; Roussel, A.; Rivière, M.; Carrière, A.; Caro, A.; Cambillau, C. & Verger, R. (2000). Digestive lipases: From three-dimensional structure to physiology. *Biochimie*, Vol. 82, pp. 973–986.

Moreau, H.; Laugier, R.; Gargouri, Y.; Ferrato, F. & Verger, R. (1988). Human pre-duodenal lipase is entirely of gastric fundic origin. *Gastroenterology,*Vol. 95, pp.1221-1226.

Mukherjee, M. (2003).Human digestive and metabolic lipases—a brief review. *Journal of Molecular Catalysis B: Enzymatic.* Vol. 22, pp. 369–376.

Mizushima, M.; Ochi, K.; Ichimura, M.; Kiura K.; Harada, H. & Koide, N. (2004). Pancreatic enzyme supplement improves dysmotility in chronic pancreatitis patients. *Journal of Gastroenterology and Hepatology*, Vol. 19, No. 9, pp. 1005–1009.

Nouri-Sorkhabi, M.H.; Chapman, B.E.; Kuchel, P.W.; Gruca, M.A. & Gaskin, K.J. (2000). Parallel Secretion of Pancreatic Phospholipase A2, Phospholipase A1, Lipase, and Colipase in Children with Exocrine Pancreatic Dysfunction. *Pediatric Research.* Vol. 48, No. 6, pp. 735-740

Nustede, R.; Köhler, H.; Fölsch, U.R. & Schafmayer, A. (1991). Plasma concentrations of neurotensin and CCK in patients with chronic pancreatitis with and without enzyme substitution. *Pancreas.* Vol. 6, No. 3, pp. 260-265.

O'Keefe, S.J.; Cariem, A.K. & Levy, M. (2001).The exacerbation of pancreatic endocrine dysfunction by potent pancreatic exocrine supplements in patients with chronic pancreatitis. *Journal of Clinical Gastroenterology*, Vol. 32, pp. 319–323.

Pasquali, C.; Fogar, P.; Sperti, C.; Bassob, D.; De Paolib, M.; Plebanib, M. & Pedrazzoli, S. (1996). Efficacy of a pancreatic enzyme formulation in the treatment of steatorrhea in patients with chronic pancreatitis. *Current Therapeutic Research & Clinical Experimentation*, Vol. 57, No. 5, pp. 358-365.

Perret, B.; Mabile, L.; Martinez, L.; Tercé, F.; Barbaras, R. & Collet, X. (2002). Hepatic lipase: structure/function relationship, synthesis, and regulation. *Journal of Lipid Research.* Vol. 43, No. 8, pp. 1163-1169.

Reboul, E.; Berton, A.; Moussa, M.; Kreuzer, C.; Crenon, I. & Borel, P. (2006). Pancreatic lipase and pancreatic lipase-related protein 2, but not pancreatic lipase-related protein 1, hydrolyze retinyl palmitate in physiological conditions. *Biochimica & Biophysica Acta*. Vol. 1761, No. 1, pp. 4–10.

Richmond, G.S. & Smith, T.K. (2011). Phospholipases A1. *International Journal of Molecular Sciences*.Vol. 12, pp. 588- 612.

Rogalska, E.; Ransac, S. &Verger, R. (1990). Stereoselectivity of lipases. II. Stereoselective hydrolysis of triglycerides by gastric and pancreatic lipases. *Journal of Biology &*. *Chemistry*.Vol. 265, pp. 20271–20276

Rosenlund, M.L.; Kim, H.K. & Kritchevsky, D. (1974). Essential fatty acids in cystic fibrosis. *Nature*. Vol. 25, pp. 251(5477):719.

Roussel, A.; Canaan, S.; Egloff, M.P.; Rivière, M.; Dupuis, L.; Verger, R. & Cambillau, C. (1999). Crystal structure of human gastric lipase and model of lysosomal acid lipase, two lipolytic enzymes of medical interest. *Journal of Biology and Chemistry*, Vol. 274, No. 24, pp. 16995–7002

Russell, R.M.; Dutta, S.K.; Oaks, E.V.; Rosenberg, I.H. & Giovetti, A.C. (1980). Impairment of folic acid absorption by oral pancreatic extracts. *Digestive Diseases and Sciences*,Vol. 25, No. 5, pp. 369-373.

Sahasrabudhe, A.V.; Solapure, S.M.; Khurana, R.; Suryanarayan, V.; Ravishankar, S.; deSousa, S.M. & Das, G. (1998) Production of Recombinant Human Bile Salt Stimulated Lipase and Its Variant in *Pichia pastoris*. *Protein expression and purification*,Vol. 14, pp. 425–433.

Safdi, M.; Bekal, P.K.; Martin, S.; Saeed, Z.A.; Burton, F.; Toskes, P.P. (2006). The effects of oral pancreatic enzymes (Creon 10 capsule) on steatorrhea: a multicenter, placebo controlled, parallel group trial in subjects with chronic pancreatitis. *Pancreas*, Vol. 33, pp.156–162.

Santamarina-Fojo, S. & Dugi, K.A. (1994). Structure, function and role of lipoprotein lipase in lipoprotein metabolism. *Current Opinion in Lipidology*. Vol. 5, pp. 117–125.

Santamarina-Fojo, S.; Gonza´lez-Navarro, H.; Freeman, L.; Wagner, E. & Nong, Z. (2004). Hepatic Lipase, Lipoprotein Metabolism, and Atherogenesis. *Arteriosclerosis Thrombosis Vascular Biology*. Vol. 24, pp.1750-1754

Schuler, C. & Schuler, E.F. (2008). Composition With a Fungal (Yeast) Lipase and Method For Treating Lipid Malabsorption in Cystic Fibrous as Well as People Suffering From Pancreatic Lipase Insufficiency. *US Patent 20080279839*.

Shama, L.M. & Peterson, R.K.D. (2008).Assessing risk of plant-based pharmaceuticals: I. human dietary exposure. *Human and Ecological Risk Assessment*, Vol. 14, pp. 179-193.

Sias, B.; Ferrato, F.; Grandval, P.; Lafont, D.; Boullanger, P.; De Caro, A.; Leboeuf, B.; Verger, R. & Carriere, F. (2004). Human pancreatic lipase-related protein 2 is a galactolipase. *Biochemistry*, Vol. 43, pp. 10138–10148.

Sims, H.F.; Jennens, M.L. & Lowe, M.E. (1993). The human pancreatic lipase-encoding gene: structure and conservation of an Alu sequence in the lipase gene family. *Gene*, Vol. 131, pp. 281–285.

Sikkens, E.C.M.; Cahen, D.L.; Kuipers, E.J. & Bruno, M.J. (2010). Pancreatic enzyme replacement therapy in chronic pancreatitis. *Best practice research Clinical gastroenterology,*Vol. 24, No. 3, pp. 337-347.

Slaff, J.; Jacobson, D.; Tillman, C.R.; Curington, C. & Toskes, P. (1984). Protease-specific suppression of pancreatic exocrine secretion. *Gastroenterology,* Vol. 87, pp. 44–52.

Smyth, R.L.; Smyth, A.R.; Lloyd, D.A.; vanVelzen, D. & Heaf D.P. (1994). Strictures of a scending colon in cystic fibrosis and high-strength pancreatic enzymes. *The Lancet,* Vol. 343, No. 8889, pp. 85- 86.

Smyth, R.L.; O'Hea, U.; Burrows, E.; Ashby, D.; Lewis, P. & Dodge, J.A. (1995). Fibrosing colonopathy in cystic fibrosis: results of a case-control study. *The Lancet,* Vol. 346, No. 8985, pp.1247-1251.

Stein, J.; Jung, M.; Sziegoleit, A.; Zeuzem, S.; Caspary, W.F. & Lembcke, B. (1996). Immunoreactive elastase I: clinical evaluation of a new noninvasive test of pancreatic function. *Clinical Chemistry,* Vol. 42, pp. 222–226.

Stern, R.C.; Eisenberg, J.D.; Wagener, J.S.; Ahrens, R.; Rock, M.; doPico, G.; Orenstein, D.M. (2000). A comparison of the efficacy and tolerance of pancrelipase and placebo in the treatment of steatorrhea in cystic fibrosis patients with clinical exocrine pancreatic insufficiency. *The American Journal of Gastroenterology.* Vol. 95, No. 8, pp. 1932-1938.

Swan, J.S.; Hoffman, M.M.; Lord, M.K. & Poechmann, J.L. (1992).Two forms of human milk bile-salt-stimulated lipase. *Biochemistry Journal,* Vol. 283, No. 1, pp. 119 –122.

Swedish Orphan Biovitrum website www. sobi.com

Taylor, C.J. (2002). Fibrosing colonopathy unrelated to pancreatic enzyme supplementation. *Journal of Pediatric Gastroenterology and Nutrition,* Vol. 35, No. 3, pp. 268-269.

Thirstrup, K.; Verger, R. & Carrière, F. (1994). Evidence for a pancreatic lipase subfamily with new kinetic properties. *Biochemistry,* Vol. 33, No. 10, pp. 2748–2756.

Trapnell, B.C.; Maguiness, K.; Graff, G.R., Boyd, D.; Beckmann, K. & Caras, S. (2009). Efficacy and safety of Creon® 24,000 in subjects with exocrine pancreatic insufficiency due to cystic fibrosis. *Journal of Cystic Fibrosis,* doi:10.1016/j.jcf.2009.08.008.

Trolli, P.A.; Conwell, D.L.; Zuccaro, G. Jr (2001). Pancreatic enzyme therapy and nutritional status of outpatients with chronic pancreatitis. Gastroenterology Nursing, Vol. 24, No. 2, pp. 84 - 87.

Turki, S.; Mrabet, G.; Jabloun Z.; Destain, J.; Thonart, P. & Kallel, H. (2010a). A highly stable *Yarrowia lipolytica* lipase formulation for the treatment of pancreatic insufficiency. *Biotechnology and Applied Biochemistry,* Vol. 57, No. 4, 134 -149.

Turki, S.; Jabloun, Z.; Mrabet, G.; Marouani, A.; Thonart, P.; Diouani, M.F.; Ben Abdallah, F.; Amra A.; Rejeb, A. & Kallel, H. (2010 b). Preliminary safety assessment of Yarrowia lipolytica extracellular lipase: Results of acute and 28-day repeated dose oral toxicity studies in rats. *Food and Chemical Toxicology,* Vol. 48, pp. 2393-2400.

U.S. Food and Drug Administration. (2004). FDA requires pancreatic extract manufacturers to submit marketing applications. FDA News. *http://www. fda.gov/bbs/topics/news/2004/NEW01058.html.* Published April 27, 2004. Accessed 8 August 2008

U.S. Food and Drug Administration (2006). Center for Drug Evaluation and Research. Guidance for Industry: Exocrine Pancreatic Insufficiency Drug Products— Submitting NDAs. *http://www.fda.gov/cder/guidance/6275fnl.htm*. Published April 13, 2006. Accessed March 9 2009.

Verheij, M.H.; Westerman, J.; Sternby, B. & de Haas, G.H. (1983). The complete primary structure of phospholipase A2 from human pancreas. *Biochimica & Biophysica Acta*. Vol. 747, No. 1-2, pp. 93–99.

Vuoristo, M.; Vaananen, H.; Miettinen, T.A. (1992). Cholesterol malabsorption in pancreatic insufficiency: effects of enzyme substitution. *Gastroenterology*. Vol. 102, pp. 647–655.

Walker-Smith, J.; Barnard, J.; Bhutta, Z.; Heubi, J.; Reeves, Z. & Schmitz, J. (2002). Chronic Diarrhea and Malabsorption (Including Short Gut Syndrome): Working Group Report of the First World Congress of Pediatric Gastroenterology, Hepatology, and Nutrition. *Journal of Pediatric Gastroenterology and Nutrition*,Vol 35, No. 2, pp. 98–105.

Walters, M.P. & Littlewood, J.M. (1996). Pancreatin preparations used in the treatment of cystic fibrosis-lipase content and in vitro release. *Alimentary Pharmacology & Therapeutics*. Vol. 10, No. 3, pp. 433-440.

Whitcomb, D.C. & Lowe, M.E (2007).Human pancreatic digestive enzymes. *Digestive Diseases & Sciences*, Vol. 52, No. 1, pp. 1-17.

Winkler, F.K.; D'Arcy, A. & Hunziker, W. (1990). Structure of Human pancreatic lipase. *Nature*, Vol. 343, pp.771-774.

Wion, K.L.; Kirchgessner, T.G.; Lusis, A.J.; Schotz, M.C. & Lawn, R.M. (1987). Human lipoprotein lipase complementary DNA sequence. *Science*, Vol. 235, pp. 1638–1641.

Wolle, J.; Jansen, H.; Smith, L.C. & Chan, L. (1993). Functional role of N-linked glycosylation in human hepatic lipase: asparagine- 56 is important for both enzyme activity and secretion. *Journal of Lipid Research*. Vol. 34, pp. 2169–2176.

Wooldridge, J.L.; Heubi, J.E.; Amaro-Galvez, R.; Boas, S.R.; Blake, K.V.; Nasr, S.Z.; Chatfield, B.; McColley, S.A.; Woo, M.S.; Hardy, K.A.; Kravitz, R.M.; Straforini, C.; Anelli, M. & Lee, C. (2010). EUR-1008 pancreatic enzyme replacement is safe and effective in patients with cystic fibrosis and pancreatic insufficiency. *Journal of Cystic Fibrosis*. Vol. 8, No. -, pp. 405- 417.

Whitcomb, D.C.; Lehman, G.A.; Vasileva, G.; Malecka-Panas, E.; Gubergrits, N.; Shen, Y.; Sander-Struckmeier, S. & Caras S. (2009). Pancrelipase Delayed-Release Capsules (CREON) for Exocrine Pancreatic Insufficiency due to Chronic Pancreatitis or Pancreatic Surgery: A Double-Blind Randomized Trial. *The American Journal of Gastroenterology*, Vol. 105, pp. 2276-2286.

Whitcomb, D.C. & Lowe, M.E. (2007). Human pancreatic digestive enzymes. *Digestive diseases & Sciences*. Vol. 52, N°. 1, pp. 1-17

Yasuda, T.; Ishida, T. & Rader, D.J. (2010). Update on the Role of Endothelial Lipase in High-Density Lipoprotein Metabolism, Reverse Cholesterol Transport, and Atherosclerosis. *Circulation Journal*, Vol. 74, pp. 2263 – 2270.

Zentler-Munro, P.L.; Fitzpatrick, W.J.; Batten, J.C. & Northfield, T.C. (1984). Effect of intrajejunal acidity on aqueous phase bile acid and lipid concentrations in pancreatic steatorrhoea due to cystic fibrosis. *Gut*. Vol.25, No. 5, pp. 500- 507.

14

Pharmacology of Traditional Herbal Medicines and Their Active Principles Used in the Treatment of Peptic Ulcer, Diarrhoea and Inflammatory Bowel Disease

Bhavani Prasad Kota[1], Aik Wei Teoh[2] and Basil D. Roufogalis[1]
[1]University of Sydney
[2]Ferngrove Pharmaceuticals
Australia

1. Introduction

The endocrine, exocrine and paracrine secretions of the gastrointestinal (GI) tract play a pivotal role in the digestion and absorption of food and orally administered drugs. The secretion of mucus by mucus-secreting cells protects the erosion of the gastric mucosa from the highly acidic gastric juice. The secretion of hydrochloric acid from parietal cells is regulated by acetylcholine, histamine and gastrin. Disturbances in secretory functions of the gastrointestinal tract can lead to several GI complications. Conventional therapies employ a range of drugs that have been pharmacologically well characterised. While these drug molecules are proven to be beneficial, the adverse effects and drug-drug interactions highlight the need for better treatment modalities for GI tract disorders.

Since ancient times, herbal medicines have been traditionally used to treat several diseases. The gastroprotective properties of these herbs and their active constituents have been experimentally demonstrated (Al Mofleh, 2010). Asian traditional medicine systems have identified several herbs and spices to treat GI tract disorders (Langmead & Rampton, 2006; Sengupta et al., 2004). In support of these traditional claims, several preclinical and clinical studies have provided the scientific basis for the effectiveness of herbal extracts (e.g. *Glycyrrhiza glabra*) and their active constituents (e.g. flavonoids) in treating GI tract disorders (Borrelli & Izzo, 2000). The discovery and development of anti-ulcer agents such as carbenoxolone from *Glycyrrhiza glabra* and gefarnate from cabbage further highlight the presence of pharmacologically active components in herbal extracts and suggests their use as an alternative therapy to treat GI tract disorders.

The effectiveness and the mechanisms of action of crude herbal extracts vary according the composition of their chemical constituents. Herbal medicine seems to fill this gap, especially when employing high manufacturing standardised forms of herbal medicine with regard to the quality and quantity of ingredients (Suzuki et al., 2009). In addition, well characterised herbal formulations may lead to the production of reliable clinical data on efficacy and safety. As several studies have shown that herbal medicines may produce adverse reactions and herb-drug interactions, the common assumption that 'herbal products are natural, they are safe' is no longer valid. Safety and quality data of herbal medicines should be made available to medical practitioners and other healthcare professionals to avoid these unwanted effects.

Several plants have been used by traditional healers around the world to treat various gastrointestinal tract diseases. Centuries ago the reliance on nature to cure human ailments was developed by great efforts of dedicated professionals by keen observation and trial and error method. This important knowledge is updated constantly and passed from generations to generations. Today traditional healing systems play important roles in several parts of the world, especially where modern pharmaceuticals are less accessible. Modern scientific research methods are invaluable to support traditional claims and also to develop traditional remedies as a viable alternative to mainstream pharmaceuticals. In recent years, a number of research papers have been published on herbal medicines to provide the experimental evidence for their traditional claims. Given the multitude of these research publications, it is not possible to cover all of them. In this chapter, we only attempted to provide the experimental (animal and human studies) evidence for the plants that have been traditionally used to treat most notable gastrointestinal diseases, namely, peptic ulcer, diarrhoea and inflammatory bowel syndrome.

2. Peptic ulcer

2.1 Animal models of gastric ulcer

Rats are commonly used animals to induce ulcers that resemble the human condition by various noxious chemical agents. NSAIDs (eg. Indomethacin and Aspirin) cause gastrointestinal ulceration, due to their ability to suppress cytoprotective prostaglandin synthesis (Wallace, 2001). The NSAIDS-induced ulcer model is important to identify mechanisms of action of plants that maintain the gastric mucosa integrity by balancing the toxic effects of NSAIDs. The widely used ethanol-induced gastric ulcer model is suitable to study gastric protective and free radical scavenging properties of plants. Stress induced gastric lesions in rats are useful to study gastric mucosal barrier strengthening properties (eg. increased mucus production) of potential plant extracts and their actives. Pylorus ligation in rats helps to screen plants for their antisecretory properties.

2.2 Plants used in the treatment of peptic ulcer

- *Diodia sarmentosa* (Rubiaceae), *Cassia nigricans* (Celsapinaceae), *Ficus exasperate* (Moraceae) and *Synclisia scabrida* (Menispermaceae) are the most popularly used antiulcer recipes in Nigeria. In vivo studies in mice and rats revealed their anti-ulcer activities by decreasing the ulcer index in aspirin-induced ulcerogenesis, delayed intestinal transit, increased pH, and decreased volume and acidity of gastric secretion (Akah et al., 1998).
- *Eruca sativa,* commonly known as Rocket, *is* a commonly used leaf vegetable in Unani, Ayurveda and Arab traditional medicine systems. Rocket is shown to possess significant anti-secretory, anti-ulcer and cytoprotective properties in rats (Alqasoumi et al., 2009). Pretreatment with ethanolic extract of Rocket attenuated gastric ulceration induced by ethanol, indomethacin and hypothermic stress. In pylorus ligated rats, Rocket dose-dependently reduced gastric acid secretion. In addition, the extract

significantly replenished gut wall mucous and reduced malondialdehyde (an indicator of lipid peroxidation) levels in ethanol treated rats. Gastroprotective effects of Rocket are attributed to the presence of flavonoids, sterols and triterpines.

- *Turnera ulmifolia* or 'chanana' (Turneraceae) is a small herb with wide geographical distribution ranging from Guyana to the North Eastern region of Brazil. It is a widely used folk medicine for its anti-inflammatory properties. The hydroalcoholic extract of *T. ulmifolia* inhibited gastric lesions induced by pylorus ligature, by indomethacin and by ethanol, but stress mediated lesions remained unaffected. As histamine plays a role in ulcerogenesis in pylorus ligation, it was postulated by the study authors that *T. ulmifolia* exerts gastroprotective actions by inhibiting histamine. The inhibition of gastric ulcers induced by indomethacin and ethanol indicate that gastroprotective effects of *T. ulmifolia* could be due to an enhancement of mucosal defensive factors such as gastric mucus (Antônio & Souza Brito, 1998).

- *Dodonaea viscosa* is a stiff bushy plant. Tribes who reside in the forest regions of South India (Kerala) use leaves of this plant for headaches and backaches. The hexane extract of *Dodonaea viscosa* dose dependently inhibited ethanol and indomethacin induced gastric lesions. Gastric secretion studies showed significant decrease of total acid in gastric juice (Arun & Asha, 2008). Furthermore, it decreased total acid content and increased gastric glutathione levels in ethanol and indomethacin treated rats.

- *Azadirachta indica* is a native tree to the Indian subcontinent. To the Indian it is commonly known as Neem and regarded as a 'village dispensary' due its multiple therapeutic properties. It has been extensively used in Ayurveda, Siddha, Unani and other local Indian folklore medicine systems (Brahmachari, 2004). Standardized aqueous extract of Neem exhibited remarkable anti-ulcer activity in restraint-cold stress and indomethacin induced gastric ulcers in rats. Animal studies suggest that the major gastroprotective effect of Neem bark extract against ulcer is mediated through inhibition of acid secretion by H+-K+-ATPase and prevention of oxidative damage (Bandyopadhyay et al., 2002).

- The aqueous extract of Neem bark when administered for 10 days at 30 mg dose twice daily significantly inhibited gastric acid secretion in patients with chronic gastric acid problem. The bark extract completely healed the duodenal ulcers at the dose of 30-60 mg twice daily for 10 weeks (Bandyopadhyay et al., 2004). Some important blood parameters for organ toxicity such as sugar, urea, creatinine, serum glutamate oxaloacetate transaminase, serum glutamate pyruvate transaminase, albumin, globulin, hemoglobin levels and erythrocyte sedimentation rate remained unaffected upon Neem exposure.

- *Pteleopsis suberosa* is traditionally used in Mali for the treatment of gastric ulcers. The aqueous extract of *P. suberosa* exhibited protective effects on gastric mucosa in ethanol and indomethacin treated rats (De Pasquale et al., 1995). It has also been shown that *Pteleopsis suberosa* decoction containing triterpenoid saponins and tannins is effective against *Helicobacter pylori* (Germano` et al., 1998).

- *Calligonum comosum* is a shrub distributed throughout Arabia and growing in sandy deserts. It is used by the local healers to treat stomach ailments. Pre-treatment with the 10% ethanolic extract displayed a significant and dose-dependent inhibition of acute gastric ulcers induced by NSAIDs (phenylbutazone and indomethacin) and necrotic agents (0.2 N NaOH and 80% ethanol) (Liu et al., 2001).

- *Solanum torvum*, a small tree, is widely used in African folk medicine to treat various diseases including gastric ulcer (Noumi et al., 2000). Aqueous and methanolic extracts from leaves of Solanum torvum produced significant anti-ulcer activity in HCl/ethanol, indomethacin, pylorus ligation and cold-restraint stress induced gastric ulcers in rats. The authors proposed that the cytoprotective activity of extracts could be due to strengthening of the mucosal barrier through the increase of mucus production (Nguelefack et al., 2008).

- *Tetrapleura tetraptera* and *Guibourtia ehie* Leonard are native trees to Ghana. The Ghanaian ethnomedical system employs these plant extracts in the management of stomach ulcers. In support of their traditional use, aqueous extracts of the barks of *Tet. Tetraprera* and *G. ethie* dose dependently inhibited HCl/ethanol induced gastric ulcers (Noamesi et al., 1994).

- *Glycyrrhiza glabra* is a legume native to southern Europe and parts of Asia. It is a well-known folk medicine for gastric ulcer (Aly et al., 2004). Gastric mucosal damage induced by NSAIDs is markedly reduced by *G. glabra* (Aly et al., 2004). Clinical data on *Gycrrhiza glabra* is inconsistent. In a double-blind clinical trial, administration of deglycyrrhizinized liquorice thrice daily at the dose of 760 mg for four weeks significantly accelerated the healing of gastric ulcer. In contrast, a cross over study at the same dose and treatment time reported no improvement in ulcer healing (Engqvist et al., 1973). A similar result was shown in a double-blind placebo- control study with administration of deglycyrrhizinized liquorice for one month at the dose of 380 mg thrice daily (Feldman et al., 1971). No side effects are reported in subjects who received deglycyrrhizinized liquorice extract in these studies.

Plant	Scientific Evidence	Active Constituent(s)	Reference
Diodia sarmentosa	Pre-clinical	Unknown	Akah et al
Cassia nigricans	Pre-clinical	Flavonoids	Akah et al
Ficus exasperate	Pre-clinical	Gallic acid & ellagic acid	Akah et al ; Sirisha et al
Synclisia scabrida	Pre-clinical	Alkaloids & flavonoids	Akah et al ; Orisakwe et al ; Obi et al
Eruca sativa	Pre-clinical	Flavonoids, sterols & triterpines	Alqasoumi et al
Turnera ulmifolia	Pre-clinical	Flavonoids	Antônio et al
Dodonaea viscosa	Pre-clinical	Flavonoids, saponins, bitter principles & phenols	Arun et al
Azadirachta indica	Pre-clinical & clinical	Phenolic glycoside	Bandyopadhyay et al
Pteleopsis suberosa	Pre-clinical	Triterpenoid saponins & tannins	De Pasquale et al ; Germanò et al
Calligonum comosum	Pre-clinical	Unknown	Liu et al
Solanum torvum		Flavonoids, sterols & triterpenes	Nguelefack et al
Tetrapleura tetraptera	Pre-clinical	Unknown	Noamesi et al
Guibourtia ehie	Pre-clinical	Unknown	Noamesi et al
Glycyrrhiza glabra	Pre-clinical & clinical	Unknown	Aly et al, Rees et al ; Engqvist et al; Feldman et al

Table 1. Plants and their active constituents with anti-ulcer activity

3. Diarrhoea

3.1 Experimental models

Rodents are commonly used to induce experimental diarrhea and to study mechanisms of action of plants and their active principles. Castor oil, Prostaglandin E2 (PG-E2) and heat-labile enterotoxin are commonly used agents to induce diarrhea in animals. The diarrhoeal effect of castor oil is mediated through ricinoleic acid which causes irritation and inflammation of intestinal mucosa, and consequesntly leads to the stimulation of intestinal motility and increased secretion of fluid and electrolytes. This model is ideal to study the antisecretory and antimotility potential of medicinal plants. Prostaglandin E2 causes enteropooling by stimulating fluid secretion and increasing propulsive activity in the colon (Pierre et al., 1991). Heat-labile enterotoxin (LT) is the virulent factor of *Escherichia coli* and diarrhea by accumulation of salt and water in the intestinal lumen (Spangler., 1992). Therefore, the LT-induced diarroheal model is suitable to study inhibitory effects of plant extracts on bacterial toxins. In addition, the charcoal meal test and charcoal-gum acacia-induced hyperperistalsis in animals are helpful to identity the effect of potential medicinal plants on intestinal motility.

3.2 Plants tested for antidiarrheal activity in animal models of diarrhoea

- *Ficus bengalensis, Eugenia jambolana, Ficus racemosa* and *Leucas lavandulaefolia* are commonly used folk medicine to treat diarrhoea by the people who live in Khatra region of West Bengal, India. Ethanolic exracts of *Ficus bengalensis* (hanging roots), *Eugenia jambolana* (bark), *Ficus racemosa* (bark) and *Leucas lavandulaefolia* (aerial parts) significantly inhibited castor oil induced diarrhoea and PGE2 induced enteropooling in rats. In addition, these extracts also showed a significant reduction in gastrointestinal motility in charcoal meal tests in rats (Mukherjee et al., 1997).
- *Geranium mexicanum* plant is a commonly used medicinal plant in Traditional Mexican Medicine for the treatment of diarrhoea. Methanolic extract of *Geranium mexicanum* (roots) remarkably inhibited charcoal–gum acacia-induced hyperperistalsis in rats. However the authors suggested that this medicinal plant should be used with care to avoid toxic effects (Clazada et al., 2009).
- *Galla chinensis and Chaenomeles speciosa* have been traditionally used in China to treat gastrointestinal disorders. These plant extracts significantly inhibited heat-labile enterotoxin-induced diarrhoea in the mouse (Chen et al., 2006, Chen et al., 2007).
- *Satureja hortensis* is an annual herb that is traditionally used in Iran for treating stomach and intestinal disorders. Essential oil isolated from *S. hortensis* exhibited antispasmodic activity in isolated rat ileum. In addition, it also inhibited castor oil-induced diarrhea in mice (Hajhashemi et al., 1999).
- *Thespesia populnea*, a large tree found in tropical regions and coastal forests of India, is traditionally used in India to treat several disorders including diarrhea and dysentery. Residue fraction of aqueous extract of *T. populnea* significantly inhibited castor oil and prostaglandin E2 (PGE$_2$)-induced diarrhea induced diarrhea in rats. In addition, it also inhibited intestinal motility in the charcoal meal test (Viswanatha et al., 2011).
- *Mitragyna speciosa* is an indigenous tree to Thailand, where it is commonly called kratom. In folk medicine, it is often used to treat diarrhea. Methanolic extract of *M. speciosa* dose dependently inhibited castor oil-induced diarrhea and intestinal transit in rats (Chittrakarn et al., 2008).

- *Punica granatum* is a deciduous shrub or small tree that is native to the Himalayas in north Pakistan and Northern India. Bark, rind of the fruit and seeds of this plant are used in folk medicine to treat diarrhea. Methanol extract of seeds of *P. granatum* dose dependently reduced castor oil induced diarrhea. It also significantly inhibited gastrointestinal motility and PGE_2 mediated enteropooling in rats (Das et al., 1999).

Plant	Scientific Evidence	Active Constituent(s)	Reference
Ficus bengalensis	Pre-clinical	Tannin	Mukherjee et al
Eugenia jambolana	Pre-clinical	Tannin	Mukherjee et al
Ficus racemosa	Pre-clinical	Tannin	Mukherjee et al
Leucas lavandulaefolia	Pre-clinical	Tannin	Mukherjee et al
Geranium mexicanum	Pre-clinical	(-)-epicatechin, tyramine	Calzada et al
Galla chinensis	Pre-clinical	Gallic acid	Chen et al
Chaenomeles speciosa	Pre-clinical	Oleanolic acid, ursolic acid & betulinic acid	Chen et al
Satureja hortensis	Pre-clinical	Carvacrol	Hajhashemi et al
Thespesia populnea	Pre-clinical	Unknown	Viswanatha et al
Mitragyna speciosa	Pre-clinical	Mitragynine & other alkaloids	Chittrakarn et al
Punica granatum	Pre-clinical	Tannin	Das et al

Table 2. Plants and their active constituent(s) with anti-diarrheal activity

4. Inflammatory Bowel Diseases (IBD)

4.1 Animal models of IBD

In IBD oxidative stress mediates disease progression by disrupting epithelial cell integrity. Acetic acid-induced colitis is helpful to screen herbs which can inhibit cytotoxic effects of reactive oxygen species (ROS). Dextran sulphate sodium (DSS)-induced colitis is also a frequently used animal colitis model in ethnopharmacological studies. This model is useful to test the effect of herbs on inflammatory cytokines mediated cellular injury (Dieleman et al., 1998). The transgenic rat model (HLA-B27) with overt chronic gastrointestinal tract inflammation also serves to screen medicinal herbs to treat IBD.

- *Zingiber officinale* is traditionally used to treat inflammatory gastrointestinal disorders. Ethanolic extract of dried rhizomes of ginger displayed protective effects against acetic acid-induced ulcerative colitis in rats (El-Abhar et al., 2008).
- *Cordia dichotoma* is a deciduous tree with many medicinal uses in Ayurveda. Traditionally bark of the plant is reported for the treatment of ulcerative colitis. Methanolic extract of C. Dichotoma improved lesions and reduced colonic myeloperoxidase (MPO) and malondialdehyde (MDA) in acetic acid induced UC in male swiss mice (Ganjare et al., 2011).
- *Patrinia scabiosaefolia* is a commonly used herbal medicine in Korea. It is used traditionally to treat colonic inflammations. Methanolic extract of P. Scabiosaefolia significantly attenuated dextran sulfate sodium induced colitis in mice. In addition, it

also suppressed colonic MPO accumulation and pro-inflammatory mediators (TNFα, IL-1, IL-6 and nitric oxide) (Cho et al., 2011).

- *Vitex negundo* is a shrub that grows in Southeast Asia. Traditionally its roots are used in the treatment of ulcerative colitis in India. Ethanolic extract of *V. negrundo* significantly inhibited acetic acid ulcerative colitis and reduced colonic MPO and MDA levels in mice (Zaware et al., 2011).

- *Pistacia lentiscus* is a dioecious shrub that grows in the Mediterranean region. Oleogum resin from *P. Lentiscus* is used in traditional Iranian medicine to treat IBD. Treatment with oleogum resin from *P. Lentiscus* improved the symptoms of dextran sulfate sodium (DSS) induced colitis in mice (Kim & Neophytou, 2009). A pilot study conducted in mild to moderate Crohn's disease patients demonstrated that mastic (resin) from *P. Lentiscus* significantly reduced disease activity index, plasma IL-6 and C-reactive protein (Kaliora et al., 2007a) and TNFα in peripheral blood mononuclear cells (Kaliora et al., 2007b). In addition, total antioxidant potential was significantly increased. No side effects are observed in mastic treated patients (Kaliora et al., 2007a). A double-blind clinical trial in patients with duodenal ulcers exhibited symptomatic relief in 80% patients on mastic and 50% patients on placebo, while endoscopically proven healing occurred in 70% patients on mastic (Al-Habbal et al., 1984).

- *Plantago ovata* is a well-known medicinal plant in the treatment of IBD. *P. ovate* seeds ameliorated the development of colonic inflammation in transgenic rats as evidenced by an improvement of intestinal cytoarchitecture, significant decrease in some of the pro-inflammatory mediators and higher production of short-chain fatty acids (Rodríguez-Cabezas et al., 2003). An open label, parallel-group, multicenter, randomized clinical trial in patients with ulcerative colitis concluded that *Plantago ovata* seeds (dietary fiber) might be as effective as mesalamine to maintain remission in ulcerative colitis (Ferna´ndez-Ban~ ares et al., 1999).

- *Boswellia serrata*, a tree which grows in the hilly areas of India, is an efficacious remedy for IBD in traditional Iranian medicine and also it has been used in the Ayurvedic medicine for the treatment of inflammatory diseases. Despite its traditional claims, *Boswellia* extracts are ineffective in ameliorating colitis in DSS-induced colitis in mice (Kiela et al., 2004). In contrast to animal studies, a double-blind, randomized, placebo-controlled, multicenter trial in colitis patients showed higher remission in Boswellia serrata extract treated group than in the pacebo group (Madisch et al., 2007). However, a recent double-blind, placebo-controlled, randomized, parallel study in patients with Crohn's disease has shown no difference between the Boswellia treated group and control group in disease remission (Holtmeier et al., 2011).

5. Quality, efficacy and safety of herbal medicines

5.1 Quality

The quality of herbal medicines is important to ensure their safe use and efficacy. In contrast to well characterized conventional medicine, assurance of the quality of herbal medicine is a major concern. The problems associated with the herbal products include deliberate or accidental inclusion of prohibited or restricted ingredients, substitution or adulteration of herbal materials, contamination with toxic substances and differences between labelled and actual contents (Barnes et al., 2nd ed). However, increased consumer awareness and

Plant	Scientific Evidence	Chemical Constituents	Reference
Zingiber officinale	Pre-clinical	Gingerols	El-Abhar et al ; Minaiyan et al
Cordia dichotoma	Pre-clinical	Apigenin	Ganjare et al
Patrinia scabiosaefolia	Pre-clinical	Oleanonic acid, oleanolic acid & ursolic acid	Cho et al
Vitex negundo	Pre-clinical	Unknown	Zaware et al
Pistacia lentiscus	Pre-clinical & clinical	Oleanolic acid	Kim et al; Kaliora et al; Al-Habbal
Plantago ovata	Pre-clinical & clinical	Unknown	Rodriguez-Cabezas et al ; Fernandez-Banares et al
Boswellia serrata	Pre-clinical & clinical	Boswellia acids	Kiela et al ; Madisch et al ; Holtmeier et al

Table 3. Plants and their active constituents for treatment of ulcerative colitis/IBD

regulatory agencies' strict guidelines on the quality and stability of herbal products has led to significant improvements in the quality control of herbal medicines. Recently the herbal manufacturing industry has focused on improving its quality assurance and quality control mechanisms to guard against the frequent episodes of substandard quality and possible adulterations. Use of high-performance liquid chromatograms, thin-layer chromatography, atomic absorption spectroscopy, gas chromatography and where necessary more sophisticated techniques such as NMR and LC/MS has now become common in complementary medicines manufacturing industries to ensure the quality of plant materials and final product (Rosenbloom et al., 2011). The emphasis on good manufacturing practice has steadily increased over years. In addition, new regulatory laws are now in place on product stability to support its shelf life. With the steady progress on different herbal quality control fronts, it is now possible to apply almost the same set of quality standards as for conventional medicines. As most of the traditional herbs listed in this chapter are not commercially manufactured, the data on the quality of these plant medicines is scarce.

5.2 Efficacy

Herbal medicines have a long history of traditional use. However, from today's stand point, traditional claims need to be verified. A well-designed randomized controlled trial is essential to determine the efficacy and safety of herbal medicines. The use of standardized herbal extracts in clinical trials is important to obtain reproducible data on the efficacy and safety of herbal medicines. Standardization of herbal extracts has become a common practice in phytomedicines. It allows the establishment of reproducible pharmaceutical quality by comparing a product with established reference substances and by defining the specific quantity of one or several compounds. As the herbs are of natural origin, their chemical composition is affected by several factors (climate, growing conditions, time of harvesting, storage conditions and processing). Therefore, the use of standardized herbal extracts in preclinical and clinical research is helpful to develop evidence based traditional therapies. Although rigorous clinical investigations are lacking at present for many herbs used in GIT disorders, there is a vast literature on the *in vitro* and *in vivo* pharmacological effects of medicinal plants. These pre-clinical observations provide a rationale for further investigation of such plants.

5.3 Safety

The positive attitude towards herbal medicines is based on the testimony that herbs have been used since antiquity and the belief that they have the advantage of being 'natural' rather than 'synthetic'. Traditional healing systems employed herbal medicines for the symptomatic management of diseases. However, these herbs are now being used extensively for health promotion and disease prevention not only in underdeveloped and developing nations, but also increasingly in developed nations. As little is known regarding adverse effects of herbal medicines and their frequencies, the chronic exposure of these herbal ingredients may pose health risks. In particular, when herbs are extracted and purified, their toxicity might be increased due to increased concentration of potential toxic compounds. Therefore, the common assumption that herbal medicines are by inference 'safe' may not be valid by today's health standards.

Generally, traditional herbal medicines lack the following pharmacological data in humans:

- pharmacologically active chemical constituents and their metabolites
- mechanisms of action of active constituents/whole extract
- pharmacokinetics
- toxicology
- adverse effects and their frequencies
- drug–herb and food–herb interactions
- use in vulnerable individuals: children, elderly, individuals with renal or hepatic disease, gender effects, individuals with a different genetic profile
- contraindications

Phytochemical and pharmacological (preclinical and clinical) studies are important to address the above issues. The majority of the herbs mentioned in this chapter are tested only in animals. The main focus of these studies has been determining the efficacy of herbal extracts to support their traditional claims. However, it is a common procedure in these animal studies to measure toxic dose of herbal extracts. These toxicological studies are important to provide in vivo data in a whole animal situation on the dose and adverse effects of herbal extracts which may be relevant when tested in humans. None of these studies have reported any major adverse events in the experimental models of various GI disorders.

6. Conclusion

The use of plants in treating diseases is a very old human tradition. This knowledge, derived from observations and experiences, has been handed over from generation to generation verbally and also in the form of ancient texts. Medicinal plants are the foundations for modern therapeutic agents. Herbal medicines are an important part of the health care system in many developing countries. The use of herbal medicines, as health promoting agents, in developed countries has also increased and this trend is continuing. Healthcare professionals need to be aware of the pharmacology of these herbal medicines in order to provide well informed advice to patients. The traditional herbal medicines field is very vast. In this chapter we attempted to provide scientific evidence for the herbs with historical use in three major GIT disorders namely: peptic ulcer, diarrhoea and IBD. Researchers successfully reproduced these human disorders in animals by employing a range of chemical agents and scientific procedures. In some cases, these models not only have supported the traditional claims, but also provided important information on the mechanism of action of the plant extracts and in some cases their components. The majority of these preclinical studies established the scientific evidence to traditional herbal medicines. Unfortunately, very few clinical trials are conducted to translate animal data into humans. As clinical trials are important to furnish efficacy and safety data, the lack of clinical data has become the main impediment in developing traditional herbal remedies into mainstream medicines. Recent progress in the quality control of herbal products is very promising in gaining consumer confidence and promoting consideration of herbal medicines as complementary and in some cases alternative approaches to conventional therapies. Medicinal plants listed in this chapter have the potential to treat peptic ulcer, diarrhoea and IBD. Additional studies on quality, efficacy and safety in animals and humans will be required to integrate them in mainstream medicine.

7. References

Al Mofleh, IA. (2010). Spices, herbal xenobiotics and the stomach: friends or foes. *World journal of gastroenterology*, Vol.16, No.22 (June 2010), pp. 2710-2719. ISSN 1007-9327

Al-Habbal, MJ.; Al-Habbal, Z. & Huwez, FU. (1984). A double-blind controlled clinical trial of mastic and placebo in the treatment of duodenal ulcer. *Clinical and experimental pharmacology & physiology*, Vol.11, No.5 (September 1984), pp. 541-544. ISSN 0305-1870

Akah, PA.; Orisakwe, OE.; Gamaniel, KS. & Shittu, A. (1998). Evaluation of Nigerian traditional medicines: II. Effects of some Nigerian folk remedies on peptic ulcer. *Journal of ethnopharmacology*, Vol. 62, No. 2 (September 1998), pp. 123-127. ISSN 0378-8741

Alqasoumi, S.; Al-Sohaibani, M.; Al-Howiriny, T.; Al-Yahya, M. & Rafatullah, S. (2009). Rocket "*Eruca sativa*": a salad herb with potential gastric anti-ulcer activity. *World journal of gastroenterology*, Vol.15, No.16 (April 2009), pp. 1958-1965. ISSN 1007-9327

Aly, AM.; Al-Alousi, L. & Salem, HA. (2005). Licorice: a possible anti-inflammatory and anti-ulcer drug. *AAPS PharmSciTech*, Vol.6, No.1 (September 2005), pp. E74-82. ISSN 1530-9932

Antônio, MA. & Souza Brito, AR. (1998). Oral anti-inflammatory and anti-ulcerogenic activities of a hydroalcoholic extract and partitioned fractions of *Turnera ulmifolia* (Turneraceae). *Journal of ethnopharmacology*, Vol. 61, No.3 (July 1998), pp. 215-228. ISSN 0378-8741

Arun, M. & Asha, VV. (2008). Gastroprotective effect of *Dodonaea viscosa* on various experimental ulcer models. *Journal of ethnopharmacology*, Vol.118, No.3 (August 2008), pp. 460-465. ISSN 0378-8741

Ayo, RG. (2010). Phytochemical constituents and bioactives of the extracts of *Cassia nigricans* Vahl: A review. *Journal of medicinal plants research*, Vol.4, No.14 (July 2010), pp. 1339-1348. ISSN 1996-0875

Bandyopadhyay, U.; Biswas, K.; Chatterjee, R.; Bandyopadhyay, D.; Chattopadhyay, I.; Ganguly, CK.; Chakraborty, T.; Bhattacharya, K. & Banerjee RK. (2002). Gastroprotective effect of Neem (*Azadirachta indica*) bark extract: possible involvement of H(+)-K(+)-ATPase inhibition and scavenging of hydroxyl radical. *Life sciences*, Vol.71, No.24 (November 2002), pp. 2845-2865. ISSN 0024-3205

Bandyopadhyay, U.; Biswas, K.; Sengupta, A.; Moitra, P.; Dutta, P.; Sarkar, D.; Debnath, P.; Ganguly, CK. & Banerjee, RK. (2004). Clinical studies on the effect of Neem (*Azadirachta indica*) bark extract on gastric secretion and gastroduodenal ulcer. *Life sciences*, Vol.75, No.24 (October 2004), pp. 2867-2878. ISSN 0024-3205

Barnes, J.; Anderson, LA. & Phillipson JD. (2002). *Herbal Medicines* (2nd edition), Pharmaceutical Press, ISBN 0853694745, Great Britain.

Borrelli, F. & Izzo, AA. (2000). The plant kingdom as a source of anti-ulcer remedies. *Phytotherapy research*, Vol.14, No.8 (December 2000), pp. 581-591. ISSN 0951-418X

Brahmachari, G. (2004). Neem--an omnipotent plant: a retrospection. *European journal of chemical biology*, Vol.5, No.4 (April 2004), pp. 408-421. ISSN 1439-4227

Calzada, F.; Arista, R. & Pérez, H. (2010). Effect of plants used in Mexico to treat gastrointestinal disorders on charcoal-gum acacia-induced hyperperistalsis in rats. *Journal of ethnopharmacology*, Vol.128, No.1 (March 2010), pp. 49-51. ISSN 0378-8741

Chen, JC.; Ho, TY.; Chang, YS.; Wu, SL. & Hsiang, CY. (2006). Anti-diarrheal effect of *Galla Chinensis* on the Escherichia coli heat-labile enterotoxin and ganglioside interaction. *Journal of ethnopharmacology*, Vol.103, No.3 (February 2006), pp. 385-391. ISSN 0378-8741

Chen, JC.; Chang, YS.; Wu, SL.; Chao, DC.; Chang, CS.; Li, CC.; Ho, TY. & Hsiang, CY. (2007). Inhibition of Escherichia coli heat-labile enterotoxin-induced diarrhea by *Chaenomeles speciosa*. *Journal of ethnopharmacology*, Vol.113, No.2 (September 2007), pp. 233-239. ISSN 0378-8741

Chittrakarn, S.; Sawangjaroen, K.; Prasettho, S.; Janchawee, B. & Keawpradub, N. (2008). Inhibitory effects of kratom leaf extract (*Mitragyna speciosa Korth.*) on the rat gastrointestinal tract. *Journal of ethnopharmacology*, Vol.116, No.1 (February 2008), pp. 173-178. ISSN 0378-8741

Cho, EJ.; Shin, JS.; Noh, YS.; Cho, YW.; Hong, SJ.; Park, JH.; Lee, JY.; Lee, JY. & Lee, KT. (2011). Anti-inflammatory effects of methanol extract of *Patrinia scabiosaefolia* in mice with ulcerative colitis. *Journal of ethnopharmacology*, Vol.136, No.3 (July 2011), pp. 428-435. ISSN 0378-8741

Das, AK.; Mandal, SC.; Banerjee, SK.; Sinha, S.; Das, J.; Saha, BP. & Pal, M. (1999). Studies on antidiarrhoeal activity of *Punica granatum* seed extract in rats. *Journal of ethnopharmacology*, Vol.68, No.1-3 (December 1999), pp. 205-208. ISSN 0378-8741

De Pasquale, R.; Germanò, MP.; Keita, A.; Sanogo, R. & Iauk, L. (1995). Antiulcer activity of *Pteleopsis suberosa*. *Journal of ethnopharmacology*, Vol.47, No.1 (June 1995), pp. 55-58. ISSN 0378-8741.

Dieleman, LA.; Palmen, MJ.; Akol, H.; Bloemena, E.; Peña, AS.; Meuwissen, SG. & Van Rees, EP. (1998). Chronic experimental colitis induced by dextran sulphate sodium (DSS) is characterized by Th1 and Th2 cytokines. *Clinical and experimental immunology*, Vol.114, No.3 (December 1998), pp. 385-391. ISSN 0009-9104

El-Abhar, HS.; Hammad, LN. & Gawad, HS. (2008). Modulating effect of ginger extract on rats with ulcerative colitis. *Journal of ethnopharmacology*, Vol.118, No.3 (August 2008), pp. 367-372. ISSN 0378-8741

Engqvist, A.; Von Feilitzen, F.; Pyk, E. & Reichard, H. (1973). Double-blind trial of deglycyrrhizinated liquorice in gastric ulcer. *Gut*, Vol.14, No.9 (September 1973), pp. 711-715. ISSN 0017-5749

Feldman, H. & Gilat, T. (1971). A trial of deglycyrrhizinated liquorice in the treatment of duodenal ulcer. *Gut*, Vol.12, No.6 (June 1971), pp. 449-451. ISSN 0017-5749

Fernández-Bañares, F.; Hinojosa, J.; Sánchez-Lombraña, JL.; Navarro, E.; Martínez-Salmerón, JF.; García-Pugés, A.; González-Huix, F.; Riera, J.; González-Lara, V.; Domínguez-Abascal, F.; Giné, JJ.; Moles, J.; Gomollón, F. & Gassull, MA. (1999). Randomized clinical trial of *Plantago ovata* seeds (dietary fiber) as compared with mesalamine in maintaining remission in ulcerative colitis. Spanish Group for the Study of Crohn's Disease and Ulcerative Colitis (GETECCU). *The American journal of gastroenterology*, Vol.94, No.2 (February 1999), pp. 427-433. ISSN 0002-9270

Ganjare, AB.; Nirmal, SA.; Rub, RA.; Patil, AN. & Pattan, SR. (2011). Use of *Cordia dichotoma* bark in the treatment of ulcerative colitis. *Pharmaceutical biology*, Vol.49, No.8 (August 2011), pp. 850-855. ISSN 1388-0209

Germanò, MP.; Sanogo, R.; Guglielmo, M.; De Pasquale, R.; Crisafi, G. & Bisignano, G. (1998). Effects of *Pteleopsis suberosa* extracts on experimental gastric ulcers and Helicobacter pylori growth. *Journal of ethnopharmacology*, Vol.59, No.3 (January 1998), pp. 167-172. ISSN 0378-8741

Hajhashemi, V.; Sadraei, H.; Ghannadi, AR. & Mohseni, M. (2000). Antispasmodic and anti-diarrhoeal effect of *Satureja hortensis L.* essential oil. *Journal of ethnopharmacology*, Vol.71, No.1-2 (July 2000), pp. 187-192. ISSN 0378-8741

Holtmeier, W.; Zeuzem, S.; Preiss, J.; Kruis, W.; Böhm, S.; Maaser, C.; Raedler, A.; Schmidt, C.; Schnitker, J.; Schwarz, J.; Zeitz, M. & Caspary, W. (2011). Randomized, placebo-controlled, double-blind trial of *Boswellia serrata* in maintaining remission of Crohn's disease: good safety profile but lack of efficacy. *Inflammatory bowel diseases*, Vol. 17, No.2 (February 2011), pp. 573-582. ISSN 1078-0998

Kaliora, AC.; Stathopoulou, MG.; Triantafillidis, JK.; Dedoussis, GV. & Andrikopoulos, NK. (2007). Chios mastic treatment of patients with active Crohn's disease. *World journal of gastroenterology*, Vol.13, No.5 (February 2007), pp.748-753. ISSN 1007-9327

Kaliora, AC.; Stathopoulou, MG.; Triantafillidis, JK.; Dedoussis, GV. & Andrikopoulos NK. (2007). Alterations in the function of circulating mononuclear cells derived from patients with Crohn's disease treated with mastic. *World journal of gastroenterology*, Vol.13, No.45 (December 2007), pp. 6031-6036. ISSN 1007-9327

Kiela, PR.; Midura, AJ.; Kuscuoglu, N.; Jolad, SD.; Sólyom, AM.; Besselsen, DG.; Timmermann, BN. & Ghishan, FK. (2005). Effects of *Boswellia serrata* in mouse models of chemically induced colitis. *American journal of physiology. Gastrointestinal and liver physiology*, Vol. 288, No.4 (April 2005), pp. G798-808. ISSN 0193-1857

Kim, HJ. & Neophytou, C. (2009). Natural anti-inflammatory compounds for the management and adjuvant therapy of inflammatory bowel disease and its drug delivery system. *Archives of pharmacal research*, Vol.32, No.7 (July 2009), pp. 997-1004. ISSN 0253-6269

Langmead, L. & Rampton, DS. (2006). Review article: complementary and alternative therapies for inflammatory bowel disease. *Alimentary pharmacology & therapeutics*, Vol.23, No.3 (February 2006), pp. 341-349, ISSN 0269-2813

Liu, XM.; Zakaria, MN.; Islam, MW.; Radhakrishnan, R.; Ismail, A.; Chen, HB.; Chan, K. & Al-Attas, A. (2001). Anti-inflammatory and anti-ulcer activity of *Calligonum comosum* in rats. *Fitoterapia*, Vol.72, No.5 (June 2001), pp. 487-491. ISSN 0367-326X

Madisch, A.; Miehlke, S.; Eichele, O.; Mrwa, J.; Bethke, B.; Kuhlisch, E.; Bästlein, E.; Wilhelms, G.; Morgner, A.; Wigginghaus, B. & Stolte, M. (2007). *Boswellia serrata* extract for the treatment of collagenous colitis. A double-blind, randomized, placebo-controlled, multicenter trial. *International journal of colorectal disease*, Vol.22, No.12 (December 2007), pp.1445-14451. ISSN 0179-1958

Minaiyan, M.; Ghannadi, A.; Mahzouni, M. & Nabi-Meibodi, M. (2008). Anti-ulcerogenic effect of ginger (rhizome of *Zingiber officinale* Roscoe) hydroalcoholic extract on acetic acid-induced acute colitis in rats. *Research in pharmaceutical sciences*, Vol.3, No.2 (October 2008), pp. 15-22. ISSN 1735-5362

Mukherjee, PK.; Saha, K.; Murugesan, T.; Mandal, SC.; Pal, M. & Saha BP. (1998). Screening of anti-diarrhoeal profile of some plant extracts of a specific region of West Bengal, India. *Journal of ethnopharmacology*, Vol.60, No.1 (February 1998), pp. 85-89. ISSN 0378-8741

Nguelefack, TB.; Feumebo, CB.; Ateufack, G.; Watcho, P.; Tatsimo, S.; Atsamo, AD.; Tane, P. & Kamanyi, A. (2008). Anti-ulcerogenic properties of the aqueous and methanol extracts from the leaves of *Solanum torvum* Swartz (Solanaceae) in rats. *Journal of ethnopharmacology*, Vol.119, No.1 (September 2008), pp. 135-140. ISSN 0378-8741

Noamesi, BK.; Mensah, JF.; Bogale, M.; Dagne, E. & Adotey, J. (1994). Antiulcerative properties and acute toxicity profile of some African medicinal plant extracts. *Journal of ethnopharmacology*, Vol.42, No.1 (March 1994), pp. 13-18. ISSN 0378-8741

Obi, E.; Emeh, JK.; Orisakwe, OE.; Afonne, OJ.; Ilondu, NA. & Agbasi, PU. (2000). Investigation of the biochemical evidence for the antiulcerogenic activity of *Synclisia scabrida*. *Indian Journal of Pharmacology*, Vol.32, No.6 (September 2000), pp. 381-383. ISSN: 0253-7613

Orisakwe, OE.; Afonne, OJ.; Dioka, CE.; Ufearo, CS.; Okpogba, AN. & Ofoefule, SI. (1996). Some pharmacological properties of *Synclisia scabrida* II. *Indian journal of medical research*, Vol.103 (May 1996), pp. 282-284. ISSN 0971-5916

Rees, WD.; Rhodes, J.; Wright, JE.; Stamford, LF. & Bennett, A. (1979). Effect of deglycyrrhizinated liquorice on gastric mucosal damage by aspirin. *Scandinavian journal of gastroenterology*, Vol.14, No.5, (1979), pp. 605-607. ISSN 0036-5521

Rodríguez-Cabezas, ME.; Gálvez, J.; Camuesco, D.; Lorente, MD.; Concha A,; Martinez-Augustin, O.; Redondo, L. & Zarzuelo, A. (2003). Intestinal anti-inflammatory activity of dietary fiber (*Plantago ovata* seeds) in HLA-B27 transgenic rats. *Clinical nutrition*, Vol.22, No. 5 (October 2003), pp. 463-471. ISSN 0261-5614

Rivière, PJ.; Farmer, SC.; Burks, TF. & Porreca, F. (1991). Prostaglandin E2-induced diarrhea in mice: importance of colonic secretion. *The Journal of pharmacology and experimental therapeutics*, Vol.256, No.2 (February 1991), pp. 547-552. ISSN 0022-3565

Rosenbloom, RA.; Chaudhary, J. & Castro-Eschenbach, D. (2011). Traditional botanical medicine: an introduction. *American journal of therapeutics*, Vol.18, No.2 (March 2011), pp. 158-161. ISSN 1075-2765

Sengupta, A.; Ghosh, S.; Bhattacharjee, S. & Das, S. (2004). Indian food ingredients and cancer prevention - an experimental evaluation of anticarcinogenic effects of garlic in rat colon. *Asian Pacific journal of cancer prevention*, Vol.5, No.2 (April 2004), pp. 126-132. ISSN 1513-7368

Sirisha, N.; Sreenivasulu, M.; Sangeeta, K. & Madhusudhana Chetty C. (2010). Antioxidant properties of Ficus species- A review. *International journal of pharmtech research*, Vol.2, No.4 (October 2010), pp. 2174-2182. ISSN 0974-4304

Spangler, BD. (1992). Structure and function of cholera toxin and the related Escherichia coli heat-labile enterotoxin. *Microbiological reviews*, Vol.56, No.4 (December 1992), pp. 622-647. ISSN 0146-0749

Suzuki, H.; Inadomi, JM. & Hibi, T. (2009). Japanese herbal medicine in functional gastrointestinal disorders. *Neurogastroenterology and motility*, Vol.21, No.7 (Jul 2009), pp. 688-696. ISSN 1350-1925

Viswanatha, GL.; Hanumanthappa, S.; Krishnadas, N. & Rangappa, S. (2011). Antidiarrheal effect of fractions from stem bark of *Thespesia populnea* in rodents: Possible antimotility and antisecretory mechanisms. *Asian Pacific journal of tropical medicine*, Vol.4, No.6 (June 2011), pp. 451-456. ISSN 1995-7645

Wallace, JL. (2001). Pathogenesis of NSAID-induced gastroduodenal mucosal injury. *Best practice & research. Clinical gastroenterology*, Vol.15, No.5 (October 2001), pp. 691-703. ISSN 1521-6918

Zaware, BB.; Nirmal, SA.; Baheti, DG.; Patil, AN. & Mandal, SC. (2011). Potential of *Vitex negundo* roots in the treatment of ulcerative colitis in mice. *Pharmaceutical biology*, Vol.49, No.8 (August 2011), pp. 874-878. ISSN 1388-0209

15

Evaluating Lymphoma Risk in Inflammatory Bowel Disease

Neeraj Prasad
Royal Albert Edward Infirmary, Wigan
University of Salford
United Kingdom

1. Introduction

The risk of lymphoma in inflammatory bowel disease (IBD) has been a topic of great interest for many years. In 1928, the first published series of colorectal malignancies in ulcerative colitis (UC) patients included a case of lymphosarcoma, the name given to an early classification of lymphoma (Bargen, 1928). Since then a huge number of case reports, case series, cohort studies, population-based studies and meta-analyses have been presented on the topic but the matter remains controversial with conflicting results based on poor quality evidence. Most recently, a type of non-Hodgkin's lymphoma (NHL) known as hepatosplenic T-cell lymphoma (HSTCL) has understandably drawn much attention despite its rarity. HSTCL has an invariably fatal outcome despite reports of early response to treatment, it almost exclusively affects young men with Crohn's disease (CD) and seems to be linked to commonly used drugs for the management of IBD, the thiopurines and tumour necrosis factor (TNF) antagonists (Kotlyar et al., 2011). A further source of concern stems from a trend by IBD physicians to use these drugs earlier in the course of disease and also in combination because recent studies suggest that these strategies may improve outcomes (Colombel et al., 2010, D'Haens, 2009).

Proving causality has been difficult because it is difficult to separate the multiple factors involved in lymphomagenesis using the evidence that is available (see Figure 1). It has long been suspected that the chronic inflammation seen in IBD itself may be the cause of lymphoma in this setting but there has been growing concern that it is in fact the drugs used in the treatment of IBD which confers this risk. One could also speculate that it is the combination of both these factors which results in the development of lymphoma.

The case of lymphosarcoma identified by Bargen in 1928 was in an era when immunomodulators were not available for the treatment of IBD suggesting that the disease itself may predispose to lymphoma development. There are other reports of lymphoma in drug-naïve IBD patients (Aydogan et al., 2010). There does appear to be an increased risk of lymphoma in other chronic inflammatory and autoimmune conditions as well including rheumatoid arthritis (RA), primary Sjögren's syndrome, systemic lupus erythematosus (SLE) and Hashimoto's thyroiditis (Smedby et al., 2006). There is some evidence that increased severity of the disease may increase the risk of lymphoma in these conditions (Baecklund et al., 2006, Theander et al., 2006, Lofstrom et al., 2007).

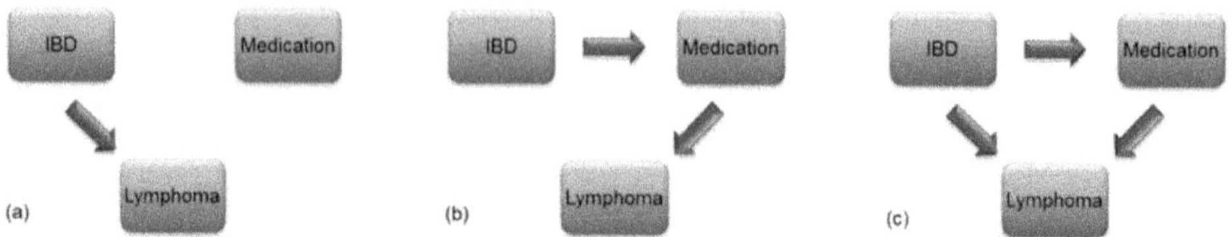

Fig. 1. Assessing the causality of lymphoma in IBD. IBD itself may be the cause of lymphoma (a), or lymphoma may be due to the medication used to treat it (b) or lymphoma may be due to a combination of the disease and the treatment (c).

Both primary and acquired immunodeficiency states have been associated with lymphoma which is important because many of the drugs used for the treatment of IBD have immunosuppressive effects. There is an increased risk of lymphoma with Human Immunodeficiency Virus (HIV) infection and in post-transplant patients treated with immunosuppressives (Serraino et al., 1992, Grulich et al., 2007b). The role of Epstein-Barr virus (EBV) is well established in lymphomagenesis in post-transplant patients and this also appears to be important in IBD patients (Dayharsh et al., 2002).

IBD is associated with significant morbidity and a small mortality (Rubin et al., 2004, Ghosh and Mitchell, 2007). It is important that IBD physicians are able to help patients weigh up the risk of lymphoma with the benefits of drugs used to treat IBD. A number of attempts have been made to quantify this risk. One of the largest population-based studies utilised a primary care database from the United Kingdom but did not find a statistically significant increased background risk of lymphoma in IBD patients (Lewis et al., 2001). A cohort study from Dublin found an alarmingly higher rate of lymphoma in their IBD patients with up to a 59-fold increase (Farrell et al., 2000). Kandiel et al performed a meta-analysis of 6 studies to evaluate the risk of lymphoma in IBD patients treated with thiopurines and found a 4-fold increased risk of lymphoma in these patients (Kandiel et al., 2005).

A number of more recent studies have been presented in the literature including large cohort studies from the United States (US) and Spain (Chiorean et al., 2010, Van Domselaar et al., 2010) as well as large population-based studies from the UK and the Netherlands (Armstrong et al., 2010, Vos et al., 2010). Most notably, the French CESAME study published in 2009 with almost 50,000 patient-years of follow up, set out to quantify the risk of lymphoma and made attempts to distinguish the background risk of lymphoma due to IBD itself from the risk conferred by its treatment (Beaugerie et al., 2009a).

This chapter aims to provide an up to date systematic review of the available literature regarding the risk of lymphoma in inflammatory bowel disease. Meta-analysis techniques have been used to pool data from multiple studies.

2. Inflammatory bowel disease

Inflammatory bowel disease (IBD) is a chronic, idiopathic, remitting and relapsing disorder of the gastrointestinal tract. It comprises of two main disease types, ulcerative colitis (UC) and Crohn's disease (CD), which have many similar but also certain distinct pathological and clinical characteristics.

2.1 Epidemiology

IBD affects 400 per 100,000 population in the United Kingdom but there is considerable variation worldwide with the highest prevalence in developed countries (Rubin et al., 2000). It most commonly presents in teenage or young adult life but it can affect any age and there is an approximate equal sex distribution.

2.2 Aetiology

The aetiology is unknown but evidence suggests an immune dysfunction which is triggered by an environmental factor in a genetically susceptible individual (Cho, 2008) leading to chronic inflammation and injury to the gastrointestinal tract. Many of the susceptibility genes identified in recent studies have been shown to have important roles in immune regulation but there is increasing evidence that these genes pertain to the innate immune system and are involved in the sensing or intracellular processing of bacteria (Packey and Sartor, 2008). Potential microbial triggers which have been studied include a form of enteroadherent *Escherichia coli* and *Mycobacterium paratuberculosis*, but more recent investigation suggests that a disturbance of normal enteric microflora may play a role in aetiology (Sartor, 2008). Additionally, a number of other potential environmental factors have also been studied including diet, smoking, appendiceal inflammation, certain drugs and stress but causality has remained difficult to establish (Bernstein, 2010). The particular combination of susceptible genes and environmental triggers probably varies between individuals with IBD and leads to different patterns and severity of disease.

Ulcerative colitis causes a continuous mucosal inflammation of the colorectum, whereas Crohn's disease can affect any part of the GI tract, characteristically with skip lesions and transmural inflammation. Additionally, chronic inflammation in Crohn's disease can lead to fistulising and stricturing disease behaviours (Satsangi et al., 2006).

2.3 Treatment

A curative treatment for inflammatory bowel disease is yet to be identified. Strategies for the management of IBD involve treatment of flares and maintenance of remission. Although a wide range of therapies including enteral nutrition (Zachos et al., 2007), antibiotics (Lal and Steinhart, 2006) and complementary medicines (Langmead and Rampton, 2006) are used in IBD, the mainstay of treatment has been with anti-inflammatory and immunomodulatory drugs. Corticosteroids, 5-aminosalicylates (5ASA), azathioprine (AZA), mercaptopurine (6MP), methotrexate (MTX) and cyclosporin A (CSA) have been the most commonly used drugs. In an attempt to reduce steroid exposure and maintain remission, immunomodulatory therapy is being used earlier, for prolonged periods and in combination. The concern is of an increased risk of side effects with this approach. Estimates suggest that up to 30% of patients may not respond to this treatment and may require more aggressive strategies. The increased understanding of the pathogenesis of IBD, has led to investigation in to a number of therapies targeted towards the abnormal cytokine expression seen in patients with IBD. Of these, only the monoclonal antibodies against tumour necrosis factor are currently in clinical use but other targets have been identified and are undergoing laboratory and clinical study. Infliximab (IXB) and adalimumab (ADA) are the two anti-tumour necrosis factor (anti-TNF) drugs available in the United Kingdom and a number of studies have proven their efficacy (Hanauer et al., 2006, Hanauer et al., 2002, Jarnerot et al., 2005). A third, pegylated anti-TNF drug, certolizumab has also been studied and appears to have equivalent clinical efficacy (Sandborn et al., 2007a). Despite medical therapy, up to 50-70% of patients with CD will undergo surgery within 5 years of diagnosis and UC patients have a 20-30% lifetime risk of colectomy (Cosnes et al., 2005).

2.4 Cancer risk in IBD

The increased risk of colonic adenocarcinoma in patients with ulcerative colitis and Crohn's colitis is well documented (Rutter et al., 2006, Jess et al., 2006). One study has suggested a protective role for thiopurines in this context (Beaugerie et al., 2009b) though these patients were not corrected for co-administration of 5ASA preparations which may also have a protective role in this setting.

There also appears to be an increased risk of certain non-colorectal malignancies amongst IBD patients. In the same cohort of patients from the CESAME study, prospective data suggested a 20-fold increased risk of small bowel adenocarcinoma and suggestion of an increased risk of skin and cervical malignancy (Beaugerie et al., 2009c). In a database of over 27,000 UC patients from Sweden, the standardised incidence ratio (SIR) for all cancers was 1.46 with increased risk of malignancy of the liver, small bowel (carcinoid), prostate and breast (Hemminki et al., 2008). In a recent review of malignancies associated with thiopurine therapy, Smith et al concluded that these drugs did not increase the risk of cervical dysplasia, colonic cancer or solid organ tumours in IBD patients (Smith et al., 2010). A retrospective cohort study of over 50,000 IBD patients from the US suggested an increased risk of non-melanomatous skin cancer and that this risk was highest in patients treated with thiopurines (Odds Ratio 4.27) and biological therapies (Odds Ratio 2.18) (Long et al., 2010).

Many of these studies have also shown an increased risk of lymphoma and this will be discussed further in this chapter.

3. Lymphoma

Lymphoma is a broad term used to describe a variety of neoplasms due to proliferation of lymphoid cells. Traditionally, lymphoid neoplasms that presented with bone marrow and blood involvement were referred to by the term *leukaemia* and those that presented with a mass would be called a *lymphoma*. However, it is now appreciated that any *lymphoma* can present with or evolve in to a leukaemic picture and occasionally, *leukaemia* can present with a mass lesion.

3.1 Classification of lymphoma

The earliest classifications of lymphoma were based entirely on the morphological features of the neoplastic cells involved. Historically, lymphomas represented by large cells were known as *reticulosarcomas* and those by small cells were *lymphosarcomas* (Diebold, 2001). Later, lymphomas began to be distinguished according to their origin from B or T lymphocytes. With the development of immunophenotyping and cytogenetics, as well as an appreciation of differences in prognosis and patient stratification, more complex classification systems have developed. The World Health Organisation (WHO)

Classification of Tumours of Haemopoietic and Lymphoid Tissues, updated in 2008 (see Table 1), is now widely accepted (Swerdlow et al., 2008) and categorises lymphoid neoplasms in to those derived from:

* B cell progenitors - bone marrow derived
* T cell progenitors - thymus derived
* Mature T lymphocytes - cytotoxic or killer T cells, helper T cells or T regulatory cells
* Mature B lymphocytes - B cells or plasma cells

Non-Hodgkin's Lymphoma	
Precursor B-cell lymphomas	**Precursor T-cell and NK-cell lymphomas**
Precursor B-cell lymphoblastic lymphoma	Precursor T-cell lymphoblastic lymphoma
	Blastic NK-cell lymphoma
Mature B-cell lymphomas	
	Mature T-cell and NK-cell lymphomas
Small lymphocytic lymphoma	
Lymphoplasmacytic lymphoma	T-cell prolymphocytic leukaemia
Splenic marginal zone lymphoma	T-cell large granular lymphocytic leukaemia
Hairy cell leukaemia	Aggressive NK-cell leukaemia
Plasma cell neoplasms	Adult T-cell lymphoma/leukaemia
Extranodal marginal zone B-cell MALT lymphoma	Extranodal NK-/T-cell lymphoma, nasal type
Nodal marginal zone B-cell lymphoma	Enteropathy-type T-cell lymphoma
Follicular lymphoma (grades 1, 2, 3a and 3b)	Hepatosplenic T-cell lymphoma
Diffuse follicle centre lymphoma	Subcutaneous panniculitis-like T-cell lymphoma
Mantle cell lymphoma	Mycosis fungoides
Diffuse large B-cell lymphoma	Peripheral T-cell lymphoma unspecified
Mediastinal (thymic) large B-cell lymphoma	Angioimmunoblastic T-cell lymphoma
Intravascular large B-cell lymphoma	Anaplastic large cell lymphoma
Primary effusion lymphoma	
Burkitt lymphoma	
B-cell proliferations of uncertain malignant potential	
Lymphomatoid granulomatosis	
Post-transplant lymphoproliferative disorder	

Hodgkin's Lymphoma
Classical Hodgkin's lymphoma
Nodular sclerosis classical HL Mixed cellularity classical HL
Lymphocyte rich classical HL Lymphocyte depleted classical HL
Nodular lymphocyte predominant HL

Table 1. WHO Classification of Non-Hodgkin's and Hodgkin's Lymphoma (Swerdlow et al, 2008). (MALT – mucosa-associated lymphoid tissue; HL – Hodgkin's Lymphoma; NK – Natural Killer).

Hodgkin's lymphoma (formerly known as Hodgkin's disease) arises from B-cells of germinal or post-germinal centres of peripheral lymph nodes. It is pathologically and clinically distinct from other lymphoid neoplasia and generally has a good prognosis. Hodgkin's lymphoma has a distinguishing cellular composition on biopsy of lymphomatous tissues with abundant inflammatory cells and only a minority of neoplastic cells, known as Reed-Sternberg cells. Reed-Sternberg cells are large, binucleated or multinucleated containing multiple eosinophilic nucleoli and have prominent cytoplasm. Hodgkin's lymphoma (HL) is classified in to *nodular lymphocyte predominant HL* and *classical HL*, which is further subdivided in to *nodular sclerosis, mixed cellularity, lymphocyte-rich* and *lymphocyte-depleted* types (see Table 1).

The term Non-Hodgkin's lymphoma encompasses all other types of lymphoma. Although the WHO classification does not distinguish NHL on the basis of disease activity, it has classically been divided in to two subtypes:

- High-grade NHL develops quickly and aggressively.
- Low-grade or indolent NHL develops slowly and there may be no symptoms for many years.

3.2 Non-Hodgkin's lymphoma

NHL can occur in children and adults but over two-thirds are diagnosed in people aged over 60 years. There is a male preponderance with a ratio of up to 1.5 in older age groups. NHL is the fifth most common cancer in the UK with over 10,000 people diagnosed with the condition in 2007 and an age-standardised rate of 14.2 per 100,000 population (Cancer-Research-UK, 2011) (see Figure 2A). In the United States, the Surveillance Epidemiology & End Results (SEER) registry provides an age-standardised rate of 19.6 per 100,000 between 2003 and 2007 (Altekruse et al., 2010). The incidence of NHL seems to be rising in the UK

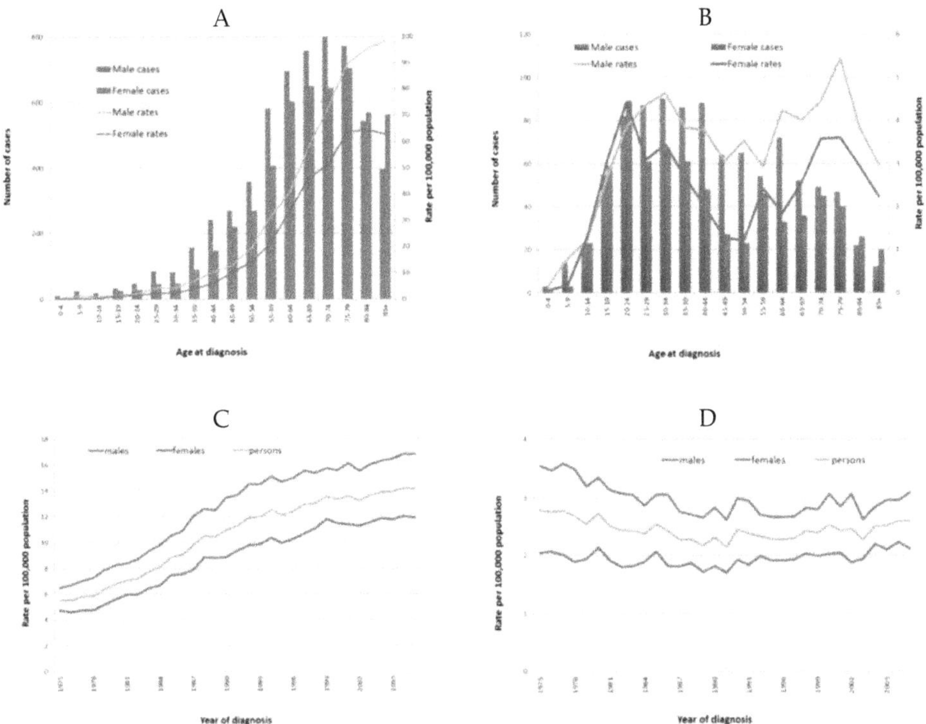

Fig. 2. Figures adapted from Cancer Research UK 2011. A: Incidence of non-Hodgkin's lymphoma by gender. B: Incidence of Hodgkin's lymphoma by gender. C: Age standardised incidence rates for non-Hodgkin's lymphoma. D: Age standardised incidence rates for Hodgkin's lymphoma.

with an increase of 35% during the 20 year interval between 1988 and 2007 (see Figure 2C). This trend seems to be reflected throughout the world. Mortality in the UK is estimated at 6.9 per 100,000 from NHL and with improvements in treatment, it is estimated that over half of patients now survive for at least 10 years following diagnosis. Up to 15% of all extra-nodal NHL presents in the GI tract (Newton et al., 1997).

A number of risk factors for the development of NHL have been studied:

- **Infectious agents** – It is thought that a proportion of the worldwide rise in incidence of NHL parallels, but is not completely explained by, the HIV epidemic. The risk of NHL in HIV and AIDS is well documented but only 3-5% of these patients will develop NHL (Serraino et al., 1992). Epstein-Barr virus has been linked to Burkitt's lymphoma and post-transplant lymphoma (Epstein et al., 1964). Other infections associated with an increased risk of NHL include *Helicobacter Pylori* (Xue et al., 2001), Hepatitis C (Dal Maso and Franceschi, 2006) and Human T-cell Lymphotropic Virus (HTLV-1) (Parkin, 2006).

- **Immunosuppression** – The use of immunosuppression following organ transplant has been shown to increase the risk of NHL and in a significant proportion of these, EBV infection has been implicated (Kawashima et al., 1994). A recent meta-analysis suggests an 8-fold increased risk of NHL in post-transplant patients (Grulich et al., 2007b).

- **Autoimmune conditions** – Conditions such as autoimmune haemolytic anaemia, systemic lupus erythematosus and Sjögren's syndrome, where there is a longstanding stimulation of the immune system have been shown to carry an increased risk of NHL but the exact mechanisms remain poorly understood (Ekstrom Smedby et al., 2008). Coeliac disease is associated with T-cell lymphoma and less frequently, B-cell lymphoma (Chandesris et al., 2010, Oruc et al., 2010). This risk can be reduced by treatment with a gluten-free diet (Silano et al., 2008).

- **Genetic susceptibility** – The sibling or progeny of an affected individual has an approximate two-fold increased risk of developing NHL and there appears to be concordance in NHL subtype (Altieri et al., 2005).

- **Exposure to chemical carcinogens** – A number of studies and meta-analyses suggest an increased risk of NHL in individuals with occupational exposure to agricultural pesticides (Merhi et al., 2007), benzene (Steinmaus et al., 2008) and aromatic hydrocarbons (Miligi et al., 2006).

- **Diet and obesity** – Dietary factors and the risk of lymphoma are controversial. A recent study from Iowa found a 31% risk reduction for women with a higher intake of fruit and vegetables (Thompson et al., 2010). However, an earlier cohort study did not corroborate this finding (Zhang et al., 2000). NHL appears to be associated with obesity with one meta-analysis showing a relative risk of 1.4 for diffuse large B-cell NHL amongst individuals with a BMI $\geq$ 30 kg/m^2 (Larsson and Wolk, 2007).

3.3 Hodgkin's lymphoma

Hodgkin's lymphoma represents 15% of all lymphomas and accounts for only 0.6% of all cancers diagnosed in the United Kingdom (Cancer-Research-UK, 2011). The age standardised incidence in 2007 was 2.6 per 100,000 population in the UK and 2.8 per 100,000 in the USA (Altekruse et al., 2010) (see Figure 2B). In the UK, age-specific peaks in incidence occur in early adult life (for men at 30 to 34 years and women at 20 to 24 years old) and in later life (over 70 years). Unlike NHL, the incidence of Hodgkin's lymphoma seems to have fallen in the 1970s and has plateaued since the 1980s (see Figure 2D). This may be explained by changes in classification of different types of lymphoma. With treatment, prognosis for Hodgkin's lymphoma is good with around 78% of patients with HL diagnosed in 2007 in the UK predicted to survive for at least 10 years according to calculations by Cancer Research UK. The overall age-standardised survival rate for patients diagnosed with HL in England between 1996 and 1999 was 80% (Coleman, 1999). The Nodular Sclerosis subtype of classical HL is the commonest occurring in 60% of cases and is associated with younger age and more affluent populations.

Many of the risk factors for Hodgkin's lymphoma are similar to those of NHL but certain factors may be more important in the development of HL:

- **Genetic susceptibility** – a family history of Hodgkin's lymphoma appears to have a much more dramatic effect on risk when compared to NHL. Monozygotic twin studies suggest a 99-fold increased risk (Mack et al., 1995) and a first degree relative diagnosed with any haematological malignancy confers a two to three-fold increased risk (Chang et al., 2005, Goldin et al., 2004). Studies from the USA suggest racial differences in susceptibility with lower risk in blacks than whites (Glaser, 1991).

- **Epstein-Barr virus** – EBV infection has long been implicated in the development of Hodgkin's lymphoma. EBV DNA can be found in 40% of cases with higher rates of association found in the paediatric population (Jarrett et al., 1996). EBV positivity is more commonly found in the Mixed Cellularity than the Nodular Sclerosis subtypes of classical HL. A previous history of infectious mononucleosis confers an increased risk of HL with an SIR of 3.49 in patients aged 15 to 34 years (Hjalgrim et al., 2000).
- **Previous non-Hodgkin's lymphoma** – Studies suggest that patients who have previously been treated for NHL are at increased risk of subsequently developing HL with a magnitude in the order of four- to twelve-fold (Travis et al., 1991, Travis et al., 1993).

4. Pathogenesis of lymphoma in IBD

Lymphoma is a clonal expansion of B- and T- lymphocytes caused by the accumulation of a series of genetic mutations affecting proto-oncogenes and tumour suppressor genes. This results in dysregulated proliferation, evasion of immune surveillance mechanisms and inhibition of apoptosis (Jaffe et al., 2001). Significant progress has been made in to the understanding of these mechanisms at a molecular level. The activation of oncogenes by aberrant chromosomal translocations as well as the inactivation of tumour suppressor genes by chromosomal deletion or mutation are both important mechanisms of lymphomagenesis (Kuppers et al., 1999). Oncogenic viruses such as EBV and HTLV1 can also introduce foreign genetic sequences into the lymphocyte genome causing disruption of normal function (Neri et al., 1991).

There are a number of genetic, environmental, infectious and iatrogenic factors amongst patients with inflammatory bowel disease which can predispose to increased susceptibility to these mechanisms for the development of lymphoma:

- **Chronic inflammation** – The pathogenesis of IBD is not completely understood but aberrations in the innate and adaptive immune response to luminal antigens has been the focus of much research. It can be postulated that the dysregulation of these immune systems seen in the chronic inflammation associated with IBD may lead to antigen-driven lymphocyte proliferation and a relatively unhindered risk of genetic and chromosomal deviations (Sokol and Beaugerie, 2009). Another possibility is that the combination of metabolites, cytokines and chemokines seen in the mucosa of IBD patients promotes mutagenesis in bystander cells. These theories may help to explain the increased risk of lymphoma seen in a variety of different auto-immune conditions and their concordance to sites of inflammation (Smedby et al., 2006). EBV related lymphoma has been reported in longstanding pyothorax of over 20 years duration (Aozasa et al., 2005). This is a condition which is regarded to be due to chronic suppuration with no autoimmunity and it is suggested that any chronic inflammatory state may predispose to lymphoma development.
- **Genetic susceptibility** – Linkage studies and genome wide association studies have identified a large array of susceptibility genes for IBD (Barrett et al., 2008). These genetic changes may also be involved in the pathogenesis of lymphoma in certain individuals. For example, the first susceptibility gene identified, IBD1, encodes for the protein

NOD1 which in its wild-type activates nuclear factor kappa B (NF-κB) (Ogura et al., 2001). NF-κB is a tightly regulated mediator of T- and B-lymphocytes and alterations in its signalling pathway have been implicated in a number of malignancies including lymphoma (Jost and Ruland, 2007). Although some plausibility exists, this link remains to be established.

- **Therapeutic immune modulation** – Immunomodulatory drugs such as the thiopurines, (azathioprine and mercaptopurine), methotrexate, and the anti-TNF drugs (infliximab, adalimumab and certolizumab) have become standard treatment for complicated IBD. These drugs exert their effects through a number of mechanisms which are incompletely understood. It is recognised that AZA and its metabolites suppress intracellular inosinic acid synthesis which interferes with intracellular purine synthesis resulting in a down regulation of B- and T-cell proliferation (Bacon and Salmon, 1987). Thiopurine nucleotides also incorporate into lymphocyte DNA disrupting structure, repair mechanisms and promoting mutagenesis (Ling et al., 1992). There is also evidence that azathioprine renders DNA highly sensitive to damage to ultraviolet (UVA) radiation and this may account for the increased risk of non-melanomatous skin cancer in patients treated with thiopurines (O'Donovan et al., 2005). A recent study showed that IBD patients on thiopurine therapy had significantly more somatic mutations in circulating T-lymphocytes than in a thiopurine-naïve control group (Nguyen et al., 2009).
The impact of anti-TNF drugs on the risk of mutagenesis has not been adequately studied. It is conceivable that interruption of TNF signalling disrupts immune surveillance mechanisms and alters the normal detection and elimination of cells with chromosomal abnormalities.
At higher doses, methotrexate is cytotoxic, whereas the lower doses used in IBD patients are known to alter T-cell derived cytokines in inflammatory states. It inhibits pro-inflammatory cytokines such as interleukin-12, interferon-γ and tumour necrosis factor-α whilst promoting anti-inflammatory cytokines such as interleukin-10 (van Dieren et al., 2006). These cytokines have fundamental effects on lymphocyte proliferation and function but the specific mechanisms which may contribute to potential lymphoma development are not known.

- **Immunosuppression** – The increased risk of lymphoma in patients with immunodeficiency states such as HIV infection (Serraino et al., 1992) and post-transplant immunosuppression (Grulich et al., 2007a) is well recognised and many of these cases are EBV positive. The increased risk of opportunistic infections amongst IBD patients on immunomodulators therapy is also well documented. Toruner et al identified 100 cases of opportunistic infections over an 8 year period on their database of IBD patients from the Mayo Clinic and found that treatment with thiopurines conferred an Odds Ratio of 3.1 (Toruner et al., 2008). The majority of these opportunistic infections were caused by viruses including cytomegalovirus, Herpes simplex virus and Epstein-Barr virus.
EBV is a widely disseminated human Herpes virus which has been associated with a number of different types of B-cell lymphoma, particularly mixed cellularity and lymphocyte depleted classical Hodgkin's lymphoma, Burkitt's lymphoma and post-transplant lymphoproliferative disorder (PTLD). EBV viral load can predict risk of PTLD (Stevens et al., 2001) and cases of infectious mononucleosis with early transformation to lymphoma have been described (Owen et al., 2010). Interestingly,

Wong et al describe a case of synchronous colonic adenocarcinoma and lymphoma and demonstrated that EBV was present in the lymphomatous tissue but not in the invasive adenomatous tissue (Wong et al., 2003). A series of IBD patients from the Mayo clinic identified 12 patients diagnosed with lymphoma between 1993 and 2000, half of whom were on azathioprine therapy. The lymphomas of five out of these six patients on azathioprine were EBV positive whereas only one out of the six azathioprine-naïve patients was EBV positive (Dayharsh et al., 2002). This study suggests a link between azathioprine therapy and EBV driven lymphoma in IBD though the numbers were too small to reach statistical significance. In the CESAME prospective study of over 21,000 French IBD patients, 9 of the 13 cases of lymphoma in patients on azathioprine were EBV positive with up to 16 years exposure to the drug (Beaugerie et al., 2009a). Reijasse et al measured EBV viral loads in patients with Crohn's disease and EBV sero-positive controls. There was no difference in viral loads between the two groups irrespective of immunomodulator or biological therapy but a minority of patients did have transient, very high EBV viral loads (Reijasse et al., 2004). It is not clear, whether these peaks in EBV viral load are associated with lymphoma risk but this does appear to be the case in post-transplant patients where EBV viral load can predict this outcome (Stevens et al., 2001).

The pathobiology of EBV and its role in lymphomagenesis is complex. The host-incorporated EBV genome encodes a number of proteins with similarities to a variety of cytokines, anti-apoptotic molecules and signal transducers that can immortalise and mutate infected cells (Sokol and Beaugerie, 2009).

The risk of other oncogenic viruses such as HLTV1 is not well described in the IBD literature. A recent meta-analysis suggested a lower prevalence of *Helicobacter Pylori* infection in IBD patients compared to control groups but its association with gastric MALT-oma is well documented (Luther et al., 2010).

5. Lymphoma risk in the literature

In order to evaluate any causality between IBD and the risk of lymphoma, it is extremely important to appreciate the quality of safety data available. Frequently, this information is flawed and difficult to interpret.

5.1 Quality of data

Randomised controlled drug trials collate information regarding adverse events but they are powered to elucidate differences in efficacy and not safety. They also tend to have relatively small numbers and a short follow up period which may not reflect the true incidence of late or delayed adverse events. Some useful safety information is available from observational studies of large populations. These have large numbers and long follow up but are susceptible to indication bias and often have other confounding factors. Case controlled series have an efficient methodology but may be hampered by the shortcomings of control selection. The most common form of safety data comes from case reports and case series which are able to identify rare risks. However, the inherent positive bias with this form of evidence, does not allow it to be utilised for risk quantification or for providing proof of causality. Post marketing surveillance, a form of *pharmaco-vigilence*, is another important source of safety data. This information may be made available through institutional reporting schemes, such as the FDA's Adverse Events Recording System (AERS) in the United States (FDA, 2011) or the MHRA's Yellow Card System in the United Kingdom (MHRA, 2011). Important information may come from drug specific data such as the TREAT registry (Lichtenstein et al., 2006), which is an on-going large-scale observational registry that was designed to examine the safety of Crohn's Disease therapies including infliximab. This type of data provides a *real world* experience with a heterogeneous group of patients suffering a variety of co-morbidities and taking concomitant medication. However, such schemes are generally voluntary systems which are prone to under-reporting and hence an under estimation of true incidence.

The low incidence of lymphoma, even in higher risk populations, poses a challenge to evaluating this risk. The incidence of all types of lymphoma diagnosed in the United Kingdom in 2007 was about 17 cases per 100,000 population (Cancer-Research-UK, 2011). A study of almost 3 million individuals would be necessary to detect an adverse event of this frequency with a confidence interval of 95%. No studies of this magnitude are available nor are likely to be available in the future.

5.2 Available data

The literature pertaining to the risk of lymphoma amongst IBD patients is dominated by case reports and case series. However, a number of large population studies have also been published over the last three decades which have been extremely valuable because they allow approximation of the risk of lymphoma (Loftus et al., 2000, Lewis et al., 2001, Beaugerie et al., 2009a, Greenstein et al., 1985). This information must be considered within the limitations of this type of study. A small number of meta-analyses have attempted to combine information from these population-based studies (Kandiel et al., 2005, Siegel et al., 2009). Post-marketing surveillance for drugs such as azathioprine, mercaptopurine and methotrexate are not available but some data regarding the newer anti-TNF therapies in IBD now exists (Lichtenstein et al., 2006).

Interest in the risk of developing lymphoma in the context of IBD and its treatment has grown exponentially (see Figure 3). This coincides with increasing use of immunomodulators in the management of IBD and concerns over their safety. Prior to the 1990s, only sporadic case reports and case series were available. More recently, a number of population based studies, review articles and meta-analyses have been published which are discussed in this report.

Additionally, changes in the classification of lymphoid neoplasia makes evaluation of the literature difficult in certain circumstances where there are overlapping features between diagnoses (Swerdlow et al., 2008).

6. Presentation of lymphoma in IBD

The presentation of lymphoma amongst IBD patients is very heterogenous and occurs in both Crohn's disease and ulcerative colitis.

There are abundant reports of lymphoma of the gastro-intestinal tract mimicking presentations of Crohn's disease (Kashi et al., 2010, Kang et al., 2007, Hurlstone, 2002, Jouini et al., 2001, Vincenzi et al., 2001, Camera et al., 1997, Maaravi et al., 1993, Scully et al., 1993,

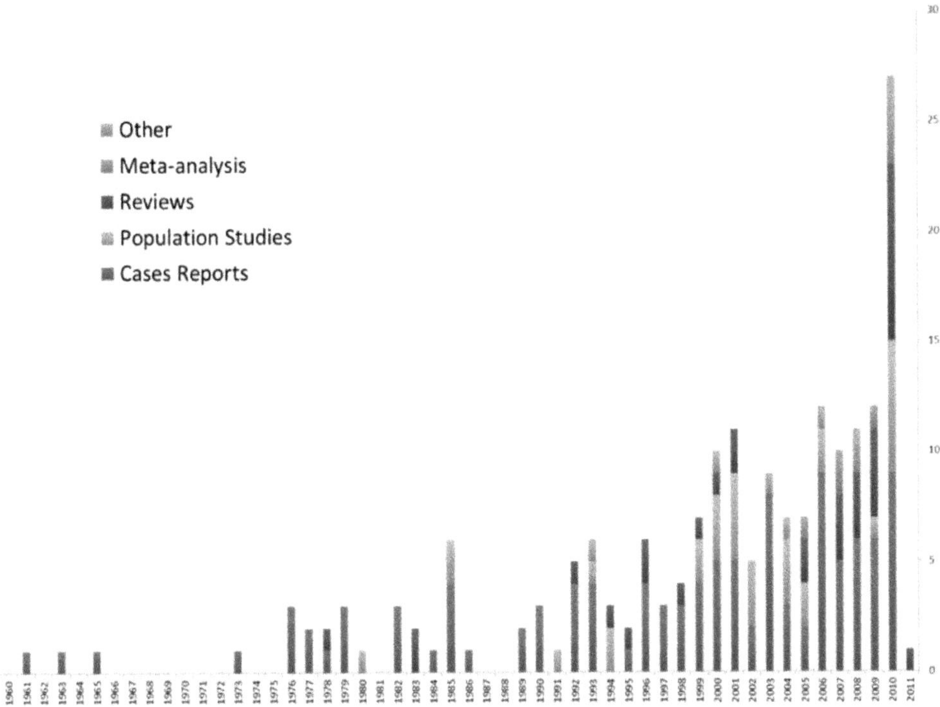

Fig. 3. Medline cited publications regarding lymphoma risk in IBD patients since 1950.

McCullough et al., 1992, Pohl et al., 1991, Bartram and Chrispin, 1973) and ulcerative colitis (Isomoto et al., 2003, Luo et al., 1997, Wagonfeld et al., 1976, Myerson et al., 1974, Parnes et al., 1974, Friedman et al., 1968, Federman et al., 1963). Clearly, lymphoma of the GI tract frequently occurs in the absence of inflammatory bowel disease. In a series from the Mayo Clinic spanning 40 years in the pre-biologic era, of the 2,332 cases of primary intestinal lymphoma identified, only 15 patients had concomitant inflammatory bowel disease (Holubar et al., 2010). These cases are not discussed further here.

6.1 Intestinal and extra-intestinal lymphoma

Lymphoma may present at a variety of sites amongst IBD patient but these can broadly be classified as intestinal and extra-intestinal.

Up to 15% of extra-nodal lymphoma involves the GI tract (Newton et al., 1997). In a series of 15 cases of intestinal lymphoma, 60% were colorectal, 27% involved the small bowel and there were individual cases in the stomach, duodenum and ileal pouch, each constituting 6.25% of this series (Holubar et al., 2010). In 80% of these cases, the location of the lymphoma was congruous to the site of IBD. In another series of 14 colorectal lymphomas, the commonest sites were the caecum and rectosigmoid but these were not IBD patients (Wong and Eu, 2006). Gastric mantle cell lymphoma has also been reported by Raderer et al in a patient with a 14 year history of Crohn's disease (Raderer et al., 2004). Ileal pouch lymphoma has also been reported in a number of other publications (Sengul et al., 2008,

Frizzi et al., 2000, Nyam et al., 1997) and one publication suggests EBV may be involved in the aetiology (Schwartz et al., 2006). Lymphoma at an ileostomy site has also been reported (Pranesh, 2002). Metachronous colonic lymphoma (Hill et al., 1993) as well as synchronous colonic adenocarcinoma and lymphoma (Hope-Ross et al., 1985, Nishigami et al., 2010) have been described in IBD patients.

In addition, a number of extra-intestinal sites of lymphoma amongst IBD patients have been reported. Hepatosplenic T-cell lymphoma (HSTCL) has become a concern amongst IBD physicians and this will be discussed in further detail. Owen et al reports a patient with UC treated with azathioprine who develops a B-cell lymphoproliferative disorder on her eyelid following a recent illness diagnosed as infectious mononucleosis (Owen et al., 2010). Deneau et al recently described the case of a child with an EBV-driven NK-cell lymphoma involving the skin and GI tract causing hepatosplenomegaly (Deneau et al., 2010). Other cutaneous lymphomas are described in the literature (Adams et al., 2004, Martinez Tirado et al., 2001). Vulval and peri-anal lymphoma has also been identified (Winnicki et al., 2009, Sivarajasingham et al., 2003). Kastner et al present a young lady with ulcerative colitis, previously treated with azathioprine, who presents with seizures and is found to have cerebral lesions of high grade B cell lymphoma (Kastner et al., 2007). Plamacytoma (a mature B-cell lymphoma) can present as a paravertebral mass (Redmond et al., 2007).

6.2 Clinical presentation

Many of the symptoms of intestinal lymphoma are very similar to those caused by inflammatory bowel disease. The most commonly presenting symptom is bloody diarrhoea occurring in almost three quarters of cases (Holubar et al., 2010, Wong and Eu, 2006). Other common symptoms include abdominal pain, weight loss and sweats. Presentation with bowel obstruction and perforation occurs less frequently (Holubar et al., 2010, Bourikas et al., 2008). Diagnosis of lymphoma is frequently made following laparotomy. Endoscopic appearances can be diverse, manifesting as ulceration, polyps or masses.

Duration of IBD before development of lymphoma appears to be very variable between individual cases. Shepherd et al reported 10 cases of colorectal lymphoma complicating inflammatory bowel disease (6 patients with UC and 4 with CD) (Shepherd et al., 1989). The duration of inflammatory bowel disease varied from 30 months to 20 years in these cases. In the CESAME study, there was between 1 to 16 years of exposure to thiopurines before lymphoma diagnosis (Beaugerie et al., 2009a).

More unusual presentations of lymphoma include jaundice due to a nodal mass at the porta hepatis in a patient with Crohn's disease (Parasher et al., 1999), spontaneous tumour lysis syndrome in a Crohn's patient with a plasmacytoma (Froilan Torres et al., 2009), nephrotic syndrome in a patient with Hodgkin's lymphoma and UC (Basic-Jukic et al., 2002), and jaundice due to vanishing bile duct syndrome in a patient with Hodgkin's lymphoma and IBD (DeBenedet et al., 2008).

7. Population and cohort studies

A number of population and cohort studies have been published and are described below. The standardised incidence ratio (SIR) is defined as the ratio between observed and expected events in a study population. This is a useful comparator to analyse the risk of lymphoma in IBD patients and has been used in much of the literature.

Incidence and Risk Factors for Lymphoma in a Single-Center Inflammatory Bowel Disease Population (Chiorean et al 2010)

A cohort study identified 3,585 patients attending a single IBD centre in Indianapolis, USA. Data was collected retrospectively between 1990 and 2005. Since 2005, the registry was updated prospectively. An electronic database was interrogated for diagnoses of Hodgkin's and non-Hodgkin's lymphoma and compared to expected age-standardised incident rates from the SEER registry. This study also used a case matched control group with a ratio of 1:10 to determine risk factors for lymphoma development. The population consisted of 2,277 Crohn's patients and 1,308 UC patients with no significant demographic differences between groups. 8 patients were identified with a diagnosis of lymphoma (6 NHL and 2 HL). Only 3 patients had thiopurine exposure but 2 of these patients had also received TNF antagonists and were EBV positive. The study did not find any statistically significant relationship between diagnosis of lymphoma with demographics, drug therapy, duration of treatment and length of diagnosis. Based on SEER statistics, the overall SIR for lymphoma was 1.6 (95% CI 0.6 to 3.0) but this was not significant. (Chiorean et al., 2010)

Risk of Cancer in Inflammatory Bowel Disease Treated with Azathioprine: A UK Population-Based Case-Control Study (Armstrong et al 2010)

This was a nested case-control study using the General Practice Research Database (GPRD) in the UK which was interrogated for patients with a diagnosis of IBD, any previous prescriptions for azathioprine or mercaptopurine and a subsequent diagnosis of any cancer. The GPRD is the largest longitudinal primary care database in the world containing approximately 50 million patient years of data. The control group consisted of all IBD patients who had not been diagnosed with a cancer. The total number of patients included in the study was 15,471 and 15 patients had diagnoses of lymphoma (2 HL, 6 NHL and 7 unspecified). The group found the risk of lymphoma for patients who had ever received thiopurines versus those that had never received such drugs was increased by an OR of 3.22 (95% CI 1.01 to 10.18). An SIR was not calculated for the risk of lymphoma compared to the background population in this study. (Armstrong et al., 2010)

Lymphoproliferative Disorders in an Inflammatory Bowel Disease Unit (Van Domselaar et al 2010)

This was a retrospective study of 911 patients attending a tertiary IBD clinic in Madrid followed up for a mean of 32.3 months. There were 7 cases of lymphoma identified in the cohort (6 NHL and 1 HL). The mean age at diagnosis was 53 years and the mean time from IBD to lymphoma diagnosis was 4.82 years (range 0 to 20 years). Three cases were associated with EBV. An SIR of 3.72 can be calculated from the figures presented though this was not calculated by the authors. (Van Domselaar et al., 2010)

Risk of Malignant Lymphoma in Patients with Inflammatory Bowel Diseases: A Dutch Nationwide Study (Vos et al)

The authors identified all IBD patients diagnosed with lymphoma between 1997 and 2004 from a Dutch nationwide histo- and cyto-pathology database known as PALGA. Age adjusted incidence of lymphoma was obtained from the Netherlands Central Bureau for

Statistics between these years. After excluding incomplete data, 44 cases of lymphoma were identified in 17,834 IBD patients. The calculated SIR was 1.27 (95% CI 0.92 to 1.68) and the authors concluded that there was no increased risk of lymphoma in IBD patients. However, the SIRs in the age groups 35-39 years and 45-49 years were 9.32 and 3.99 respectively and these did reach significance. Only 43% of patients were exposed to thiopurines. Of the patients in whom EBV status could be obtained, 92% (11/12) with EBV positive lymphoma were taking a thiopurine compared to 19% (4/21) who were EBV negative (p<0.001). (Vos et al., 2010)

Lymphoproliferative Disorders in Patients Receiving Thiopurines for Inflammatory Bowel Disease: A Prospective Observational Cohort Study (Beaugerie et al 2009)

This is a frequently quoted study which set out to objectively clarify the risk of cancer in IBD patients. 19,486 patients were enrolled into a prospective French nationwide database called CESAME (Cancers et Surrisque Associé aux Maladies inflammatoires intestinales En France) between May 2004 and June 2005 and followed up until 31st December 2007. This equated to almost 50,000 patient-years of follow up. Details regarding patient demographics, type of IBD, date of diagnosis, disease location, history of malignancy and exposure to immunosuppressive therapy including thiopurines, methotrexate and anti-TNF agents were collected. A total of 23 patients were identified who developed lymphoma (22 NHL, 1 HL). The SIR is not presented in this study but later discussed in a review article by the same author at 1.86 (95% CI 1.1 to 3.0) (Sokol and Beaugerie, 2009). The HR for patients taking AZA versus those who were not was 5.28 (95% CI 2.01 to 13.9). There was a trend towards increased risk of lymphoma with anti-TNF therapy but this did not reach statistical significance. No patients taking methotrexate developed lymphoma in this study. (Beaugerie et al., 2009a)

Risk of Haematopoietic Cancer in Patients with Inflammatory Bowel Disease (Askling et al 2005)

This was a huge population based cohort study using prospectively recorded data from a number of large Swedish IBD databases (Uppsala cohort, Stockholm County cohort, Stockholm pan-colitis register and Swedish in-patient register). 47, 679 patients were recruited in total and 180 lymphomas were detected. Compared to national Swedish cancer statistics, the calculated SIR was 1.09 in this study. (Askling et al., 2005)

Intestinal and Extra-Intestinal Cancer in Crohn's Disease: Follow-up of a Population-based Cohort in Copenhagen, Denmark (Jess et al 2004)

374 patients with a diagnosis of Crohn's disease were followed up for a median of 17 years in Copenhagen County. No lymphomas were observed in this population. (Jess et al., 2004)

Long-term Risk of Cancer in Ulcerative Colitis : A Population-based Cohort Study from Copenhagen County (Winther et al 2004)

This study is from the same cohort of patients investigated in the above study by Jess et al. In the sample of 1160 UC patients, the median follow up was 19 years. A total of 124 malignancies were observed including only 1 lymphoma. The SIR for lymphoma risk works out at 0.5 (95% CI 0.1 to 0.8) in this study. This suggests a protective role of UC in lymphomagenesis which is not demonstrated in any other studies. This result is likely to be artefactual due to the finding of only 1 case of lymphoma in the study. (Winther et al., 2004)

Inflammatory Bowel Disease is not Associated with an Increased Risk of Lymphoma (Lewis et al 2001)

This is an important large retrospective cohort study utilising the General Practice Research Database that was also used by Armstrong et al above. All patients coded with a diagnosis of UC or CD were eligible for inclusion and cross-matched for a diagnosis of HL and NHL. Prescriptions for AZA and 6MP were also analysed and an average dose per day was calculated. A control cohort was randomly selected but matched for age, sex and primary care practice. The study identified 6,605 patients with CD, 10,391 patients with UC and there were 60,506 patients in the control group. 18 patients were identified with lymphoma in this cohort compared with an expected 13.6 cases and an SIR of 1.32 (95% CI 0.78 to 2.10). The relative risk compared to the control group was 1.20 (96% CI 0.67 to 2.06). The authors concluded that IBD was not associated with an increased risk of lymphoma. Even on sub-analysis of patients prescribed thiopurines, there was no significant increased risk of lymphoma. (Lewis et al., 2001)

Cancer Risk in Patients with Inflammatory Bowel Disease – A Population-based Study (Bernstein et al 2001)

Population-based data was obtained from the University of Manitoba IBD database which was extracted from the Manitoba Health administrative databases in Winnipeg, Canada. An age and gender matched non-IBD control group was randomly selected with a ratio of 1:10. 5,529 patients were included in the study and the overall incidence of cancer was 690.2 per 100,000 population. 16 cases of NHL were identified but no cases of HL. This study found an incident rate ratio of 1.59 (95% CI 0.6 to 3.3) for the risk of lymphoma. The risk of developing lymphoma was highest in male patients with Crohn's disease where the IRR was calculated at 3.63 (95% CI 1.53 to 8.62). (Bernstein et al., 2001)

The Incidence of Lymphoid and Myeloid Malignancies Among Hospitalized Crohn's Disease Patients (Arseneau et al 2001)

This was a retrospective cohort study. Discharge data for all in-patients in the Commonwealth of Virginia and the State of California was analysed to identify patients who were admitted to hospital with a diagnosis code for Crohn's disease. These patients were then followed up for 2 years examining for new diagnostic codes for lymphoma. The patients were matched with a control group who had admissions to hospital over the same period with no history of CD. 5,426 patients were discharged from hospital in the study period with a diagnosis of CD. 10 cases of NHL were identified and an OR of 2.04 (95% CI 1.33 to 3.14) was calculated. (Arseneau et al., 2001)

Hodgkin's Disease Risk is Increased in Patients with Ulcerative Colitis (Palli et al 2000)

This is a population based study of all patients with IBD residing in Florence, Italy between 1978 and 1992. A total of 920 patients were followed up for a median of 11 years. An increased risk of Hodgkin's disease was observed in patients with UC with 6 cases identified and an SIR calculated at 9.3 (95% CI 2.5 to 23.8). The broad confidence interval makes it difficult to assess the validity of these findings in this study. (Palli et al., 2000)

Risk of Lymphoma in Inflammatory Bowel Disease (Loftus et al 2000)

This was a retrospective study of all incidence cases of IBD in Olmsted County, Minnesota between 1950 and 1993 examined for the diagnosis of lymphoma. The authors comment that the use of immunomodulators during this time frame was rare and hoped to be able to demonstrate the baseline risk of lymphoma in IBD patients. Expected cases of lymphoma were derived from published Olmsted County age-standardised incidence rates. 454 patients were diagnosed with IBD in the study period. Only 1 case of NHL was identified in the entire cohort and an SIR of 1.0 (95% CI 0.03 to 5.6) was calculated. The observed number of patients with lymphoma is so small in this study that the results are very difficult to interpret. (Loftus et al., 2000)

Increased Incidence of non-Hodgkin's Lymphoma in Inflammatory Bowel Disease Patients on Immunosuppressive Therapy but Overall Risk is Low (Farrell et al 2000)

This study interrogated an IBD database of 782 IBD patients in Dublin. 30% of patients were taking immunomodulators therapy with the majority on azathioprine. A total of 30 cancers were identified with 4 cases of NHL compared with the expected 0.53 cases. These figures produced an SIR of 31.2 (95% CI 2.0 to 85.0). All these patients were on immunosuppressive therapy (2 on MTX and 2 on AZA). Calculating an SIR for patients on immunosuppressive therapy, the authors found a 58.8 –fold increased risk. These rather alarming results have not been duplicated. The confidence intervals are very broad and difficult to interpret. A possible explanation for these outlying results is that this retrospective study was initiated shortly after two new cases of lymphoma had been identified in this cohort. This clustering of cases may have had a significant impact on risk calculations. (Farrell et al., 2000)

Increased Risk of Cancer in Ulcerative Colitis: A Population-based Cohort Study (Karlén et al 1999)

A cohort of 1547 patients with UC in Stockholm County diagnosed between 1955 and 1984 were followed on the National Cancer Register and the National Cause of Death Register until 1989. Comparisons were made with regional cancer statistics. 3 lymphomas were identified in the cohort with an SIR of 1.2 (95% CI 0.3 to 2.5). (Karlen et al., 1999)

Long-term Neoplasia Risk after Azathioprine Treatment in Inflammatory Bowel Disease (Connell et al 1994)

This study from St Mark's Hospital in London followed up 755 IBD patients taking azathioprine for a median of 12.5 months. The overall risk of cancer was similar to that of the background population with an SIR of 1.27 but there was an increased risk of colorectal malignancy with an SIR of 6.7. No cases of lymphoma were identified in this cohort. (Connell et al., 1994)

Crohn's Disease and Cancer: A Population-based Cohort Study (Persson et al 1994)

This study was performed by the same group and used similar methodology to the Karlén study from Stockholm described above. 1251 patients with Crohn's disease were followed up. There was an increased incidence of small bowel and upper GI tract malignancies. 4 cases of lymphoma were identified with an SIR of 1.4 (95% CI 0.4 to 3.5). (Persson et al., 1994)

Extracolonic Malignancies in Inflammatory Bowel Disease (Ekbom et al 1991)

This was a population based cohort with IBD consisting of 4776 patients from the Uppsala Health Care Region in central Sweden. All patients were followed up in the Swedish Cancer Registry and the Registry of Causes of Death for a diagnosis of malignancy. 9 cases of lymphoma were found in this cohort with an expected 8.9 cases. The SIR was 1.0 (95% CI 0.5 to 1.6). (Ekbom et al., 1991)

Extraintestinal Cancers in Inflammatory Bowel Disease (Greenstein et al 1985)

This was a retrospective case note review of patients with a diagnosis of IBD at the Mount Sinai Hospital, New York. 1961 patients were studied with a total of 8 lymphomas (6 NHL and 2 HL). The expected frequency of lymphoma expected was 1.67 giving an SIR of 4.79. (Greenstein et al., 1985)

8. Baseline risk of lymphoma in IBD

An estimate of the baseline lymphoma risk has been made for this chapter using a meta-analysis technique. Populations and cohort studies were identified using the MEDLINE database provided by the US National Library of Medicine (NLM). Statistical analysis was carried out using the Review Manager (RevMan) Version 5 software which is provided by The Cochrane Collaboration, Copenhagen, for preparing and maintaining Cochrane reviews and meta-analyses. Dichotomous data was entered and analysed using the Mantel-Haentszel statistical technique and a 95% confidence interval assuming a Poisson distribution of lymphoma incidence. Studies were only weighted by their size. Graphical representation of results is performed with a Forest plot indicating 95% confidence intervals.

A total of 145,208 patients from 16 trials were included in the meta-analysis (see Figure 4). This produced a cumulative Risk Ratio of 1.29 (95% CI of 1.10 to 1.51, p=0.002). However, this included hospital-based and specialist clinic cohorts which can introduce selection bias. The meta-analysis was repeated only including the 12 population-based studies (see Figure 5). 133,463 patients were included. This did not have a very large effect on the results and the Risk Ratio falls slightly to 1.23 (95% CI 1.05 to 1.45, p=0.01). In both analyses, the test for heterogeneity was not significant and the test for overall effect was 3.15 and 2.52 respectively.

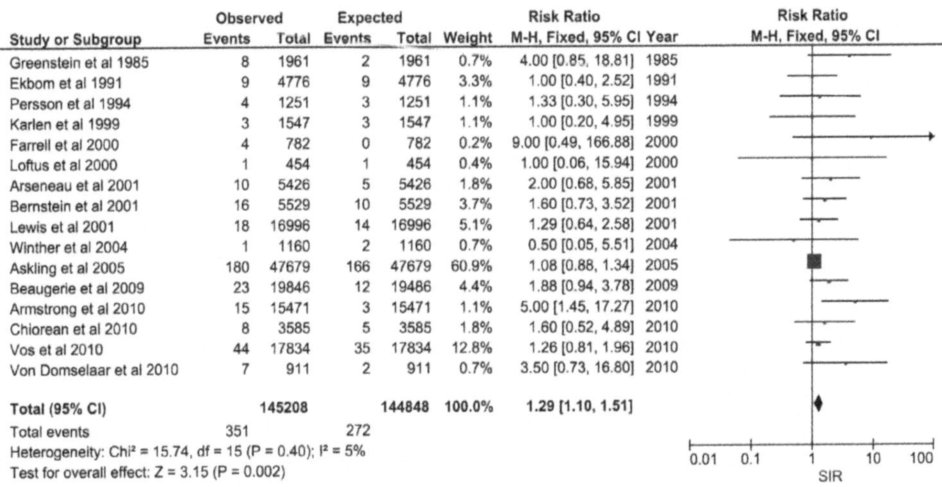

Fig. 4. Meta-analysis of population and cohort studies to evaluate the baseline risk of lymphoma.

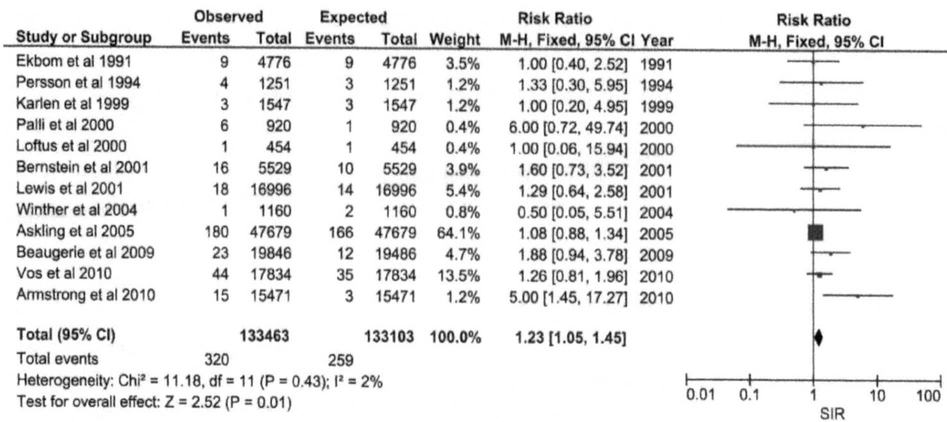

Study or Subgroup	Observed Events	Total	Expected Events	Total	Weight	Risk Ratio M-H, Fixed, 95% CI	Year	Risk Ratio M-H, Fixed, 95% CI
Ekbom et al 1991	9	4776	9	4776	3.5%	1.00 [0.40, 2.52]	1991	
Persson et al 1994	4	1251	3	1251	1.2%	1.33 [0.30, 5.95]	1994	
Karlen et al 1999	3	1547	3	1547	1.2%	1.00 [0.20, 4.95]	1999	
Palli et al 2000	6	920	1	920	0.4%	6.00 [0.72, 49.74]	2000	
Loftus et al 2000	1	454	1	454	0.4%	1.00 [0.06, 15.94]	2000	
Bernstein et al 2001	16	5529	10	5529	3.9%	1.60 [0.73, 3.52]	2001	
Lewis et al 2001	18	16996	14	16996	5.4%	1.29 [0.64, 2.58]	2001	
Winther et al 2004	1	1160	2	1160	0.8%	0.50 [0.05, 5.51]	2004	
Askling et al 2005	180	47679	166	47679	64.1%	1.08 [0.88, 1.34]	2005	
Beaugerie et al 2009	23	19846	12	19486	4.7%	1.88 [0.94, 3.78]	2009	
Vos et al 2010	44	17834	35	17834	13.5%	1.26 [0.81, 1.96]	2010	
Armstrong et al 2010	15	15471	3	15471	1.2%	5.00 [1.45, 17.27]	2010	
Total (95% CI)		133463		133103	100.0%	1.23 [1.05, 1.45]		
Total events	320		259					

Heterogeneity: Chi² = 11.18, df = 11 (P = 0.43); I² = 2%
Test for overall effect: Z = 2.52 (P = 0.01)

Fig. 5. Meta-analysis of population studies only to evaluate risk of lymphoma.

These findings would suggest that there is only a small (if any) increased risk of lymphoma in IBD patients compared to the general population.

9. Risk of lymphoma with thiopurines

The risk of lymphoma in patients treated with thiopurines has been analysed by including all cohort and population-based studies (see Figure 6). There were 35805 patients included from 7 studies. The test for heterogeneity was not significant and the test for overall effect was 4.03. Overall Risk Ratio is calculated at 3.54 (95% CI 1.91 to 6.54, p<0.0001) confirming the suspected increased risk of lymphoma in patients treated with azathioprine or mercaptopurine.

Study or Subgroup	Observed Events	Total	Expected Events	Total	Weight	Risk Ratio M-H, Fixed, 95% CI	Risk Ratio M-H, Fixed, 95% CI
Armstrong et al 2010	15	15471	5	15456	38.5%	3.00 [1.09, 8.24]	
Beaugerie et al 2009	15	16659	2	16659	15.4%	7.50 [1.72, 32.79]	
Connell et al 1994	0	755	1	755	11.5%	0.33 [0.01, 8.17]	
Farrell et al 2000	4	238	0	238	3.8%	9.00 [0.49, 166.24]	
Fraser et al 2002	8	626	2	626	15.4%	4.00 [0.85, 18.76]	
Korelitz et al 1999	2	591	1	591	7.7%	2.00 [0.18, 22.00]	
Lewis et al 2001	1	1465	1	1465	7.7%	1.00 [0.06, 15.97]	
Total (95% CI)		35805		35790	100.0%	3.54 [1.91, 6.54]	
Total events	45		12				

Heterogeneity: Chi² = 4.63, df = 6 (P = 0.59); I² = 0%
Test for overall effect: Z = 4.03 (P < 0.0001)

Fig. 6. Meta-analysis to evaluate the risk of lymphoma in patients treated with thiopurines.

10. Comparison to other published meta-analyses

Only three meta-analyses have investigated the background risk and the thiopurine-associated risk of lymphoma in IBD patients. Results from Von Roon et al and Kandiel et al support the findings of the meta-analyses produced here but the work by Masunaga et al shows some disparity.

The Risk of Cancer in Patients with Crohn's Disease (Von Roon et al 2007)

Meta-analytical techniques were used to quantify the risk of intestinal, extra-intestinal and haemopoietic malignancies in Crohn's patients. 34 studies were included with a total of 61,122 patients. Overall pooled estimates were obtained using a random-effects model. The relative risk of lymphoma was 1.42 (95% CI 1.16 to 1.73). This publication, similar to the meta-analysis presented in this dissertation, suggests only a slight increased baseline risk of lymphoma compared to the general population. (von Roon et al., 2007)

Increased Risk of Lymphoma among Inflammatory Bowel Disease Patients Treated with Azathioprine and 6-Mercaptopurine (Kandiel et al 2005)

This meta-analysis sought to provide an estimate of the relative risk of lymphoma among IBD patients treated with thiopurine therapy. Inclusion criteria were strict with only cohort studies in the English language, where the exposed group had received AZA or 6MP and the study had been specifically designed to evaluate the risk of cancer. 6 studies were included with a total of 3891 IBD patients. Similar methodology was used to the presented meta-analysis in this dissertation. Results were also pooled using a Mantzel-Haenszel method but weighting was proportioned to the inverse variance rather than the population size.

The pooled data identified 11 cases of lymphoma whilst the expected number of cases was 2.63, resulting in an SIR of 4.18 (95% CI 2.07 to 7.51). This is similar in magnitude to the SIR in the meta-analysis presented here at 3.54. However, Kandiel et al found a significant test of heterogeneity explained by the substantially higher rates of lymphoma in two of the included studies (Farrell et al 2000 and Connell et al 1994). Exclusion of these studies did not produce a large impact on the pooled SIR. (Kandiel et al., 2005)

Meta-Analysis of Risk of Malignancy with Immunosuppressive Drugs in Inflammatory Bowel Disease (Masunaga et al 2007)

This group aimed to compare the risks of developing malignancy in IBD patients receiving immunosuppressants with those who were not. 9 cohort studies met the inclusion criteria. Where a control group for comparison was not available in these studies, Masunaga et al compared incidence of lymphoma with that of the University of Manitoba IBD Database used by Bernstein et al in their population study. The meta-analysis technique calculated a Weighted Mean Difference (WMD) rather than SIR at 0.0 (95% CI -0.8 to 0.7). These results were not significant and the authors concluded that there was no increased risk of lymphoma in IBD patients treated with immunosuppressives. This result seems to deviate from the findings of the larger recent population studies (such as the CESAME study), that of the meta-analysis performed by Kandiel et al and the meta-analysis presented in this dissertation. This may be due to bias introduced by the arbitrary control method used to calculate expected lymphoma rates in control groups in this meta-analysis. (Masunaga et al., 2007)

11. Risk of lymphoma in patients treated with methotrexate

There is virtually no data for the risk of lymphoma in IBD patients taking methotrexate. Only 2 cases of lymphoma associated with MTX treatment for inflammatory bowel disease have been reported in the literature (Farrell et al., 2000). In this study, 31 patients were receiving methotrexate and two of them were subsequently diagnosed with lymphoma. One of these patients had also received cyclosporin A. As discussed earlier, the authors of this study found risk of lymphoma in their IBD cohort to be much higher than is reported elsewhere and this deviation may have resulted from a clustering of lymphoma diagnosis at the time of investigation. No reliable determination of risk can be obtained from this study.

In the large CESAME study, almost 700 patients (4%) had on-going or previous MTX use but no cases of lymphoma were identified in these patients (Beaugerie et al., 2009a).

Some information can be extrapolated from studies of other inflammatory conditions though this data must be applied with caution in IBD because the risk of the drug cannot be easily separated from the risk of the disease itself. Lymphoma associated with methotrexate has been reported in the rheumatology literature.

A large observational study of rheumatoid arthritis patients treated with methotrexate and/or anti-TNF drugs followed up 18,572 patients biannually found an SIR of 1.7 (95% CI 0.9 to 3.2). The authors concluded that there was no significant increased risk of lymphoma with methotrexate therapy over baseline (Wolfe and Michaud, 2004). A French 3 year prospective population study of RA patients treated with methotrexate identified 18 cases of NHL and 7 cases of HL. Compared to national population statistics, the authors found no increased risk of NHL but a Standardised Mortality Ratio of 7.4 (95% CI 3.0 to 15.3) for HL in their cohort (Mariette et al., 2002).

There are no similar studies in IBD and it is not possible to evaluate a relative or absolute risk of lymphoma with methotrexate therapy. However, it would appear that the risk of lymphoma in this patient group is low.

12. Risk of lymphoma in patients treated with anti-TNF drugs

It is difficult to assess the specific risk of anti-TNF drugs in IBD patients because most patients will have had thiopurine or methotrexate exposure prior to using this modality of treatment. The bulk of the literature regarding anti-TNF drugs is for the use of infliximab in Crohn's disease and little is known regarding differences in safety when used in UC.

A meta-analysis has recently been carried out by Siegel et al with very comprehensive methodology (Siegel et al., 2009). In this meta-analysis, 26 studies with a total of 8905 patients with 21,178 patient-years of exposure to anti-TNF drugs were included (see Table 2). 22 studies were regarding infliximab, 3 regarding adalimumab and only one regarding certolizumab. All the included studies were for the treatment of Crohn's disease through randomised controlled trials, cohort studies and case series. There were 13 cases of NHL with a mean age at presentation of 52 years and 62% male. 10 out of the 13 patients with NHL had received dual therapy with immunomodulators and anti-TNFs. The SIR for the risk of lymphoma in patients treated with anti-TNF drugs was 3.23 (95% CI 1.5 to 6.9) compared to SEER statistics (see Table 3). However, the majority of the lymphoma patients had previously had exposure to immunomodulators and the SIR calculated for anti-TNF therapy should actually be referred to as the risk of combination therapy. This numerical result is in the same order of magnitude as the risk for immunomodulator therapy alone (as calculated by the meta-analysis in this dissertation and other studies). This may suggest that immunomodulator therapy may play the dominant role in lymphoma risk even in settings where combination therapy is used.

Study	Year	Setting	Drug	N	Median f/u (weeks)	NHL cases
Colombel et al	2007	PRECISE RCT	CTZ	905	53	0
Colombel et al	2007	OLE of GAIN and CHARM	ADA	1169	58	0
Sandborn et al	2007	CLASSIC II RCT	ADA	276	56	1
Lemann et al	2006	RCT IXB + AZA	IXB	57	52	0
Schroder et al	2006	Controlled pilot study of IXB + MTX	IXB	19	48	0
Mantzaris et al	2004	RCT IXB + AZA	IXB	45	60	0
Sands et al	2004	IXB for fistulising CD	IXB	282	54	0
Hanauer et al	2002	ACCENT I	IXB	573	54	1
Rutgeerts et al	1999	RCT	IXB	73	48	6
Lichtenstein et al	2007	TREAT registry	IXB	3396	201	0
Biancome et al	2006	Matched pair study	IXB	404	109	1
Doumit et al	2004	Cohort study	IXB	322	104	0
Carbone et al	2007	Case series	IXB	34	52	0
Peyrin-Biroulet et al	2007	Case series for switch to ADA	ADA	52	52	0
Hyder et al	2006	Case series for fistulising CD	IXB	22	91	0
Pacault et al	2006	Case series	IXB	137	150	0
Talbot et al	2005	Case series for perianal CD	IXB	21	87	0
Choi et al	2005	Case series from Korea	IXB	13	57	0
Ardizzone et al	2004	Case series for perianal CD	IXB	20	67	0
Colombel et al	2004	Case series from Mayo Clinic	IXB	500	74	1
Rodrigo et al	2004	Case series for fistulising CD	IXB	44	72	0
Schroder et al	2004	Case series IXBMTX in fistulising CD	IXB	12	57.6	0
Sciderer et al	2004	Cohort study	IXB	92	113	0
Ljung et al	2003	Population-based cohort	IXB	191	52	3
Kinney et al	2003	Case series	IXB	117	52	0
Cohen et al	2000	Case series	IXB	129	52	0

Table 2. Studies included in meta-analysis By Siegel et al 2009. (ADA adalimumab; CTZ certolizumab, MTX methotrexate, AZA azathioprine, CD Crohn's disease, RCT randomised controlled trial, f/u follow up, OLE open label extension).

	NHL rate per 10,000 patient-years	SIR	95% CI
SEER (all ages)	1.9		
IM alone	3.6		
Anti-TNF vs SEER	6.1	3.23	1.5 to 6.9
Anti-TNF vs IM alone	6.1	1.7	0.5 to 7.1

Table 3. Results of meta-analysis by Siegel et al 2009.

The majority of these studies have relatively small numbers of patients, short follow up and were not designed to evaluate efficacy. However, the TREAT registry data includes the largest number of patients and has the longest follow up. The TREAT (Crohn's Therapy, Resource, Evaluation and Assessment Tool) registry is a large prospective, observational, multi-centre, long-term registry of Crohn's disease patients designed to evaluate the safety of infliximab and is a form of post-marketing surveillance. The TREAT registry is hoped to represent *real world* patients without the biases inherent to patients included in trials. No cases of lymphoma were reported in the registry.

The CESAME study data was not included in the meta-analysis by Siegel et al. Beaugerie et al calculated SIRs depending on anti-TNF and thiopurine combination or mono-therapy as well as whether drugs were continued or discontinued (Beaugerie et al., 2009a). These results are presented in Table 4. The results cannot confirm an increased risk of lymphoma in those continuing anti-TNF therapy because the confidence interval crosses 1.0. However, there does appear to be an increased risk when anti-TNF drugs have been used with thiopurines, particularly when combination therapy is continued.

	NHL cases	SIR	95% CI
Continuing anti-TNF therapy	2	4.53	0.55 to 16.4
Discontinued anti-TNF therapy	3	6.92	1.43 to 20.2
Continuing thiopurines and anti-TNF therapy	2	10.2	1.24 to 36.9
Continuing thiopurines but discontinued or never anti-TNFs	13	6.53	3.48 to 11.2

Table 4. SIRs in patients treated with thiopurines and anti-TNF drugs (Beaugerie et al 2009)

13. Hepatosplenic T-cell lymphoma

Hepatosplenic T-cell lymphoma (HSTCL) is a rare form of peripheral non-Hodgkin's lymphoma. In the majority of incidences, it results from a clonal expansion of γ/δ T-cells but α/β T-cell receptors can also be expressed in some cases (Gaulard et al., 1990). Only 100 to 200 cases of HSTCL in the entire medical literature have been reported (Belhadj et al., 2003) but there has been recent concern regarding the safety of thiopurines and anti-TNF therapy, particularly when used in combination, for the management of IBD. To date, 36 cases of HSTCL have been reported in IBD patients (Kotlyar et al., 2011), mostly affecting young men and the prognosis has been invariably fatal. Despite treatment with chemotherapy and stem cell transplantation, median survival is only 11 months (Falchook et al., 2009) but novel treatment strategies have shown some promise in isolated cases (Jaeger et al., 2008, Tey et al., 2008). Diagnosis is made by liver, splenic or bone marrow biopsy exhibiting atypical medium-sized lymphoid cells with round nuclei, small distinct nucleoli, loosely condensed chromatin, moderate pale cytoplasm and particular immunophenotypic expression which will be discussed further (Swerdlow et al., 2008).

13.1 Clinical presentation

The aberrant cells infiltrate into the sinusoids of the spleen, liver and bone marrow resulting in the classical presentation of hepatosplenomegaly with thrombocytopenia but no lymphadenopathy. Systemic B symptoms of fever, night sweats and weight loss may affect up to 80% of patients. Other findings may include anaemia, abnormal liver function tests and less frequently atypical lymphocytes on peripheral blood film (Falchook et al., 2009).

13.2 Immunophenotypic and genetic features

The tumour cells express CD2, surface CD3, CD7 and CD16 but there is absence of CD4, CD5, CD8 and the B-cell surface marker CD20 (Swerdlow et al., 2008). Most cases express the γ/δ T-cell receptor (TCR-γ positive) but rarer cases express the α/β T-cell receptor (TCR-β positive) and studies demonstrate clonal rearrangements of the TCR gene.

A recent systematic review investigating chromosomal abnormalities in IBD patients diagnosed with HSTCL identified the development of isochrome 7q in 57.1%, aberrations of chromosome 8 in 35.7%, trisomy 8 in 21.4% and loss of the Y chromosome in 14.3 % of cases (Kotlyar et al., 2010). The group were intrigued by the cases with loss of the Y chromosome as almost all cases of HSTCL have presented in men. These chromosomal abnormalities are not specific to IBD patients.

13.3 HSTCL in IBD

HSTCL is not linked to EBV infection. However, the risk of HSTCL does seem to be related to thiopurine and anti-TNF therapy. DNA damage specific to chromosome 7 has been seen in a dose dependent manner with thiopurine agents (Piccin et al., 2010) and inhibition of TNF may result in decreased effectiveness of immune surveillance eliminating cells with aberrant abnormal chromosomal pattern (Shale et al., 2008).

Early concern was regarding a risk of HSTCL in IBD patients who had previous exposure to both thiopurines and anti-TNF drugs but more and more cases have been identified with only thiopurine exposure. Anti-TNF drugs are frequently used in non-IBD conditions, such as rheumatoid arthritis, ankylosing spondylitis and psoriasis, but they are rarely used in combination with other immunomodulators. It is interesting that, HSTCL has only been reported in a single non-IBD patient who received adalimumab for rheumatoid arthritis (Shale et al., 2008). Conversely, there are a number of case reports of patients developing HSTCL whilst on immunosuppression in the post-transplant setting (Roelandt et al., 2009, Tey et al., 2008, Steurer et al., 2002) where anti-TNF drugs are not used.

Kotlyar et al recently presented a systematic review investigating medications, duration of therapy and ages of IBD patients diagnosed with HSTCL (Kotlyar et al., 2011). 36 cases of HSTCL have occurred in IBD patients since 1996, all of whom had a history of thiopurine exposure. 20 of these patients also had also received anti-TNF therapy. Four patients had previously received both infliximab and adalimumab and an additional patient had received a third biologic, natalizumab. There were no patients who had received an anti-TNF drug alone. Most patients had received at least 2 years therapy with a thiopurine and of those patients who had received infliximab, the number of previous infusions ranged from 1 to 20 up to 5 years prior to the diagnosis of HSTCL. The age range of patients was 12 to 58 years with a median of 23 years. The majority of patients were under 35 years old and the older patient appears to be an isolated case. Of the 31 patients in whom gender was known, only two were female.

13.4 Clinical application

From the limited information available, HSTCL seems to be linked to previous prolonged thiopurine exposure and the risk may be higher in those who have also received an anti-TNF drug. This seems to compete with conclusions drawn from recent efficacy trials. The SONIC trial found that combination therapy with azathioprine and infliximab reached significantly higher rates of steroid-free clinical remission than either of these drugs as monotherapy for a cohort of naïve patients with moderate to severe Crohn's disease (24.1% vs 34.9% vs 46.2% AZA vs IXB vs AZA+IXB at 50 weeks) (Colombel et al., 2010).

Whilst it is not possible to estimate the relative risk of HSTCL in IBD patients, Kotlyar et al attempted to derive the absolute risk of HSTCL in men using epidemiology data from the US and Europe as well as an estimate of thiopurine use in IBD patients from the French CESAME trial (Beaugerie et al., 2009a, Kotlyar et al., 2010). The group concluded that more than 99.99% of patients in immunomodulatory treatment will not develop HSTCL. Further reassurance comes from the CESAME study in that no cases of HSTCL were found despite analysis of over 50,000 patient-years follow up.

A vigilant approach must be taken when using thiopurines for the treatment of male patients under 35 years. Kotlyar et al recommended careful monitoring in patients who have been on thiopurine treatment for more than 2 years but this may be difficult to put in to practice as no pre-malignant markers have been identified. Decisions between the use of combination or monotherapy must be made in the context of clinical severity of disease and poor prognostic markers for complicated IBD. The risk of HSTCL is extremely low and patients should be made aware of this when making choices regarding their treatment. Highly efficacious therapeutic strategies should not be rejected based entirely on the low risk of HSTCL. Somewhat reassuringly, despite the rapidly increasing number of patients on anti-TNF drugs, exceeding 5 million patient-years exposure, the rate at which new cases of HSTCL have been diagnosed has not changed over the last 15 years.

14. Confounding factors and limitations

There are a number of limitations to the data which has been pooled for the meta-analyses presented in this chapter. There are also confounding factors which are not taken in to account by the source studies.

14.1 Age

Data from the US and UK clearly demonstrates that the incidence of non-Hodgkin's lymphoma, the predominant form of lymphoid neoplasm seen in IBD patients, increases with advancing age (see Figure 2). Most of the studies reviewed in this chapter use age standardised statistics to estimate risk of lymphoma in IBD patients. An earlier meta-analysis carried out by Kandiel et al, found a relative risk for the development of lymphoma in IBD patients treated with thiopurines of 4.18 (95% CI 2.07 to 7.51) which is comparable to the findings of the meta-analysis presented here. The authors went on to calculate the number of patients that would need to be treated for each new diagnosis of lymphoma i.e. the number needed to harm (NNH). Approximating to a relative risk of 4, the NNH varied from 4357 in 20-29 year olds to just 355 in 70-79 year olds (Kandiel et al., 2005). The risk of lymphoma is not uniform across all age groups and this needs to be taken in to account when this information is applied to a clinical setting.

14.2 Gender

Gender also appears to be a further factor when analysing the risk of both Hodgkin's and non-Hodgkin's lymphoma. Although other autoimmune conditions tend to affect more women, the gender difference for IBD is small. Men have an increased risk of lymphoma (see Figure 2 and Figure 3) but the magnitude of the gender difference varies with age and type of lymphoma. In NHL there is only a slight preponderance for males but in HL, the incidence is three times greater in males in certain age groups. As discussed, HSTCL occurs almost exclusively in young men. Many of the studies in this analysis did not separate results for male and female patients but this may have made analysis difficult because of the generally small number of cases of lymphoma detected in these cohorts. Vos et al, in their nationwide Dutch study, calculated SIRs for male and female patients separately but did not find a substantial difference when they took both groups as a whole. However, in the 35-39 years age range, males had an SIR of 10.25 (95% CI 2.56 to 23.05) and females, 6.74 (95% CI 1.20 to 16.77) and this difference was significant (Vos et al., 2010).

14.3 Type of lymphoma

Non-Hodgkin's lymphoma appears to be the predominant lymphoid malignancy detected in IBD patients, particularly diffuse large B-cell lymphoma (DLBCL). The CESAME study group found 22 cases of NHL and only 1 HL in their large cohort of patients from France (Beaugerie et al., 2009a). Few studies have attempted to separate findings for HL and NHL. Palli et al did find an increased risk of HL in patients with UC but the confidence interval was large and the validity of these results has been put in to question (Palli et al., 2000).

14.4 Type of IBD

Whether Crohn's disease or ulcerative colitis confers a higher risk of lymphoma has not been established. Two publications from the same population-based cohort in Copenhagen, Denmark distinguished their analysis between CD and UC patients. In the CD group no lymphomas were identified and only 1 lymphoma was found in the UC group (SIR 0.5) (Winther et al., 2004, Jess et al., 2004). A further population-based cohort from Stockholm, Sweden also analysed UC and CD separately in two different publications. Again no cases of lymphoma were seen in the CD group but there were 3 in the UC group (SIR 1.2) (Persson et al., 1994, Karlen et al., 1999). Interpreting these findings with such small numbers is fraught with difficulty. In the CESAME study, 16 of the 23 lymphomas were in patients with Crohn's disease (Beaugerie et al., 2009a).

14.5 Exposure to immunomodulators

Not all studies have attempted to evaluate the risk of lymphoma associated with immunomodulator therapy. The studies which have attempted to make this estimation are heterogenous and frequently there is a lack of distinction between lifetime exposure to these drugs, the cumulative doses received and whether cessation of a drug returns any lymphoma risk back to baseline. The CESAME study group attempted to answer some of these questions (Beaugerie et al., 2009a) by analysing patients who have *continuing*, *discontinued* or *never received* thiopurines. The SIRs for these three groups were 6.86 (95% CI 3.94 to 11.31), 1.44 (95% CI 0.17 to 5.20) and 1.43 (CI 95% 0.53 to 3.12) respectively. This may suggest that discontinuation of thiopurines returns risk to baseline but the results were not statistically significant.

14.6 Disease severity

It is not clear whether it is the disease itself, its treatment or a combination of the two which might put IBD patients at increased risk of lymphoma. It is possible that the use of drugs such as thiopurines and biologics are a marker of more aggressive disease and it is disease severity which disposes to lymphoma development. However, modern management of IBD has led to earlier use of these drugs, often in patients who do not have severe disease but possess risk factors for complicated disease, in an attempt to alter the natural history of the condition.

Severity of disease as a risk factor for lymphoma has not been analysed in any depth in IBD patients but there is some evidence available from other autoimmune diseases. A study of 378 RA patients diagnosed with lymphoma found no significant association with individual drugs but a marked increased risk with high disease activity which conferred a 70-fold increased risk (Baecklund et al., 2006). The authors concluded that it was the disease activity, not its treatment that was important in lymphomagenesis. In the CESAME study, some data regarding disease activity was collated but was not linked to lymphoma risk (Beaugerie et al., 2009a).

15. Other risk factors for lymphoma development

It is important to recognise a number of other risk factors for lymphoma development which are relevant to the IBD population but have not been well studied yet.

15.1 Pharmacogenomics of thiopurine therapy

Azathioprine is a pro-drug which is metabolised to 6-mercaptopurine and then to a number of further metabolites including 6-thioguanine (6TG) and 6-methylmercaptopurine (6MMP) which are associated with myelo- and hepato-toxicity when they accumulate at high levels. Important enzymes in this pathway include thiopurine methyl transferase (TPMT) and hypoxanthine phosphoribosyltransferase (HPRT). It is recognised that polymorphisms of TPMT can influence TPMT activity and hence levels of 6TG and 6MMP. About 1 in 300 individuals have homozygote TPMT mutations and AZA or 6MP therapy results in very high levels of 6TG causing myelo-toxicity. Those with heterozygote mutations have intermediate TPMT activity and dose adjustment of AZA and 6MP may be required.

Thiopurines are also commonly used drugs for the management of acute lymphoblastic leukaemia (ALL) in paediatric patients. Following treatment, these patients have an increased risk of subsequently developing secondary myelodysplasia or acute myeloid leukaemia but it had been thought that this risk is associated with alkylating agents, epipodophyllotoxins or radiation therapy rather than due to AZA. However, Bo et al showed that paediatric patients with allelic variations of the TPMT gene (and lower TPMT levels) had a higher rate of secondary leukaemias in this setting (Bo et al., 1999). Thiopurines result in the incorporation of 6TG, a purine analogue, into lymphocyte DNA which can activate DNA repair mechanisms. This introduces the risk of point mutations and chromosomal abnormalities during repair processes. It follows that higher levels of 6TG may increase this risk further, possibly explaining the link with lymphomagenesis in IBD patients treated with thiopurines.

Disanti et al made an interesting observation in a cohort of IBD patients treated with 6MP over a 37 year period. The investigators divided the group of over 600 patients in to those who developed a sustained leukopenia of $<4.0 \times 10^9/l$ for 20 or more days and those who did not. They found that there was an increased risk of haematological malignancies in the group with sustained leukopenia (p=0.014) (Disanti et al., 2006).

Although, the TPMT levels were not known in these patients, further investigation in to the association between TPMT and lymphoma risk may be intriguing.

15.2 Radiation exposure

The use of imaging modalities such as computed tomography and fluoroscopy have been an important component for the diagnosis and assessment of IBD but there has been increasing concern regarding the cancer risk associated with diagnostic ionising radiation (Brenner and Hall, 2007). Much of the risk of medical radiation exposure is extrapolated from studies of populations near nuclear explosions and occupational exposure but there is some evidence in certain medical settings (Brenner et al., 2003). For example, young patients with scoliosis who have had repeated chest x-rays were at increased risk of breast malignancy (Doody et al., 2000).

Recent evidence suggests that CT imaging is being used more frequently in IBD patients, particularly those with Crohn's disease (Newnham et al., 2007, Kroeker et al., 2011). Leukaemia is well recognised as a long term consequence of radiation exposure and this risk is higher in children (Darby et al., 1992, Shimizu et al., 1990). However, there is little evidence to confirm an increased risk of lymphoma in patients exposed to diagnostic ionising radiation though the mechanisms of oncogenesis may be similar. There was no increased risk of lymphoma seen in patients receiving radiotherapy for uterine cancer nor amongst tuberculosis patients with repeated pneumothorax who had an average of 77 chest x-rays on follow up (Boice, 1992). A study including 318 NHL patients found no increased exposure to diagnostic radiation compared to controls if imaging from the 12 months immediately prior to lymphoma diagnosis was excluded. The authors felt that radiological procedures within this period were performed to investigate the lymphoma rather than a causative factor (Boice et al., 1991).

15.3 Vitamin D and sunlight exposure

Vitamin D deficiency is common amongst IBD patients. Recent studies have shown suboptimal levels of Vitamin D in 57 to 78% of recently diagnosed patients with IBD (Leslie et al., 2008, Bours et al., 2010). The protective role of Vitamin D has been investigated in a number of malignancies including prostate, colon, lung, pancreatic, endometrial, breast and even skin cancer (Schwartz and Skinner, 2007). The paracrine and autocrine effects of extra-renal 25-hydroxy-Vitamin-D_3 via the nuclear Vitamin D Receptor (VDR) include regulation of cell cycle proliferation, induction of apoptosis and increased cell differentiation signalling.

Recent epidemiologic studies demonstrate a reduction in NHL risk with increased sunlight exposure (Armstrong and Kricker, 2007). As sunlight is a major vitamin D source, it has been suggested that vitamin D status may mediate this observed association. A recent review of the literature could not conclude or dismiss a link between vitamin D insufficiency and lymphoma due to confounding findings in a number of studies and the limitations on the accuracy of dietary history taking which was the most frequent methodology in these studies (Kelly et al., 2009).

The role of Vitamin D in lymphomagenesis in the IBD population has not been investigated and warrants further study.

16. Summary of findings and application to clinical practice

This systematic review and the meta-analyses carried out in this chapter have made some key findings:

- There is only a small (if any) increased overall risk of lymphoma in IBD patients.
- Thiopurine therapy results in a 3 to 4-fold increased risk of lymphoma in IBD patients.
- The risk of lymphoma with methotrexate therapy cannot be evaluated adequately but appears to be low.
- Treatment with anti-TNF drugs appears to confer an increased risk of lymphoma in IBD patients. However, this may reflect previous or concurrent immunomodulator exposure rather than the risk of anti-TNFs alone.
- HSTCL is associated with long term thiopurine therapy. Additionally, anti-TNF therapy may increase this risk.

It is the role of the IBD physician to help patients balance up the risks and benefits of these drugs and make the right choice for themselves. Due to the significant morbidity associated with IBD, simply avoiding these drugs is frequently not an option. It is mandatory to provide clear communication of risks and benefits and to individualise this to the patient because lymphoma risk in IBD patients is not uniform nor is the risk of complicated disease. A recent study found that patients were more likely to tolerate the risk of adverse events due to IBD drug therapy for moderately symptomatic Crohn's disease than gastroenterologists would choose for their patients (Johnson et al., 2010).

Patient selection is paramount. The risk of most forms of lymphoma appears to be higher in males and in older age groups. HSTCL is particularly relevant to men under the age of 35 years. Special consideration of the risks must be made in these groups. A number of predictors for severe or complicated disease are now being identified which should allow selection of patients who are most likely to gain from aggressive treatment (Beaugerie et al., 2006).

There is ample evidence that immunomodulators and anti-TNF drugs are very effective for the treatment of IBD. In a 30 year review, Fraser et al found that there were 64% and 87% remission rates at 6 months for patients treated with AZA for Crohn's disease and ulcerative colitis respectively (Fraser et al., 2002). Feagan et al found 65% remission at 40 weeks with MTX for Crohn's disease (Feagan et al., 2000). In the SONIC study, there was 57% remission at 1 year for combined AZA and IXB therapy (Colombel et al., 2010). The CHARM study and its open label extension, ADHERE, for adalimumab in Crohn's disease found improved fistula healing rates, 57% decreased hospitalisation and improved Work Productivity Scores (Panaccione et al., 2010). A Markov model found that the benefits of azathioprine for the treatment of Crohn's disease outweighed the risk of lymphoma but such calculations are inherently based on estimations and assumptions (Lewis et al., 2000).

Additionally, there is evidence that stopping these drugs may be harmful to patients. Azathioprine withdrawal leads to relapse within 18 months at 21% vs 8% (p=0.02, NNH=8) (Lemann et al., 2005). Methotrexate withdrawal leads to relapse within 40 weeks in 61% vs 35% (p=0.04, NNH=4) (Feagan et al., 2000). Infliximab withdrawal leads to hospitalisation within 1 year in 38% vs 23% (p=0.05, NNH=7) (Rutgeerts et al., 2004). However, the CESAME study did suggest that stopping immunomodulator therapy did return the risk of lymphoma back to baseline.

No form of screening is able to predict lymphoma development. Although, the role of vitamin D status and TPMT expression on lymphoma risk is intriguing, there is insufficient evidence to recommend the routine testing of these parameters to guide patient management. Prophylactic use of antivirals in renal transplant recipients has been shown to reduce the risk of post-transplant lymphoproliferative disorders by as much as 83% and the use of this strategy in IBD patients on immunosuppression is warranted (Funch et al., 2005).

The morbidity associated with IBD, the efficacy of these drugs and the risks of stopping them are important factors in making management decisions with patients. In many patients, the benefits will outweigh the risks.

17. References

Adams, A. E., Zwicker, J., Curiel, C., Kadin, M. E., Falchuk, K. R., Drews, R. & Kupper, T. S. 2004. Aggressive cutaneous T-cell lymphomas after TNFalpha blockade. *J Am Acad Dermatol*, 51, 660-2.

Altekruse, S., Kosary, C., Krapcho, M., Neyman, N., Aminou, R., Waldron, W., Ruhl, J., Howlander, N., Tatalovich, Z., Cho, H., Mariotto, A., Eisner, M., Lewis, D., Cronin, K., Chen, H., Feuer, E., Stinchcomb, D. & Edwards, B. 2010. SEER Cancer Statistics Review, 1975-2007. National Cancer Institute.

Altieri, A., Bermejo, J. L. & Hemminki, K. 2005. Familial risk for non-Hodgkin lymphoma and other lymphoproliferative malignancies by histopathologic subtype: the Swedish Family-Cancer Database. *Blood*, 106, 668-72.

Aozasa, K., Takakuwa, T. & Nakatsuka, S. 2005. Pyothorax-associated lymphoma: a lymphoma developing in chronic inflammation. *Adv Anat Pathol*, 12, 324-31.

Ardizzone, S., Maconi, G., Colombo, E., Manzionna, G., Bollani, S. & Bianchi Porro, G. 2004. Perianal fistulae following infliximab treatment: clinical and endosonographic outcome. *Inflamm Bowel Dis*, 10, 91-6.

Armstrong, B. K. & Kricker, A. 2007. Sun exposure and non-Hodgkin lymphoma. *Cancer Epidemiol Biomarkers Prev*, 16, 396-400.

Armstrong, R. G., West, J. & Card, T. R. 2010. Risk of cancer in inflammatory bowel disease treated with azathioprine: a UK population-based case-control study. *Am J Gastroenterol*, 105, 1604-9.

Arseneau, K. O., Stukenborg, G. J., Connors, A. F., Jr. & Cominelli, F. 2001. The incidence of lymphoid and myeloid malignancies among hospitalized Crohn's disease patients. *Inflamm Bowel Dis*, 7, 106-12.

Askling, J., Brandt, L., Lapidus, A., Karlen, P., Bjorkholm, M., Lofberg, R. & Ekbom, A. 2005. Risk of haematopoietic cancer in patients with inflammatory bowel disease. *Gut*, 54, 617-22.

Aydogan, A., Corapcioglu, F., Elemen, E. L., Oncel, S., Gurbuz, Y. & Tugay, M. 2010. Childhood non-Hodgkin's lymphoma arising as a complication early in the course of Crohn's disease. *Turk J Pediatr*, 52, 411-5.

Bacon, P. A. & Salmon, M. 1987. Modes of action of second-line agents. *Scand J Rheumatol Suppl*, 64, 17-24.

Baecklund, E., Iliadou, A., Askling, J., Ekbom, A., Backlin, C., Granath, F., Catrina, A. I., Rosenquist, R., Feltelius, N., Sundstrom, C. & Klareskog, L. 2006. Association of chronic inflammation, not its treatment, with increased lymphoma risk in rheumatoid arthritis. *Arthritis Rheum*, 54, 692-701.

Bargen, J. 1928. Chronic ulcerative colitis associated with malignant disease. *Arch Surg*, 17, 561-576.

Barrett, J. C., Hansoul, S., Nicolae, D. L., Cho, J. H., Duerr, R. H., Rioux, J. D., Brant, S. R., Silverberg, M. S., Taylor, K. D., Barmada, M. M., Bitton, A., Dassopoulos, T., Datta, L. W., Green, T., Griffiths, A. M., Kistner, E. O., Murtha, M. T., Regueiro, M. D., Rotter, J. I., Schumm, L. P., Steinhart, A. H., Targan, S. R., Xavier, R. J., Libioulle, C., Sandor, C., Lathrop, M., Belaiche, J., Dewit, O., Gut, I., Heath, S., Laukens, D., Mni, M., Rutgeerts, P., Van Gossum, A., Zelenika, D., Franchimont, D., Hugot, J. P., De Vos, M., Vermeire, S., Louis, E., Cardon, L. R., Anderson, C. A., Drummond, H., Nimmo, E., Ahmad, T., Prescott, N. J., Onnie, C. M., Fisher, S. A., Marchini, J., Ghori, J., Bumpstead, S., Gwilliam, R., Tremelling, M., Deloukas, P., Mansfield, J., Jewell, D., Satsangi, J., Mathew, C. G., Parkes, M., Georges, M. & Daly, M. J. 2008. Genome-wide association defines more than 30 distinct susceptibility loci for Crohn's disease. *Nat Genet*, 40, 955-62.

Bartram, C. & Chrispin, A. R. 1973. Primary lymphosarcoma of the ileum and caecum. *Pediatr Radiol*, 1, 28-33.

Basic-Jukic, N., Radman, I., Roncevic, T. & Jakic-Razumovic, J. 2002. Hodgkin s disease with nephrotic syndrome as a complication of ulcerative colitis: case report. *Croat Med J*, 43, 573-5.

Beaugerie, L., Brousse, N., Bouvier, A. M., Colombel, J. F., Lemann, M., Cosnes, J., Hebuterne, X., Cortot, A., Bouhnik, Y., Gendre, J. P., Simon, T., Maynadie, M.,

Hermine, O., Faivre, J. & Carrat, F. 2009a. Lymphoproliferative disorders in patients receiving thiopurines for inflammatory bowel disease: a prospective observational cohort study. *Lancet,* 374, 1617-25.

Beaugerie, L., Seksik, P. & Carrat, F. 2009b. Thiopurine therapy is associated with a three-fold decrease in the incidence of advanced neoplaisa in IBD patients with longstanding extensive colitis: the CESAME prospective data. *Journal of Crohn's and Colitis,* 3.

Beaugerie, L., Seksik, P., Nion-Larmurier, I., Gendre, J. P. & Cosnes, J. 2006. Predictors of Crohn's disease. *Gastroenterology,* 130, 650-6.

Beaugerie, L., Sokol, H. & Seksik, P. 2009c. Noncolorectal malignancies in inflammatory bowel disease: more than meets the eye. *Dig Dis,* 27, 375-81.

Belhadj, K., Reyes, F., Farcet, J. P., Tilly, H., Bastard, C., Angonin, R., Deconinck, E., Charlotte, F., Leblond, V., Labouyrie, E., Lederlin, P., Emile, J. F., Delmas-Marsalet, B., Arnulf, B., Zafrani, E. S. & Gaulard, P. 2003. Hepatosplenic gammadelta T-cell lymphoma is a rare clinicopathologic entity with poor outcome: report on a series of 21 patients. *Blood,* 102, 4261-9.

Bernstein, C. N. 2010. Epidemiologic clues to inflammatory bowel disease. *Curr Gastroenterol Rep,* 12, 495-501.

Bernstein, C. N., Blanchard, J. F., Kliewer, E. & Wajda, A. 2001. Cancer risk in patients with inflammatory bowel disease: a population-based study. *Cancer,* 91, 854-62.

Biancone, L., Orlando, A., Kohn, A., Colombo, E., Sostegni, R., Angelucci, E., Rizzello, F., Castiglione, F., Benazzato, L., Papi, C., Meucci, G., Riegler, G., Petruzziello, C., Mocciaro, F., Geremia, A., Calabrese, E., Cottone, M. & Pallone, F. 2006. Infliximab and newly diagnosed neoplasia in Crohn's disease: a multicentre matched pair study. *Gut,* 55, 228-33.

Bo, J., Schroder, H., Kristinsson, J., Madsen, B., Szumlanski, C., Weinshilboum, R., Andersen, J. B. & Schmiegelow, K. 1999. Possible carcinogenic effect of 6-mercaptopurine on bone marrow stem cells: relation to thiopurine metabolism. *Cancer,* 86, 1080-6.

Boice, J. D., Jr. 1992. Radiation and non-Hodgkin's lymphoma. *Cancer Res,* 52, 5489s-5491s.

Boice, J. D., Jr., Morin, M. M., Glass, A. G., Friedman, G. D., Stovall, M., Hoover, R. N. & Fraumeni, J. F., JR. 1991. Diagnostic x-ray procedures and risk of leukemia, lymphoma, and multiple myeloma. *JAMA,* 265, 1290-4.

Bourikas, L. A., Tzardi, M., Hatzidakis, A. & Koutroubakis, I. E. 2008. Small bowel perforation due to non-Hodgkin-lymphoma in a patient with ulcerative colitis and systemic lupus erythematosus. *Dig Liver Dis,* 40, 144.

Bours, P. H., Wielders, J. P., Vermeijden, J. R. & Van De Wiel, A. 2010. Seasonal variation of serum 25-hydroxyvitamin D levels in adult patients with inflammatory bowel disease. *Osteoporos Int.*

Brenner, D. J. & Hall, E. J. 2007. Computed tomography--an increasing source of radiation exposure. *N Engl J Med,* 357, 2277-84.

Brenner, D. J., Doll, R., Goodhead, D. T., Hall, E. J., Land, C. E., Little, J. B., Lubin, J. H., Preston, D. L., Preston, R. J., Puskin, J. S., Ron, E., Sachs, R. K., Samet, J. M., Setlow, R. B. & Zaider, M. 2003. Cancer risks attributable to low doses of ionizing radiation: assessing what we really know. *Proc Natl Acad Sci U S A,* 100, 13761-6.

Camera, L., Della Noce, M. & Cirillo, L. C. 1997. [Primary ileo-cecal lymphoma mimicking Crohn's disease. Report of a case]. *Radiol Med,* 94, 122-4.

Cancer-Research-UK. 2011. *Cancer Research UK* [Online]. Available: http://www.cancerresearchuk.org/.

Carbone, J., Gonzalez-Lara, V., Sarmiento, E., Chean, C., Perez, J. L., Marin, I., Rodriguez-Molina, J. J., Gil, J. & Fernandez-Cruz, E. 2007. Humoral and cellular monitoring to predict the development of infection in Crohn's disease patients beginning treatment with infliximab. *Ann N Y Acad Sci,* 1107, 346-55.

Chandesris, M. O., Malamut, G., Verkarre, V., Meresse, B., Macintyre, E., Delarue, R., Rubio, M. T., Suarez, F., Deau-Fischer, B., Cerf-Bensussan, N., Brousse, N., Cellier, C. & Hermine, O. 2010. Enteropathy-associated T-cell lymphoma: a review on clinical presentation, diagnosis, therapeutic strategies and perspectives. *Gastroenterol Clin Biol,* 34, 590-605.

Chang, E. T., Smedby, K. E., Hjalgrim, H., Porwit-Macdonald, A., Roos, G., Glimelius, B. & Adami, H. O. 2005. Family history of hematopoietic malignancy and risk of lymphoma. *J Natl Cancer Inst,* 97, 1466-74.

Chiorean, M. V., Pokhrel, B., Adabala, J., Helper, D. J., Johnson, C. S. & Juliar, B. 2010. Incidence and Risk Factors for Lymphoma in a Single-Center Inflammatory Bowel Disease Population. *Dig Dis Sci.*

Cho, J. H. 2008. The genetics and immunopathogenesis of inflammatory bowel disease. *Nat Rev Immunol,* 8, 458-66.

Cohen, R. D. 2001. Efficacy and safety of repeated infliximab infusions for Crohn's disease: 1-year clinical experience. *Inflamm Bowel Dis,* 7 Suppl 1, S17-22.

Coleman, J. R. 1999. Cancer Survival Trends in England & Wales, 1971-1995 by deprivation and NHS region. *The Stationary Office.*

Colombel, J. F., Loftus, E. V., Jr., Tremaine, W. J., Egan, L. J., Harmsen, W. S., Schleck, C. D., Zinsmeister, A. R. & Sandborn, W. J. 2004. The safety profile of infliximab in patients with Crohn's disease: the Mayo clinic experience in 500 patients. *Gastroenterology,* 126, 19-31.

Colombel, J. F., Sandborn, W. J., Reinisch, W., Mantzaris, G. J., Kornbluth, A., Rachmilewitz, D., Lichtiger, S., D'haens, G., Diamond, R. H., Broussard, D. L., Tang, K. L., Van Der Woude, C. J. & Rutgeerts, P. 2010. Infliximab, azathioprine, or combination therapy for Crohn's disease. *N Engl J Med,* 362, 1383-95.

Connell, W. R., Kamm, M. A., Dickson, M., Balkwill, A. M., Ritchie, J. K. & Lennard-Jones, J. E. 1994. Long-term neoplasia risk after azathioprine treatment in inflammatory bowel disease. *Lancet,* 343, 1249-52.

Cosnes, J., Nion-Larmurier, I., Beaugerie, L., Afchain, P., Tiret, E. & Gendre, J. P. 2005. Impact of the increasing use of immunosuppressants in Crohn's disease on the need for intestinal surgery. *Gut,* 54, 237-41.

Dal Maso, L. & Franceschi, S. 2006. Hepatitis C virus and risk of lymphoma and other lymphoid neoplasms: a meta-analysis of epidemiologic studies. *Cancer Epidemiol Biomarkers Prev,* 15, 2078-85.

Darby, S. C., Olsen, J. H., Doll, R., Thakrar, B., Brown, P. D., Storm, H. H., Barlow, L., Langmark, F., Teppo, L. & Tulinius, H. 1992. Trends in childhood leukaemia in the

Nordic countries in relation to fallout from atmospheric nuclear weapons testing. *BMJ*, 304, 1005-9.

Dayharsh, G. A., Loftus, E. V., Jr., Sandborn, W. J., Tremaine, W. J., Zinsmeister, A. R., Witzig, T. E., Macon, W. R. & Burgart, L. J. 2002. Epstein-Barr virus-positive lymphoma in patients with inflammatory bowel disease treated with azathioprine or 6-mercaptopurine. *Gastroenterology*, 122, 72-7.

Debenedet, A. T., Berg, C. L., Enfield, K. B., Woodford, R. L., Bennett, A. K. & Northup, P. G. 2008. A case of vanishing bile duct syndrome and IBD secondary to Hodgkin's lymphoma. *Nat Clin Pract Gastroenterol Hepatol*, 5, 49-53.

Deneau, M., Wallentine, J., Guthery, S., O'gorman, M., Bohnsack, J., Fluchel, M., Bezzant, J. & Pohl, J. F. 2010. Natural killer cell lymphoma in a pediatric patient with inflammatory bowel disease. *Pediatrics*, 126, e977-81.

D'haens, G. R. 2009. Top-down therapy for Crohn's disease: rationale and evidence. *Acta Clin Belg*, 64, 540-6.

Diebold, D. 2001. World Health Organisation Classification of Malignant Lymphomas. *Experimental Oncology*, 23, 101-103.

Disanti, W., Rajapakse, R. O., Korelitz, B. I., Panagopoulos, G. & Bratcher, J. 2006. Incidence of neoplasms in patients who develop sustained leukopenia during or after treatment with 6-mercaptopurine for inflammatory bowel disease. *Clin Gastroenterol Hepatol*, 4, 1025-9.

Doody, M. M., Lonstein, J. E., Stovall, M., Hacker, D. G., Luckyanov, N. & Land, C. E. 2000. Breast cancer mortality after diagnostic radiography: findings from the U.S. Scoliosis Cohort Study. *Spine (Phila Pa 1976)*, 25, 2052-63.

Ekbom, A., Helmick, C., Zack, M. & Adami, H. O. 1991. Extracolonic malignancies in inflammatory bowel disease. *Cancer*, 67, 2015-9.

Ekstrom Smedby, K., Vajdic, C. M., Falster, M., Engels, E. A., Martinez-Maza, O., Turner, J., Hjalgrim, H., Vineis, P., Seniori Costantini, A., Bracci, P. M., Holly, E. A., Willett, E., Spinelli, J. J., La Vecchia, C., Zheng, T., Becker, N., De Sanjose, S., Chiu, B. C., Dal Maso, L., Cocco, P., Maynadie, M., Foretova, L., Staines, A., Brennan, P., Davis, S., Severson, R., Cerhan, J. R., Breen, E. C., Birmann, B., Grulich, A. E. & Cozen, W. 2008. Autoimmune disorders and risk of non-Hodgkin lymphoma subtypes: a pooled analysis within the InterLymph Consortium. *Blood*, 111, 4029-38.

Epstein, M. A., Achong, B. G. & Barr, Y. M. 1964. Virus Particles in Cultured Lymphoblasts from Burkitt's Lymphoma. *Lancet*, 1, 702-3.

Falchook, G. S., Vega, F., Dang, N. H., Samaniego, F., Rodriguez, M. A., Champlin, R. E., Hosing, C., Verstovsek, S. & Pro, B. 2009. Hepatosplenic gamma-delta T-cell lymphoma: clinicopathological features and treatment. *Ann Oncol*, 20, 1080-5.

Farrell, R. J., Ang, Y., Kileen, P., O'briain, D. S., Kelleher, D., Keeling, P. W. & Weir, D. G. 2000. Increased incidence of non-Hodgkin's lymphoma in inflammatory bowel disease patients on immunosuppressive therapy but overall risk is low. *Gut*, 47, 514-9.

FDA. 2011. *FDA* [Online]. Available: http://www.fda.gov/.

Feagan, B. G., Fedorak, R. N., Irvine, E. J., Wild, G., Sutherland, L., Steinhart, A. H., Greenberg, G. R., Koval, J., Wong, C. J., Hopkins, M., Hanauer, S. B. & Mcdonald, J.

W. 2000. A comparison of methotrexate with placebo for the maintenance of remission in Crohn's disease. North American Crohn's Study Group Investigators. *N Engl J Med*, 342, 1627-32.

Federman, J., Goldstein, M. E. & Weingarten, B. 1963. Malignant lymphoma of over fifteen years' duration masquerading as ulcerative colitis. *Am J Roentgenol Radium Ther Nucl Med*, 89, 771-8.

Fraser, A. G., Orchard, T. R. & Jewell, D. P. 2002. The efficacy of azathioprine for the treatment of inflammatory bowel disease: a 30 year review. *Gut*, 50, 485-9.

Friedman, H. B., Silver, G. M. & Brown, C. H. 1968. Lymphoma of the colon simulating ulcerative colitis. Report of four cases. *Am J Dig Dis*, 13, 910-7.

Frizzi, J. D., Rivera, D. E., Harris, J. A. & Hamill, R. L. 2000. Lymphoma arising in an S-pouch after total proctocolectomy for ulcerative colitis: report of a case. *Dis Colon Rectum*, 43, 540-3.

Froilan Torres, C., Castro Carbajo, P., Pajares Villarroya, R., Plaza Santos, R., Gomez Senent, S., Martin Arranz, M. D., Adan Merino, L., Martin Arranz, E., Mancenido Marcos, N., Peces, R. & Benito Lopez, D. 2009. Acute spontaneous tumor lysis syndrome in a patient with Crohn's disease taking immunosuppressants. *Rev Esp Enferm Dig*, 101, 288-94.

Funch, D. P., Walker, A. M., Schneider, G., Ziyadeh, N. J. & Pescovitz, M. D. 2005. Ganciclovir and acyclovir reduce the risk of post-transplant lymphoproliferative disorder in renal transplant recipients. *American journal of transplantation : official journal of the American Society of Transplantation and the American Society of Transplant Surgeons*, 5, 2894-900.

Gaulard, P., Bourquelot, P., Kanavaros, P., Haioun, C., Le Couedic, J. P., Divine, M., Goossens, M., Zafrani, E. S., Farcet, J. P. & Reyes, F. 1990. Expression of the alpha/beta and gamma/delta T-cell receptors in 57 cases of peripheral T-cell lymphomas. Identification of a subset of gamma/delta T-cell lymphomas. *Am J Pathol*, 137, 617-28.

Ghosh, S. & Mitchell, R. 2007. Impact of inflammatory bowel disease on quality of life: Results of the European Federation of Crohn's and Ulcerative Colitis Associations (EFCCA) patient survey. *J Crohns Colitis*, 1, 10-20.

Glaser, S. L. 1991. Black-white differences in Hodgkin's disease incidence in the United States by age, sex, histology subtype and time. *Int J Epidemiol*, 20, 68-75.

Goldin, L. R., Pfeiffer, R. M., Gridley, G., Gail, M. H., Li, X., Mellemkjaer, L., Olsen, J. H., Hemminki, K. & Linet, M. S. 2004. Familial aggregation of Hodgkin lymphoma and related tumors. *Cancer*, 100, 1902-8.

Greenstein, A. J., Gennuso, R., Sachar, D. B., Heimann, T., Smith, H., Janowitz, H. D. & Aufses, A. H., JR. 1985. Extraintestinal cancers in inflammatory bowel disease. *Cancer*, 56, 2914-21.

Grulich, A. E., Vajdic, C. M. & Cozen, W. 2007a. Altered immunity as a risk factor for non-Hodgkin lymphoma. *Cancer Epidemiol Biomarkers Prev*, 16, 405-8.

Grulich, A. E., Van Leeuwen, M. T., Falster, M. O. & Vajdic, C. M. 2007b. Incidence of cancers in people with HIV/AIDS compared with immunosuppressed transplant recipients: a meta-analysis. *Lancet*, 370, 59-67.

Hanauer, S. B., Feagan, B. G., Lichtenstein, G. R., Mayer, L. F., Schreiber, S., Colombel, J. F., Rachmilewitz, D., Wolf, D. C., Olson, A., Bao, W. & Rutgeerts, P. 2002. Maintenance infliximab for Crohn's disease: the ACCENT I randomised trial. *Lancet,* 359, 1541-9.

Hanauer, S. B., Sandborn, W. J., Rutgeerts, P., Fedorak, R. N., Lukas, M., Macintosh, D., Panaccione, R., Wolf, D. & Pollack, P. 2006. Human anti-tumor necrosis factor monoclonal antibody (adalimumab) in Crohn's disease: the CLASSIC-I trial. *Gastroenterology,* 130, 323-33; quiz 591.

Hemminki, K., Li, X., Sundquist, J. & Sundquist, K. 2008. Cancer risks in ulcerative colitis patients. *Int J Cancer,* 123, 1417-21.

Hill, D. H., Mills, J. O. & Maxwell, R. J. 1993. Metachronous colonic lymphomas complicating chronic ulcerative colitis. *Abdom Imaging,* 18, 369-70.

Hjalgrim, H., Askling, J., Sorensen, P., Madsen, M., Rosdahl, N., Storm, H. H., Hamilton-Dutoit, S., Eriksen, L. S., Frisch, M., Ekbom, A. & Melbye, M. 2000. Risk of Hodgkin's disease and other cancers after infectious mononucleosis. *J Natl Cancer Inst,* 92, 1522-8.

Holubar, S. D., Dozois, E. J., Loftus, E. V., Jr., Teh, S. H., Benavente, L. A., Harmsen, W. S., Wolff, B. G., Cima, R. R. & Larson, D. W. 2010. Primary intestinal lymphoma in patients with inflammatory bowel disease: A descriptive series from the prebiologic therapy era. *Inflamm Bowel Dis.*

Hope-Ross, M., Magee, D. J., O'donoghue, D. P. & Murphy, J. J. 1985. Ulcerative colitis complicated by lymphoma and adenocarcinoma. *Br J Surg,* 72, 22.

Hurlstone, D. P. 2002. Early phase mantle cell lymphoma: macroscopic similarities to terminal ileal Crohn's disease. *Am J Gastroenterol,* 97, 1577-8.

Isomoto, H., Furusu, H., Onizuka, Y., Kawaguchi, Y., Mizuta, Y., Maeda, T. & Kohno, S. 2003. Colonic involvement by adult T-cell leukemia/lymphoma mimicking ulcerative colitis. *Gastrointest Endosc,* 58, 805-8.

Jaeger, G., Bauer, F., Brezinschek, R., Beham-Schmid, C., Mannhalter, C. & Neumeister, P. 2008. Hepatosplenic gammadelta T-cell lymphoma successfully treated with a combination of alemtuzumab and cladribine. *Ann Oncol,* 19, 1025-6.

Jaffe, E., Harris, N., Stein, H. & Vardiman, J. (eds.) 2001. *World Health Organisation Classification of Tumours. Pathology and Genetics of Tumours of Haemopoietic and Lymphoid Tissues*: IARC Press, Lyon.

Jarnerot, G., Hertervig, E., Friis-Liby, I., Blomquist, L., Karlen, P., Granno, C., Vilien, M., Strom, M., Danielsson, A., Verbaan, H., Hellstrom, P. M., Magnuson, A. & Curman, B. 2005. Infliximab as rescue therapy in severe to moderately severe ulcerative colitis: a randomized, placebo-controlled study. *Gastroenterology,* 128, 1805-11.

Jarrett, A. F., Armstrong, A. A. & Alexander, E. 1996. Epidemiology of EBV and Hodgkin's lymphoma. *Ann Oncol,* 7 Suppl 4, 5-10.

Jess, T., Loftus, E. V., Jr., Velayos, F. S., Harmsen, W. S., Zinsmeister, A. R., Smyrk, T. C., Schleck, C. D., Tremaine, W. J., Melton, L. J., 3rd, Munkholm, P. & Sandborn, W. J. 2006. Risk of intestinal cancer in inflammatory bowel disease: a population-based study from olmsted county, Minnesota. *Gastroenterology,* 130, 1039-46.

Jess, T., Winther, K. V., Munkholm, P., Langholz, E. & Binder, V. 2004. Intestinal and extra-intestinal cancer in Crohn's disease: follow-up of a population-based cohort in Copenhagen County, Denmark. *Aliment Pharmacol Ther*, 19, 287-93.

Johnson, F. R., Hauber, B., Ozdemir, S., Siegel, C. A., Hass, S. & Sands, B. E. 2010. Are gastroenterologists less tolerant of treatment risks than patients? Benefit-risk preferences in Crohn's disease management. *J Manag Care Pharm*, 16, 616-28.

Jost, P. J. & Ruland, J. 2007. Aberrant NF-kappaB signaling in lymphoma: mechanisms, consequences, and therapeutic implications. *Blood*, 109, 2700-7.

Jouini, S., Ayadi, K., Mokrani, A., Wachuku, E., Hmouda, H. & Gourdie, R. 2001. [Mediterranean lymphoma mimicking Crohn's disease]. *J Radiol*, 82, 855-8.

Kandiel, A., Fraser, A. G., Korelitz, B. I., Brensinger, C. & Lewis, J. D. 2005. Increased risk of lymphoma among inflammatory bowel disease patients treated with azathioprine and 6-mercaptopurine. *Gut*, 54, 1121-5.

Kang, H. Y., Hwang, J. H., Park, Y. S., Bang, S. M., Lee, J. S., Chung, J. H. & Kim, H. 2007. Angioimmunoblastic T-cell lymphoma mimicking Crohn's disease. *Dig Dis Sci*, 52, 2743-7.

Karlen, P., Lofberg, R., Brostrom, O., Leijonmarck, C. E., Hellers, G. & Persson, P. G. 1999. Increased risk of cancer in ulcerative colitis: a population-based cohort study. *Am J Gastroenterol*, 94, 1047-52.

Kashi, M. R., Belayev, L. & Parker, A. 2010. Primary extranodal Hodgkin lymphoma of the colon masquerading as new diagnosis of Crohn's disease. *Clin Gastroenterol Hepatol*, 8, A20.

Kastner, F., Paulus, W., Deckert, M., Schlegel, P., Evers, S. & Husstedt, I. W. 2007. [Primary CNS lymphoma in azathioprine therapy for autoimmune diseases: review of the literature and case report]. *Nervenarzt*, 78, 451-6.

Kawashima, K., Hayashi, K., Ohnoshi, T., Teramoto, N. & Kimura, I. 1994. Epstein-Barr virus-associated post-transplant non-Hodgkin's lymphoma: establishment and characterization of a new cell line. *Jpn J Cancer Res*, 85, 1080-6.

Kelly, J. L., Friedberg, J. W., Calvi, L. M., Van Wijngaarden, E. & Fisher, S. G. 2009. Vitamin D and non-Hodgkin lymphoma risk in adults: a review. *Cancer Invest*, 27, 942-51.

Kinney, T., Rawlins, M., Kozarek, R., France, R. & Patterson, D. 2003. Immunomodulators and "on demand" therapy with infliximab in Crohn's disease: clinical experience with 400 infusions. *Am J Gastroenterol*, 98, 608-12.

Kotlyar, D. S., Blonski, W., Diamond, R. H., Wasik, M. & Lichtenstein, G. R. 2010. Hepatosplenic T-cell lymphoma in inflammatory bowel disease: a possible thiopurine-induced chromosomal abnormality. *Am J Gastroenterol*, 105, 2299-301.

Kotlyar, D. S., Osterman, M. T., Diamond, R. H., Porter, D., Blonski, W. C., Wasik, M., Sampat, S., Mendizabal, M., Lin, M. V. & Lichtenstein, G. R. 2011. A systematic review of factors that contribute to hepatosplenic T-cell lymphoma in patients with inflammatory bowel disease. *Clin Gastroenterol Hepatol*, 9, 36-41 e1.

Kroeker, K. I., Lam, S., Birchall, I. & Fedorak, R. N. 2011. Patients with IBD are exposed to high levels of ionizing radiation through CT scan diagnostic imaging: a five-year study. *J Clin Gastroenterol*, 45, 34-9.

Kuppers, R., Klein, U., Hansmann, M. L. & Rajewsky, K. 1999. Cellular origin of human B-cell lymphomas. *N Engl J Med*, 341, 1520-9.

Lal, S. & Steinhart, A. H. 2006. Antibiotic therapy for Crohn's disease: a review. *Can J Gastroenterol*, 20, 651-5.

Langmead, L. & Rampton, D. S. 2006. Review article: complementary and alternative therapies for inflammatory bowel disease. *Aliment Pharmacol Ther*, 23, 341-9.

Larsson, S. C. & Wolk, A. 2007. Obesity and risk of non-Hodgkin's lymphoma: a meta-analysis. *Int J Cancer*, 121, 1564-70.

Lemann, M., Mary, J. Y., Colombel, J. F., Duclos, B., Soule, J. C., Lerebours, E., Modigliani, R. & Bouhnik, Y. 2005. A randomized, double-blind, controlled withdrawal trial in Crohn's disease patients in long-term remission on azathioprine. *Gastroenterology*, 128, 1812-8.

Lemann, M., Mary, J. Y., Duclos, B., Veyrac, M., Dupas, J. L., Delchier, J. C., Laharie, D., Moreau, J., Cadiot, G., Picon, L., Bourreille, A., Sobahni, I. & Colombel, J. F. 2006. Infliximab plus azathioprine for steroid-dependent Crohn's disease patients: a randomized placebo-controlled trial. *Gastroenterology*, 130, 1054-61.

Leslie, W. D., Miller, N., Rogala, L. & Bernstein, C. N. 2008. Vitamin D status and bone density in recently diagnosed inflammatory bowel disease: the Manitoba IBD Cohort Study. *Am J Gastroenterol*, 103, 1451-9.

Lewis, J. D., Bilker, W. B., Brensinger, C., Deren, J. J., Vaughn, D. J. & Strom, B. L. 2001. Inflammatory bowel disease is not associated with an increased risk of lymphoma. *Gastroenterology*, 121, 1080-7.

Lewis, J. D., Schwartz, J. S. & Lichtenstein, G. R. 2000. Azathioprine for maintenance of remission in Crohn's disease: benefits outweigh the risk of lymphoma. *Gastroenterology*, 118, 1018-24.

Lichtenstein, G. R., Feagan, B. G., Cohen, R. D., Salzberg, B. A., Diamond, R. H., Chen, D. M., Pritchard, M. L. & Sandborn, W. J. 2006. Serious infections and mortality in association with therapies for Crohn's disease: TREAT registry. *Clin Gastroenterol Hepatol*, 4, 621-30.

Ling, Y. H., Chan, J. Y., Beattie, K. L. & Nelson, J. A. 1992. Consequences of 6-thioguanine incorporation into DNA on polymerase, ligase, and endonuclease reactions. *Mol Pharmacol*, 42, 802-7.

Ljung, T., Karlen, P., Schmidt, D., Hellstrom, P. M., Lapidus, A., Janczewska, I., Sjoqvist, U. & Lofberg, R. 2004. Infliximab in inflammatory bowel disease: clinical outcome in a population based cohort from Stockholm County. *Gut*, 53, 849-53.

Lofstrom, B., Backlin, C., Sundstrom, C., Ekbom, A. & Lundberg, I. E. 2007. A closer look at non-Hodgkin's lymphoma cases in a national Swedish systemic lupus erythematosus cohort: a nested case-control study. *Ann Rheum Dis*, 66, 1627-32.

Loftus, E. V., Jr., Tremaine, W. J., Habermann, T. M., Harmsen, W. S., Zinsmeister, A. R. & Sandborn, W. J. 2000. Risk of lymphoma in inflammatory bowel disease. *Am J Gastroenterol*, 95, 2308-12.

Long, M. D., Herfarth, H. H., Pipkin, C. A., Porter, C. Q., Sandler, R. S. & Kappelman, M. D. 2010. Increased risk for non-melanoma skin cancer in patients with inflammatory bowel disease. *Clin Gastroenterol Hepatol*, 8, 268-74.

Luo, J. C., Hwang, S. J., Li, C. P., Liu, J. H., Chen, P. M., Liu, S. M., Chiang, J. H., Chang, F. Y. & Lee, S. D. 1997. Primary low grade B-cell lymphoma of colon mimicking inflammatory bowel disease: a case report. *Zhonghua Yi Xue Za Zhi (Taipei)*, 59, 367-71.

Luther, J., Dave, M., Higgins, P. D. & Kao, J. Y. 2010. Association between Helicobacter pylori infection and inflammatory bowel disease: a meta-analysis and systematic review of the literature. *Inflamm Bowel Dis*, 16, 1077-84.

Maaravi, Y., Wengrower, D. & Leibowitz, G. 1993. A unique presentation of lymphoma of the colon. *J Clin Gastroenterol*, 17, 49-51.

Mack, T. M., Cozen, W., Shibata, D. K., Weiss, L. M., Nathwani, B. N., Hernandez, A. M., Taylor, C. R., Hamilton, A. S., Deapen, D. M. & Rappaport, E. B. 1995. Concordance for Hodgkin's disease in identical twins suggesting genetic susceptibility to the young-adult form of the disease. *N Engl J Med*, 332, 413-8.

Mariette, X., Cazals-Hatem, D., Warszawki, J., Liote, F., Balandraud, N. & Sibilia, J. 2002. Lymphomas in rheumatoid arthritis patients treated with methotrexate: a 3-year prospective study in France. *Blood*, 99, 3909-15.

Martinez Tirado, P., Redondo Cerezo, E., Gonzalez Aranda, Y., M, J. C. T., Nogueras Lopez, F. & Gomez Garcia, M. 2001. [Ki-1 lymphoma of the skin in a patient with Crohn's disease undergoing treatment with azathioprine]. *Gastroenterol Hepatol*, 24, 271-2.

Masunaga, Y., Ohno, K., Ogawa, R., Hashiguchi, M., Echizen, H. & Ogata, H. 2007. Meta-analysis of risk of malignancy with immunosuppressive drugs in inflammatory bowel disease. *Ann Pharmacother*, 41, 21-8.

Mccullough, J. E., Kim, C. H. & Banks, P. M. 1992. Mantle zone lymphoma of the colon simulating diffuse inflammatory bowel disease. Role of immunohistochemistry in establishing the diagnosis. *Dig Dis Sci*, 37, 934-8.

Merhi, M., Raynal, H., Cahuzac, E., Vinson, F., Cravedi, J. P. & Gamet-Payrastre, L. 2007. Occupational exposure to pesticides and risk of hematopoietic cancers: meta-analysis of case-control studies. *Cancer Causes Control*, 18, 1209-26.

MHRA. 2011. *MHRA* [Online]. Available: http://www.mhra.gov.uk/index.htm.

Miligi, L., Costantini, A. S., Benvenuti, A., Kriebel, D., Bolejack, V., Tumino, R., Ramazzotti, V., Rodella, S., Stagnaro, E., Crosignani, P., Amadori, D., Mirabelli, D., Sommani, L., Belletti, I., Troschel, L., Romeo, L., Miceli, G., Tozzi, G. A., Mendico, I. & Vineis, P. 2006. Occupational exposure to solvents and the risk of lymphomas. *Epidemiology*, 17, 552-61.

Myerson, P., Myerson, D., Miller, D., Deluca, V. A., Jr. & Lawson, J. P. 1974. Lymphosarcoma of the bowel masquerading as ulcerative colitis: report of a case. *Dis Colon Rectum*, 17, 710-5.

Neri, A., Barriga, F., Inghirami, G., Knowles, D. M., Neequaye, J., Magrath, I. T. & Dalla-Favera, R. 1991. Epstein-Barr virus infection precedes clonal expansion in Burkitt's and acquired immunodeficiency syndrome-associated lymphoma. *Blood*, 77, 1092-5.

Newnham, E., Hawkes, E., Surender, A., James, S. L., Gearry, R. & Gibson, P. R. 2007. Quantifying exposure to diagnostic medical radiation in patients with inflammatory bowel disease: are we contributing to malignancy? *Aliment Pharmacol Ther*, 26, 1019-24.

Newton, R., Ferlay, J., Beral, V. & Devesa, S. S. 1997. The epidemiology of non-Hodgkin's lymphoma: comparison of nodal and extra-nodal sites. *Int J Cancer*, 72, 923-30.

Nguyen, T., Vacek, P. M., O'neill, P., Colletti, R. B. & Finette, B. A. 2009. Mutagenicity and potential carcinogenicity of thiopurine treatment in patients with inflammatory bowel disease. *Cancer Res*, 69, 7004-12.

Nishigami, T., Kataoka, T. R., Torii, I., Sato, A., Tamura, K., Hirano, H., Hida, N., Ikeuchi, H. & Tsujimura, T. 2010. Concomitant adenocarcinoma and colonic non-Hodgkin's lymphoma in a patient with ulcerative colitis: a case report and molecular analysis. *Pathol Res Pract*, 206, 846-50.

Nyam, D. C., Pemberton, J. H., Sandborn, W. J. & Savcenko, M. 1997. Lymphoma of the pouch after ileal pouch-anal anastomosis: report of a case. *Dis Colon Rectum*, 40, 971-2.

O'donovan, P., Perrett, C. M., Zhang, X., Montaner, B., Xu, Y. Z., Harwood, C. A., Mcgregor, J. M., Walker, S. L., Hanaoka, F. & Karran, P. 2005. Azathioprine and UVA light generate mutagenic oxidative DNA damage. *Science*, 309, 1871-4.

Ogura, Y., Bonen, D. K., Inohara, N., Nicolae, D. L., Chen, F. F., Ramos, R., Britton, H., Moran, T., Karaliuskas, R., Duerr, R. H., Achkar, J. P., Brant, S. R., Bayless, T. M., Kirschner, B. S., Hanauer, S. B., Nunez, G. & Cho, J. H. 2001. A frameshift mutation in NOD2 associated with susceptibility to Crohn's disease. *Nature*, 411, 603-6.

Oruc, N., Ozutemiz, O., Tekin, F., Sezak, M., Tuncyurek, M., Krasinskas, A. M. & Tombuloglu, M. 2010. Celiac disease associated with B-cell lymphoma. *Turk J Gastroenterol*, 21, 168-71.

Owen, C. E., Callen, J. P. & Bahrami, S. 2010. Cutaneous Lymphoproliferative Disorder Complicating Infectious Mononucleosis in an Immunosuppressed Patient. *Pediatr Dermatol*.

Packey, C. D. & Sartor, R. B. 2008. Interplay of commensal and pathogenic bacteria, genetic mutations, and immunoregulatory defects in the pathogenesis of inflammatory bowel diseases. *J Intern Med*, 263, 597-606.

Palli, D., Trallori, G., Bagnoli, S., Saieva, C., Tarantino, O., Ceroti, M., D'albasio, G., Pacini, F., Amorosi, A. & Masala, G. 2000. Hodgkin's disease risk is increased in patients with ulcerative colitis. *Gastroenterology*, 119, 647-53.

Panaccione, R., Colombel, J. F., Sandborn, W. J., Rutgeerts, P., D'haens, G. R., Robinson, A. M., Chao, J., Mulani, P. M. & Pollack, P. F. 2010. Adalimumab sustains clinical remission and overall clinical benefit after 2 years of therapy for Crohn's disease. *Aliment Pharmacol Ther*, 31, 1296-309.

Parasher, G., Jaswal, S., Golbey, S., Grinberg, M. & Iswara, K. 1999. Extraintestinal non-Hodgkin's lymphoma presenting as obstructive jaundice in a patient with Crohn's disease. *Am J Gastroenterol*, 94, 226-8.

Parkin, D. M. 2006. The global health burden of infection-associated cancers in the year 2002. *Int J Cancer*, 118, 3030-44.

Parnes, I. H., Warner, R. R., Berman, R. & Sanders, M. 1974. Diffuse lymphosarcoma of the colon simulating ulcerative colitis. *Mt Sinai J Med*, 41, 802-6.

Persson, P. G., Karlen, P., Bernell, O., Leijonmarck, C. E., Brostrom, O., Ahlbom, A. & Hellers, G. 1994. Crohn's disease and cancer: a population-based cohort study. *Gastroenterology,* 107, 1675-9.

Peyrin-Biroulet, L., Laclotte, C. & Bigard, M. A. 2007. Adalimumab maintenance therapy for Crohn's disease with intolerance or lost response to infliximab: an open-label study. *Aliment Pharmacol Ther,* 25, 675-80.

Piccin, A., Cortelazzo, S., Rovigatti, U., Bourke, B. & Smith, O. P. 2010. Immunosuppressive treatments in Crohn's disease induce myelodysplasia and leukaemia. *Am J Hematol,* 85, 634.

Pohl, C., Eidt, S., Ziegenhagen, D. & Kruis, W. 1991. [Immunoproliferative disease of the small intestine. A rare differential diagnosis of Crohn's disease]. *Dtsch Med Wochenschr,* 116, 1265-9.

Pranesh, N. 2002. Lymphoma in an ileostomy. *Postgrad Med J,* 78, 368-9.

Raderer, M., Puspok, A., Birkner, T., Streubel, B. & Chott, A. 2004. Primary gastric mantle cell lymphoma in a patient with long standing history of Crohn's disease. *Leuk Lymphoma,* 45, 1459-62.

Redmond, M., Quinn, J., Murphy, P., Patchett, S. & Leader, M. 2007. Plasmablastic lymphoma presenting as a paravertebral mass in a patient with Crohn's disease after immunosuppressive therapy. *J Clin Pathol,* 60, 80-1.

Reijasse, D., Le Pendeven, C., Cosnes, J., Dehee, A., Gendre, J. P., Nicolas, J. C. & Beaugerie, L. 2004. Epstein-Barr virus viral load in Crohn's disease: effect of immunosuppressive therapy. *Inflamm Bowel Dis,* 10, 85-90.

Rodrigo, L., Perez-Pariente, J. M., Fuentes, D., Cadahia, V., Garcia-Carbonero, A., Nino, P., De Francisco, R., Tojo, R., Moreno, M. & Gonzalez-Ballina, E. 2004. Retreatment and maintenance therapy with infliximab in fistulizing Crohn's disease. *Rev Esp Enferm Dig,* 96, 548-54; 554-8.

Roelandt, P. R., Maertens, J., Vandenberghe, P., Verslype, C., Roskams, T., Aerts, R., Nevens, F. & Dierickx, D. 2009. Hepatosplenic gammadelta T-cell lymphoma after liver transplantation: report of the first 2 cases and review of the literature. *Liver Transpl,* 15, 686-92.

Rubin, G. P., Hungin, A. P., Chinn, D. J. & Dwarakanath, D. 2004. Quality of life in patients with established inflammatory bowel disease: a UK general practice survey. *Aliment Pharmacol Ther,* 19, 529-35.

Rubin, G. P., Hungin, A. P., Kelly, P. J. & Ling, J. 2000. Inflammatory bowel disease: epidemiology and management in an English general practice population. *Aliment Pharmacol Ther,* 14, 1553-9.

Rutgeerts, P., D'haens, G., Targan, S., Vasiliauskas, E., Hanauer, S. B., Present, D. H., Mayer, L., Van Hogezand, R. A., Braakman, T., Dewoody, K. L., Schaible, T. F. & Van Deventer, S. J. 1999. Efficacy and safety of retreatment with anti-tumor necrosis factor antibody (infliximab) to maintain remission in Crohn's disease. *Gastroenterology,* 117, 761-9.

Rutgeerts, P., Van Assche, G. & Vermeire, S. 2004. Optimizing anti-TNF treatment in inflammatory bowel disease. *Gastroenterology,* 126, 1593-610.

Rutter, M. D., Saunders, B. P., Wilkinson, K. H., Rumbles, S., Schofield, G., Kamm, M. A., Williams, C. B., Price, A. B., Talbot, I. C. & Forbes, A. 2006. Thirty-year analysis of a colonoscopic surveillance program for neoplasia in ulcerative colitis. *Gastroenterology*, 130, 1030-8.

Sandborn, W. J., Feagan, B. G., Stoinov, S., Honiball, P. J., Rutgeerts, P., Mason, D., Bloomfield, R. & Schreiber, S. 2007a. Certolizumab pegol for the treatment of Crohn's disease. *N Engl J Med*, 357, 228-38.

Sandborn, W. J., Hanauer, S. B., Rutgeerts, P., Fedorak, R. N., Lukas, M., Macintosh, D. G., Panaccione, R., Wolf, D., Kent, J. D., Bittle, B., Li, J. & Pollack, P. F. 2007b. Adalimumab for maintenance treatment of Crohn's disease: results of the CLASSIC II trial. *Gut*, 56, 1232-9.

Sands, B. E., Anderson, F. H., Bernstein, C. N., Chey, W. Y., Feagan, B. G., Fedorak, R. N., Kamm, M. A., Korzenik, J. R., Lashner, B. A., Onken, J. E., Rachmilewitz, D., Rutgeerts, P., Wild, G., Wolf, D. C., Marsters, P. A., Travers, S. B., Blank, M. A. & Van Deventer, S. J. 2004. Infliximab maintenance therapy for fistulizing Crohn's disease. *N Engl J Med*, 350, 876-85.

Sartor, R. B. 2008. Microbial influences in inflammatory bowel diseases. *Gastroenterology*, 134, 577-94.

Satsangi, J., Silverberg, M. S., Vermeire, S. & Colombel, J. F. 2006. The Montreal classification of inflammatory bowel disease: controversies, consensus, and implications. *Gut*, 55, 749-53.

Schroder, O., Blumenstein, I. & Stein, J. 2006. Combining infliximab with methotrexate for the induction and maintenance of remission in refractory Crohn's disease: a controlled pilot study. *Eur J Gastroenterol Hepatol*, 18, 11-6.

Schroder, O., Blumenstein, I., Schulte-Bockholt, A. & Stein, J. 2004. Combining infliximab and methotrexate in fistulizing Crohn's disease resistant or intolerant to azathioprine. *Aliment Pharmacol Ther*, 19, 295-301.

Schwartz, G. G. & Skinner, H. G. 2007. Vitamin D status and cancer: new insights. *Curr Opin Clin Nutr Metab Care*, 10, 6-11.

Schwartz, L. K., Kim, M. K., Coleman, M., Lichtiger, S., Chadburn, A. & Scherl, E. 2006. Case report: lymphoma arising in an ileal pouch anal anastomosis after immunomodulatory therapy for inflammatory bowel disease. *Clin Gastroenterol Hepatol*, 4, 1030-4.

Scully, C., Eveson, J. W., Witherow, H., Young, A. H., Tan, R. S. & Gilby, E. D. 1993. Oral presentation of lymphoma: case report of T-cell lymphoma masquerading as oral Crohn's disease, and review of the literature. *Eur J Cancer B Oral Oncol*, 29B, 225-9.

Seiderer, J., Goke, B. & Ochsenkuhn, T. 2004. Safety aspects of infliximab in inflammatory bowel disease patients. A retrospective cohort study in 100 patients of a German University Hospital. *Digestion*, 70, 3-9.

Sengul, N., Berho, M., Baig, M. K. & Weiss, E. 2008. Ileal pouch lymphoma following restorative proctocolectomy for ulcerative colitis. *Inflamm Bowel Dis*, 14, 584.

Serraino, D., Salamina, G., Franceschi, S., Dubois, D., La Vecchia, C., Brunet, J. B. & Ancelle-Park, R. A. 1992. The epidemiology of AIDS-associated non-Hodgkin's lymphoma in the World Health Organization European Region. *Br J Cancer*, 66, 912-6.

Shale, M., Kanfer, E., Panaccione, R. & Ghosh, S. 2008. Hepatosplenic T cell lymphoma in inflammatory bowel disease. *Gut*, 57, 1639-41.

Shepherd, N. A., Hall, P. A., Williams, G. T., Codling, B. W., Jones, E. L., Levison, D. A. & Morson, B. C. 1989. Primary malignant lymphoma of the large intestine complicating chronic inflammatory bowel disease. *Histopathology*, 15, 325-37.

Shimizu, Y., Kato, H. & Schull, W. J. 1990. Studies of the mortality of A-bomb survivors. 9. Mortality, 1950-1985: Part 2. Cancer mortality based on the recently revised doses (DS86). *Radiat Res*, 121, 120-41.

Siegel, C. A., Marden, S. M., Persing, S. M., Larson, R. J. & Sands, B. E. 2009. Risk of lymphoma associated with combination anti-tumor necrosis factor and immunomodulator therapy for the treatment of Crohn's disease: a meta-analysis. *Clin Gastroenterol Hepatol*, 7, 874-81.

Silano, M., Volta, U., Vincenzi, A. D., Dessi, M. & Vincenzi, M. D. 2008. Effect of a gluten-free diet on the risk of enteropathy-associated T-cell lymphoma in celiac disease. *Dig Dis Sci*, 53, 972-6.

Sivarajasingham, N., Adams, S. A., Smith, M. E. & Hosie, K. B. 2003. Perianal Hodgkin's lymphoma complicating Crohn's disease. *Int J Colorectal Dis*, 18, 174-6.

Smedby, K. E., Hjalgrim, H., Askling, J., Chang, E. T., Gregersen, H., Porwit-Macdonald, A., Sundstrom, C., Akerman, M., Melbye, M., Glimelius, B. & Adami, H. O. 2006. Autoimmune and chronic inflammatory disorders and risk of non-Hodgkin lymphoma by subtype. *J Natl Cancer Inst*, 98, 51-60.

Smith, M. A., Irving, P. M., Marinaki, A. M. & Sanderson, J. D. 2010. Review article: malignancy on thiopurine treatment with special reference to inflammatory bowel disease. *Aliment Pharmacol Ther*, 32, 119-30.

Sokol, H. & Beaugerie, L. 2009. Inflammatory bowel disease and lymphoproliferative disorders: the dust is starting to settle. *Gut*, 58, 1427-36.

Steinmaus, C., Smith, A. H., Jones, R. M. & Smith, M. T. 2008. Meta-analysis of benzene exposure and non-Hodgkin lymphoma: biases could mask an important association. *Occup Environ Med*, 65, 371-8.

Steurer, M., Stauder, R., Grunewald, K., Gunsilius, E., Duba, H. C., Gastl, G. & Dirnhofer, S. 2002. Hepatosplenic gammadelta-T-cell lymphoma with leukemic course after renal transplantation. *Hum Pathol*, 33, 253-8.

Stevens, S. J., Verschuuren, E. A., Pronk, I., Van Der Bij, W., Harmsen, M. C., The, T. H., Meijer, C. J., Van Den Brule, A. J. & Middeldorp, J. M. 2001. Frequent monitoring of Epstein-Barr virus DNA load in unfractionated whole blood is essential for early detection of posttransplant lymphoproliferative disease in high-risk patients. *Blood*, 97, 1165-71.

Swerdlow, S., Campo, E., Harris, N., Jaffe, E., Pileri, S., Stein, H., Thiele, J. & Vardiman, J. (eds.) 2008. *World Health Organisation Classification of Tumours of the Haemopoietic and Lymphoid Tissues*, Lyon: IARC Press.

Talbot, C., Sagar, P. M., Johnston, M. J., Finan, P. J. & Burke, D. 2005. Infliximab in the surgical management of complex fistulating anal Crohn's disease. *Colorectal Dis*, 7, 164-8.

Tey, S. K., Marlton, P. V., Hawley, C. M., Norris, D. & Gill, D. S. 2008. Post-transplant hepatosplenic T-cell lymphoma successfully treated with HyperCVAD regimen. *Am J Hematol*, 83, 330-3.

Theander, E., Henriksson, G., Ljungberg, O., Mandl, T., Manthorpe, R. & Jacobsson, L. T. 2006. Lymphoma and other malignancies in primary Sjogren's syndrome: a cohort study on cancer incidence and lymphoma predictors. *Ann Rheum Dis*, 65, 796-803.

Thompson, C. A., Habermann, T. M., Wang, A. H., Vierkant, R. A., Folsom, A. R., Ross, J. A. & Cerhan, J. R. 2010. Antioxidant intake from fruits, vegetables and other sources and risk of non-Hodgkin's lymphoma: the Iowa Women's Health Study. *Int J Cancer*, 126, 992-1003.

Toruner, M., Loftus, E. V., Jr., Harmsen, W. S., Zinsmeister, A. R., Orenstein, R., Sandborn, W. J., Colombel, J. F. & Egan, L. J. 2008. Risk factors for opportunistic infections in patients with inflammatory bowel disease. *Gastroenterology*, 134, 929-36.

Travis, L. B., Curtis, R. E., Boice, J. D., Jr., Hankey, B. F. & Fraumeni, J. F., JR. 1991. Second cancers following non-Hodgkin's lymphoma. *Cancer*, 67, 2002-9.

Travis, L. B., Curtis, R. E., Glimelius, B., Holowaty, E., Van Leeuwen, F. E., Lynch, C. F., Adami, J., Gospodarowicz, M., Wacholder, S., Inskip, P. & Et Al. 1993. Second cancers among long-term survivors of non-Hodgkin's lymphoma. *J Natl Cancer Inst*, 85, 1932-7.

Van Dieren, J. M., Kuipers, E. J., Samsom, J. N., Nieuwenhuis, E. E. & Van Der Woude, C. J. 2006. Revisiting the immunomodulators tacrolimus, methotrexate, and mycophenolate mofetil: their mechanisms of action and role in the treatment of IBD. *Inflamm Bowel Dis*, 12, 311-27.

Van Domselaar, M., Lopez San Roman, A., Bastos Oreiro, M. & Garrido Gomez, E. 2010. [Lymphoproliferative disorders in an inflammatory bowel disease unit]. *Gastroenterol Hepatol*, 33, 12-6.

Vincenzi, B., Finolezzi, E., Fossati, C., Verzi, A., Santini, D., Tonini, G., Arullani, A. & Avvisati, G. 2001. Unusual presentation of Hodgkin's disease mimicking inflammatory bowel disease. *Leuk Lymphoma*, 42, 521-6.

Von Roon, A. C., Reese, G., Teare, J., Constantinides, V., Darzi, A. W. & Tekkis, P. P. 2007. The risk of cancer in patients with Crohn's disease. *Dis Colon Rectum*, 50, 839-55.

Vos, A. C., Bakkal, N., Minnee, R. C., Casparie, M. K., De Jong, D. J., Dijkstra, G., Stokkers, P., Van Bodegraven, A. A., Pierik, M., Van Der Woude, C. J., Oldenburg, B. & Hommes, D. W. 2010. Risk of malignant lymphoma in patients with inflammatory bowel diseases: A Dutch nationwide study. *Inflamm Bowel Dis*.

Wagonfeld, J. B., Baker, A. L., Reed, J. S., Platz, C. E. & Kirsner, J. B. 1976. Acute dilation of the colon in malignant lymphoma. *Gastroenterology*, 70, 264-7.

Winnicki, M., Gariepy, G., Sauthier, P. G. & Funaro, D. 2009. Hodgkin lymphoma presenting as a vulvar mass in a patient with crohn disease: a case report and literature review. *J Low Genit Tract Dis*, 13, 110-4.

Winther, K. V., Jess, T., Langholz, E., Munkholm, P. & Binder, V. 2004. Long-term risk of cancer in ulcerative colitis: a population-based cohort study from Copenhagen County. *Clin Gastroenterol Hepatol*, 2, 1088-95.

Wolfe, F. & Michaud, K. 2004. Lymphoma in rheumatoid arthritis: the effect of methotrexate and anti-tumor necrosis factor therapy in 18,572 patients. *Arthritis Rheum,* 50, 1740-51.

Wong, M. T. & Eu, K. W. 2006. Primary colorectal lymphomas. *Colorectal Dis,* 8, 586-91.

Wong, N. A., Herbst, H., Herrmann, K., Kirchner, T., Krajewski, A. S., Moorghen, M., Niedobitek, F., Rooney, N., Shepherd, N. A. & Niedobitek, G. 2003. Epstein-Barr virus infection in colorectal neoplasms associated with inflammatory bowel disease: detection of the virus in lymphomas but not in adenocarcinomas. *J Pathol,* 201, 312-8.

Xue, F. B., Xu, Y. Y., Wan, Y., Pan, B. R., Ren, J. & Fan, D. M. 2001. Association of H. pylori infection with gastric carcinoma: a Meta analysis. *World J Gastroenterol,* 7, 801-4.

Zachos, M., Tondeur, M. & Griffiths, A. M. 2007. Enteral nutritional therapy for induction of remission in Crohn's disease. *Cochrane Database Syst Rev,* CD000542.

Zhang, S. M., Hunter, D. J., Rosner, B. A., Giovannucci, E. L., Colditz, G. A., Speizer, F. E. & Willett, W. C. 2000. Intakes of fruits, vegetables, and related nutrients and the risk of non-Hodgkin's lymphoma among women. *Cancer Epidemiol Biomarkers Prev,* 9, 477-85.

16

Development, Optimization and Absorption Mechanism of DHP107, Oral Paclitaxel Formulation for Single-Agent Anticancer Therapy

In-Hyun Lee, Jung Wan Hong, Yura Jang,
Yeong Taek Park and Hesson Chung
*Korea Institute of Science and Technology
and Daehwa Pharmaceutical
Korea*

1. Introduction

Paclitaxel, administered as intravenous infusion currently, is an effective anticancer drug belonging to the taxane family (Figure 1) and used in the treatment of a wide variety of cancers including breast and ovarian cancers (Rowinsky et al., 1995). Researchers have been looking for more effective and convenient ways to administer paclitaxel with less formulation-related toxicities than the commercially available formulations like Taxol® by Bristol-Meyers Squibb. It is well known that some of the limitations of the current formulation come from Cremophor EL, a polyoxyethylated castor oil. This particular component is known to cause hypersensitivity (Weiss et al., 1990), to be responsible for nonlinear pharmacokinetic behavior (Kearns et al., 1995; Gianni, 1995) and to cause paclitaxel precipitation oftentimes when diluted during the infusion process (Pfeifer, 1993). Formulations for paclitaxel and its analogs have been prepared in many different ways for various administration procedures (Kim et al., 2006; Xie et al., 2007; Sugahara et al., 2007; Singla et al., 2002; Hennenfent & Govindan, 2006). Several years ago, Abraxane®, a suspension of albumin nanoparticles containing paclitaxel, obtained approval to treat metastatic breast cancer patients (Ibrahim et al., 2002; Garber, 2004). Abraxane®, a solvent-

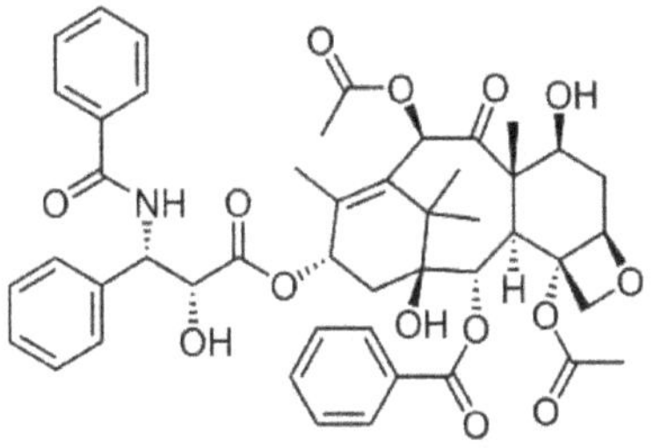

Fig. 1. Structure of paclitaxel

Formulation	AUC (µg·h/ml)	Cmax (µg/ml)	Dose (mg/kg)	Rodent species	Ref
Without inhibitors					
Taxol	0.50 (0-8*)	0.14	10	mice	Sparreboom et al., 1997
Taxol	0.37 (0-4)	0.13***	10	mice	Bardelmeijer et al., 2004
Taxol	1.89 (0-∞)	0.11	50	rat	Choi & Li, 2005
Taxol	0.41 (0-6)	0.12	10	mice	Bardelmeijer et al., 2000
Cremophor/ethanol	0.51 (0-24)	0.10	5	mice	Asperen et al., 1998
Supersaturable-SEDDS	0.44 (0-∞)	0.28	10	rat	Gao et al., 2003
SMEDDS	0.81 (0-24)	0.05	2	rat	Yang et al., 2004
SMEDDS	0.97 (0-24)	0.05	10	rat	Yang et al., 2004
microemulsion	0.45 (0-24)	0.05	25	rat	Woo et al., 2003
Suspension in Tween 80	1.65 (0-24)	0.11	40	rat	Choi et al., 2004a, 2004b
Lipid nanocapsule	1.05 (0-∞)	0.37	10	rat	Peltier et al., 2006
With inhibitors					
Cremophor/Ethanol +Cyclosporine A (50**)	6.68 (0-24)	0.73	10	mice	Asperen et al., 1998
Supersaturable-SEDDS +cyclosporine A (30)	1.05 (0-∞)	0.31	10	rat	Gao et al., 2003
SMEDDS+cyclosporine A (40)	1.14 (0-24)	0.16	2	rat	Yang et al., 2004
Taxol+verapamil (15)	4.27 (0-∞)	0.19	50	rat	Choi & Li, 2005
Microemulsion+KR-30031 (20)	3.37 (0-24)	0.22	25	rat	Woo et al., 2003
Surfactant mix + KR30031 (5)	0.39 (0-12)	0.06	5	rat	Kim et al., 2004
Suspension in Tween 80 + quercetin (20)	5.00 (0-24)	0.28	40	rat	Choi et al., 2004b
Taxol+cyclosporine A (50)	3.61 (0-4)	0.82***	10	mice	Bardelmeijer et al., 2004
Taxol+PSC 833 (50)	2.71 (0-4)	1.47***	10	mice	Bardelmeijer et al., 2004
Taxol+GF120918 (25)	1.39 (0-4)	0.55***	10	mice	Bardelmeijer et al., 2004
Taxol+LY335979 (80)	1.41 (0-4)	0.42***	10	mice	Bardelmeijer et al., 2004
Taxol+R101933 (80)	0.93 (0-4)	0.32***	10	mice	Bardelmeijer et al., 2004
Taxol+GF120918 (25)	2.65 (0-10)	0.77	10	mice	Bardelmeijer et al., 2000
Taxol+PSC 833 (50)				mice	Asperen et al., 1997

* Time-interval used for the calibration of AUC,
** Dose of the inhibitor in mg/kg, and
*** Estimated concentration

Table 1. Mini-review: Selective pharmacokinetic data of paclitaxel after oral administration to rodents.

free formulation has a number of improved features such as shorter infusion time and no hypersensitivity without premedication (Garber, 2004).

Since an oral route would clearly be an attractive alternative to injection for patients as well as for medical personnel, there have been many attempts to prepare effective oral paclitaxel formulations. Paclitaxel, however, is known to be absorbed poorly in the gastrointestinal tract when administered orally (Sparreboom et al., 1997; Bardelmeijer et al., 2004; Choi & Li, 2005; Bardelmeijer et al., 2000). The reasons for poor absorption were identified to be drug metabolism by cytochrome P450 (CYP) and the existence of the efflux system, such as P-glycoproteins in intestinal epithelial cells and liver (Schellens et al., 2000). Tellingen and co-workers identified that the epithelial efflux system composed of P-glycoproteins lowered the drug absorption by demonstrating that orally administered paclitaxel can be absorbed well in mice with a homozygously disrupted mdr1a gene (mdr1a(-/-) mice) (Sparreboom et al., 1997). Proof-of-concept experiments in mice and man have also shown that oral absorption of paclitaxel could be increased dramatically by concomitant administration of a P-glycoprotein inhibitor, cyclosporine A (Schellens et al., 2000; Asperen et al., 1998; Meerum Terwogt et al., 1999). Other P-glycoprotein blockers that could also serve as CYP 450 inhibitors also boosted the oral absorption of paclitaxel (Sparreboom et al., 1997; Bardelmeijer et al., 2004; Choi & Li, 2005; Kim et al., 2004; Asperen et al., 1997). Formulations that do not contain Cremophor EL, that could lower the *in vivo* toxicity and increase solubilization of paclitaxel, were shown to deliver paclitaxel efficiently via oral administration especially when P-glycoprotein inhibitors were given simultaneously (Kim et al., 2004; Gao et al., 2003; Yang et al., 2004; Woo et al., 2003; Choi et al., 2004a, 2004b; Peltier et al., 2006).

In Table 1, we reviewed the literature on oral paclitaxel formulations and summarized the pharmacokinetic data of paclitaxel obtained from the small-animal experiments (FVB mice and Sprague-Dawley rats). In the Table, we have listed Area under the plasma concentration vs. time curve (AUC) value, maximum drug concentration in the blood (C_{max}) and oral dose. One has to keep in mind that the data from different papers may not be compared directly since the AUC values in the literature were estimated for different time intervals and drug doses while the pharmacokinetics of paclitaxel is known to be non-linear (Kearns et al., 1995; Gianni, 1995). Different time intervals could not be normalized due to lack of information in the pharmacokinetics data to make such estimations and thus must be viewed with caution. Another important point to note is that Cremophor EL in Taxol®, used for intravenous administration in some cases (Sparreboom et al., 1997; Bardelmeijer et al., 2004; Asperen et al., 1998; Gao et al., 2003; Yang et al., 2004; Peltier et al., 2006), causes nonlinear pharmacokinetic behavior (Sparreboom et al., 1996). Also, paclitaxel dissolved in Tween 80, also used for intravenous controls in others (Choi & Li, 2005; Bardelmeijer et al., 2000; Woo et al., 2003; Choi et al., 2004a, 2004b), does show linear pharmacokinetic behavior, but has *ca.* 5~10 times lower AUC values when compared to diluted Taxol® (Sparreboom et al., 1996). For these reasons, it was impossible to list the bioavailability values in Table 1.

In the past several years, we have been developing paclitaxel formulations with biocompatible oils, lipids and emulsifiers (Lee et al. Hong et al., 2004; I. H. Lee et al., 2005; S. J. Lee et al., 2005). Paclitaxel dissolved in a stable Lipiodol formulation was shown to retard the growth of hepatocellular carcinoma efficiently when transcatheter arterial chemoembolization was performed in rabbits (Yoon et al., 2003). Also, a paclitaxel formulation prepared with monoolein, tricaprylin and Tween 80 was mucoadhesive when given intravesically (S. J. Lee et al., 2005). Paclitaxel in this formulation penetrated to lamina propria and close to the muscle layer of the bladder while the paclitaxel concentration was low throughout the depth of the bladder tissue when Taxol® was used. We also have shown that this mucoadhesive formulation can deliver paclitaxel effectively when given by oral route without additional active pharmaceutical ingredient as an absorption enhancer (Lee et al., 2004; Hong et al., 2004; I. H. Lee et al., 2005, Shin et al., 2009). As an endeavor to formulate more efficient oral paclitaxel formulations, we have prepared oil-based paclitaxel formulations with monoolein, saturated triglycerides and emulsifiers. Monoolein was included in the formulation as a main ingredient due to its high bioadhesiveness (Nielsen et al., 1998) and its ability to release the encapsulated drug in a controlled fashion (Clogston et al., 2005a, 2005b). Triglycerides were added since they can solubilize paclitaxel efficiently (Kan et al., 1999). To access the effectiveness of the formulations, pharmacokinetic and anti-tumor efficacy studies were performed in mice models.

2. Materials and methods

2.1 Materials

Distilled monoolein (RYLO™ MG 19, > 90 % pure) was purchased from Danisco Ingredients, Denmark. Paclitaxel was obtained from Samyang Genex (Korea) and Indena S.P.A. (Italy). Cremophor EL, Tween 80 and triglycerides (triacetin, tributyrin, tricaproin, tricaprylin, tricaprin and trilaurin) were purchased from Sigma Chemical Co. (St. Louis, MO).

2.2 Preparation of oral paclitaxel formulations

The compositions of the oral paclitaxel formulations used in the experiments are summarized in Tables 2 and 3. Paclitaxel formulations with various triglycerides (Table 2) were prepared as follows: Paclitaxel in amorphous form was dissolved completely at 10 mg/ml in mixtures of oils consisting of monoolein, triglycerides and Tween 80 by sonication for 30 s. Some of the oral paclitaxel formulations were semi-solid or solid wax at ambient temperatures with the melting points of 30 ~ 50 °C, and therefore had to be warmed before oral feeding.

In Table 3, Paclitaxel, amorphous or crystalline, was dissolved completely in excess amount of methylene chloride and mixed subsequently with tricaprylin. Methylene chloride was evaporated completely to prepare paclitaxel/tricaprylin solution by vacuum evaporation (BUCHI rotavapor R-200, Germany) at 40 °C for 1 h. The content of methylene chloride was determined by gas chromatography and was less than 100 ppm in the paclitaxel/tricaprylin solution. Monoolein and Tween 80 were added to the paclitaxel/tricaprylin solution and mixed completely by sonication for 30 s. A formulation that does not contain paclitaxel, eG2, was also prepared for control. The oral paclitaxel formulations were semi-solid wax with the melting temperature of 33 ~ 35 °C, and were warmed to body temperature before feeding.

Dispersions of the oral paclitaxel formulations (G8, G9, and G10) were prepared by adding 2.3 times (by volume) of distilled water or syrup to the formulation G2 (also will be referred to as DHP107) and by vortexing or sonicating for 1 min.

2.3 Animals

Male ICR and Balb/c athymic mice, 7 weeks old, were purchased from Orient Bio Co. (Seoul, Korea) and Japan SLC (Japan), respectively, and maintained 1 week. Animal care and handling followed institutional guidelines (Korea Institute of Science and Technology). Mice were maintained with free access to food and water under a 12-h light/dark cycle.

2.4 Differential scanning calorimetry

Differential scanning calorimetry (DSC) was performed to obtain the heating thermograms of paclitaxel and the formulations in Table 2 (DSC 821e, Mettler Toledo, Columbus, OH, equipped with Intracooler, Haake EK90/MT, Haake, Denmark) at a heating scan rate of 5 °C/min. Scans were made with samples contained in hermetically sealed aluminum crucibles (ME-27331, Mettler Toledo). Initial heating scans were reported for paclitaxel and the formulations in Table 2. In case of the formulations, thermal history did not alter the heating thermograms if the samples were cooled to − 20 °C before reheating.

2.5 Determination of the particle size in the dispersion

The average particle size in the dispersions G8, G9 and G10 in Table 3 was determined by quasielastic laser light scattering with a Malvern Zetasizer® (Malvern Instruments Limited, England). The dispersions were diluted by 300 times in water before the measurement. The size determination was repeated 3 times/sample. The average size and the size distribution were estimated from the log-normal size distribution function as shown previously (Chung et al., 2001)

2.6 Oral administration of paclitaxel formulations

Paclitaxel formulations in Tables 2 and 3 were liquefied at 37 ~ 50 °C and administered orally at doses of 25, 50, 75, and 100 mg/kg with a blunt needle via the esophagus into the stomach. The male ICR mice were fasted for 8 h prior to oral administration except for the group G3. Taxol® prepared by dissolving paclitaxel in an equivolume mixture of Cremophor EL and ethanol at 6 mg/ml (Taxol®) was diluted by 6 times with the saline solution, and was administered via bolus tail-vein injection at a dose of 10 mg/kg as a positive control. Blood samples were collected at various time points (n=6) after drug administration, and were stored at -70 °C until analysis.

2.7 Analysis of paclitaxel concentrations in blood

Whole blood (200 µl) was spiked with irbesartan (0.5 µg/ml; internal standard), mixed and added to acetonitrile (400 µl) to precipitate proteins. After centrifugation at 14,000 RCF for 20 min, the supernatant was collected and mixed with the mobile phase to adjust the volume to 0.6 ml. Ten microliters of the blood was injected into the LC/MS/MS system. Analyses were performed with a Thermo-Finnigan Discovery Max LC/MS/MS (San Jose, CA, USA). The LC system was performed at 35 °C on a Capcellpak C18 column (150 X 2.0 mm i.d., 5 µm particle size, Shisheido, Japan) equipped with a Zorbax SB-Aq (12.5 X 2.1 mm i.d.) guard column. The mobile phase consisted of 55 % acetonitrile, 0.08 % formic acid and 44.92 % water, and the flow rate was 0.4 ml/min. The instrument was operated in SRM mode (positive ion), monitoring the ion transitions from m/z 854 → 285 (paclitaxel) and m/z 429 → 195 (internal standard). The paclitaxel LC/MS/MS assay was linear over the range of 2 ~ 1000 ng/ml with a lower quantitation limit of 2 ng/ml in blood. Paclitaxel concentrations in blood were calculated based on a standard curve of paclitaxel in blank pooled animal blood with the internal standard.

2.8 Tumor experiment

Suspension of NCI-H358 human non-small cell lung cancer cells (1.2×10^7 cells/mouse), purchased from American Type Culture Collection (ATCC, Manassas, VA), was injected subcutaneously to the dorsal flank of male Balb/c athymic mice (8 weeks). When the tumor volume (length × width × height × 0.5236) reached *ca.* 100 mm³ in 10 days after the injection (day 0), the experimental groups were divided at random into three groups (n=8). On days 1, 2, 3, 4 and 5, G2 formulation (DHP107) was administered orally at a dose of 50 mg/kg (G2). For controls, mice injected intravenously with diluted Taxol® (Taxol, 10 mg/kg) and fed orally with the vehicle only (eG2) on days 1, 2, 3, 4 and 5 were also observed.

2.9 Characterization of crystalline forms of paclitaxel

X-Ray diffraction (XRD) measurements were made by using an x-ray diffractometer (D8 Discover, Bruker, Karlsruhe, Germany) with the general area detector diffraction system (GADDS, Bruker, Karlsruhe, Germany). The Cu K_α radiation of wavelength 1.542 Å was provided by the x-ray generator (FL CU 4 KE, Bruker, Karlsruhe, Germany) operating at 40 kV and 45 mA. Sample-to-detector distance was 300 mm. Exposure time was 1 ~ 5 h. To avoid air scattering, the beam path was filled with helium. The surface morphology of paclitaxel was observed by scanning electron microscopy (SEM; Hitachi S-2460N, Japan) at an accelerating voltage of 15 kV after Pt/Au sputter coating (Hitachi E1010 Ion sputter, Japan).

3. Results

3.1 Characterization of crystalline forms of paclitaxel

Crystalline forms of paclitaxel obtained from different sources were determined by DSC, x-ray diffraction and scanning electron microscopy. Paclitaxel can exist as different polymorphs having distinct physical properties, which could influence the manufacturing process of the formulations (Liggins et al., 1997; Lee et al., 2001). Paclitaxel obtained from Samyang Genex (Genexol, Korea) had the glass transition temperature at 150 °C and an exothermic transition at 220 °C whereas paclitaxel obtained from Indena had the melting transition at 210 °C as shown in Figure 2, corresponding to amorphous and anhydrous crystalline forms, respectively, as shown in the literature (Liggins et al., 1997). X-ray diffraction data revealed the differences in the crystallinity of paclitaxel. Diffraction pattern of Genexol showed two broad scattering peaks centered at *ca.* 10° and 20° characteristic of the amorphous form. Paclitaxel from Indena, on the other hand, revealed a pattern with strong and sharp diffraction peaks at 5.7° and 12.6° indicating a highly ordered structure. Surface morphology was also visualized by SEM. Genexol was observed to be in the powder form with highly contoured surfaces. We note that the grain size or the surface area of the powder varied depending on the lot numbers of Genexol (data not shown). For instance, Genexol 131 was composed of powders with wrinkled surfaces whereas Genexol 183 contained smooth and round particles as well when observed by SEM. Needle-like crystals were observed for paclitaxel from Indena. Based on DSC, XRD and SEM experiments,

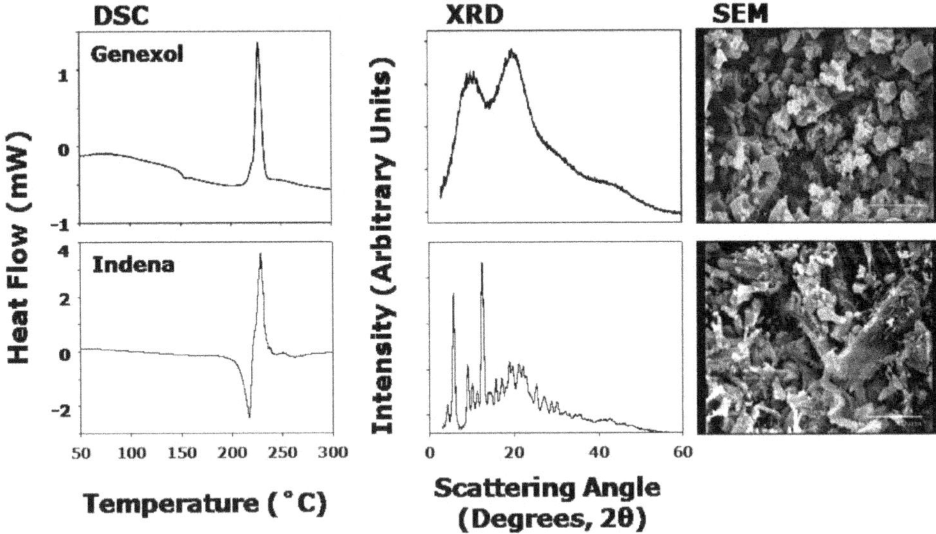

Fig. 2. Differential Scanning calorimetry, x-ray diffraction and scanning electron microscopy of paclitaxel obtained from of Genexol (upper panels) and Indena (lower panels).

we confirmed that Paclitaxel from Samyang Genex and Indena were in amorphous and anhydrous crystalline forms, respectively.

Due to the differences in the grain size and crystalline forms, we used two different procedures in preparing the oral formulations. Genexol 131 was readily soluble in all of the lipid mixtures in Table 2 when sonicated for *ca.* 30 s. Genexol 183, which had larger grains than Genexol 131, and paclitaxel from Indena did not dissolve in the lipid mixture. In these cases, paclitaxel was solubilized completely in the mixture of methylene chloride and triglyceride. Methylene chloride was evaporated completely from the mixture before other ingredients were added to prepare the formulations in Table 3.

3.2 Physical properties of oral paclitaxel formulations

Oral paclitaxel formulations existed as oil/wax mixtures at ambient temperatures, but formed clear liquid at 37 °C except for the Formulation T12 (Table 2). The T12 formulation existed as solid wax at ambient temperatures. Thermal behavior of the formulations containing different triglycerides was investigated by performing DSC (Figure 3A).

The thermograms were identical with or without paclitaxel in the formulations, and those with paclitaxel are shown in the Figure. Tween 80, liquid at room temperature, did not show any phase transition in the temperature range from 0 to 60 °C. Lamellar crystalline-to-fluid isotropic, or the chain melting, phase transition of monoolein was observed at 32 °C, which is similar to the values reported for pure monoolein (Briggs et al., 1996; Qiu & Caffrey, 2000) or Myverol 18-99K (Clogston, 2000) in the literature. The chain melting transition of monoolein for the monoolein/Tween 80 (55.0:16.5 by weight) mixture was observed at 26 °C, since Tween 80 lowered the transition temperature of monoolein. In the formulations T2, T4 and T6, only the chain melting transition of monoolein was observed because triacetin,

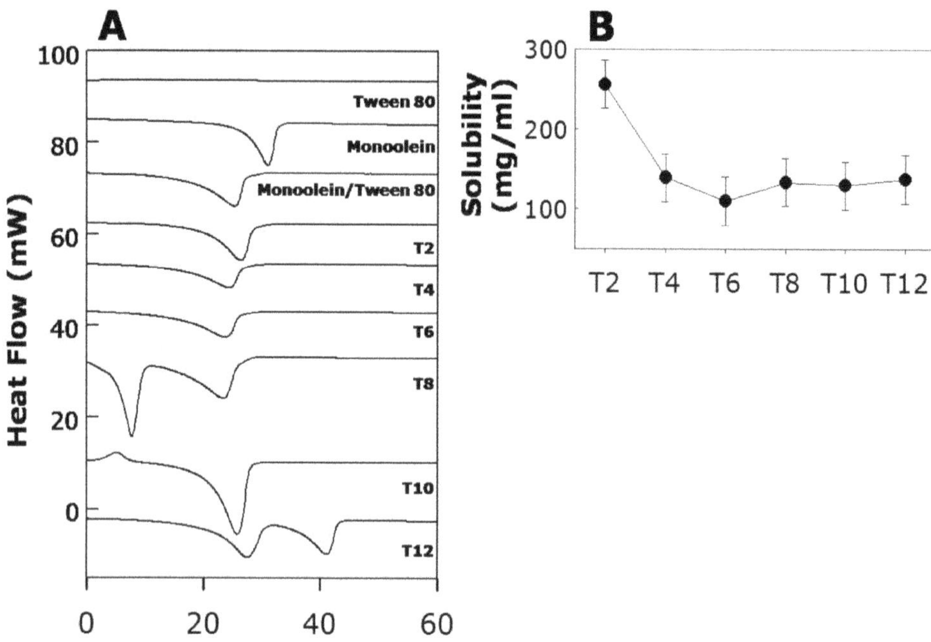

Fig. 3. A) Heating thermograms obtained from the formulations prepared with different triglycerides (T2 ~ T12, in Table 2), Tween 80, monoolein and monoolein/Tween 80 mixture (55.0:16.5 by weight). The concentration of paclitaxel was 1 %(w/w) in all formulations. B) Solubility of paclitaxel in the formulations containing monoolein, triglyceride and Tween 80 at 55.0:27.5:16.5 by weight at 37 °C.

tributyrin and tricaprin were immiscible with solid monoolein. We could identify visually the phase separation of these triglycerides below *ca.* 26 °C. In T8 formulation, chain melting transitions of tricaprylin and monoolein were observed at 8 and 23 °C, respectively. In case of T10 formulation, single transition peak from the melting transition of the eutectic mixture of monoolein and tricaprin (2:1 by weight) was observed at 26 °C (Roh et al., 2004). The chain melting transitions of monoolein and trilaurin were observed at 32 and 41 °C, respectively, for T12 formulation. Results show that all the formulations existed as solid/liquid or solid/solid mixtures at room temperature, but transforms into the single-phase liquid when heated to the body temperature for T2 ~ T10 formulations or above 45 °C for T12 formulation. Paclitaxel was solubilized well inside all of the formulations in the temperature range studied when observed by polarized light microscopy (data not shown).

3.3 Solubility of paclitaxel in oral formulations

The solubility of paclitaxel in the oral formulations with different triglycerides was determined at 37 °C. Mixtures of monoolein/triglyceride/Tween 80 were prepared at 55.0:27.5:16.5 by weight and warmed to melt. Paclitaxel in powder form (Genexol, Samyang Genex, lot G131) was added stepwise to these mixtures until undissolved aggregates were observed. The mixtures were vortexed for 10 s and sonicated for 3 min after each addition at 37 °C. The formulation containing trilaurin was heated to 60 °C and cooled to 37 °C to obtain the undercooled liquid for the measurement. Solubility of paclitaxel was *ca.* 250 ± 30 mg/ml for the formulation containing triacetin, but was *ca.* 120 ± 40 mg/ml for those with other triglycerides (Figure 3B).

3.4 Pharmacokinetics of oral paclitaxel administration and intravenous Taxol injection

Oral paclitaxel formulations were warmed to body temperature and administered to male ICR mice. We note that not the dispersions but the oily formulations were administered, and no other active pharmaceutical ingredients were given to the animals. Diluted Taxol® was given intravenously as a control. Paclitaxel concentration in blood after oral administration of formulation G2 (DHP107, paclitaxel dose of 50 mg/kg) and intravenous injection of Taxol® (10 mg/kg) was plotted as a function of time in Figure 4A (normal scale) and Figure 4B (logarithmic scale). Paclitaxel concentration in blood was 60.2 µg/ml in 1 min after intravenous injection, and dropped to *ca.* 6.2 and 0.8 µg/ml and in 0.5 and 3 h, respectively. Paclitaxel concentration in blood increased and became 1.2 and 2.1 µg/ml at 1 and 3 h, respectively, after oral administration of DHP107. Pharmacokinetic parameters are listed in Table 2. The bioavailability [(BA) (%) = (AUC_{oral} / AUC_{iv}) · ($Dose_{iv}$/ $Dose_{oral}$) ×100] of DHP107 in mice was *ca.* 14 %. Since the plasma concentration of paclitaxel above a threshold value of 85.3 ng/ml (dashed line in Figure 4B) was proven to be pharmacologically active, DHP107 could be effective for more than 8 h (Huizing et al., 1997).

Treatment group	Triglyceride type	T_{max} (h)	C_{max} (µg/ml)	AUC_{0-9} (µg·h /ml)
T2	Triacetin	3	0.4	1.6
T4	Tributyrin	3	1.5	5.4
T6	Tricaproin	3	3.1	12.0
T8	Tricaprylin	1	2.7	8.9
T10	Tricaprin	1	2.2	8.4
T12	Trilaurin	1	1.5	4.9

Table 2. Pharmacokinetic parameters of paclitaxel after oral administration (50 mg/kg dose) of the formulations containing different triglycerides to Balb/c mice. The composition of the formulations was paclitaxel:monoolein:triglyceride:Tween 80 = 1.0:55.0:27.5:16.5 by weight.

3.5 Oral administration of formulations with different triglycerides

Paclitaxel formulations prepared with various triglycerides (paclitaxel: monoolein: triglyceride:Tween 80 = 1.0:55.0:27.5:16.5 by weight) were administered orally at 50 mg/kg dose to male ICR mice (Table 2, Figure 4C). AUC values were 12.1 ± 2.6, 8.9 ± 1.8 and 8.4 ± 2.7 µg·h/ml for T6, T8 and T10 groups, respectively, with no statistical differences (p<0.15 by Student *t*-test). In case of T2, T4 and T12 groups, AUC of paclitaxel was 1.6 ± 0.5 (p<0.003 compared the AUC with T6 formulation), 5.4 ± 0.7 (p<0.01) and 4.9 ±1.6 µg·h/ml (p<0.01), respectively. Maximum concentration of paclitaxel in blood (C_{max}) was also the highest for the formulation with tricaproin (T6) and was 3.2 ± 0.7 µg·h/ml. Interestingly, the time to reach C_{max} (T_{max}) was 3 h for the formulations with shorter chain triglycerides (T2, T4 and T6) and 1 h for T8, T10 and T12 groups.

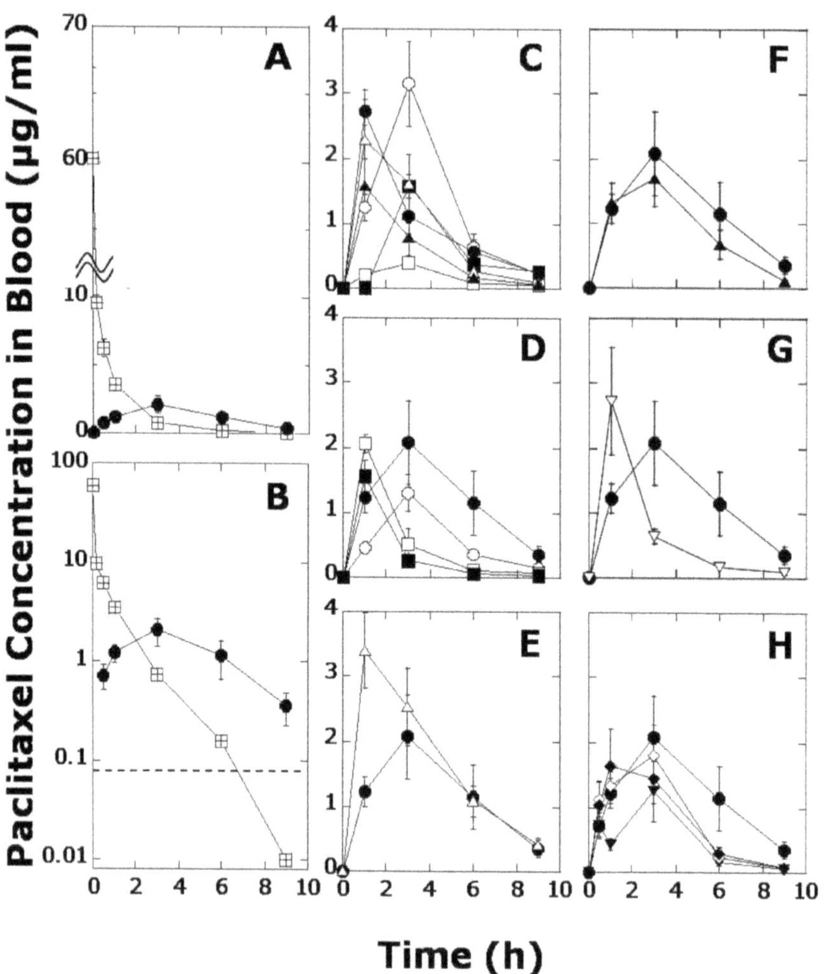

Fig. 4. Mean blood concentration of paclitaxel after intravenous administration of Taxol® and administration of oral formulations. Comparison between intravenous Taxol (⊞, 10 mg/kg) and oral DHP107 (G2, ●, 50 mg/kg) is shown in normal (A) and logarithmic (B) scales. The dashed line in B) indicates the pharmacologically effective concentration (85.3 ng/ml). Oral administration of paclitaxel formulations C) with different triglycerides (T2: □, T4: ■, T6: ○, T8: ●, T10: △, T12: ▲), D) with different paclitaxel contents (G1: ○, 5 mg paclitaxel/ml formulation, G2, DHP107: ●, 10 mg/ml, G3: □, 15 mg/kg, G4: ■, 20 mg/ml), E) under the fasting (G2, DHP107: ●) and non-fasting (G5: △) conditions, F) prepared with crystalline (G6: ▲) and amorphous (G2, DHP107: ●) paclitaxel, G) with (G2, DHP107: ●) or without (G7: ▽) Tween 80, and H) dispersed in syrup (G8: ▼) or in water (G9: ◇) by vortexing and in water by sonication (G10: ◆) or given per se (G2, DHP107: ●). The oral dose of paclitaxel was 50 mg/kg except for G1 (25 mg/kg), G3 (75 mg/kg) and G4 (100 mg/kg).

Treatment group	Paclitaxel Dose (mg/kg)	Composition [%(w/w)]						T_{max} (h)	C_{max} (µg/ml)	AUC_{0-9} (µg h /ml)	Crystallinity of paclitaxel
		Paclitaxel	Monoolein	Tricaprylin	Tween 80	Cremophor EL	Ethanol				
G1	25 (p.o.)	0.5	55.5	27.5	16.5	-	-	3	1.3	5.2	Amorphous
G2 (DHP107)	50 (p.o.)	1.0	55.0	27.5	16.5	-	-	3	2.0	11.0	Amorphous
G3	75 (p.o.)	1.5	54.5	27.5	16.5	-	-	1	2.0	4.7	Amorphous
G4	100 (p.o.)	2.0	54.0	27.5	16.5	-	-	1	1.5	3.1	Amorphous
G5 (DHP107, Non-fasting)	50 (p.o.)	1.0	55.0	27.5	16.5	-	-	1	3.4	15.3	Amorphous
G6	50 (p.o.)	1.0	55.0	27.5	16.5	-	-	3	1.6	8.3	Crystalline
G7	50 (p.o.)	1.0	66.0	33.0	-	-	-	1	2.7	6.3	Amorphous
eG2	0 (p.o.)	0.0	56.0	27.5	16.5	-	-	-	-	-	-
Taxol	10 (i.v.)	0.6	-	-	-	57.0	42.4	0.016	60.2	15.7	Amorphous

Treatment group	Paclitaxel Dose (mg/kg)	Composition [%(w/w)]						T_{max} (h)	C_{max} (µg/ml)	AUC_{0-9} (µg h /ml)	Dispersing method
		Paclitaxel	Monoolein	Tricaprylin	Tween 80	Syrup	Water				
G8	50 (p.o.)	0.3	16.2	8.0	5.5	70	-	3	1.2	4.6	Vortex
G9	50 (p.o.)	0.3	16.2	8.0	5.5	-	70	3	1.8	7.5	Vortex
G10	50 (p.o.)	0.3	16.2	8.0	5.5	-	70	1	1.6	7.1	Sonication

Table 3. Compositions of paclitaxel formulations and pharmacokinetic parameters of paclitaxel after intravenous or oral administration in Balb/c mice.

3.6 Oral administration of formulations with different paclitaxel contents

We prepared the formulations with different Paclitaxel contents while fixing the weight ratio of monoolein:tricaprylin:Tween 80 to 55.0:27.5:16.5 by weight (G1, G2, G3 and G4 in Table 3, Figure 4D). Bioavailability was 13 % and 14 % when the concentration of paclitaxel was 0.5 and 1 %(w/w), respectively, in the formulation. When the concentration was 1.5 and 2.0 %(w/w), bioavailability decreased with increasing paclitaxel dose and was 4 % and 2 %, respectively.

3.7 Fasting vs. non-fasting conditions

When the formulation is given orally, the fullness of stomach can influence the pharmacokinetics of the administered drug. Throughout the experiments, we administered the oral formulations after 8 h of fasting. In G5, however, we fed DHP107 to mice with free access to food and water before and after the drug administration in order to observe the influence of stomach emptiness on the absorption of the drug. Under the non-fasting condition, C_{max} increased to 3.4 µg/ml when compared to the fasting condition (2.0 µg/ml) and T_{max} was reduced to 1 h (Figure 4E). The AUC values for non-fasting and fasting conditions were 15.3 (20 % BA) and 11.0 µg·h /ml (14 % BA), respectively. We could conclude that the food in the gastrointestinal tract did not interfere with, but rather helped the absorption of paclitaxel.

3.8 Crystalline vs. amorphous paclitaxel

The formulations made with crystalline and amorphous paclitaxel were administered orally to mice (Figure 4F). The pharmacokinetic profiles were virtually identical for these two formulations. We expected that the crystallinity of the drug would not affect the degree of oral absorption since paclitaxel was dissolved completely in tricaprylin/dichloromethane mixture before adding other ingredients, and therefore, the final products would be identical.

3.9 Formulation without Tween 80

Oral formulations with (G2, DHP107, Table 3) or without Tween 80 (G7) were prepared. Pharmacokinetic profiles were different for these two formulations (Figure 4G). When the formulation without Tween 80 was administered, T_{max} was 1 h instead of 3, and the AUC value was reduced to 6.3 µg·h /ml, which was *ca.* 56 % of that for DHP107.

3.10 Oral administration of the aqueous dispersions of DHP107

Even though our oral paclitaxel formulations including DHP107 can be taken *per se*, they can also be mixed with water or taste-masking syrups for administration. To examine how the absorption of paclitaxel changes upon feeding the dispersion, DHP107 was mixed with water or syrup at 3:7 by weight. DHP107 was dispersed spontaneously in water to produce emulsion droplets having average diameter of 6-8 µm. By vortexing the mixture of DHP107 and water or syrup for 1 min, the diameters of emulsion droplets were reduced to 6 (polydispersity = 1) or 3 (polydispersity = 1) µm, respectively. By sonicating DHP107/water mixture at 180 KW for 1 min, we also obtained the dispersion with the oil droplets having 1.4 µm (polydispersity = 1) in diameter.

When the dispersions were orally administered, pharmacokinetic profiles did not change significantly except for the fact that the AUC values were reduced to *ca.* 40 ~ 70 % of the original G2 formulation.

3.11 Antitumor efficacy of DHP107 in experimental animals

To evaluate the antitumor activity of DHP107 in mice, suspension of NCI-H358 cells was injected subcutaneously to Balb/c athymic mice. All of the mice inoculated with the human non-small cell lung cancer cells developed progressively growing tumors. The mice were administered orally with DHP107 (G2, 50 mg/kg) or intravenously with Taxol® (10 mg/kg) for 5 consecutive days 10 days after the inoculation. The entire tumor tissue was removed surgically after the experiment and photographed as shown in Figure 5A. In the group administered with oral DHP107 and intravenous Taxol®, the tumor size was reduced gradually from *ca.* 100 to 15 ± 3 and 19 ± 5 mm³, respectively, in *ca.* 25 days after the administration of the drug and remained unchanged for the duration of the experiment (Figure 5B). The tumor size data for these two groups were indifferent statistically. In the control group administered orally with the vehicle only, the tumor grew continuously to *ca.* 360 ± 20 mm³ in 45 days.

4. Discussion

In current study, we prepared oil formulations for oral administration of paclitaxel and examined their physical properties, pharmacokinetic profiles and antitumor activities.

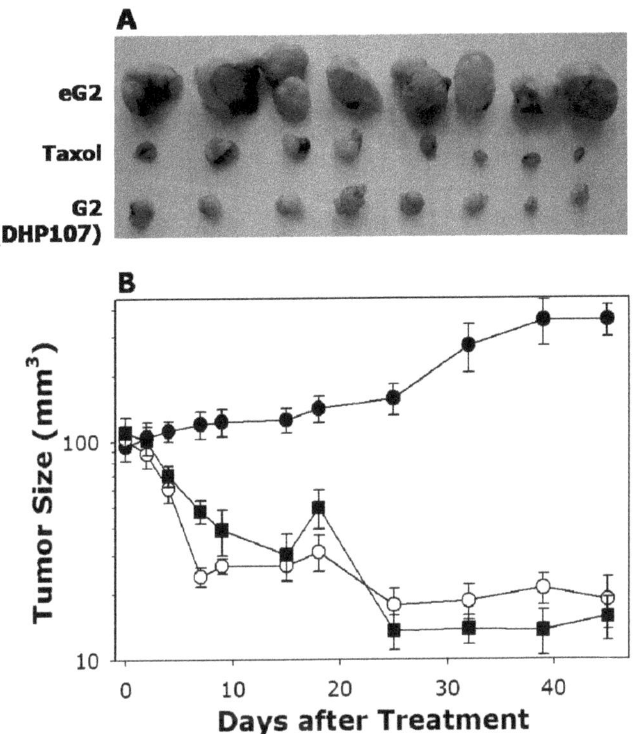

Fig. 5. Antitumor activity of DHP107 in male Balb/c athymic mice, subcutaneously injected with suspension of NCI-H358 cells (1.2×10⁷ cells/mouse). A) The entire tumor tissue removed surgically after the experiment. B) The volume of tumor for the oral vehicle control (eG2, ●), intravenous Taxol® (○, 10mg/kg) and oral DHP107 (G2, ■, 50 mg/kg).

Paclitaxel was commercially available in at least two different polymorphs. Amorphous paclitaxel was readily soluble in our oral formulations at 10 mg/ml when sonicated for 30 s. Crystalline paclitaxel, on the other hand, did not dissolve in the oily formulations directly. We had to dissolve crystalline paclitaxel in the tricaprylin/methylene chloride mixture completely, and to remove the solvent in turn to obtain the oily solution of paclitaxel/tricaprylin before adding monoolein and Tween 80. Even though paclitaxel could also be dissolved in methylene chloride/tricaprylin/monoolein/Tween 80 as well as in methylene chloride/tricaprylin, monoolein and Tween 80 were not added to the mixture until after evaporating the solvent to minimize the oxidation of these materials containing unsaturated hydrocarbons. Pharmacokinetic study showed that AUC values were identical statistically when paclitaxel from different vendors or different preparation processes was used (Figure 4F).

DSC study was performed for the formulations with different triglycerides. In the heating thermograms, two endothermic transitions were observed corresponding to the chain melting transitions of monoolein and triglycerides for T8 and T12 formulations. Chain melting transition of triacetin, tributyrin and tricaproin were not observed since the phase transition temperatures of these triglycerides were below 0 °C. There was only a single endothermic transition for the tricaprin/monoolein mixture at the weight ratio of 2:1 since they formed a eutectic mixture (Roh et al., 2004). The phase behavior of monoolein and triglycerides could be explained by the classical binary eutectic phase diagram of two immiscible solid phases and a completely miscible melt.

We could conclude from the DSC data that monoolein and tricaprylin do not mix below *ca.* 30 °C where monoolein exists as lamellar crystalline phase. Monoolein and Tween 80 did not mix in this temperature range either. Above 30 °C, however, all three ingredients, tricaprylin, monoolein and Tween 80 existed as liquid and mixed homogeneously. Two important things to note were that paclitaxel precipitates were not observed even at 0 °C by microscopy in any of the oral formulations and that the formulations could be heated and cooled in cycles between -20 and 40 °C without compromising the effectiveness of the drug. These results are significant in that the oral formulation (possibly in a soft capsule) can be stored in the shelf and orally administered in the phase-separated form, but transforms into a homogenous liquid solution by the body heat while traveling inside the gastrointestinal tract.

In our oral formulations, monoolein was included due to its well-known mucoadhesive property (Nielsen et al., 1998). Monoolein and other monoglycerides have been used in oral drug delivery formulations since they can enhance absorption of small molecules and even proteins through the epithelial cells (Ganem-Quintanar et al., 2000; Chung et al., 2002). The absorption enhancing mechanism is not clearly known. Nanopore induction or the membrane perturbation (Anderson, 2005), and the intermediate phases formed in the intestine (Kossena et al., 2005) were considered important. *In vitro* study showed that monoglycerides can enhance the cellular absorption of drugs by inhibition of P-glycoproteins (Konishi et al., 2004). Further studies are required to explain the absorption enhancing mechanism of monoolein unequivocally.

In the previous study, we administered intravesically the dispersion of DHP107 in water to experimental rabbits and observed that the formulation adhered tightly to the bladder mucosa, and paclitaxel penetrated through the physical barrier imposed by the uroepithelium (S. J. Lee et al., 2005). Histological examination of the bladder and other tissues did not reveal any local or systemic toxicity to the rabbits.

Oral administration of formulations containing different triglycerides showed that those with tricaproin, tricaprylin and tricaprin had higher AUC values than others. The formulation with tricaproin had the highest AUC value. We must note that paclitaxel was mixed directly with the vehicles and sonicated for 30 s to obtain the formulations in Table 2. When the preparation process was changed to add and to remove methylene chloride in turn in order to solubilize crystalline as well as amorphous paclitaxel, the AUC value of tricaprylin/monoolein/Tween 80/paclitaxel formulation (G2, DHP107) increased from 8.9 to 11.0 µg·h/ml, which was similar to that of tricaproin/monoolein/Tween 80/paclitaxel formulation in Table 2 (T6) statistically. We proceeded with the tricaprylin/monoolein/Tween 80/paclitaxel formulation for further experiments because the toxicity of tricaprylin (LD50 = 3700 mg/kg; intravenous and 26600 mg/kg; oral) was much lower than that of tricaproin (LD50 = 122 mg/kg; intravenous) for mice according to the Material Safety Data Sheets for tricaprylin (T9126) and tricaproin (T4137) provided by Sigma (www.sigma-aldrich.com).

We also performed the pharmacokinetic study with the formulations having different contents of the drug, under fasting or non-fasting conditions, by changing the commercial source of paclitaxel, with or without the emulsifier, Tween 80 and in the form of dispersions in syrup or in water. From these experiments, we could conclude that the optimum concentration of paclitaxel in the formulation was 10 mg/ml, and the tricaprylin/monoolein/Tween 80/paclitaxel formulation was the most effective when given directly to the non-fasting animals. Under the fasting conditions, T_{max} was 3 h. T_{max}, however, was 1 h when the animal had free access to food and water. In a separate experiment, we observed that the bile salts helped the micronization and micellization of DHP107. It is possible that the micronization process of DHP107 was fastened by the secreted bile salts already existing under the non-fasting condition. When the formulation was fed to the empty stomach, on the other hand, bile salt secretion would start after the oily DHP107 reaches the upper intestine.

Our liquid type formulations were very effective in delivering paclitaxel orally, easy to prepare, biocompatible, and physically stable. Preclinical studies have demonstrated superior antitumor efficacy and high bioavailability. Most notably, the blood paclitaxel concentration was high after the oral administration even though the P-glycoprotein inhibitors were not co-administered when compared to the formulations reported in the literature (Table 1). The results show that the blood paclitaxel concentration reached as high as *ca.* 3 µg/ml and higher than 1 µg/ml for 4~6 hours in Balb/c mice after oral administration of 50 mg/kg of paclitaxel dose. Also the bioavailability of paclitaxel was *ca.* 14 % and 20 % when compared to Taxol® injection under fasting and non-fasting conditions, respectively.

Antitumor experiment also showed that the tumor regression rate of the oral DHP107 group (50 mg/kg) was similar to that of the intravenous Taxol® group (10 mg/kg). Also, the tumor size of an established non-small cell lung cancer was significantly reduced after the oral treatment. Considering that the bioavailability of DHP107 was *ca.* 14 ~ 20 % compared to Taxol® injection, similar regression rate was expected to a degree.

5. Conclusions

In conclusion, we prepared oral paclitaxel formulations that do not contain P-glycoprotein inhibitors as active pharmaceutical ingredients. The formulations are liquid at body temperature and can solubilize paclitaxel effectively. The oral bioavailability of paclitaxel was 14 ~ 20 % when compared to the intravenous Taxol® formulation without concomitant administration of P-glycoprotein inhibitors. Preclinical efficacy study on mice showed that the tumor size was reduced significantly for the human non-small cell lung carcinoma. In separate studies, we have determined the tissue distribution of paclitaxel after oral administration (manuscript in preparation) and performed pre-clinical antitumor efficacy studies in mice with several tumor types (manuscript in preparation). Regulatory preclinical experiments to initiate the clinical evaluations of DHP107 have also been carried out.

6. References

Anderson, D. (2005) Reversed liquid crystalline phases with non-paraffin hydrophobes. European Patent 1539099A2, 2005

Bardelmeijer, H. A., Beijnen, J. H., Brouwer, K. R., Rosing, H., Nooijen, W. J., Schellens, J. H. M., & van Tellingen, O. (2000) Increased oral bioavailability of paclitaxel by GF120918 in mice through selective modulation of P-glycoprotein. *Clin. Cancer Res.*, Vol. 6. pp. 4416-4421

Bardelmeijer, H. A., Ouwehand, M., Beijnen, J. H., Schellens, J. H. M,. & van Tellingen, O. (2004) Efficacy of novel P-glycoprotein inhibitors to increase the oral uptake of paclitaxel in mice. *Inves. New Drugs,* Vol. 22. pp. 219–229

Briggs, J., Chung, H., & Caffrey, M. (1996) The temperature-composition phase diagram and mesophase structure characterization of the monoolein/water system. *J. Phys. II France,* Vol. 6. pp. 723-751

Choi, J. S., & Li, X. (2005) The effect of verapamil on the pharmacokinetics of paclitaxel in rats. Eur. *J. Pharm. Sci.,* Vol. 24. pp. 95-100

Choi, J. -S., Choi, H. -K., & Shin, S. -C. (2004) Enhanced bioavailability of paclitaxel after oral coadministration with flavone in rats. *Int. J. Pharm.,* Vol. 275. pp. 165–170

Choi, J. -S., Jo, B. -W., & Kim, Y. -C. (2004) Enhanced paclitaxel bioavailability after oral administration paclitaxel or prodrug to rats pretreated with quercetin. *Eur. J. Pharm. Biopharm.,* Vol. 57. pp. 313–318

Chung, H., Kim, J.-s., Um, J. Y., Kwon, I. C., & Jeong, S. Y. (2002) Self-assembled "nanocubicle" as a carrier for peroral insulin delivery. *Diabetologia,* Vol. 45. pp. 448-451

Chung, H., Kim, T. W., Kwon, M., Kwon, I. C., & Jeong, S. Y. (2001) Oil components modulate physical characteristics and function of the natural oil emulsions as drug or gene delivery system. *J. Control. Rel.,* Vol. 71. pp. 339-350

Clogston, J., Craciun, G., Hart D.J., & Caffrey, M. (2005) Controlling release from the lipidic cubic phase by selective alkylation. *J. Cont. Rel.,* Vol. 102. pp. 441-461

Clogston, J., & Caffrey, M. (2005) Controlling release from the lipidic cubic phase. Amino acids, peptides, proteins and nucleic acids. *J. Cont. Rel.,* Vol. 107. pp. 97-111

Clogston, J., Rathman, J., Tomasko, D., Walker, H., & Caffrey, M. (2000) Phase behavior of a monoacylglycerol (Myverol 18-99K)/water system. *Chem. Phys. Lipids,* Vol. 107. pp. 191–220

Ganem-Quintanar, A., Quintanar-Guerrero, & D., Buri, P. (2000) Monoolein: A review of pharmaceutical applications. *Drug Dev. Indust. Pham.,* Vol. 26. pp. 809–820

Gao, P., Rush, B. D., Pfund, W. P., Huang, T., Bauer, J. M., Morozowich, W., Kuo, M. -S., & Hageman, M. J. (2003) Development of a supersaturable SEDDS (S-SEDDS) formulation of paclitaxel with improved oral bioavailability. *J. Pharm. Sci.,* Vol. 92. pp. 2386-2398

Garber, K. (2004) Improved paclitaxel formulation hints at new chemotherapy approach. *J. Natl. Cancer Inst.,* Vol. 96. pp. 90-91

Gianni, L., Kearns, C. M., Giani, A., Capri, G., Vigano, L., Lacatelli, A., Bonadonna, G., & Egorin, M. J. (1995). Nonlinear pharmacokinetics and metabolism of paclitaxel and its pharmacokinetic/pharmacodynamic relationships in humans. *J. Clin. Oncol.,* Vol. 13. pp. 180-190

Hennenfent, K. L., & Govindan, R. (2006) Novel formulations of taxanes: a review. Old wine in a new bottle? *Ann. Oncol.,* Vol. 17. pp. 735 - 749

Hong, J. W., Lee, I. H., Kwok, Y. H., Park, Y. T., Kwon, I. C., Jeong, S. Y., & Chung, H. (2004) The tissue distribution of paclitaxel after peroral administration of mucoadhesive formulation, *Proceedings of Controlled Release Society 31st Annual Meeting,* Honolulu, HA, 2004

Huizing, M. T., Giaccone, G., Van Warmerdam, L. J. C., Rosing, H., Bakker, P. J. M., Vermorken, J. B., Postmus, P. E., Zandwijk, N., van Koolen, M. G. J., ten Bokkel Huinink, W. W., van der Vijgh, W. J., Bierhorst, F. J., Lai, A., Dalesio, O., Pinedo, H. M., Veenhof, C. H., & Beijnen, J. H. (1997) Pharmacokinetics of paclitaxel and carboplatin in a dose escalating and dose sequencing study in patients with non small cell lung cancer. *J. Clin. Oncol.*, Vol. 15. pp. 317–329

Ibrahim, N. K., Desai, N., Legha, S., Soon-Shiong, P., Theriault, R. L., Rivera, E., Esmaeli, B., Ring, S. E., Bedikian, A., Hortobagyi, G. N., & Ellerhorst, J. A. (2002) Phase I and pharmacokinetic study of ABI-007, a Cremophor-free, protein-stabilized, nanoparticle formulation of paclitaxel. *Clin. Cancer Res.*, Vol. 8. pp. 1038-1044

Kan, P., Chen, Z. B., Lee, C. J., & Chu, I. M. (1999) Development of nonionic surfactant/ phospholipids o/w emulsion as a paclitaxel delivery system. *J. Control. Rel.*, Vol. 58. pp. 271– 278

Kearns, C. M., Gianni, L., & Egorin, M. J. (1995). Paclitaxel pharmacokinetics and pharmacodynamics. *Semin. Oncol.*, Vol. 3. pp. 16-23

Kim, D. W., Kwon, J. S., Kim, Y. G., Kim, M. S., Lee, G. S., Youn, T. J., & Cho, M. -C. (2004) Novel oral formulation of paclitaxel inhibits neointimal hyperplasia in a rat carotid artery injury model. *Circulation*, Vol. 109. pp. 1558-1563

Kim, J.-H., Kim, Y.-S., Kim, S., Park, J. H., Kim, K., Choi, K., Chung, H., Jeong, S. Y., Park, R.-W., Kim, I.-S., & Kwon, I. C. (2006) Hydrophobically modified glycol chitosan nanoparticles as carriers for paclitaxel. *J. Cont. Rel.*, Vol. 111. pp. 228-234

Konishi, T., Satsu, H., Hatsugai, Y., Aizawa, K., Inakuma, T., Nagata, S., Sakuda, S.-h., Nagasawa, H., & Shimizu, M. (2004) Inhibitory effect of a bitter melon extract on the P-glycoprotein activity in intestinal Caco-2 cells. *Brit. J. Pharm.*, Vol. 143. pp. 379-387

Kossena, G. A., Charman, W. N., Boyd, B. J., & Porter, C. J. H. (2005) Influence of the intermediate digestion phases of common formulation lipids on the absorption of a poorly water-soluble drug. *J. Pharm. Sci.*, Vol. 94. pp. 481-492

Lee, I. H., Hong, J. W., Y. H., Kwak, Y. H., Park, Y. T., Kwon, I. C., Jeong, S. Y., & Chung, H. (2004) Oral paclitaxel delivery systems, *Proceedings of Controlled Release Society 31st Annual Meeting*, Honolulu, HA, 2004

Lee, I.-H., Park, Y. T., Roh, K., Chung, H., Kwon, I. C., & Jeong, S. Y. (2005) Stable paclitaxel formulations in oily contrast medium. *J. Cont. Rel.*, Vol. 102. pp. 415–425

Lee, J. H., Gi, U.-S., Kim, J.-H., Kim, Y., Kim, S.-H., Oh, H., & Min, B. (2001) Preparation and characterization of solvent induced dihydrated, anhydrous, and amorphous paclitaxel. *Bull. Korean Chem. Soc.*, Vol. 22. pp. 925-928

Lee, S.-J., Kim, S. W., Chung, H., Park, Y. T., Choi, Y. W., Cho, Y.-H., & Yoon, M. S. (2005) Bioadhesive drug delivery system using glyceryl monooleate for the intravesical administration of paclitaxel. *Chemotherapy*, Vol. 51. pp. 311–318

Liggins, R.T., Hunter, W. L., & Burt, H. M. (1997) Solid-state characterization of paclitaxel. *J. Pharm. Sci.*, 86 pp. 1458-1463

Meerum Terwogt, J. M., Malingre, M. M., Beijnen, J. H., ten Bokkel Huinink, W. W., Rosing, H., Koopman, F. J., van Tellingen, O., Swart, M., & Schellens, J. H. M. (1999) Coadministration of oral cyclosporin A enables oral therapy with paclitaxel. *Clin. Cancer Res.*, Vol. 5. pp. 3379– 3384

Nielsen, L. S., Schubert, L., & Hansen, J. (1998) Bioadhesive drug delivery systems. I. Characterisation of mucoadhesive properties of systems based on glyceryl mono-oleate and glyceryl monolinoleate. *Eur. J. Pharm. Sci.*, Vol. 6. pp. 231-239

Peltier, S., Oger, J.-M., Lagarce, F., Couet, W., Benoît, J.-P. (2006) Enhanced oral paclitaxel bioavailability after administration of paclitaxel-loaded lipid nanocapsules. *Pharm. Res.*, Vol. 23. pp. 1243-1250

Pfeifer, R.W., Hale, K.N., Cronquist, & S. E., Daniels, M. (1993) Precipitation of paclitaxel during infusion by pump. *Am. J. Hosp. Pharm.*, Vol. 50. pp. 2518–2521

Qiu, H., & Caffrey, M. (2000) The phase diagram of the monoolein/water system: metastability and equilibrium aspects. *Biomaterials,* Vol. 21. pp. 223-234

Roh, K. H., Lee, S. Y., Kwon, I. C., Jeong, S. Y., & Chung, H. (2004) Hydrophilic polymers stabilize eutectic mixture of monoglyceride and triglyceride. *Proceedings of Biophysical Society 48th Annual Meeting,* Baltimore, MD, 2004

Rowinsky, E. K. & Donehower, R. C. (1995). Paclitaxel (Taxol), *N. Engl. J. Med.,* Vol. 332. pp. 1004-1014

Schellens, J. H. M., Malingre, M. M., Kruijtzer, C. M. F., Bardelmeijer, H. A., van Tellingen, O., Schinkel, A. H., & Beijnen, J. H. (2000) Modulation of oral bioavailability of anticancer drugs: from mouse to man. *Eur. J. Pharm. Sci.,* Vol. 12. pp. 103-110

Shin, B. S., Kim, H. J., Hong, S. H., Lee, J. B., Hwang, S. W., Lee, M. H., & Yoo, S. D. (2009) Enhanced absorption and tissue distribution of paclitaxel following oral administration of DHP 107, a novel mucoadhesive lipid dosage form. Cancer Chemoth. Pharm. Vol. 64. Pp. 87-94

Singla, A. K., Garg, A., & Aggarwal, D. (2002) Paclitaxel and its formulations. *Int. J. Pharm.,* Vol. 235. pp. 179–192

Sparreboom, A., Van Asperen, J., Mayer, U., Schinkel, A. H., Smit, J. W., Meijer, D. K. F., Borst, P., Nooijen, W. J., Beijnen, J. H., & Van Tellingen, O. (1997) Limited oral bioavailability and active epithelial excretion of paclitaxel (Taxol) caused by P-glycoprotein in the intestine. *Proc. Natl. Acad. Sci. USA,* Vol. 94. pp. 2031–2035

Sparreboom, A., van Tellingen, O., Nooijen, W. J., & Beijnen, J. H. (1996) Nonlinear pharmacokinetics of paclitaxel in mice results from the pharmaceutical vehicle Cremophor EL. *Cancer Res.,* Vol. 56. pp. 2112-2115

Sugahara, S.-i., Kajiki, M., Kuriyama, H., & obayashi, T.-r. (2007) Complete regression of xenografted human carcinomas by a paclitaxel–carboxymethyl dextran conjugate (AZ10992). *J. Cont. Rel.,* Vol. 117. pp. 40-50

van Asperen, J., van Tellingen, O., Sparreboom, A., Schinkel, A. H., Borst, P., Nooijen, W. J., Beijnen, J. H. (1997) Enhanced oral bioavailability of paclitaxel in mice treated with the P-glycoprotein blocker SDZ PSC 833. *Br. J. Cancer,* Vol. 76. pp. 1181-1183

Van Asperen, J., van Tellingen, O., van der Valk, M. A., Rozenhart, M., & Beijnen, J. H. (1998) Enhanced oral absorption and decreased elimination of paclitaxel in mice cotreated with cyclosporine A. *Clin. Cancer Res.,* Vol. 4. pp. 2293–2297

Weiss, R. B., Donehower, R. C., Wiernik, P. H. T., Ohnuma, R. J., Trump, D. L., Baker Jr, J. R., Van Echo, D. A., Von Hoff, D. D. & Leyland-Jones, B. (1990). Hypersensitivity reactions from taxol, *J. Clin. Oncol.,* Vol. 8. pp. 1263-1268

Woo. J. S., Lee, C. H., Shim, C. K., & Hwang, S. -J. (2003) Enhanced oral bioavailability of paclitaxel by coadministration of the P-glycoprotein inhibitor KR30031. *Pharm. Res.,* Vol. 20. pp. 24-30

Xie, Z., Guan, H., Chen, X., Lu, C., Chen, L., Hu, X., Shi, Q., & Jing, X. A (2007) novel polymer–paclitaxel conjugate based on amphiphilic triblock. *J. Cont. Rel.,* Vol. 117. pp. 210-216

Yang, S., Gursoy, R. N., Lambert, G., & Benita, S. (2004) Enhanced oral absorption of paclitaxel in a novel self-microemulsifying drug delivery system with or without concomitant use of P-glycoprotein inhibitors. *Pharm. Res.,* Vol. 21. pp. 261-270

Yoon, C. J., Chung, J. W., Park, J. H., Yoon, Y. H., Lee, J. W., Jeong, S. Y., & Chung, H. (2003) Transcatheter arterial chemoembolization with paclitaxel-lipiodol solution in rabbit VX2 liver tumor. *Radiology,* Vol. 229. pp. 126-131

17

Differences in the Development of the Small Intestine Between Gnotobiotic and Conventionally Bred Piglets

Soňa Gancarčíková
University of Veterinary Medicine and Pharmacy, Košice
Slovakia

1. Introduction

The health quality of human population is strongly connected to the decrease of environmental burden and increase of quality and safety of food. The production of high-quality and safe food and materials of animal origin is conditioned by the good health of raised animals. Diseases of the gastrointestinal tract can be considered the most important health and economic problem of rearing young animals, since they may cause extremely high losses due to morbidity, mortality, cost of treatment and weight loss. At an early age, diseases debilitate the animal organism and cause delays in development which can subsequently become evident as health problems and decreased productivity. For this reason, it is extremely important to ensure optimum development of the digestive tract in young animals. These relations are determined by digestive juice and enzyme secretion, morphological development and microbial colonization of the digestive tract as well as by absorption capacity of the latter. The pig gut is exposed to a variety of stress factors particularly in the early postnatal period and just after weaning. This is the period of significant growth, morphological changes and maturation of the gastrointestinal tract (Godlewski et al., 2005; Trahair & Sanglid, 2002; Xu, 1996). Prior to birth, the alimentary tract is exposed to substances from the ingested amniotic fluid which seems to be of importance to its development (Trahair & Sanglid, 2002). The colostrum, however, differs from the amniotic fluid by the density of nutrients and high immunoglobulin, enzyme, hormone, growth factor and neuroendocrine peptide levels. Widdowson & Crabb (1976) were the first to demonstrate the effect of the colostrum upon development of the alimentary tract by comparing the colostrums-suckling piglets with watered animals. Maternal colostrums contained high levels of several hormones and growth promoting peptides like insulin, epidermal growth factor (EGF), insulin-like growth factor-I and II (IGF-I and II), transforming growth factor-β (TGF- β), glucagon-like peptide-2 (GLP-2) and leptin. It was proved that colostral growth factors play an important role in the postnatal development of the digestive tract in newborn animals (Guilloteau et al., 2002; Xu, 1996). During the several initial days of life of newborns, their small intestine increases its weight by about 70%, length by approx. 20%, diameter by 15%. Its absorption area increases by about 50% during the first postnatal day and by 100% during the first 10 postnatal days (Marion et al., 2003; Xu, 1996). A large luminal surface area with optimal enterocyte functional maturity is important to young growing pigs so they may attain maximum digestive and absorptive capability. Consequently, suboptimal or adverse environmental factors, influencing the morphological development of intestinal tissue, may have critical functional consequences for the young growing pig. The marked and abrupt morphological responses to weaning in the small intestine, characterized by the transformation from a dense finger-like villi population to a smooth, compact, tongue-shaped luminal villi surface may indicate critical consequences for the young pig digestive capacity and subsequent use of nutrients during the starter phase (Skrzypek et al., 2005). The changes at weaning which include shortening of villi, hyperplasia of crypts, decrease in absorption capacity and certain loss of carbohydrate activity may, in combination with changes in the number and type of enterobacteria, induce various degree of post-weaning diarrhoea (Pluske et al., 1997). By now, the prevention and therapy of diseases of sucklings and weanlings was implemented by means of synthetic substances, which enormously burden not only the organisms, but also the living environment as a whole. The extensive use of antibiotics has increased the risk of development of resistance in human and animal pathogens and chemical residues in meat of animals. In progress is the research and development of new methods of biotechnological and natural character that with their complex influence will maximally make efficient the prevention of diseases of animals by the stabilisation of physiological function of biological barriers of the gastrointestinal tract ecosystem. Biological barriers of digestive tract represent the prime and basal protection of organism from negative impacts of external and internal environment, and therefore it is possible to decrease a health risk by its sophisticated modulation. The indigenous microbiota suppresses colonization of incoming bacteria by a process named colonization resistance that is a first line of defence against invasion by exogenous, potential pathogenic organisms or indigenous opportunists. Beneficial microbiota prevent bacterial colonization by competing for epithelium receptors and enteric nutrients, producing antimicrobial compounds such as bacteriocins and metabolizing nutrients to create a restrictive environment which is generally unfavourable for the growth of many enteric pathogens (Bomba et al., 2002; Marinho et al., 2007). Probiotics as natural bioregulators assist the maintenance of the homeostasis of the gastrointestinal tract ecosystem and, during the critical periods of animal life, can play an important role in prevention of diarrhoeic diseases of dietetic and bacterial origin (Bomba et al., 2002; Marinho et al., 2007). Gastrointestinal microflora may be affected by adding probiotic micro-organisms of genera *Lactobacillus*, *Bifidobacterium* (Bomba et al., 2002), *Bacillus*, *Enterococcus* and *Streptococcus* (Scharek et al., 2005) to feed or by their combinations (Bomba et al., 2002; Mathew et al., 1998). Enterococci belong to those lactic-acid bacteria which inhabit human and animal intestines (Devriese et al., 1991). It was observed that *Enterococcus faecium* prevents adherence of enterotoxigenic *Escherichia coli* K 88[+] to the surface of intestinal mucosa of piglets (Scharek et al., 2005). In terms of exactitude and interpretability of results, gnotobiotic piglets are an ideal experimental model for the study of digestive processes and their development. The presence of normal microflora influences the structure of the host intestinal mucous membrane, its function and short-chain fatty acids (SCFAs) production. By means of gnotobiotic conditions, we excluded the influence of the normal microflora and sow's milk. The changes in the small intestine, observed under the specific controlled conditions, were compared to the development of the gut in conventionally bred piglets.

The aim of the study was to evaluate the effects of piglet´s age and diet (natural feeding, artificial feeding and gnotobiotic conditions) on the development of microflora, production of short-chain fatty acids (SCFAs), postnatal morphological development and disaccharidase enzymes activity in the small intestine in piglets reared under the sow, piglets fed on milk replacement, as well as in gnotobiotic piglets.

2. Materials and methods

The experiments on growing and weaned piglets were carried out at the Institute of Microbiology and Gnotobiology, University of Veterinary Medicine and Pharmacy, Košice, Slovakia. The State Veterinary and Food Administration of the Slovak Republic approved the experimental protocols and the animals were handled and sacrificed in a humane manner in accordance with the guidelines established by the relevant commission.

2.1 Animal, housing and diets

2.1.1 Gnotobiotic piglets - 1st experiment

The experiment was carried out in 4 gnotobiotic units, each consisting of reserve, waste and rearing isolator (Velaz s.r.o., Prague, Czech Republic). All experimental materials, including milk substitute, distilled water, saline solution and glass and metal materials were sterilised by autoclaving at 121°C and pressure 1.3 MPa for 30 minutes and cellulose wadding and other sanitary material was gamma-irradiated (Bioster, Veverská Bitýška, Czech Republic). The isolators were sterilized with a 2% solution of peracetic acid (36%, Merci s.r.o., Brno, Czech Republic), sealed for 24 hrs, and vented for a minimum of 72 hrs prior to placing pigs inside. Isolators were maintained under positive pressure, the filtering unit consisting of a fan with preliminary EU 3 filter and two-stage filtering chamber (Velaz s.r.o., Prague, Czech Republic). The first stage of filtration consisted of a frame filter type KS-W, filtration class F 7, the second stage used a KS MIKRO S filter, filtration class H 13, for removing of microparticles. The vented air passed through a frame filter KS W/48, filtration class F 5. The filtration unit assured a minimum of 10 exchanges of air per hour at overpressure of 50-70 kPa and air flow 8-30 m³.

The experiment was carried out on 18 gnotobiotic piglets of Slovak white × Landrace breed. Gnotobiotic sucklings were obtained using the method of open hysterotomy on day 112 of pregnancy. After opening the abdominal cavity and uterus the piglets were immediately transferred through a disinfectant bath containing 2% Incidur® (Ecolab GmbH & Co. OHG, Düsseldorf, Germany) into a hysterectomy box were they were subjected to preliminary treatment and then were placed into 1 of 4 gnotobotic rearing isolators. The floor of isolators was heated by electric underfloor heating system to ensure floor temperature of 34°C for new born piglets and 30°C for 7-14 days old piglets. The piglets were non-colostral and were fed autoclaved milk substitute (Sanolac Ferkel, Germany, in 1 kg dry matter: fat 18.0%, N-free extract 20.0%, lysine 1.7%, Ca 0.9%, P 0.7%, Na 1.0%, Mg 0.2%, fibre 1.5%, ash 10.0%, ME 17.5 MJ, vitamin A 50 000 IU, vitamin D_3 5 000 IU, vitamin E 100 mg, biotin 200 µg, Fe 100 mg, vitamin B_1 4 mg, vitamin B_2 4 mg, vitamin B_6 2 mg, vitamin B_{12} 20 µg, calcium pantothenate 10 mg, nicotinic acid 20 mg, folic acid 1 mg, vitamin C 100 mg, choline chloride 250 mg), diluted 1 : 5 with distilled water. The milk substitute was fed to piglets individually from a glass bottle six times daily (2, 6, 10, 14, 18, 22 h), *ad libitum*. A total of 18 gnotobiotic animals derived from 2 litters were divided into 4 isolators. From the first day of life, a probiotic strain of *Enterococcus faecium* isolated from non autoclaved milk substitute (Sanolac Ferkel, Germany) was administered continuously at a dose of 2 ml of inoculum;

1 ml contained 1×10^4 cfu (data analysed in the Laboratory of Gnotobiology). From the 5th day of life, autoclaved water was available to piglets *ad libitum* and they were fed irradiation-sterilized rations intended for early weaning of piglets. At the age of 28 days, the suckling piglets were weaned and fed irradiation-sterilized starter feedstuff *ad libitum* (OŠ-02®, Tajba Čaňa, Slovak Republic, in 1 kg dry matter: crude protein 180 g, fibre 45 g, lysine 11.5 g, methionine and cysteine 6.3 g, threonine 7.5 g, Ca 7 g, P 5.8 g, Na 1.5 g, Cu 10 mg, Zn 100 mg, Mn 30 mg, ME 13 MJ, vitamin A 8 000 IU, vitamin D_3 1 000 IU, vitamin E 20 mg, Fe 125 mg, vitamin B_2 3 mg, vitamin B_{12} 20 µg, choline 600 mg). A routine microbiological control of gnotobiotic isolators was performed throughout the experiment. Microbiological swabs were taken from isolator walls, surface of animals and from their rectum. The samples were cultivated in PYG medium (Imuna, Slovak Republic). The microbiological control was verified every day on TSA agar with 5% ram's blood (BBL, Microbiology systems, Cockeysville, USA).

2.1.2 Conventional suckled piglets - 2nd experiment

In the experiment, 24 piglets of both sexes (Large white breed x Landrace) from two litters were included. The pigs were housed in two pens, 12 piglets in each, equipped with automatic heating, forced ventilation and completely slatted floors. The suckling piglets had access to sows 6 times daily (2, 6, 10, 14, 18, 22 h.) and from day 5 onwards the animals were provided commercial mixed feed OŠ-01® (Tajba Čaňa, Slovak Republic, in 1 kg dry matter: crude protein 200 g, fibre 40 g, lysine 14 g, methionine and cysteine 6.3 g, threonine 9.1 g, Ca 8 g, P 6.7 g, Na 2 g, Cu 10 mg, Zn 100 mg, Mn 30 mg, ME 13.3 MJ, vitamin A 8 000 IU, vitamin D_3 1 000 IU, vitamin E 20 mg, Fe 125 mg, vitamin B_2 3 mg, vitamin B_{12} 20 µg, choline 300 mg) *ad libitum*. The piglets were weaned at 28 days of age, fed starter feedstuff *ad libitum* (OŠ-02®, Tajba Čaňa, Slovak Republic) and moved to 2 pens (375 x 165 cm) where three piglets were housed per pen. The temperature in the nursery was maintained at 32°C during the first week, and was gradually reduced to 25°C between weeks two and six. The animals had free access to water throughout the experiment (42 days).

2.1.3 Conventional replacer-fed piglets - 3rd experiment

The experiment included 26 piglets of both sexes (Large white breed x Landrace) from two litters. The experiment was carried out in two blocks, 13 piglets in each. The piglets were separated from the sow immediately after birth and had no contact with sow faeces. They were born naturally, were non-colostral, and were fed a commercial milk replacer diluted with distilled water 1:5 (Sanolac Ferkel, Germany), enriched by *Enterococcus faecium* 0.1×10^4 cfu/g of feed. Milk was given to piglets individually from a glass bottle 6 times daily (2, 6, 10, 14, 18, 22 h.), *ad libitum*. Starting from day 5, the suckling piglets were offered the same commercial mixed feed OŠ-01® (Tajba Čaňa, Slovak Republic) and were housed under the same hygiene conditions as those in the second experiment.

2.2 Experimental procedure

All pigs were sacrificed by intracardial euthanasia with 1 ml/kg BW T61® (Intervet International B.V. Boxmeer, The Netherlands). In the first experiment, three hours after birth and at the age of two and seven days, two piglets of each indicated age were sacrificed. Three piglets of each indicated age were sacrificed at the age of 14, 21, 28 and 35 days. In the course of conventional experiments, three piglets from each group were sacrificed at 3 hours post partum and at 2, 7, 14, 21, and 28 days of age. In the second experiment the piglets were slaughtered also on days 35 and 42 of age. The gastrointestinal tract was immediately removed and divided into six segments as follows: stomach, three equal segments of the small intestine, caecum and colon. The total content of each segment was weighed, pH was immediately measured. Intestinal tissue (1 cm^2) were taken from the duodenum (5 cm distal to the orifice of the pancreatic duct) and the medial part of both the jejunum and ileum. The samples were fixed in 4% formalin solution for microscopic assessment of mucosal morphology. Sections of jejunum, ileum and caecum (1 g) were collected and processed for microbial counting and short-chain fatty acids (SCFAs) determinations were carried out in the contents from jejunum, ileum and colon. The intestinal segments (duodenum, jejunum and ileum) were rinsed thoroughly with ice-cold saline solution, opened lengthwise and blotted dry. The mucosa was scraped using a glass slide and immediately frozen in liquid nitrogen. Samples of mucosa were then stored at -70°C until the analysis of digestive enzyme activities.

2.2.1 Microbiological analysis

For microbial analysis, about 1 g of samples (jejunum, ileum, caecum) was placed in a sterile polyethylene stomacher Lab Blender bag (Seward Medical Limited, London, UK) with 9 ml of sterile anaerobic diluent (0.4 g Na HCO$_3$, 0.05g L-cysteine HCl, 1 ml resazurine 0.1%), 7.5 ml mineral solution I (0.6% K$_2$HPO$_4$), 7.5 ml mineral solution II (1.2% NaCl, 1.2% (NH$_4$)$_2$SO$_4$, 0.6% KH$_2$PO$_4$, 0.12% CaCl$_2$, 0.25% MgSO$_4$ and 84 ml distilled water, pH 6.8) and stomached (Stomacher Lab Blender 80, Seward Medical Limited, London, UK) for 5 min under a CO$_2$ atmosphere. A series of 10-fold dilutions (10^{-2} to 10^{-8}) were made in the same diluents. From appropriate dilutions, 0.1 ml aliquots were spread onto one non-selective agar plate: trypticase soy blood agar with 10% sheep blood (BBL, Microbiology systems, Cockeysville, USA) for aerobes. Aliquots (0.1 ml) were also spread on 5 selective agar media as follows: Beerens medium (Beerens, 1990) for *Bifidobacterium*, Rogosa agar (Imuna, Šarišské Michaľany, Slovak Republic) for *Lactobacillus*, Enterococcosel agar (BBL) for *Enterococcus*, MacConkey agar (Imuna) for *Coliforms* and Endo agar (Imuna) for *Enterobacteriaceae*. Plates for the enumeration of *aerobic* bacteria were incubated for 2 days at 37°C. Colonies were counted and bacteria were Gram stained and visualized under a microscope for morphological characterization. The viable counts are expressed as the log 10 of colony forming units (cfu)g^{-1} of sample.

2.2.2 Biochemical analysis

After the collection, 1 g of digesta (jejunum, ileum, colon) was diluted in 50 ml of deionized H$_2$O and applied at a volume of 30 µl for analysis of SCFAs. The concentration of formic, acetoacetic, lactic, succinic, acetic, propionic, butyric and valeric acids in the intestinal content was determined by capillary isotachophoresis (ITP). The measurements were done on an „Isotachophoretic analyser ZKI 01" (SR). In the pre-separation capillary, a leading electrolyte of the following composition was used: 10^{-2} M HCl + 2.2. 10^{-2} M ε-aminocaproic acid + 0.1% methylhydroxyethylcellulosic acid, pH 4.3. As finishing electrolyte, a solution of 5.10^{-3} M caproic acid + histidine was used. This electrolytic system worked at 250µA in pre-separation and 50 µA in the analytic capillary. pH was measured by a pH meter (LP Prague, Czech Republic).

2.2.3 Disaccharidase activity

The lactase (EC 3.2.1.23), maltase (EC 3.2.1.20) and saccharase (EC 3.2.1.26) activities were measured according to Mir et al. (1997). Mucosa samples (200 mg) were homogenized for 3 min with 1 mL saline solution at 0°C. The homogenate was transferred to a test tube together with 2.5 mL (2 × aliquot) of saline solution. Three reaction tubes were filled with 100 µL of the homogenate and placed in a 37°C water bath, and then 400 µL of 56 mM lactose, maltose, saccharose in citrate buffer (pH 6.6, 0.01 mM) were added, respectively. After shaking and incubation for 30 min enzyme activity was stopped in boiling water. The reaction tubes were centrifuged at 2000 × g (30 min, 5°C). The individual enzymes were determined using enzymatic UV method (Boehringer Mannheim, Germany). Protein content in homogenate was started according to Bradford et al. (1976) and the results were expressed as µmol/ mg protein/ hour.

2.2.4 Small intestinal morphology

Fixed intestinal segments were rinsed with water, the samples were dehydrated in a graded series of absolute ethanol (30%, 50%, 70%, 90%), cleared with benzene, saturated with and embedded in paraffin. Sections of 7 µm thickness (10 slices of each sample) were stained with haematoxylin/eosin and observed under a light microscope. The length of 10 villi and depth of 10 crypts was determined by a computer operated Image C picture analysis system (Intronic GmbH, Berlin, Germany) and the IMES analysis software, using a colour video camera (Sony 3 CCD) and a light microscope (Axiolab, Carl Zeiss Jena, Germany).

2.2.5 Statistical analysis

Statistical analysis was performed using Statistic software PRIZMA (version 3.0). All the data were presented as means ± SEM. To estimate the effect of age and weaning on the concentration of SCFAs, bacterial count, disaccharidase activity and intestinal morphology, the data were evaluated statistically by one-way analysis of variance (ANOVA) followed by a multiple comparison Tukey's test. Significant differences between the two groups of piglets were tested using analysis of variance and Student's t-test. Probability values less than 0.05 were used as the criterion for statistical significance.

3. Results

3.1 Health status of animals

The deficit of colostral feeding on day 4 of life caused clinical symptoms of disease in 8 replacer-fed piglets (i.e. 30.8 % of the total number of 26 piglets). The other piglets from this group were healthy. The sick piglets were apathic and did not show any interest in feeding. The disease was peracute and proceeded with physiological temperature. Even though antibiotics were administered, the piglets died within 8 hrs of the first appearance of symptoms. Rectal smears and blood for hematological examination were taken from the piglets and both pathological and anatomical dissections were carried out. In the piglets, lymphocytic leukocytosis as well as hypochromic anaemia were diagnosed, and *E. coli* K88 was isolated from rectal swabs. The colonies from the final dilutions were verified by slide agglutination with K88ab antiserum (Imuna Šarišské Michaľany, Slovakia). The pathological and anatomical dissection for peracuteness of the course of the disease revealed only petechial bleeding on seroses and mucoses of the gastrointestinal tract. Transudate in the abdominal cavity was of a deep-red colour, and the blood was uncoagulated. In the groups of suckled piglets (natural feeding) and gnotobiotic piglets the health status was good.

3.2 Acidity

The actual acidity of stomach digesta in replacer-fed piglets ranged more widely - i.e. from pH 1.7 to 3.8. During the period of observation, only on day 2 of age the pH of stomach contents of these piglets was significantly lower (p<0.01, p<0.05) than in suckled piglets with pH ranging from 2.9 to 3.7 and gnotobiotic piglets with 2.7 - 4.1 pH range (Table 1). In the proximal segment of GIT (content of duodenum and jejunum) of gnotobiotic piglets we recorded between days 7 and 28 days of age the lowest levels of pH which differed significantly on day 14 of age (p<0.001) in duodenum and on day 21 of age (p<0.01) in jejunum in comparison with replacer-fed piglets. The pH level in the caudal segment of GIT (ileal content) of suckled piglets was lower in comparison with replacer-fed piglets and significantly lower on days 2 (p<0.05) and 21 (p<0.01) of age. The ileal and colonic pH were on average lower by 0.08 to 0.5 in the group of suckled piglets and the pH values ranged from 6.27 to 7.17 and from 6.50 to 7.21 compared to replacer-fed piglets in which the pH of the ileal content ranged from 6.93 to 7.64 and the pH of the colonic content ranged from 6.24 to 7.53.

3.3 Effect of age and weaning on production of SCFAs in the intestinal tract of gnotobiotic and conventionally bred piglets

3.3.1 Conventional suckled piglets (natural feeding)

Concentration of both acetoacetic and acetic acid in the jejunal content of suckled piglets (Table 2) within the period of milk nutrition was the highest at 7 days of age (p < 0.001 and p < 0.01, respectively). Subsequently the values declined at 2 weeks of age to 14.76 mmol/l of acetoacetic and to 28.02 mmol/l of acetic acid. This decline continued in acetoacetic acid by day 35 of age to 6.10 mmol/l and in acetic acid by week 4 of life to 7.71 mmol/l (p < 0.01). The concentration of lactic acid in jejunal contents was comparable to that of both acetoacetic and acetic acid, with a mean decline of 11.85 mmol lactic acid/l between day 2 and day 21. But a pronounced increase in the concentration of lactic acid was recorded at 1st week post-weaning - i.e. 53.91 mmol/l. The course of the concentration of both acetoacetic and lactic acid in the ileal content (Table 3) was largely similar to that recorded in the jejunal content. Under the influence of more diverse populations of microorganisms, the conditions in the colonic content changed. Propionic acid concentration (Table 4) increased gradually up to weaning (28 days) and then markedly after weaning (day 35: p < 0.01 and on day 42: p < 0.05). The most pronounced production of acids in the colonic content was observed in acetoacetic acid with highest concentrations at day 14 and 28 of age (p < 0.001 and p < 0.001) and a sudden 4-fold decline at 1st week post-weaning (p < 0.01). In acetic acid, a gradual increase in values was recorded from 7 days of age (11.91 mmol/l), with its highest concentration at 2 weeks post-weaning (p < 0.001).

3.3.2 Conventional replacer-fed piglets (artificial feeding)

In both acetoacetic and lactic acid, the highest levels in the jejunal content in replacer-fed piglets (Table 2) were recorded at 7 days of age (19.89 mmol/l and 24.92 mmol/l, p < 0.01,

	Segments of GIT						p - value	
	St	D	J	Ile	C	SEM	SC × RFP	GP × RFP
Day 2								
Suckled piglets	3.7	5.5	6.1	6.6a	7.2	0.27	p < 0.05	-
Replacer-fed piglets	1.7ba	5.7	6.8	7.4	7.4	0.12	p < 0.01	p < 0.05
Gnotobiotic piglets	4.1	ND	7.2	8.0	7.7	0.39	-	-
Day 7								
Suckled piglets	2.9	5.6	6.2	6.3	6.5	0.09	NS	-
Replacer-fed piglets	3.8	5.8	6.0	6.9	6.3b	0.22	NS	p < 0.01
Gnotobiotic piglets	4.1	4.5	5.9	7.4	7.0	0.56	-	-
Day 14								
Suckled piglets	3.4	5.4	6.1	7.2	6.7	0.09	NS	-
Replacer-fed piglets	2.5	5.5	5.9	7.1	7.5	0.18	NS	-
Gnotobiotic piglets	3.5	4.2c	5.4	7.0	6.4	0.23	-	p < 0.001
Day 21							p < 0.05	
Suckled piglets	3.3	5.2	6.2a	6.8b	7.4	0.15	p < 0.01	-
Replacer-fed piglets	3.4	5.4	6.7	7.5	7.5	0.23	-	-
Gnotobiotic piglets	3.1	4.2	5.9b	6.9	6.7	0.34	-	p < 0.01
Day 28								
Suckled piglets	3.2	5.8	5.9	6.6	6.5	0.18	NS	-
Replacer-fed piglets	2.9	6.0	6.7	7.6	6.2	0.25	NS	NS
Gnotobiotic piglets	2.7	4.4	5.8	6.7	6.6	0.34	-	NS

ND- not detectable, NS- not significant, SP- suckled piglets, GP- gnotobiotic piglets, RFP- replacer-fed piglets, St- stomach, D- duodenum, J- jejunum, Ile- ileum, C- colon, GIT- gastrointestinal tract
Significantly different (SP,GP vs RFP): a (p < 0.05), b (p < 0.01), c (p < 0.001)

Table 1. The pH along the gastrointestinal tract of gnotobiotic and conventionally bred piglets

respectively), with a slight decline in the concentration up to the end of observation. Concentrations of acetoacetic acid in the colonic content (Table 4) were similar to those in the jejunal content except on day 7 of age when a value of 24.09 mmol/l was recorded (p < 0.05). With lactic acid, the highest concentration was seen on day 7 of age (31.17 mmol/l), with a sudden 10-fold decline from day 14 of age (3.15 mmol/l) up to 28 days of life. Acetic acid concentration was relatively stable from 2 to 21 days of life. Thereafter, a marked increase in the concentration was observed at 4 weeks of life (p < 0.01).

3.3.3 Gnotobiotic piglets

The concentration of acetoacetic acid in the jejunal content of gnotobiotic piglets (Table 2) reached the highest level at the age of 7 days, in the period of milk nutrition (p < 0.05), in comparison with the concentration recorded three hours after birth (3.35 mmol/l). A more

	Age (days)									p - value					
	0	2	7	14	21	28	35	42	SEM	0 × 7	2 × 7	7 × 28	28 × 35	SC × RFP	GP × RFP
Formic acid															
Suckled piglets	ND	4.86	5.09	5.77	7.82	8.49	11.74	8.49	1.37	NS	NS	NS	NS	NS	-
Replacer-fed piglets	ND	7.00a	10.85a	11.50	7.21a	ND	ND	ND	1.82	NS	NS	-	-	p < 0.05	p < 0.05
Gnotobiotic piglets	1.00	6.64	7.54	4.46	3.62	10.67	4.58	ND	1.20	NS	NS	NS	NS	-	NS
Acetoacetic acid															
Suckled piglets	ND	18.12	28.69***	14.76	9.11	10.51	6.10	13.51	2.96	NS	p< 0.001	NS	NS	NS	-
Replacer-fed piglets	ND	9.11a	19.89	9.05	12.24	ND	ND	ND	1.81	NS	NS	-	-	NS	p < 0.05
Gnotobiotic piglets	3.35	6.47	17.78*	17.70	12.93	13.26	8.02*	ND	2.40	p < 0.05	NS	NS	p < 0.05	-	NS
Lactic acid															
Suckled piglets	ND	22.98	27.52*	18.18	11.13	17.89	53.91	30.26	8.17	NS	p < 0.05	NS	NS	NS	-
Replacer-fed piglets	ND	17.61	24.92**	23.75	21.98b	ND	ND	ND	1.10	NS	p < 0.01	-	-	p < 0.01	NS
Gnotobiotic piglets	14.22	16.57	23.59	19.96	21.94	21.38	31.25	ND	3.22	NS	NS	NS	NS	-	NS
Succinic acid															
Suckled piglets	ND	9.05	15.10	11.74c	5.36	4.24	5.92	11.74	1.77	NS	NS	NS	NS	p < 0.001	-
Replacer-fed piglets	ND	2.68	6.44	4.59	6.87	ND	ND	ND	0.89	NS	NS	-	-	NS	NS
Gnotobiotic piglets	2.01	2.01	2.67	4.09	5.79	6.03	4.40	ND	0.66	NS	NS	NS	NS	-	NS
Acetic acid															
Suckled piglets	8.50	21.14a	33.05**	28.02c	10.17	7.71**	11.45	11.69	2.99	NS	p < 0.01	p < 0.01	NS	p< 0.05, p< 0.001	-
Replacer-fed piglets	ND	6.71	21.43	13.49a	14.08	ND	ND	ND	2.49	NS	NS	-	-	NS	p < 0.05
Gnotobiotic piglets	6.57	5.20	8.18	5.80	12.86	22.11**	15.95	ND	1.75	NS	NS	NS	(0×28) p < 0.01	-	NS

Table 2. Effect of age, weaning and diets on production of SCFAs in the jejunum (mmol/l) of gnotobiotic and conventionally bred piglets. ND- not detectable, NS- not significant, SP- suckled piglets, GP- gnotobiotic piglets, RFP- replacer-fed piglets. Significantly different (SC,GP vs RFP): a (p < 0.05), b (p < 0.01), c (p < 0.001)

pronounced post-weaning decrease in the level of acetoacetic acid was recorded one week after weaning (p < 0.05). The proportion of lactic acid was relatively stable from day 7 to 28 of life and ranged between 19.96 and 23.59 mmol/l. Afterwards, in the 5th week of life, the lactic acid level increased to 31.25 mmol/l. Similarly, acetic acid level was relatively stable during the first two weeks of life of piglets, then increased significantly (p < 0.01) at the age of 28 days compared to the level at 3 hours after birth (6.57 mmol/l). The most important production of acids in the colon of gnotobiotic piglets (Table 4) was the production of acetic acid which remained relatively stable between days 7 and 35 of life and the difference between its concentration recorded at 3 hours after the birth (6.94 mmol/l) and that determined on day 7 of life (41.98 mmol/l) was significant (p < 0.05). A significant difference in concentration of lactic acid was recorded on day 28 of age (p < 0.001, p < 0.01) compared to the level on the second day (8.18 mmol/l) and 21st day (14.49 mmol/l). Subsequently, we recorded a non-significant, 3-fold increase in the level of this acid at 5 weeks of age (to 76.30 mmol/l). A similar tendency was recorded for acetoacetic and propionic acid in the colonal content with the exception of the level recorded at 3 hours after the birth. The level of acetoacetic acid was significantly higher on day 21 of age (16.22 mmol/l, p < 0.01) compared to the second day of life (6.71 mmol/l).

3.4 Effect of diets on production of SCFAs in the intestinal tract of gnotobiotic and conventionally bred piglets

The concentration of acetoacetic acid in the jejunal content (Table 2) was higher in suckled piglets at 7 days of life (28.69 mmol/l) compared to the replacer-fed animals in which the level of the above acid represented 19.89 mmol/l. In both groups of piglets observed, well-balanced levels of the above acid were recorded thereafter. The course of the concentration of lactic acid up to day 7 of age was the same in 3 groups of piglets with a subsequent increase in replacer-fed piglets at 21 days of age (p < 0.01) compared to suckled animals. In the acetic acid of suckled piglets, significantly higher levels were recorded at day 2 and 14 of age compared to the replacer-fed piglets (p < 0.05, p < 0.001). The proportion of acetic acid in gnotobiotic piglets was up to two weeks of life considerably lower in comparison with both investigated groups and the decrease on day 14 of life was significant (p < 0.05) in comparison with replacer-fed piglets. The course of the concentration of acetoacetic acid in the ileal content (Table 3) was the same in all 3 observed groups except at 3 weeks of age of replacer-fed piglets. While the content of acetoacetic acid represented 17.11 mmol/l in suckled piglets at 3 weeks of life, in the non-colostral group a decline to 8.78 mmol/l was observed. The level of acetic acid in the ileal contents of suckled piglets was higher throughout the period of investigation ranging from about 7 to 21.5 mmol/l compared with the replacer-fed piglets which showed the highest concentration on day 2 (p < 0.001) and 14 of life (p < 0.05). Insignificantly higher concentrations of acetic acid in the ileal content were observed also in gnotobiotic piglets (2.05 - 13.69 mmol/l) compared to replacer-fed piglets. A similar tendency was recorded in lactic acid, in the ileal content up to 14 days of age, with higher concentrations in suckled piglets as compared to the replacer-fed piglets in which the values later ranged about 8.2 till 21.4 mmol/l and a significantly higher level of the acid was recorded at 7 days of age (p < 0.001). Higher production of lactic acid by gnotobiotic piglets (0.6 - 10.14 mmol/l) was observed throughout the observation period in comparison with replacer-fed piglets with a significant increase on day 7 of age (p < 0.01).

	Age (days)									p - value		
	0	2	7	14	21	28	35	42	SEM	28 × 35	SC × RFP	GP × RFP
Formic acid												
Suckled piglets	ND	6.37	6.70	4.79	9.23	14.65	12.19	13.08	1.50	NS	NS	-
Replacer-fed piglets	ND	9.66	8.38	14.35a	8.55	7.41	ND	ND	1.20	-	p < 0.05	NS
Gnotobiotic piglets	3.28	9.02	26.17	22.82	20.84a	12.68	21.47	ND	3.57	NS	-	p < 0.05
Acetoacetic acid												
Suckled piglets	ND	9.06	26.17	13.58	17.11	14.16	4.18*	5.14	3.48	p < 0.05	NS	-
Replacer-fed piglets	ND	5.39	22.48	10.12a	8.78	9.13	ND	ND	2.75	-	NS	p < 0.05
Gnotobiotic piglets	6.37	6.84	13.42	6.14	13.08	7.68	6.17	ND	2.00	NS	-	NS
Lactic acid												
Suckled piglets	ND	25.63	26.91c	21.64	15.52	37.58	60.11	55.90	12.61	NS	p < 0.001	-
Replacer-fed piglets	ND	6.27	14.42	13.41	20.30	16.17	ND	ND	1.79	-	NS	NS
Gnotobiotic piglets	8.72	6.87	24.56b	12.25	24.40	20.67	23.73	ND	7.34	NS	-	p < 0.01
Succinic acid												
Suckled piglets	ND	7.24	23.62	11.07c	11.07	9.72	4.85	5.47	1.97	NS	p < 0.001	-
Replacer-fed piglets	ND	4.72	2.91	3.40	8.38	7.51	ND	ND	0.85	-	NS	NS
Gnotobiotic piglets	1.87	2.91	3.69	4.56	5.02	5.03	2.50	ND	0.79	NS	-	NS
Acetic acid												
Suckled piglets	ND	35.23c	21.81	27.18a	25.00	34.00	11.34	15.83	5.74	NS	p < 0.05, p < 0.001	-
Replacer-fed piglets	ND	15.10	10.47	20.13	19.86	13.43	ND	ND	2.03	-	NS	NS
Gnotobiotic piglets	7.71	11.14	24.16	22.18	32.08	21.58	25.41	ND	5.48	NS	-	NS
Propionic acid												
Suckled piglets	ND	ND	3.18	6.71	8.38	ND	ND	ND	1.06	-	NS	-
Replacer-fed piglets	ND	ND	5.30	4.57	5.03	7.24	ND	ND	1.36	-	NS	NS
Gnotobiotic piglets	ND	2.21	6.17	ND	1.84	3.52	1.17	ND	0.48	NS	-	NS
Butyric acid												
Suckled piglets	ND	2.68	ND	ND	1.67	ND	2.25	3.48	0.68	-	NS	-
Replacer-fed piglets	ND	2.51	ND	ND	ND	3.02	ND	ND	0.84	-	NS	NS
Gnotobiotic piglets	ND	2.01	ND	3.52	3.38	7.24	1.71	ND	1.03	NS	-	NS

Table 3. Effect of age, weaning and diets on production of SCFAs in the ileum (mmol/l) of gnotobiotic and conventionally bred piglets. ND - not detectable, NS- not significant, SP- suckled piglets, GP- gnotobiotic piglets, RFP- replacer-fed piglets. Significantly different (SP,GP vs RFP): a (p < 0.05), b (p < 0.01), c (p < 0.001)

The value of acetoacetic acid in the colonic content (Table 4) was significantly higher in the group of suckled piglets from day 14 to 28 of age ($p < 0.01$), compared to replacer-fed

	Age (days)								SEM	p - value						
	0	2	7	14	21	28	35	42		2 × 7	7 × 14	21 × 28	28 × 35	28 × 42	SC × RFP	GP × RFP
Formic acid																
Suckled piglets	9.22	3.85	4.12	5.03	6.59	6.04	9.29	8.04	0.67	NS	NS	NS	NS	NS	NS	-
Replacer-fed piglets	5.36	7.21b	10.77c	6.94	6.20b	5.36	ND	ND	0.83	NS	NS	NS	NS	-	p < 0.01, p < 0.001	p < 0.01
Gnotobiotic piglets	3.08	9.73	5.56	5.90	2.76	2.48	2.01	ND	1.43	NS	NS	NS	NS	-	-	NS
Acetoacetic acid																
Suckled piglets	3.18	7.55	12.91	71.3b***	54.58b	67.2b***	16.95**	18.00	4.39	NS	p<0.001	NS	p < 0.01	p<0.001	p < 0.01	-
Replacer-fed piglets	3.55	11.50a	24.09*	12.41	8.58	8.69	ND	ND	1.37	p < 0.05	NS	NS	-	-	p < 0.05	NS
Gnotobiotic piglets	9.09	6.71	10.57	22.85	16.22c**	18.29	12.84	ND	3.12	NS	NS	NS	p < 0.01 (2×21)	-	-	p < 0.001
Lactic acid																
Suckled piglets	5.09	5.19	3.01	3.23	2.23	3.35	4.36	4.02	0.42	NS	NS	NS	NS	NS	NS	-
Replacer-fed piglets	6.94	4.96	31.17	3.15	4.19	4.69	ND	ND	2.96	NS	NS	NS	-	-	NS	NS
Gnotobiotic piglets	21.61	8.18a	19.09	19.39b	14.49b	26.34b ** ***	76.3	ND	6.42	NS	NS	p < 0.01	p < 0.001 (2×28)	-	-	p<0.05, p<0.01
Acetic acid																
Suckled piglets	27.17b	15.17	11.91	46.81***	57.22	71.14	89.99*	95.3 ***	2.39	NS	p<0.001	NS	p < 0.05	p<0.001	p < 0.01	-
Replacer-fed piglets	11.47	44.86bb	46.03	46.06	49.66	64.13a**	ND	ND	6.95	NS	NS	p < 0.01	NS	NS	p < 0.01	p<0.01, p<0.05
Gnotobiotic piglets	6.94	10.06	41.98*	44.96	44.20**	44.90	46.95	ND	8.05	p < 0.05	NS	NS	NS		-	NS
Propionic acid																
Suckled piglets	8.72	ND	ND	16.27	13.08	22.59	59.63**	71.14*	4.46	NS	NS	NS	p < 0.01	p < 0.05	NS	-
Replacer-fed piglets	6.37	ND	11.07	14.76	18.28b	21.81b	ND	ND	4.18	NS	NS	NS	-	-	NS	p < 0.01
Gnotobiotic piglets	1.34	4.69	5.02	9.73	5.52	7.37	6.54	ND	1.28	NS	NS	NS	NS	-	-	NS
Butyric acid																
Suckled piglets	ND	3.39	2.01	11.74	14.76	14.43	11.40	14.65	3.74	NS	NS	NS	NS	NS	-	-
Replacer-fed piglets	2.55	11.12a	17.11	14.93	3.35	3.35	ND	ND	2.25	NS	NS	NS	-	-	p < 0.05	NS
Gnotobiotic piglets	3.02	ND	3.01	8.21	6.28	3.35	2.14	ND	1.27	-	NS	NS	NS		-	NS
Valeric acid																
Suckled piglets	ND	ND	ND	ND	5.53	3.91	6.71	5.20	0.68	-	-	NS	NS	NS	NS	-
Replacer-fed piglets	ND	5.03	2.01	2.14	ND	ND	ND	ND	0.60	NS	NS	-	-	-	NS	-
Gnotobiotic piglets	ND	ND	ND	ND	ND	5.26	ND	2.93	1.57	-	-	-	-	-	-	-

Table 4. Effect of age, weaning and diets on production of SCFAs in the colon (mmol/l) of gnotobiotic and conventionally bred piglets. ND- not detectable, NS- not significant, SP- suckled piglets, GP- gnotobiotic piglets, RFP- replacer-fed piglets. Significantly different (SP,GP vs RFP): a ($p < 0.05$), b ($p < 0.01$), c ($p < 0.001$)

piglets. In the period between weeks 2 to 4 of life, production of this acid by gnotobiotic piglets was also higher in comparison with replacer-fed piglets with significant increase at 3 weeks of life ($p < 0.001$). While the dynamics of lactic acid in the colon of suckled and replacer-fed piglets was similar with the exception of week 1, and its levels were low and did not exceed 7 mmol/l, gnotobiotic piglets produced higher level of this acid with peaks at 2 days ($p < 0.05$) and 14, 21 and 28 days of age ($p < 0.01$) compared to the replacer-fed animals. Dynamics of acetic acid in colonal content of suckled piglets resembled that in jejunal and ileal contents and reached higher levels with the exception of days 2 and 7 of age. Significant difference ($p < 0.01$) was observed at 3 hours after the birth in comparison with replacer-fed piglets. Acetic acid in replacer-fed piglets showed an opposite trend in the proximal section of the intestinal tract where we recorded a gradual increase in concentrations up to the end of observation with highest levels at 2 days ($p < 0.01$) and 28 days of age ($p < 0.05$) compared to the gnotobiotic piglets. In the colon of replacer-fed piglets we recorded also higher production of propionic acid on days 21 and 28 of age ($p < 0.01$) compared to the gnotobiotic piglets and butyric acid at 2 days of age ($p < 0.05$) compared to suckled piglets.

3.5 Effect of diets on development of microflora in the digestive tract of suckling piglets and replacer-fed piglets

In suckled piglets, an increase in the followed microflora population was recorded towards the caudal part of the intestine. Bacterial populations ranged from 4 to 8 log cfu/g in the jejunum, from 4 to 9 log cfu/g in the ileum, and from 6 to 9 log cfu/g in the caecum. The lactobacilli in the ileum slightly increased within the period of observation ranging from 1 to 2 log. The cfu of *E. coli* and *Enterobacteriaceae* in the ileum remained more or less stable over time, while they declined in the caecum. The course of development of total aerobes was similar in the jejunum and ileum throughout the period of observation, in the colon, however, total aerobes populations maintained at a constant level of 9 log cfu/g.

Likewise, in conventional piglets fed on milk replacement, an increase in the microflora population was observed towards the caudal part of the intestine. Bacterial populations ranged from 4 to 8 log cfu/g in the jejunum, from 4 to 9 log cfu/g in the ileum and from 6 to 9 log cfu/g in the caecum. In all parts of the intestine, *E. coli* and *Enterobacteriaceae* increased by 1 to 3 log units between days 2 and 14, and decreased thereafter until day 28. In the jejunum and ileum lactobacilli and enterococci slightly increased throughout the period of observation, in the colon, however, lactobacilli populations persisted at a constant level of 9 log cfu/g. *Enterococcus* spp. in colon contents declined by about 2 log units until 28 days of age. The course of the development of total aerobes was the same throughout the period of observation in all parts of the intestine.

Total lactobacilli populations in the jejunal content were significantly higher in the group of conventional replacer-fed piglets with highest counts on days 21 and 28 of age ($p < 0.001$ and $p < 0.001$) compared to the group of suckled piglets (Figure 1). The course of *E. coli* development in the jejunal content was the same in both observed groups except at 2 weeks of age. Whereas total *E. coli* populations were lower in the group of suckled piglets at 2 weeks of life, i.e. 3.78 log cfu/g, a significant increase was observed in group of replacer-fed piglets ($p < 0.001$). In conventional piglets fed on milk replacement, an increase in enterococci populations (Table 5) in the jejunal content was seen throughout the period of

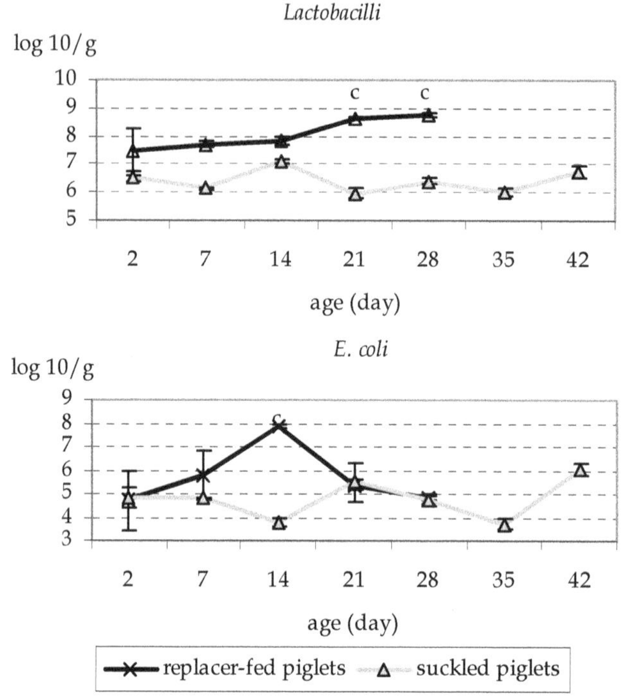

Each bar represents the mean ± SE of 3 piglets.
Significantly different (SP vs RFP): c (p < 0.001)

Fig. 1. Effect of diets on bacterial population (lactobacilli and *E.coli*) in the jejunum of suckling piglets and replacer-fed piglets

observation. In suckled piglets, on the other hand, total enterococci populations were by 0.5 - 2.5 log lower. The highest enterococci populations in the jejunal content of replacer-fed piglets were recorded at 21 and 28 d of age (p < 0.001 and p < 0.001, respectively). Total counts of *Enterobacteriaceae* in the jejunal content were the highest in replacer-fed piglets at 2 (6.95 log cfu/g) and 14 days of age (p < 0.001) compared to the group of suckled piglets in which lower numbers (by 3 logs) were seen at 2 days of life (4.00 log cfu/g) and at 14 days of age the populations were by 3.6 log lower (4.11 log cfu/g). The course of the development of total aerobes in the jejunal content was the same in both groups of piglets, however, with the difference that in replacer-fed piglets, the total numbers of observed bacteria were by 0.5 to 1.2 log higher with significantly higher numbers at 7 (p < 0.001), 14 (p < 0.05), and 21 days of age (p < 0.001).

In the ileal content of replacer-fed piglets we detected higher lactobacilli populations (Figure 2) compared to the suckled animals throughout the period of observation except at 14 days of age with significantly higher numbers at 7 and 21 days of age (p < 0.01 and p < 0.05). The course of development of *E. coli* was the same in both groups, however, with the difference that in the group of suckled piglets the total numbers were higher by 0.5 log except at 14 days of age when an increase in the total *E. coli* populations was recorded (p < 0.001). Total enterococci populations in the ileal content (Table 5) were higher by 1 to 3.5 log in replacer-

| | Content | | | | | | |
| | Jejunum | | Ileum | | Caecum | | |
	SP	RFP	SP	RFP	SP	RFP	SEM
Day 2							
Enterococci	6.36	6.83	6.10	7.70***	8.08	8.69*	0.31
Enterobacteiaceae	4.00	6.95	6.89***	4.55	8.95	7.92	0.25
Total aerobes	7.35	7.97	9.04	8.31	9.33	9.35	0.19
Day 7							
Enterococci	6.19	7.22	3.96	7.42***	7.49	8.73*	0.29
Enterobacteiaceae	4.43	4.02	7.24***	5.27	8.51	8.35	0.19
Total aerobes	6.56	8.15***	7.76	8.45**	9.24	9.57	0.14
Day 14							
Enterococci	5.12	6.80	5.06	7.49***	6.82	7.41	0.31
Enterobacteiaceae	4.11	7.72***	7.16***	8.17	7.37	9.42	0.26
Total aerobes	7.51	8.13*	7.46	8.83**	9.15	9.43	0.19
Day 21							
Enterococci	4.93	7.42***	6.01	6.93***	6.91	6.57	0.14
Enterobacteiaceae	5.38	4.69	6.69	6.57	7.10	8.13	0.19
Total aerobes	6.93	8.22***	8.77	9.35	9.13	9.12	0.29
Day 28							
Enterococci	5.52	7.46***	6.38	8.95***	7.17	6.94	0.16
Enterobacteiaceae	4.81	4.74	6.71**	5.96	6.07	6.53	0.28
Total aerobes	7.95	7.65	8.89	9.20	9.05	8.79	0.21
Day 35							
Enterococci	4.45	ND	5.15	ND	7.17	ND	0.39
Enterobacteiaceae	3.00	ND	5.79	ND	5.98	ND	0.19
Total aerobes	6.61	ND	9.26	ND	9.38	ND	0.14
Day 42							
Enterococci	6.75	ND	7.94	ND	8.91	ND	0.19
Enterobacteiaceae	5.38	ND	5.30	ND	5.36	ND	0.14
Total aerobes	7.80	ND	8.07	ND	9.13	ND	0.51

SP- suckled piglets (n=3), RFP- replacer-fed piglets (n=3), ND- not detectable
*p < 0.05, **p < 0.01, ***p < 0.001

Table 5. Effect of diets on bacterial population ($\log_{10}$ cfu/g of digesta) at various locations along the intestinal tract of suckling piglets and replacer-fed piglets

fed piglets than those in suckled piglets throughout the period of observation with significant difference between days 7 and 28 of age (p < 0.001). In suckled piglets, total *Enterobacteriaceae* populations were by 2 log higher by 1 week of life compared to the

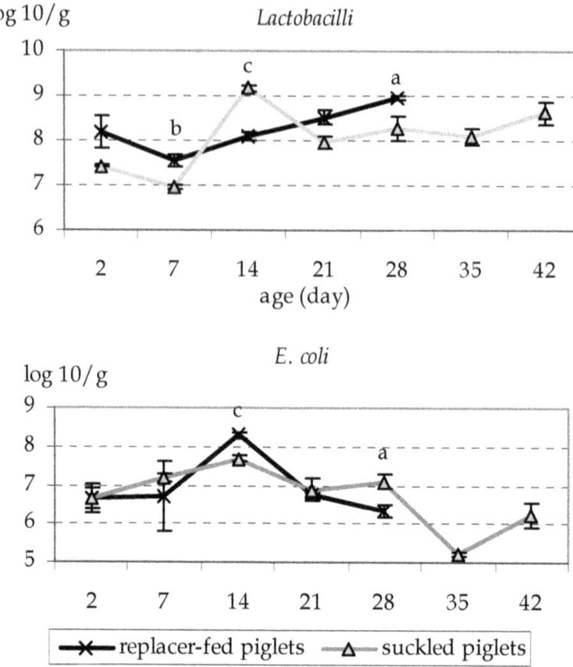

Each bar represents the mean ± SE of 3 piglets
Significantly different (SP vs RFP): a (p < 0.05), b (p < 0.01), c (p < 0.001)

Fig. 2. Effect of diets on bacterial population (lactobacilli and *E.coli*) in the ileum of suckling piglets and replacer-fed piglets

replacer-fed piglets. Thereafter, the populations of observed bacteria slightly declined up to the end of the period of observation. A significant increase in the *Enterobacteriaceae* populations in replacer-fed piglets was recorded at 14 days of age (p < 0.001). Numbers of total aerobes in the ileal content were by 0.5 - 1.5 log higher in replacer-fed piglets compared to colostral animals with significant difference on day 7 (p < 0.01) and 14 of age (p < 0.01).

In the caecum of suckled piglets, *E. coli* populations gradually declined throughout the period of observation (Figure 3) compared with replacer-fed piglets in which a significant increase in numbers was recorded at 14 and 21 days of age (p < 0.001 and p < 0.01, respectively). The course of the development of lactobacilli and total aerobes in the content of the caecum was the same. Total enterococci populations in replacer-fed piglets (Table 5) were by 0.6 - 1.2 log higher by day 14 of age, with significant enterococci populations at 2 and 7 days of age (p < 0.05 and p< 0.05). After day 14, the cfu of *Enterococcus* spp. in the caecum contents of replacer-fed piglets were about 0.3 log units lower than those of suckled piglets. A significant increase in the *Enterobacteriaceae* populations in replacer-fed piglets compared to the second group was recorded from day 14 of age (p < 0.001) to the end of the period of observation (p < 0.01) at 21 days of age and (p < 0.05) at 28 days of age.

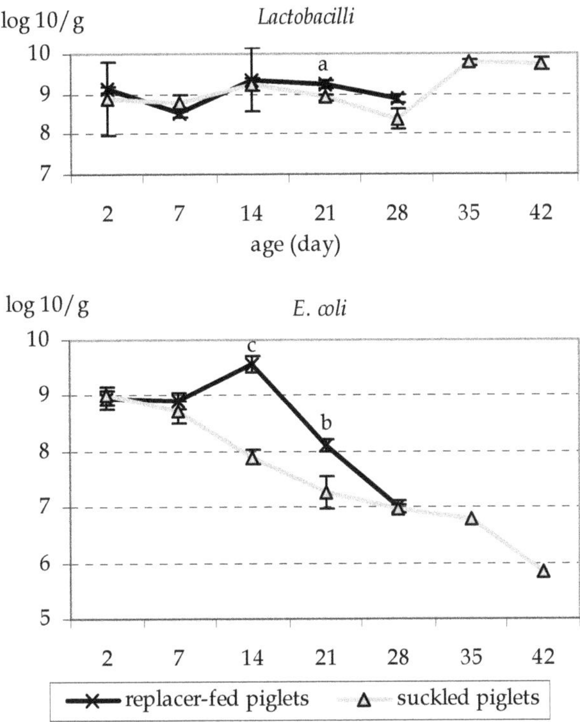

Each bar represents the mean ± SE of 3 piglets.
Significantly different (SP vs RFP): a (p < 0.05), b (p < 0.01), c (p < 0.001)

Fig. 3. Effect of diets on bacterial population (lactobacilli and *E.coli*) in the colon of suckling piglets and replacer-fed piglets

3.6 Effect of age, weaning and diets on development of intestinal morphology in gnotobiotic and conventionally bred piglets

From day 2 of age we recorded a gradual increase in body weight of gnotobiotic piglets from 0.75 kg up to 1.80 kg (p < 0.05) on day 14 of age and 3.90 kg (p < 0.01) on day 21 of age. On day 28 (day of weaning) and one week after weaning the body weight of piglets was decreased insignificantly (Table 6). The increase in relative weight of the small intestine resembled that of the large intestine throughout the period of investigation with the exception that the relative weight of the large intestine in comparison with the weight on day 2 of age was increased significantly on day 21 (p < 0.05), 28 (p < 0.05) and 35 of age (p < 0.001). Similar trend of body weight increase as that recorded in gnotobiotic piglets was observed also in conventional piglets, increasing from 1.41 kg at 2 days of age to 3.50 kg at 14 days of age (p < 0.05). The body weight of piglets increased gradually up to the end of observation with significant increase on day 35 of life (p < 0.01) in comparison with the day of weaning (Table 6).

The development of relative weight of the small and large intestine of suckled piglets was similar and the relative weights decreased gradually between days 2 and 21 of age. On day

	Age (day)						
	2	7	14	21	28	35	SEM
Suckled piglets							
Weight (kg)	1.41	2.05	3.50*a	4.30	5.35	8.55**a	0.39
Small intestinal weight (g/kg)	67.88	64.59	43.59	41.88	44.27	156.6***a	7.08
Large intestinal weight (g/kg)	25.52	24.65	15.68	15.53	23.38	125.4***a	2.38
Gnotobiotic piglets							
Weight (kg)	0.75	1.29	1.80*	3.90**	3.65	3.25	0.46
Small intestinal weight (g/kg)	42.47	52.59	53.02	64.68b	55.41	60.67	6.14
Large intestinal weight (g/kg)	13.89	18.31	20.07	47.41*b	42.1*	85.63***	4.07

Significantly different (SP vs GP): a (p < 0.05), b (p < 0.01)
*p < 0.05, **p < 0.01, ***p < 0.001

Table 6. Effect of age, weaning and diets on weight, gut weight of suckling piglets and gnotobiotic piglets

28 of age the relative weights showed an insignificant increase but in the first week post-weaning the relative weights of both small and large intestine increased significantly (p < 0.001) in comparison with all periods of investigation. The weight of conventional piglets was greater throughout the experiment and significant differences (p < 0.05) were recorded on days 14 and 35. Completely opposite trend was recorded for relative weights of small and large intestines of these piglets (Table 6). While relative weights of intestines of gnotobiotic piglets gradually increased throughout the experiment with the exception of day 28 of life, the weight of small and large intestine in suckled piglets decreased gradually between days 2 and 21 of life. Between days 2 and 28 of life the relative weight of the intestines of gnotobiotic piglets was higher compared to conventional piglets with significant difference on day 21 of life (p < 0.01). In the post-weaning period (one week post-weaning), the weight of small and large intestine of suckled piglets was significantly higher (p < 0.05) in comparison with gnotobiotic piglets in the same period of observation.

The development of the height of villi in individual segments of the small intestine of gnotobiotic piglets is shown in Table 7. On day 21, the height of villi in the duodenum was decreased significantly (p < 0.01). A decrease in their length was also recorded on day 28 but the difference was insignificant. In the duodenum of suckled piglets, the height of villi (Table 7) increased significantly (p < 0.001) in the period between birth and day 14 of age. Subsequently, their length decreased gradually up to the weaning (p < 0.01). Throughout the experiment, the willi in the duodenum of gnotobiotic piglets were higher and their height differed significantly from that of conventional piglets at 3 hours after birth, days 2 and 7 of age (p < 0.01) and day 14 of age (p < 0.05) (Figure 4).

The length of jejunal villi of gnotobiotic piglets (Table 7) increased from day 0 up to day 2 of age reaching maximum of 725.18 μm. In the subsequent 5 weeks, the length of villi decreased gradually down to 387.44 μm in the week after weaning and the decrease was significant on days 14 (p < 0.05) and 21 of age (p < 0.001). In the jejunum of suckled piglets we observed a gradual but insignificant increase in villi height in the period from birth up to day 7 of life. In the following period, from day 14 of age till one week post-weaning we recorded gradual decrease in the height of villi, significant on days 21 (p < 0.001) and 35 of

	Content						
	Duodenum		Jejunum		Ileum		
	SP	GP	SP	GP	SP	GB	SEM
Day 0							
Villus height, μm	253.67	371.29	689.68	679.43	574.80	587.37	47.11
Crypt depth, μm	129.13	81.63	53.67	67.12	48.14	79.43	1.96
Day 2							
Villus height, μm	308.42***	424.81	701.57	725.18	588.29	455.05	45.66
Crypt depth, μm	140.23	104.15	69.77	72.66	77.77	82.54	2.73
Day 7							
Villus height, μm	374.98***	502.63	718.21	691.74	401.54***	393.00	28.60
Crypt depth, μm	188.00	124.10	83.82	90.97	71.18	111.35	5.03
Day 14							
Villus height, μm	547.83***	605.14	661.59	581.23*	369.52	424.16	29.03
Crypt depth, μm	151.79	119.27	92.53	103.47	178.96	118.22	3.96
Day 21							
Villus height, μm	454.48**	478.43**	492.42***	442.86***	351.01	423.29	34.21
Crypt depth, μm	168.54	162.33*	129.44	136.17	134.26	176.15*	3.60
Day 28							
Villus height, μm	351.81**	349.21	447.67	401.93	361.69	358.57	31.64
Crypt depth, μm	220.94	197.82	164.80	145.50	165.94	157.69	3.70
Day 35							
Villus height, μm	364.13	396.07	324.23**	387.44	310.00	336.54	25.33
Crypt depth, μm	343.56***	205.10	230.11**	164.23	206.80*	166.91	5.83
Day 42							
Villus height, μm	379.44	ND	440.08	ND	358.65	ND	18.32
Crypt depth, μm	322.66	ND	223.39	ND	174.81	ND	4.22

SP- suckled piglets, GP- gnotobiotic piglets, ND- not detectable
*p < 0.05, **p < 0.01, ***p < 0.001

Table 7. Effect of age and weaning on small intestinal morphology at various locations along the intestinal tract of suckling piglets and gnotobiotic piglets

age (p < 0.01). Comparison of both animal groups showed that villi in the jejunum of conventional piglets were higher between days 14 and 28 of age, the difference being significant on day 14 (p < 0.05). In the post-weaning period, villi were significantly higher (p < 0.05) in gnotobiotic piglets on day 35 (Figure 4).

When comparing both mentioned groups, higher villi were observed in ileum of gnotobiotic piglets, resembling the situation in duodenum, with significant difference (p < 0.05) on days

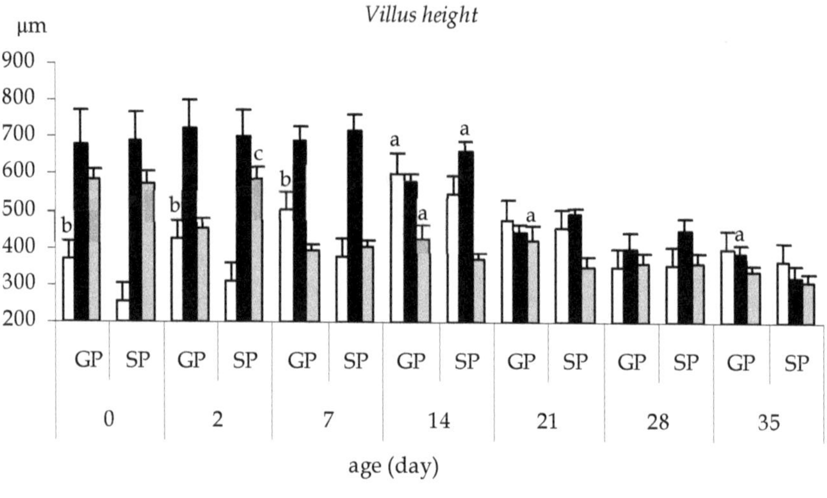

SP- suckled piglets, GP- gnotobiotic piglets
Significantly different (SP vs GP): a (p < 0.05), b (p < 0.01), c (p < 0.001)

Fig. 4. Effect of diets on small intestinal morphology at various locations along the intestinal tract of suckling and gnotobiotic piglets

14 and 21 of age with the exception of day 2 of life when ileal villi were significantly higher (p < 0.001) in conventional piglets (Figure 4).

The postnatal changes in the depth of crypts (Table 7) were the same in all small intestinal segments of gnotobiotic piglets. From the birth up to day 35 of life the crypts in the jejunal segment gradually deepened and reached 164.23 μm on day 35 of life. Similar development was observed also in the duodenal segment of the small intestine, where, with the exception of slight decrease on day 14 of age, the depth of crypts gradually increased throughout the observation period with significant difference on day 21 of age (p < 0.05). One week after weaning the depth of crypts in the duodenum reached 205.1 μm. A significant increase in the depth of crypts (p < 0.05) was recorded on day 21 of age also in the ileal segment of gnotobiotic piglets. Also dynamics of development of the depth of crypts was similar in all small intestine segments of colostral piglets. In the first post-weaning week we recorded a significant deepening of crypts in duodenal (p < 0.001), jejunal (p < 0.01) and ileal (p < 0.05) segments.

Staining with haematoxylin/eosin showed that the small intestinal mucosa of gnotobiotic piglets and suckled piglets at 3 h after birth (Figure 5/a,b) and on day 2 of age (Figure 5/c,d) was covered by population of dense, finger-like villi of the same height. While on the surface of villi of gnotobiotic piglets we were able to observe enterocytes with apically located nucleus, in suckled piglets the enterocytes had apically to medially located nucleus. The fibrous base of intestinal villi was poorly differentiated and the intestinal crypts were small. By day 7 of age of gnotobiotic piglets (Figure 5/e) the height of villi decreased but their diameter increased. In the same period the villi in suckled piglets preserved their finger-like shape with medially to basally located nucleus in enterocytes (Figure 5/f). At the

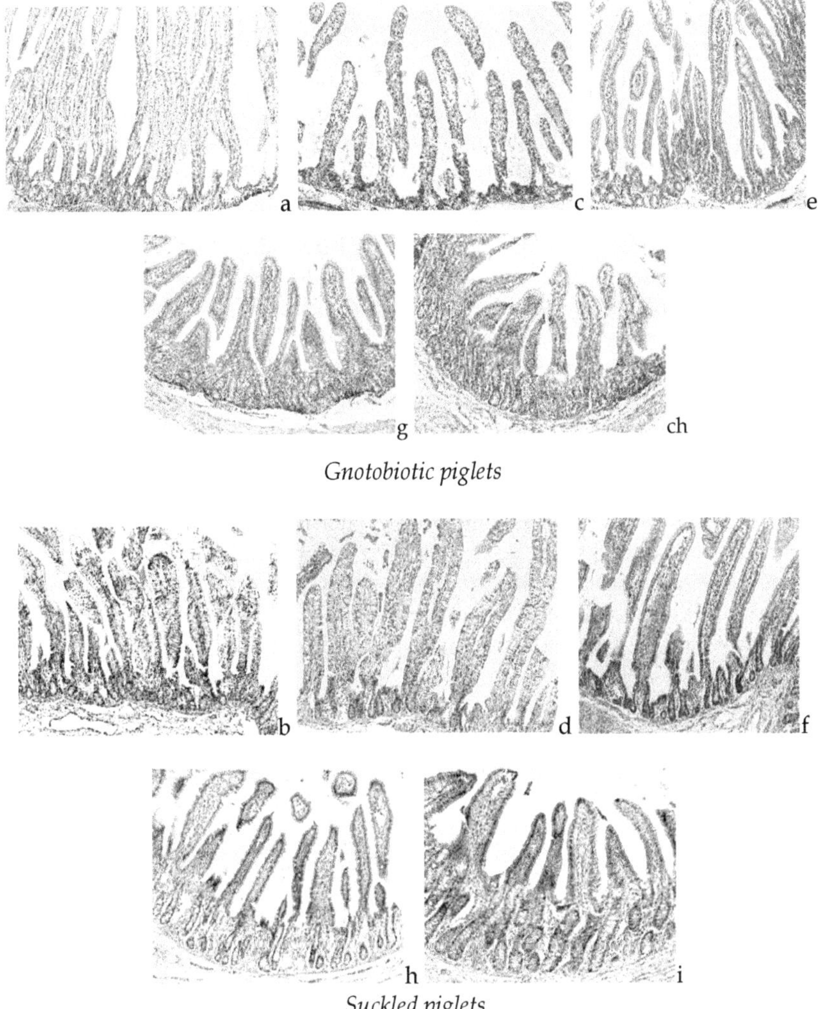

Gnotobiotic piglets

Suckled piglets

(a, b) 3 hours after birth, (c, d) 2 days of age, (e, f) 7 days of age, (g, h) 28 days of age, (ch) 35days of age of GP, (i) 42 days of age of SP, SP- suckled piglets, GP- gnotobiotic piglets, Magnification x 125.

Fig. 5. Light micrograph of hematoxylin and eosin-stained jejunal mucosa of gnotobiotic and suckling piglets

time of weaning (day 28 of age) the differentiated basis of intestinal villi in both observed groups of piglets consisted of thin fibrous tissue containing fascicles of smooth muscle cells. On the surface of the villi we were able to observe goblet cells interspersed among enterocytes (Figure 5/g, h). The enterocyte nuclei were located in the medial part of the cytoplasm. The villi stroma was infiltrated with small number of lymphocytes and plasmatic cells. By day 35 of life, the jejunal villi acquired tongue-like shape (Figure 5/ch). On day 42 of age intestinal crypts of suckled piglets (Figure 5/i) almost completely filled up *lamina propria* of the small intestine and their bases almost reached *lamina muscularis mucosae.*

Intestinal villi were shorter and acquired tongue-like shape. Such characteristic development was observed in all investigated segments of the small intestine which, however, differed by morphometric parameters of villi height.

3.7 Effect of age, weaning and diets on development of specific activity of disaccharidases in the small intestine of gnotobiotic and conventionally bred piglets

In our study we registered that development of lactase activity of gnotobiotic piglets was similar in the duodenum and jejunum in the period from day 0 to 35 of age. The specific activity of lactase (Figure 6) in the duodenum reached at birth the level of 3.4 µmol/mg protein/hour. From the 2nd day of life the increasing enzyme activity was noticed with a measured maximum on day 7 of life ($p < 0.001$). High enzyme levels were observed until the 21th day of life (5.80 µmol/mg protein/hour), after which the enzyme activity decreased in the weeks 4 ($p < 0.001$) and 5 ($p < 0.001$) to levels similar to those noticed at birth. In terms of lactase activity distribution throughout the small intestine, higher activity in the duodenum and jejunum were noticed than in distal parts of the small intestine, where the incidence of enzyme was 4 times lower. The specific activity of lactase in the duodenum of conventional piglets (Figure 6) reached at birth 3.6 µmol/mg protein/hour. The course of activity of this enzyme during our observations resembled that of gnotobiotic piglets with maximum recorded on day 7 of age ($p < 0.001$), gradual decrease from day 14 of life and significant decrease ($p < 0.001$) on the day of weaning and in the 1st post-weaning weak. As far as the distribution of lactase in the small intestine was concerned, the highest activity of lactase

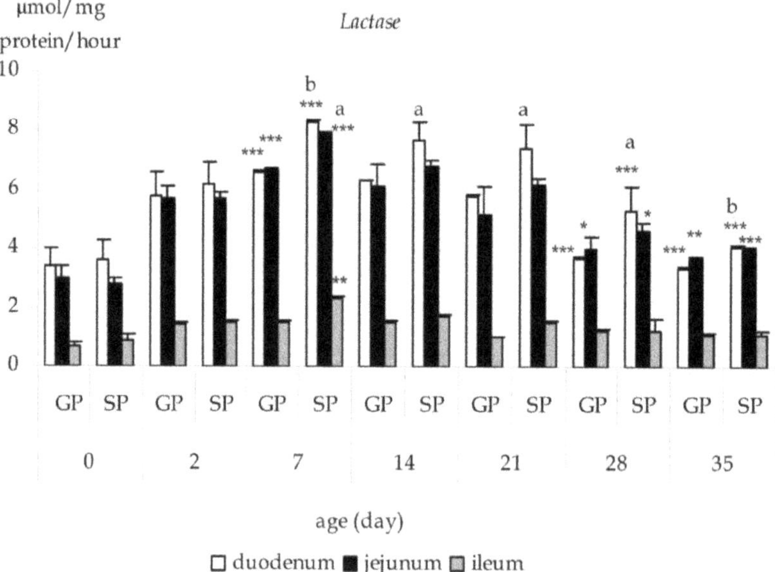

Significantly different (SP vs GP): a ($p < 0.05$), b ($p < 0.01$), *$p < 0.05$, **$p < 0.01$, ***$p < 0.001$

Fig. 6. Effect of age, weaning and diets on specific activity of lactase at various locations along the intestinal tract of suckling and gnotobiotic piglets, SP- suckled piglets, GP-gnotobiotic piglets

was recorded in duodenum and the lowest in ileum where lactase levels were 4-fold lower compared to proximal small intestine segments. Significant increase in the activity of enzyme was observed in jejunum ($p < 0.001$) and ileum ($p < 0.01$) of conventional piglets on day 7 of age. Comparison of both animal groups (Figure 6) showed that specific activity of lactase in the intestinal tract was higher in conventional piglets throughout the experiment with significantly higher lactase activity in duodenum from day 7 to 35 of age ($p < 0.05$, $p < 0.01$) and significantly higher level in the jejunum ($p < 0.05$) on day 7 of age.

The post-natal dynamics of maltase (Figure 7) and saccharase (Figure 8) in gnotobiotic piglets took a completely different course. Very low levels of maltase in the jejunum detected at birth (0.3 µmol/mg protein/hour) and during the 1st week of life slightly increased in the following period and on the 14th day reached 1.2 µmol/mg protein/hour. The slightly increased specific activity of maltase persisted also in the following period. Maltase distribution (Figure 7) throughout the small intestine changed depending on the age with a predominant concentration of maltase activity in the jejunum at the age of 1-2 weeks, through a higher activity in the duodenal part at the age of 21 days, until a balanced distribution in the proximal and medial part of the small intestine was achieved at the age of 4-5 weeks. Similarly also very low specific saccharase activity in the jejunum (Figure 8) recorded until the 1st week of life (1.12 µmol/mg protein/hour) progressively increased with a maximum on the 21st day of life ($p < 0.001$), sustained values were reached in the 4th and 5th week of the life of piglets. Saccharase activity distribution throughout the small intestine of gnotobiotic piglets was higher in the jejunum during the entire period of observation. Specific activities of maltase (Figure 7) and saccharase (Figure 8) in newborn

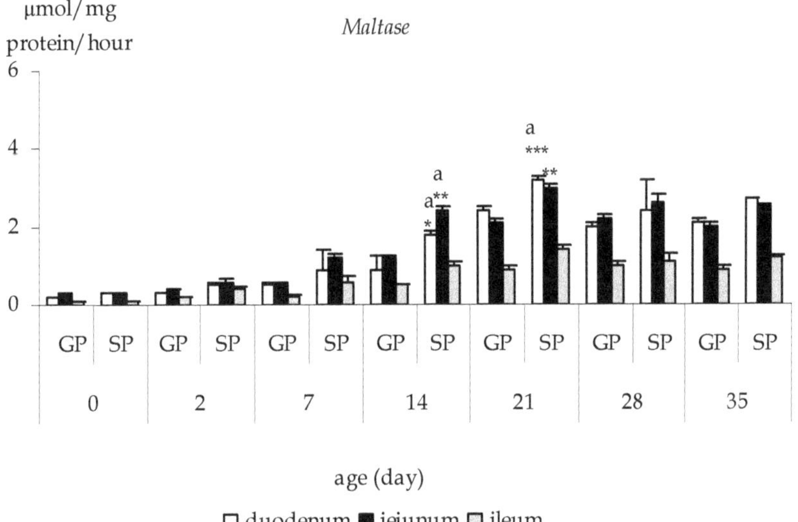

Significantly different (SP vs GP): a ($p < 0.05$), *$p < 0.05$, **$p < 0.01$, ***$p < 0.001$

Fig. 7. Effect of age, weaning and diets on specific activity of maltase at various locations along the intestinal tract of suckling and gnotobiotic piglets, SP- suckled piglets, GP- gnotobiotic piglets.

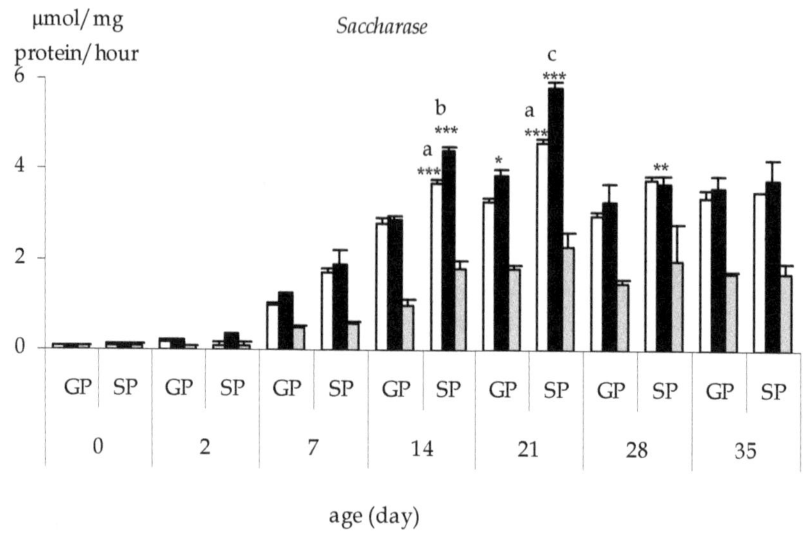

SP- suckled piglets, GP- gnotobiotic piglets.
Significantly different (SP vs GP): a (p < 0.05), b (p < 0.01), c (p < 0.001), *p < 0.05, **p < 0.01, ***p < 0.001

Fig. 8. Effect of age, weaning and diets on specific activity of saccharase at various locations along the intestinal tract of suckling and gnotobiotic piglets

and 2-day old conventional piglets were very low and did not exceed 0.6 μmol/mg protein/hour. After one week of age of piglets, activities of both enzymes increased. The maximum specific activity of maltase peaked on days 14 and 21 (p < 0.05, p < 0.001) in the duodenum and significant difference was observed (p < 0.05) in the jejunal segment. Similarly, activity of saccharase reached highest values on days 14 and 21 of age and differed significantly (p < 0.001) in both the duodenal and jejunal segment. On day 28 of age we observed a decrease in the specific activity of both enzymes with significant difference in saccharase (p < 0.01) in the jejunum. Observation of distribution of maltase in the small intestine of conventional piglets showed that in the direction of terminal ileum, up to the age of 2 weeks the highest activity was detected in the jejunum and the lowest in the ileum. In the following period activity of this enzyme was higher in proximal to medial segments of the intestine than in the distal ones. Throughout the experiment saccharase reached the highest activity in the jejunum and the lowest in the ileum.

The postnatal development of specific activity of enzymes maltase and saccharase showed a similar trend with higher activities of both enzymes in suckled piglets in all digestive tract segments throughout the observation. The highest activity of the enzymes in comparison with gnotobiotic piglets was recorded on days 14 and 21 of age with significant differences in the level of maltase (p < 0.05, p < 0.001) in the duodenum and significantly different activity of the enzyme (p < 0.05) in jejunum. Significantly different activities of saccharase compared to the other group of piglets were observed in the same period (days 14 and 21) in duodenum (p < 0.05) and jejunum (p < 0.01, p < 0.001).

4. Discussion

4.1 Effect of age and diets on development of the small intestine – Intestinal microflora

At birth, a young pig which is axenic during its uterine life is suddenly confronted with a complex bacterial environment. Beginning with birth, the young are in contact with several microbial ecosystems - i.e. faeces, contaminated vagina and perineum, but also from the skin and teats of the sow which are usually contaminated as well. It could be assumed that each of these ecosystems contributes to constituting the gut flora of the newborn (Siggers et al., 2007). However, in the following days, simplified microbiota profiles have been characterized, which will become more complex with time, increasing its diversity as the animal grows (Inoue at al., 2005). The population level of the microbiota in various parts of the gastrointestinal tract of monogastric animals depends on the attachment ability, replication period of the microorganism under the physicochemical tract conditions and the emptying rhythm in the part of the gastrointestinal tract under investigation. Swords et al. (1993) studied pig faecal microbiota evolution within the first four months of life, and concluded that the establishment of the adult faecal flora is a large and complex process with three different marked phases in the bacterial succession. The first phase corresponds with the first week of life, the second one, from the end of the first week to conclusion of suckling, and the third phase from weaning to final adaptation to dry food. In this first phase, aerobes and facultative anaerobes from the sow and the environment become the predominant bacterial groups, comprising 80% of the total flora by three hours after birth. The gut colonization is extremely fast, only twelve hours after birth, total bacteria in distal colon reaches counts of 10^9 cfu/g colonic content (Jensen et al., 1998; Swords et al., 1993). First colonizers modify the gastrointestinal environment (by consumption of molecular oxygen and reduction of the redox potential), making it more favourable for the following colonization by anaerobes. As a result, aerotolerant bacteria are gradually supplanted by strict anaerobes, and 48h after birth, piglets already show 90% of anaerobic bacteria (Swords et al., 1993). Of these bacterial groups, lactobacilli and streptococci become the dominant bacteria at the end of the first week of life and will be maintained for the whole suckling period with counts of around 10^7-10^9 cfu/g digesta (Swords et al., 1993). Microbiota remains fairly stable in terms of species composition during the second phase when the piglets receive milk from their mother (Mathew et al., 1996). The diversity of anaerobic bacteria increases in this period (Inoue et al., 2005) and supplantation of aerobic and facultative anaerobic bacteria by anaerobic bacteria become almost completed in this phase. As has been mentioned before, lactobacilli and streptococci continue being dominant bacteria, which are well adapted to utilize substrate from the milk diet. *Clostridium, Bacteroides, bifidobacteria,* and low densities *Eubacterium, Fusobacterium, Propionibacterium* and *Streptococcus* spp. are also usually found in this second phase (Swords et al., 1993). In our experiment with piglets fed maternal milk, the gut flora developed very quickly post partum. As early as within 48 hrs post partum, *Escherichia coli,* enterococci and lactobacilli were detected in the content of digesta in suckled piglets, the populations of which represented 10^5 - 10^9 bacteria/g per sample. The gut flora of piglets in the proximal part (jejunum) consisted of facultatively anaerobic bacteria (enterococci, *E. coli*) and aerotolerant anaerobes (lactobacilli) counting 10^4 - 10^6 bacteria/g per sample. These numbers increased progressively in the ileum and the dominant flora in the posterior portions of the digestive tract (caecum) was facultatively anaerobic bacteria (*E. coli,* enterococci, *Enterobacteriaceae* and lactobacilli) counting 10^8 - 10^9 bacteria/g per sample. As the piglets grew, the flora progressively changed. The replacement of maternal milk by a milk replacement diet in our third experiment resulted at 2 and 14 days of age in increased numbers of bacterial flora, of the family *Enterobacteriaceae* in the proximal small intestine (jejunum) by 3 log compared to suckled piglets. At the same time a gradual increase in the numbers of coliform bacteria (p < 0.001) in the proximal (jejunum) and terminal (caecum) part of the intestine occurred reaching numbers as much as by 4 log higher in the jejunum at 14 d of age compared to colostral piglets. Similar findings were obtained by (Franklin et al. 2002; Jensen et al., 1998; Pluske et al., 1997) which observed, in addition to higher populations of anaerobic and coliform bacteria, a significant decline in lactobacilli populations in piglets fed replacement milk. The mechanism of the selection has not yet been determined, although feeding may be a primary factor. According to different authors it is almost impossible to prevent neonatal *E. coli* diarrhoea in piglets which do not receive maternal colostrum (Pluske et al., 1997; Xu et al., 1996). Colostrum and also maternal milk contain highly digestible nutrients and components such as immunoglobulins and lysozymes and have both bacteriostatic and antiadhesive properties towards the pathogen *E. coli* (Xu et al., 1996). This protective effect, however, does not seem to be accompanied by an elimination of *E. coli* from the digestive tract. In addition, in both the jejunal and ileal part (p < 0.001) of the small intestine of replacer-fed piglets, high numbers of enterococci were recorded, being by 1-3.5 log higher compared to the colostrum-fed piglets throughout the period of observation. It is likely, however, that this result was influenced by the milk replacement having been enriched by *Enterococcus faecium* counting 10^4 cfu/g of feed. The human intestinal microbiota is a complex ecosystem, consisting of several hundred (more than 800) different bacterial species. This microbiota plays an important role in human health and nutrition by producing nutrients, preventing colonization of the gut by potential pathogenic microorganisms (Guarner & Malagelada, 2003), and preserving the health of the host through interactions with the developing immune system. The microbiota in early life has been linked to allergy risk (Penders et al., 2007). Major changes in the intestinal microbial composition occur in early life. Sterile *in utero*, the gastrointestinal tract of the newborn infant is rapidly colonized at birth by a myriad of maternal vaginal and faecal bacteria and other sources from its environment. The first few weeks after birth correspond to critical stages of gut colonization. Bacterial colonization of the gastrointestinal tract is influenced by numerous factors including diet, environment, antibiotic treatment, mucosal maturation, and age. Naturally delivered babies experienced a period of 2-3 days in which, as a consequence of the low selective potential of their stomach and small bowel, bacteria invading and reproducing within the gut belong to aerobic species as *Enterobacteriaceae*, streptococci, and staphylococci. These bacteria, arriving from the external environment, belong to species with a pathogenic potential, and therefore, it might seem that they would not be the best choice for the health of neonates. However, the metabolisms of these bacteria are believed to be positive factors in preparing the path to a beneficial enteric flora. In the study of Fallani et al. (2010) they confirmed previously published work (Hopkins et al., 2005; Penders et al., 2007) that bifidobacteria are the predominant group detected in the faeces of pre-weaned infants, followed by *Bacteroides* and enterobacteria.

4.2 Production of SCFAs and pH

Organic acids are the main metabolites of intestinal fermentation. The degree of their concentration in the digesta reflects the level of intestinal fermentation (Piva et al., 2002). It is well known that organic acids exhibit antibacterial activity (Piva et al., 2002), increase intestinal absorption of minerals and improve ileal digestion of proteins and amino acids. Their relative levels vary depending on location (stomach, small intestine, large intestine) and diet composition (dietary lactose level, fibre level, etc). Lactic acid is in the greatest concentration in the stomach and small intestine while other organic acids, acetic along with propionic and butyric, are predominant in the large intestine. In our study, in suckled piglets we recorded higher level of acetic acid in the ileal contents in comparison with the replacer-fed piglets throughout the observation, ranging from about 7 to 21.5 mmol/l. Higher concentrations of this acid were observed in the same segment also in gnotobiotic piglets compared to replacer-fed piglets, ranging from 2.05 to 13.69 mmol/l. A similar tendency was recorded in lactic acid, in the ileal content, with higher concentrations in suckled piglets compared to the replacer-fed piglets in which the values later ranged from about 8.2 to 21.4 mmol/l. Higher production of lactic acid in gnotobiotic piglets in comparison with replacer-fed piglets was recorded throughout the observation and ranged from 0.6 to 10.14 mmol/l. Increasing concentrations of lactate in ileal digesta should therefore reflect an increased population and activity of lactic acid bacteria (Pluske et al., 2002). These findings are of importance relative to the management of growing pigs, because lactate has been shown to have antibacterial effects on *E. coli* and *Salmonella* species, and lactobacilli have been shown to inhibit adhesion of enterotoxigenic *E. coli* to the ileal epithelium (Pluske et al., 2002). The ability to generate organic acids, particularly lactic and acetic acid, present one of the mechanisms by which lactobacilli perform their inhibitory effect upon pathogens. With decreasing pH values, the inhibitory activity of the above acids increases, their molecular form being toxic for bacteria. The increased toxicity of acetic acid is attributed to its higher pKa in comparison to lactic acid. Increased lactic acid levels intensify the toxicity of acetic acid. Comparison of lactic acid levels in the jejunal and ileal contents of one week old gnotobiotic piglets (Bomba et al., 1998) and conventional suckling piglets (Zitnan et al., 2001) revealed that the highest levels were found in conventional animals (29.30 and 27.90 mmol/l, resp.) and in *Lactobacillus plantarum* inoculated gnotobiotic piglets (26.60 and 14.20 mmol/l, resp.). High levels of lactic acid were recorded in our study in jejunal and ileal contents of conventional suckling piglets (27.52 and 26.91 mmol/l, resp.) and piglets inoculated with *Enterococus faecium* at the age of 1 week (23.59 and 24.56 mmol/l, resp.). Lower concentrations of this acid were found in replacer-fed piglets (24.92 and 14.42) and the lowest levels of lactic acid in the jejunal and ileal contents (Bomba et al., 1998) were seen in germ-free piglets (4.40 and 6.45 mmol/l, resp.). At the age of 3 weeks, the level of lactic acid in the jejunum of piglets inoculated with *Enterococcus faecium* was lower in comparison with that in the jejunum of piglets inoculated with *Lactobacillus plantarum* (21.94 and 33.15 mmol/l, resp.) but in the ileum of *Enterococcus faecium* inoculated piglets we found the highest level of this acid (24.40 mmol/l) in comparison with all other groups of piglets. The mentioned authors presented different results also with regard to acetic acid, as the highest concentrations of acetic acid in the jejunum and ileum (30.05 and 23.61 mmol/l, resp.) were observed in conventional piglets by Zitnan et al. (2001) and in conventional suckling piglets investigated in our study (33.05 and 21.81 mmol/l, resp.). Lower levels were observed in replacer-fed piglets (21.43 and 10.47 mmol/l, resp.) and in gnotobiotic piglets (Bomba et al. 1998) inoculated with lactobacilli (11.80 and 11.85 mmol/l, resp.) and in those inoculated with *Enterococcus faecium* (8.18 and 24.16 mmol/l, resp.). Similarly low levels were detected also in germ-free piglets (13.15 and 3.9 mmol/l, resp.). On the contrary, at the age of 3 weeks, we recorded higher levels of acetic acid in the jejunal and ileal content of gnotobiotic piglets inoculated with *Enterococcus faecium* (12.86 and 32.08 mmol/l, resp.) in comparison with all other groups of piglets (10.7 and 25.9 mmol/l, resp.) of conventional suckling piglets (Zitnan, 2001), (5.36 and 25.00 mmol/l, resp.) of conventional suckling piglets in our study, (6.87 and 19.86 mmol/l, resp.) of replacer-fed piglets and gnotobiotic piglets inoculated with *Lactobacillus plantarum* (11.85 and 14.2 mmol/l, resp.). Under the influence of more diverse populations of microorganisms the conditions in the colonic content changed with gradual occurrences of propionic, butyric, and valeric acids. Organic acids and ammonia concentrating in the colon were according to Kiare et al. (2007) 5-10-fold bigger than those in the ileum and their increased concentrations resulted in additional fermentation activity of short-chain organic acids. This indicates higher microbial activity and considerable N-metabolism in the caudal segment of the intestine. The most significant increase in production of organic acids in the colonic segment observed in our study involved acetoacetic, acetic, propionic and butyric acids in the group of suckled piglets compared to replacer-fed piglets, at important concentrations of acetoacetic acid from 14 to 28 days of age (p < 0.01). Significant increase was observed also in production of lactic acid in gnotobiotic piglets compared to the replacer-fed animals throughout the observation period with the highest concentrations reached on days 2 (p < 0.05), 14, 21 and 28 of age (p < 0.01). Decreased pH of the gut content and increased production of lactic and acetic acids affects positively optimisation of digestive processes. Bomba et al. (1998) investigated intestinal metabolism of gnotobiotic piglets and recorded significantly lower pH (p<0.05) in the jejunal content in piglets inoculated with *Lactobacillus plantarum* in the 1st week of life in comparison with germ-free piglets. Zitnan et al. (2001) observed pH in the jejunal and ileal content of conventional piglets of the same age. When comparing the actual acidity in individual segments of the small intestine, pH of the jejunum content of germ-free piglets was higher in the first week of life (7.49) in comparison with pH of conventional piglets (6.23) of the same age. Contrary to that, pH of the jejunal content of gnotobiotic piglets inoculated with *Lactobacillus plantarum* was considerably lower (5.63). Similar low pH was recorded in our study in gnotobiotic piglets of the same age inoculated with *Enterococcus faecium* (6.02). Bomba et al. (1998) conducted two experiments to investigate the influence of short-term and continuous preventive administration of *Lactobacillus casei* subs.casei against *E.coli* on actual acidity, production of organic acids and colonisation of jejunum with *E.coli* O8:K88 in gnotobiotic piglets. After the short-term administration of *L.casei* they recorded lower pH in the jejunal content of experimental piglets (L-E) while pH of the ileal content of these piglets increased significantly (7.63) in comparison with the control (7.03). After continuous administration, the authors recorded lower pH in the experimental group L-E (6.1) in comparison with the control group (6.28). In our experiment we observed a positive influence of *Enterococcus faecium* on intestinal metabolism in replacer-fed piglets in terms of increased production of organic acids (formic acid, acetoacetic, propionic and butyric acid). However, production of lactic acid responsible for decrease in pH was lower in our observations and their concentrations ranged between 6.27 and 20.30 mmol/l in the ileal segment of replacer-fed piglets in comparison with suckled piglets (15.52 to 60.11mmol/l) and failed to induce the corresponding pH reduction. pH in the ileum of non-colostral piglets ranged from 6.9 to 7.6. Although acetic acid reached higher levels in the colon segment, it could become toxic only at low pH of the environment dependent on sufficient concentration of lactic acid in the gut. According to Mufandaedza et al. (2006), decreased active acidity, pH < 5.0, limits even stops growth and multiplication of *E. coli*. Similar conclusions were drawn from our study. Production of organic acids by replacer-fed piglets was low and resulted in their low concentrations which did not decrease pH so effectively as it was observed in gnotobiotic piglets inoculated with *Enterococcus faecium*. Deficit of colostral nutrition in these piglets resulted in worsened health in 8 out of total 26 piglets. The disease was peracute and proceeded with physiological temperature. Even though antibiotics were administered, the piglets died within 8 hrs of appearing of the first symptoms. In the piglets, lymphocytic leukocytosis as well as hypochromic anemia were diagnosed, and *E. coli* K88 was isolated from rectal swabs.

4.3 Intestinal morphology and disaccharidase activity

Due to numerous similarities of the physiology and anatomy of the gastrointestinal tract of man and pigs, the pig model is a very attractive model for human nutritional studies (Miller & Ullrey, 1987). Investigations performed in humans and pigs showed that the portions of total life required to reach chemical maturity for both these species are nearly identical, 4.4% and 4.6, respectively. Even though there are species-specific differences of the placenta and immunological system of pigs and human, the piglets are optimum experimental model for investigations concerning physiology and pathology of the gastrointestinal tract of human newborn (Miller & Ullrey, 1987). The postnatal development of the gastrointestinal (GI) system is a very dynamic process. In the neonatal pig with the mean birth body weight of 1.45kg, the small intestine and pancreas weight contribute to 3.1% and 0.14% of the total body weight, respectively (Zabielski et al., 2008). Within the first four postnatal weeks weight of the piglet is increased >5-fold, with the GI organs growing faster than many other organs of the body (Zabielski et al., 2008). Can we suspect the same changes in human neonates? Presumably yes, but the intensity of the remodelling is not as dramatic. The development in humans is slower, and the growth rate is slower in comparison to pigs. In humans the birth weight is doubled within ca. 170 days. Nevertheless, a number of similarities pig and human in the process of the development can be seen. In the study of Len et al. (2009), similar to our investigations of conventional piglets, the absolute weight of visceral organs and GI tract increased with piglet age. However, when expressed as g/kg empty body weight, the weight of visceral organs decreased with age (Len et al., 2009), which is in agreement with Pluske et al. (2002), who found that the relative weight of the visceral organs of piglets had a tendency to decrease between 14 and 28 days of age. In our study we observed a gradual decrease in the weight of small and large intestine between days 2 and 21 of age in suckled piglets while in gnotobiotic piglets the relative weight of intestines increased gradually throughout the period of observation. In germ-free and monoassociated pigs (Shirkey et al., 2006), the relative small intestine length was reduced compared with conventional pigs. The mechanisms affecting intestinal length are unknown, however, it can be hypothesized that increased small intestine length in conventionalized pigs is a compensatory response to the decreased absorptive capacity associated with decreased surface area (decreased villi length) and/or to direct competition with the microbiota for dietary nutrients. Shirkey et al. (2006) observed that in the proximal region of the small intestine, the relative weights for segments from conventional pigs tended to be higher than those from germ-free and monoassociated pigs. This is consistent with our study, as well as with the previous reports indicating that compared with germ-free animals, conventionally reared animals experience intestinal "thickening" associated primarily with increased *lamina propria* cellularity (Miniats & Valli, 1973) as well as thickening of the submucosa and muscular layers (Furuse & Okumura, 1994). On the contrary, higher relative weight of the distal part of the intestine was reported in germ-free piglets (Shirkey et al., 2006). Similar results were obtained in our study which showed higher relative weight of the large intestine in gnotobiotic piglets inoculated with *Enterococcus faecium* in comparison with conventional piglets starting from the second week of age up to the weaning (day 28 of age). In addition to an intensive growth of the GI system, during the first month of life an intense rebuilding of the tissues takes place. The most intensive processes are observed in the epithelium of the small intestine (Zabielski et al., 2008). The weight of small intestinal mucosa doubles during the first postnatal day due to a complex of processes involving, accumulation of colostrum proteins in the enterocytes as a result of an open „gut barrier", increase of local blood flow concurrently with a reduction in basal vascular resistance (Nankervis et al., 2001), and finally changes in epithelial cell turnover, namely, increased mitosis accompanied by the inhibition of apoptosis which result in a 2-fold increase in the mitosis/apoptosis ratio within the first 2 postnatal days (Zabielski et al., 2008). The regulation of small intestine development (especially the tissue growth) is in a positive feed-back to colostrum and milk intake (Marion et al., 2003). Currently none artificial feeding system (milk, artificial milk formula, nor feeding with any other compositions like lactose, glucose solutions) could reproduce the developmental characteristics obtained with maternal colostrum feeding (Zabielski et al., 2008). Furthermore, high specificity of colostrum, especially concerning the composition of hormones and bioactive compounds prevents utilization of colostrum of other species as the replacement. In the study of Meslin et al. (1973), the overall mass of the small intestine in germ-free species was decreased, and its surface area was smaller, whereas the villi of the small intestine were unusually uniform in shape and appear slender, with crypts, which were shorter and less populated than in the respective conventional control animals. Our study showed that the jejunal part of the intestinal tract in gnotobiotic pigs was characterized up to 14 days of life by relatively short crypts, extremely long villi and narrow *lamina propria* containing few cells. Reduced crypt depth and increased villus length agree with the previous observations in germ-free pigs (Shirkey et al., 2006; Shurson et al., 1990). In the present study in gnotobiotic piglets villi were the longest in the jejunum and shortest in the duodenum and ileum, whereas crypt depth was shortest in the jejunum and deepest in the duodenum throughout the observation period. These morphological characteristics suggested that the rates of enterocyte proliferation and exfoliation were the highest in the proximal small intestine, as indicated by deep crypts and shorter villi, respectively, with rates decreasing distally along the small intestine (Hampson & Kidder, 1986). In agreement with our morphological findings, Miniats & Valli (1973) reported longer jejunal villi in germ-free pigs but did not measure villi in other regions. Shurson et al. (1990) reported that germ-free pigs had longer ileal and duodenal villi but shorter jejunal villi compared to their conventional counterparts. Similar results were obtained also in our study as the villi in the duodenum and ileum of gnotobiotic piglets were higher in comparison with conventional piglets throughout the experiment. The difference was significant at 3 hours after birth, on days 2 and 7 of age (p < 0.01) and day 14 of age (p < 0.05) in the duodenum and on days 14 and 21 in the ileum (p < 0.05). Shirkey et al. (2006) suggested that regional variation in morphology, especially in the proximal small intestine, is not entirely dependent on microbial colonization but is also influenced by such non-microbial factors as bile salts, pancreatic secretions, and compounds of dietary origin which would be expected to be in higher concentration and have more contact with mucosal surface in the duodenum.

The gastrointestinal tract goes through substantial structural and functional changes in the early postnatal period (Walthall et al., 2005). As the piglets grow, functional changes occur in the expression and kinetics (Fan et al., 2002) of brush border digestive enzymes. Each brush border enzyme shows a specific developmental pattern as the animal ages, which have been associated with the maturation of enterocytes (Walthall et al., 2005). Specifically, changing disaccharidasae activities have been used as an indicator of intestinal maturation. Measurable lactase levels were detected in bush border homogenates and membrane vesicles of the small intestine in the 7th week of pregnancy (Buddington & Malo, 1996). For comparison, activity of lactase in human foetuses was confirmed only later and only in the 34th week of gravidity (Menard & Basque, 2001). Aumaitre & Corring (1978) measured lactase in small intestine homogenates from pig foetuses at 105th day of gravidity and observed that the total activity of lactase in the intestine amounted to only 10% of the activity determined at birth. It was stated that specific activities of lactase in homogenates or membrane vesicles of the small intestine brush border were high at birth and stayed at this level during the first 7-10 days of postnatal life (Torp et al., 1993). In suckling pigs, lactase activity was observed to undergo an initial marked decrease sometime during the second to fifth week of age which was followed by a period when it remained relatively constant or continued to decrease gradually up to 8 weeks of age (Kelly et al., 1991). In terms of enzyme distribution throughout the intestine, neonatal and 1-day old piglets show the highest specific lactase activity in the proximal part of the small intestine and the lowest in the distal part, but at the age of 6-10 days its distribution throughout the intestine was more regular (Buddington & Malo, 1996). The intestinal microbiota has been shown to affect brush border enzyme expression, as the intestine of a germ-free mouse has a different pattern of brush border enzymes than a conventional mouse (Kozakova et al., 2001). The mechanism by which bacteria induce changes in brush border enzyme activities or which bacteria are responsible has not been elucidated. According to (Willing & Kessel, 2009), conventionalization in pigs reduced enterocyte brush border enzyme activity compared with germ-free without a concomitant reduction in gene expression in the case of lactase phlorizin hydrolase. Because of the reduced villus height and increased enterocyte replacement rate observed in conventional as compared with germ-free animals (Furuse & Okumura, 1994), it has been postulated that the higher disaccharidase activity in the small intestine of germ-free as compared with conventional rats is because of an increased number of mature enterocytes (Willing & Kessel, 2009). These reports were confirmed by Reddy & Wostmann (1966) who observed that disaccharidase activity was higer in the small intestine of the germ-free as compared with conventional rats. However, in our study, contrary to previous studies, specific activities of lactase along the entire intestinal tract were higher in conventional piglets throughout the experiment. Kozakova et al. (2001) concluded that individual bacteria can stimulate a similar response, as monoassociation of gnotobiotic mice with *Bifidobacteria bifidum* induces a shift in enzyme activity to a pattern similar to that of a conventional mouse. Aumaitre & Corring (1978) reported that the intestinal tract of foetal (105th day of gravidity) and newborn piglets contained maltase but saccharase was present in one week old piglets. Similar observations for saccharase were presented by Buddington & Malo (1996). However, the studies by James et al. (1987) and Sangild et al. (1991) revealed low activities of saccharase and maltase in the small intestine of newborn piglets. Starting from 1 week of age specific activities of maltase and saccharase abruptly increased reaching maximum at the age of 10 - 16 days and sustained values at the age of approximately 3 weeks (James et al., 1987; Sangild et al., 1991). Similar tendencies of specific activity of maltase and saccharase were observed also in our study. When comparing the postnatal development of specific activities of enzymes maltase and saccharase in gnotobiotic and conventional piglets we observed a similar trend but higher activities of both enzymes in all segments of digestive tract of conventional piglets throughout the observation period. In 6 - 7 days old piglets, the distribution of activities of saccharase and maltase was similar along the small intestine but the activities of both enzymes were higher in the proximal to medial parts of the jejunum compared to distal part of the small intestine (Aumaitre & Corring, 1978; Buddington & Malo, 1996). In our study, saccharase activity distribution throughout the small intestine of gnotobiotic and conventional piglets was higher in the jejunum during the entire period of observation. Distribution of maltase along the small intestine changed depending on age, from predominant concentration of the activity in the proximal half of the small intestine at the age of 1-2 weeks (Aumaitre & Corring, 1978) through uniform distribution along the small intestine at the age of 2-3 weeks (Kelly et al., 1991) up to higher activity in the range of 10-15% along 80-90% of the intestine length at the age of 5 - 8 weeks (Hampson & Kidder, 1986). Similar distribution of maltase along the small intestine was observed also in our study in both gnotobiotic and conventional piglets. Transition from milk nutrition to definitive nutrition in children is accompanied with induction of maltase and decreasing activity of lactase as an adaptation of GIT to changes in nutrition with age (Menard & Basque, 2001). Other factors besides age which affect development of disaccharidases activities in the small intestine include: feed offered to piglets in the period of suckling (Hampson & Kidder, 1986), weaning to dry or liquid feed, growth factors, for example epidermal growth factor (James et al., 1987) and hormones, for example insulin (Shulman, 1990), corticosteroids (Kreikemeier et al., 1990), ACTH - adrenocorticotropin (Sangild et al.,1991). Willing & Kessel (2009) concluded that enterocyte upregulation of brush border enzyme expression occurs as either a direct response to microbial colonization or as a feedback mechanisms in response to reduced enzyme activity through microbial degradation. This mechanism may play a role in ensuring effective competition of the host with the intestinal microbiota for available nutrients.

4.4 Effect of weaning on development of the small intestine of conventionally and gnotobiotic bred piglets

Another critical phase in the gastrointestinal tract development of young animals is the weaning period. The weaning of piglets usually takes place between 3 and 4 week of life, when the majority of nutrients are ingested with milk. Weaning for farm animals occurs in an early age, when the gastrointestinal system motility, digestive and absorptive functions are not yet matured and prepared for food other than milk. In a wild boar, domestic pig ancestor, the offspring is weaned in much older age and change of the diet is gradual, therefore weaning disorders are nearly nonexistent. In intensive livestock production shorter suckling period benefits in increased number of piglets born per year, but at the negative side is an increased number of weaning disorders (Zabielski et al., 2008). Weaning is associated with mixing of piglets from different litters and sometimes also with the transport of animals from the place of birth to specialized nursery units. This results in profound social and environmental stress which is a caused also by the changes in the diet. The gastrointestinal tract has to adapt to the new type of feed, which leads to changes in myenteron motility, enzymes secretion and activity, and the composition of bacterial flora (Barszcz & Skomial, 2011). According to Lalles et al. (2007) weaning is a critical phase for piglets, it is associated with a variable period of anorexia during the first days after weaning, the deterioration of the digestive function and accumulation of undigested feed as a result of inefficient digestion. During this period, piglets are more susceptible to suffer from post-weaning diarrhoea with the proliferation and attachment to the intestinal mucosa of β-haemolytic strains of *E. coli* (Fairbrother et al., 2005). Nabuurs (1998) and Pluske et al. (1997) stated that predisposition to infections with eneterotoxigenic bacteria depends on a number of factors. Miller et al. (1986) concluded that the problems induced by weaning were caused rather by the changes in the structure of the intestines and specific loss of digestive enzymes than by any great changes in absorption function despite the fact that the data of Nabuurs et al. (1998) were contradictory. Nabuurs (1998) concluded that piglets suffering from post-weaning diarrhoea excreted enterotoxigenic *E. coli* strains and *rotavirus,* and that these piglets developed a hyperregenerative villus atrophy, and subsequently a severe loss of net absorption of fluid and electrolytes in the small intestine. A simulated halving of the absorption in the large intestine of weaned piglets aggravates the adverse effects of an enterotoxigenic *E. coli* in the small intestine (Nabuurs, 1998). Franklin et al. (2002) recorded no post-weaning increase in *E.coli* in pigs weaned at 17 days of age, in agreement with the studies of Etheridge et al. (1984) and Mathew et al. (1998), but in contrast with others (Mathew et al., 1996) who reported increase in *E.coli* populations after weaning. We have observed changes during the first week post-weaning in the jejunal part of the digestive tract of colostral piglets that pointed to a decrease in all observed groups of bacteria with the highest decrease by 1-1.8 log for enterococci, *E. coli* and *Enterobacteriaceae.* Mathew et al. (1998) postulated the absence of an *E.coli* increase may be due to weaning pigs into a highly sanitized, environmentally controlled room with limited contact among pigs. Franklin et al. (2002) also observed *E.coli* populations to be lower in pigs remaining on the sow, as have other investigators (Etheridge et al., 1984; Mathew et al., 1996). Jensen (1998) reported that lactobacilli are inversely proportionate to coliform bacteria during 1 week post-weaning. This is also confirmed by the results of Risley et al. (1992), but however, has not been confirmed in our experiments. In the study by Franklin et al. (2002) faecal populations of lactobacilli and *E.coli* followed patterns typical of those observed in the more anterior portions of the gastrointestinal tract. However, faecal bifidobacteria populations increased post-weaning, possibly due to the decrease in lactobacilli and *E.coli* in the posterior gastrointestinal tract. The loss of direct competition may benefit other bacterial populations, including bifidobacteria. The infant's microbiota initially shows low diversity and instability, but evolves into a more stable adult-type microbiota over the first 24 months of life (Zoetendal et al., 1998). *Bifidobacterium* populations are dominant in the first months of life, especially in breast-fed infants due to the bifinogenic effect of breast milk, while a more diverse microbiota is found in formula-fed infants, weaning children and adults (Gueimonde et al., 2006). In adults and weaned children the major constituents of the colonic microbiota are *Bacteroides,* followed by several genera belonging to the division *Firmicutes,* such as *Eubacterium, Ruminococcus* and *Clostridium,* and the genus *Bifidobacterium.* By contrast, in infants the genus *Bifidobacterium* is predominant and also a few genera from the family *Enterobacteriaceae,* as a *Escherichia, Raoultella,* and *Klebsiella* (Kurokawa et al., 2007). It is well know that weaning has a dramatic negative impact on the intestinal mucosal morphology of piglets. Significant post-weaning reduction in villus height has been observed by study (Berkeveld et al., 2007). In study of Hedemann et al. (2003) villus height decreased to a minimum during the first 3 days post-weaning and this is in accordance with the other studies showing that villous height is minimal 2-5 days post-weaning (Hampson & Kidder, 1986; Kelly et al., 1991). In the jejunum and ileum of conventional piglets, investigated in our study, we observed a post-weaning decrease in the height of villi significant on day 35 of age in the jejunum (p < 0.01). Elongation of the crypts post-weaning has been observed in several studies (Hampson & Kidder, 1986; Hedemann et al., 2003) and was confirmed in the present experiment. In our study, in the first week after weaning, conventional piglets showed significant deepening of crypts in duodenal (p < 0.001), jejunal (p < 0.01) and ileal (p < 0.05) segments. Villous atrophy may result both from increased rate of cell loss leading to higher rate of mitosis in crypts and their hyperplasia and from slower rate of cell renewal resulting from the reduction of cell division, i.e. in case of underfeeding. During the time of weaning villous shape also undergoes modifications. The marked and abrupt morphological response to weaning in the small intestine, characterized by transformation from a dense finger-like villi population to a smooth, compact, tongue-shaped luminal villi was observed in previous study (Skrzypek et al., 2005) and in the present study. The morphological changes observed in the small intestine around weaning are closely related to changes in the mucosal enzyme activity observed at the same time. When shortening of the villi is associated with cell loss, loss of mature enterocytes where digestive enzymes are located also occurs. The disaccharidases have been the most commonly investigated mucosal enzymes in relation to weaning of piglets (Kelly et al., 1991). Morphological changes in the small intestine of piglets after weaning are accompanied by smaller activity of brush border enzymes, lactase and sucrase (Pacha, 2000). In our study we registered that of lactase activity of gnotobiotic piglets decreased in the weeks 4 (p < 0.001) and 5 (p < 0.001) to levels similar to those noticed at birth. Similarly, we recorded a post-weaning decrease in lactase specific activity also in conventional piglets. The results of these studies have been used to interpret the digestive and absorptive capacity of the small intestine as well as the maturity of the enterocytes.

5. Conclusion

Gnotobiotic animals are a very useful model in studying the physiology of the digestive tract. The gnotobiotic model allowed us to carry out systematic examination of the effect of a defined microbial population on postnatal intestinal development. We characterized regional variations in morphological and functional responses of the small intestine. We also identified that morphological and functional responses were affected differently by respective bacterial species, supporting the assumption that postnatal bacterial colonization patterns play an important role in neonatal intestinal development. Very good application of gnotobiotic animals is anticipated in the field of study of mutual interaction of natural microflora and pathogens in the digestive tract, mechanisms of probiotic effects of micro-organisms. We can conclude that the development of the intestinal mucosa membrane is in direct junction to breeding conditions. In connection with postnatal differentiation and the development of the small intestine in piglets, currently there is increasingly high interest in the explanation of the important role that can be played by colostrum and by milk containing growth factors, hormones and other bio-active compounds. It is likely that removal of milk will have a profound influence upon the processes regulating the growth of cells in the small intestine, their differentiation and function.

6. Acknowledgments

This study was supported by the project SK0021, co-financed through the EEA financial mechanism, the Norwegian financial mechanism and the state budget of the Slovak

Republic and by the project from the Research and Development Support Agency APVV-20-062505.

7. References

Aumaitre, A. & Corring, T. (1978). Development of digestive enzymes in the piglet from birth to 8 weeks. II. Intestine and intestinal disaccharidases. *Nutrition and Metabolism*, Vol.22, No.4, (July-August 1978), pp.244-255, ISSN 0029-6678

Barszcz, M. & Skomial, J. (2011). The development of the small intestine of piglets-chosen aspects. *Journal of Animal and Feed Sciences*, Vol.20, No.1, (January 2011), pp.3-15, ISSN 1230-1388

Beerens, H. (1990). An elective and selective isolation medium for *Bifidobacterium spp. Letters in Applied Microbiology*, Vol.11, No.3, (September 1990), pp. 155-157, ISSN 1472-765X

Berkeveld, M.; Langendijk, P.; van Beers-Schreurs, H.M.G.; Koets, A.P.; Taverne, M.A.M.; Verheijden, J.H.M. (2007). Intermittent suckling during an extended lactation period: Effects on piglet behavior. *Journal of Animal Science*, Vol.85, No.12, (December 2007), pp.3415-3424, ISSN 0021-8812

Bomba, A.; Gancarcikova, S.; Nemcova, R.; Herich, R.; Kastel, R.; Depta, A.; Demeterova, M.; Ledecky, V.; Zitnan, R. (1998). The effect of lactic acid bacteria on intestinal metabolism and metabolic profile of gnotobiotic pigs. *Deutsche Tierarztliche Wochenschrift*, Vol.105, No.10, (October 1998), pp. 384-389, ISSN 0341-6593

Bomba, A.; Nemcova, R.; Gancarcikova, S.; Herich, R.; Guba, P.; Mudronova, D. (2002). Improvement of the probiotic effect of microorganisms by their combination with maltodextrins, fructo-oligosacharides and polyunsaturated acids. *British Journal of Nutrition*, Vol.88, No.1, (September 2002), pp. 95-99, ISSN 0007-1145

Buddington, R. K. & Malo, CH. (1996). Intestinal brush-border membrane enzyme activities and transport functions during prenatal development of pigs. *Journal of Pediatric Gastroenterology and Nutrition*, Vol.23, No.1, (July 1996), pp.51-64, ISSN 0277-2116

Bradford, M.M. (1976). A rapid and sensitive method for the quantitation of microgram quantities of protein utilizing the principle of protein-dye binding. *Analytical Biochemistry*, Vol.72, No.7, (May 1976), pp. 248-254, ISSN 003-2697

Devriese, L.A.; Hommez, J.; Wijfels, R.; Haesebrouck, F. (1991). Composition of the enterococcal and streptococcal intestinal flora of poultry. *Journal of Applied Bacteriology*, Vol.71, No.1, (July 1991), pp. 46-50, ISSN 0021-8847

Etheridge, R.D.; Seerley, R.W. & Wyatt, R.D. (1984). The effect of diet on performance, digestibility, blood composition and intestinal microflora of weaned pigs. *Journal of Animal Science*, Vol.58, No.6, (June 1984), pp.1396-1402, ISSN 0021-8812

Fairbrother, J.M.; Nadeau, E. & Gyles, C.I. (2005). *Escherichia coli* in postweaning diarrhea in pigs: an update on bacterial types, pathogenesis, and prevention strategies. *Animal Health Research Reviews*, Vol.6, No.1, (June 2005), pp.17-39, ISSN 1466-2523

Fallani, M.; Young, D.; Scott, J.; Norin, E.; Amarri, S.; Adam, R.; Aguilera, M.; Khanna, S.; Gil, A.; Edwards, C.A.; Dore, J. (2010). Intestinal microbiota of 6-week-old infants across Europe: geographic influence beyond delivery mode, breast-feeding, and antibiotics. *Journal of Pediatric Gastroenterology and Nutrition*, Vol.51, No.1, (July 2010), pp.77-84, ISSN 0277-2116

Franklin, M.A.; Mathew, A.G.; Vickers, J.R.; Clift, R.A. (2002). Characterization of microbial populations and volatile fatty acid concentrations in the jejunum, ileum and cecum, of pigs weaned at 17 vs. 24 days of age. *Journal of Animal Science*, Vol.80, No.11, (November 2002), pp. 2904-2910, ISSN 0021-8812

Furuse, M. & Okumura, J. (1994). Nutritional and physiological characteristics in germ-free chickens. *Comparative Biochemistry and Physiology A - Physiology*, Vol.109, No.3, (November 1994), pp. 547-556, ISSN 1096-4940

Godlewski, M.M.; Slupecka, M.; Wolinski, J.; Skrzypek, T.; Skrzypek, H.; Motyl, T.; Zabielski, R. (2005). Into the unknown - the death pathways in the neonatal gut epithelium. *Journal of Physiology and Pharmacology*, Vol.56, No.3, (June 2005), pp. 7-24, ISSN 0867-5910

Guarner, F. & Malagelada, J.R. (2003). Gut flora in health and disease. *Lancet*, Vol.361, No.9356, (February 2003), pp. 512-519, ISSN 0140-6736

Gueimonde, M.; Salminen, S. & Isolauri, E. (2006). Presence of specific antibiotic (tet) resistance genes in infant faecal microbiota. *FEMS Immunology and Medical Microbiology*, Vol.48, No.1, (October 2006), pp.21-25, ISSN 0928-8244

Guilloteau, P.; Biernat, M.; Wolinski, J.; Zabielski, R. (2002). Gut regulatory peptides and hormones of the small intestine, In: *Biology of the Intestine in Growing Animals*, R. Zabielski; P.C. Gregory & B. Westrom, (Eds.), 325-362, Elsevier, ISBN 978-044-4509-28-4, Amsterdam, The Netherlands

Hampson, D.J. & Kidder, D.E. (1986). Alteration in piglet small intestinal structure at weaning. *Research in Veterinary Science*, Vol.40, (1986), pp.32-40, ISSN 0034-5288

Hedemann, M.S.; Hojsgaard, S. & Jensen, J.J. (2003). Small intestinal morphology and activity of intestinal peptidases in piglets aroun weaning. *Journal of Animal Physiology and Animal Nutrition*, Vol.87, No.1-2, (February 2003), pp.32-41, ISSN 0931-2439

Hopkins, M.J.; Macfarlane, G.T.; Furrie, E.; Fite, A.; Macfarlane, S. (2005). Characterisation of intestinal bacteria in infant stools using real-time PCR and northern hybridisation analyses. *FEMS Microbiology Ecology*, Vol.54, No.1, (September 2005), pp. 77-85, ISSN 1574-6941

Inoue, R.; Tsukahara, T.; Nakanishi, N.; Ushida, K. (2005). Development of the intestinal microbiota in the piglet. *Journal of General and Applied Microbiology*, Vol.51, No.1, (August 2005), pp. 257-265, ISSN 0022-1260

James, P.S.; Smith, M.W.; Tivey, D.R. & Wilson, T.J.G. (1987). Epidermal growth factor selectively increases maltase and sucrase activities in neonatal piglet intestine. *Journal of Physiology*, Vol.393, (December 1987), pp.583-594, ISSN 0022-3751

Jensen, B.B. (1998). The impact of feed additives on the microbial ecology of the gut in young pigs. *Journal of Animal and Feed Sciences*, Vol.7, No.1, (1998), pp. 45-64, ISSN 1230-1388

Kelly. D.; Smyth, J.A. & McCracken, K.J. (1991). Digestive development in the earlyweaned pig. I. Effect of continuous nutrient supply on the development of the digestive tract and on changes in digestive enzyme activity during the first week post-weaning. *British Journal of Nutrition*, Vol.65, No.2, (March 1991), pp. 169-180, ISSN 0007-1145

Kiarie, E.; Nyachoti, C.M.; Slominski, B.A.; Blank, G. (2007). Growth performance, gastrointestinal microbial activity and nutrient digestibility in early-weaned pigs fed diets containing flaxseed and carbohydrase enzyme. *Journal of Animal Science*, Vol.85, No.11, (November 2007), pp. 2982-2993, ISSN 0021-8812

Kozakova, H.; Rehakova, Z. & Kolinska, J. (2001). *Bifidobacterium bifidum* monoassociation of gnotobiotic mice: effect on enterocyte brush-border enzymes. *Folia Microbiologica (Praha)*, Vol.46, No.6, (November-December 2001), pp.573-576, ISSN 0015-5632

Kreikemeier, K.K.; Harmon, D.L. & Nelssen, J.L. (1990). Influence of hydrocortisone acetate on pancreas and mucosal weight, amylase and disaccharidase activities in 14-day-old pigs. *Comparative Biochemistry and Physiology*, Vol.97, No.1, (January 1990), pp.45-50, ISSN 0300-9629

Kurokawa, K.; Itoh, T.; Kuwahara, T.; Oshima, K.; Toh, H.; Toyoda, A.; Takami, H.; Morita, H.; Sharma, V.K.; Srivastava, T.P.; Taylo, T.D.; Noguchi, H.; Mori, H.; Ogura, Y.; Ehrlich, D.; Itoh, K.; Takag, T.; Sakaki, Y.; Hayashi, T.; Hattori, M. (2007). Comparative metagenomics revealed commonly enriched gene sets in human gut microbiomes. *DNA Research*, Vol.14, No.4, (October 2007), pp. 169-181, ISSN 1340-2838

Lalles, J.P.; Bosi, P.; Smidt, H.; Stokes, C.R. (2007). Weaning-a challenge to gut physiologists. *Livestock Science*, Vol.108, No.1-3, (May 2007), pp.82-93, ISSN 1871-1413

Len, N.T.; Hong, T.T.T.; Ogle, B.; Lindberg, J.E. (2009). Comparison of total tract digestibility, development of visceral organs and digestive tract of Mong cai and Yorkshire × Landrace piglets fed diets with different fibre sources. *Journal of Animal Physiology and Animal Nutrition*, Vol.93, No.2, (April 2009), pp.181-191, ISSN 0931-2439

Marinho, M.C.; Lordelo, M.M.; Cunha, L.F.; Freire, J.P.B. (2007). Microbial activity in the gut of piglets: I. Effect of prebiotic and probiotic supplementation. *Livestock Science*, Vol. 108, No.1, (May 2007), pp. 236-9, ISSN 1871-1413

Marion, J.; Rome,V.; Savary, G.; Thomas, F.; Le Dividich, J.; Le Huerou-Luron, I. (2003). Weaning and feed intake alter pancreatic enzyme activities and coresponding mRNA levels in 7-d-old piglets. *Journal of Nutrition*, Vol.133, (February 2003), pp. 362-368, ISSN 0022-3166

Mathew, A.G.; Franklin, M.A.; Upchurch, W.G.; Chattin, S.E. (1996). Effect of weaning on ileal short-chain fatty acid concentrations in pigs. *Nutrition Research*, Vol.16, No.10, (October 1996), pp.1689-1698, ISSN 0271-5317

Mathew, A.G.; Chattin, S.E.; Robbins, C.M.; Golden, D.A. (1998). Effects of a direct-fed yeast culture on enteric microbial populations, fermentations acids, and performance of weanling pigs. *Journal of Animal Science*, Vol.76, No.8, (August 1998), pp. 2138-2145, ISSN 0021-8812

Menard, D. & Basque, J.R. (2001). Gastric digestive function, In: *Nestle´ Nutrition Workshop Series. Gastrointestinal Functions*, E.E. Delvin & M.J. Lentze, (Eds.), 147-164, Lippincott Williams & Wilkins, ISBN 0-7817-3208-5, Philadelphia, USA

Meslin, J.C.; Sacquet, E.; Guenet, J.L. (1973). Action of bacterial flora on the morphology and surface mucus of the small intestine of the rat. *Annales de Biologie Animale Biochimie Biophysique*, Vol.13, No.2, (April-June 1973), pp. 334-335, ISSN 0003-388X

Miller, B.G.; James, P.S.; Smith, M.W.; Bourne, F.J. (1986). Effect of weaning on the capacity of pig intestinal villi to digest and absorb nutrients. *Journal of Agricultural Science*, Vol.107, No.3, (April 1986), pp.579-589, ISSN 0021-8596

Miller E.R. & Ullrey, D.E.(1987). The pig as a model for human nutrition. *Annual Review of Nutrition*, Vol.7, (1987), pp. 361-382, ISSN 0199-9885

Miniats, O.P. & Valli, V.E. (1973). The gastrointestinal tract of gnotobiotic pigs, In: *Germfree Research: Biological Effects of Gnotobiotic Environments*, J.B. Henegan, (Ed.), 575-588, Academic Press, ISBN 978-012-3406-50-7, New York, USA

Mir, P.S.; Bailey, D.R.C.; Mir, Z.; Morgan Jones, S.D.; Douwes, H.; Mc Allister, T.A.; Weselake, R.J.; Lozeman, F.J. (1997). Activity of intestinal mucosal membrane carbohydrases in cattle of different breeds. *Canadian Journal of Animal Science*, Vol.77, No.3, (May 1997), pp. 441-444, ISSN 0008-3984

Mufandaedza, J.; Viljoen, B.C.; Feresu, S.B.; Gadaga, T.H. (2006). Antimicrobial properties of lactic acid bacteria and yeast-LAB cultures isolated from traditional fermented milk against pathogenic *Escherichia coli* and *Salmonella enteritidis* strains. *International Journal of Food Microbiology*,Vol.108,No.1, (April 2006), pp.147-152, ISSN 0168-1705

Nabuurs, M.J.A. (1998). Weaning piglets as a model for studying pathophysiology of diarrhoea. *The Veterinary Quarterly*, Vol.20, No.3, (1998), pp.42-45, ISSN 0165-2176

Nankervis, C.A.; Reber, K.M. & Nowicki, P.T. (2001). Age-dependent changes in the postnatal intestinal microcirculation. *Microcirculation*, Vol.8, No.6, (December 2001), pp. 377-387, ISSN 1073-9688

Pacha, J. (2000). Development of intestinal transport function in mammals. *Physiological Reviews*, Vol.80, No.4, (October 2000), pp.1633-1667, ISSN 0031-9333

Penders, J.; Thijs, C.; van de Brandt, P.A.; Kummeling, I.; Snijders, B.; Stelma, F.; Adams, H.; van Ree, R.; Stobberingh, E.E. (2007). Gut microflora composition and development of atopic manifestations in infancy: the KOALA birth cohort study. *Gut*, Vol.56, No.5, (May 2007), pp. 661-667, ISSN 0017-5749

Piva, A.; Prandini, A.; Fiorentini, L.; Morlacchini, M.; Galvano, F.; Luchansky, J.B. (2002). Tributyrin and lactitol synergistically enhanced the trophic status of the intestinal mucosa and reduced histamine levels in the gut of nursery pigs. *Journal of Animal Science*, Vol.80, No.3, (March 2002), pp. 670-680, ISSN 0021-8812

Pluske, J.R.; Hampson, D.J. & Williams, I.H. (1997). Factors influencing the structure and function of the small intestine in the weaned pig. *Livestock Production Science*, Vol.51, No.1-3, (November 1997), pp. 215-236, ISSN 0301-6226

Pluske, J.R.; Pethick, D.W.; Hopwood, D.E. & Hampson, D.J. (2002). Nutritional influences on some major enteric bacterial diseases of pigs. *Nutrition Research Reviews*, Vol.15, No.2, (December 2002), pp. 333-371, ISSN 0954-4224

Reddy, B.S. & Wostmann, B.S. (1966). Intestinal disaccharidase activities in the growing germfree and conventional rats. *Archives of Biochemistry and Biophysics*, Vol.113, No.3, (March 1966), pp.609-616, ISSN 0003-9861

Risley, C.R.; Kornegay, E.T.; Lindemann, H.D.; Wood, C.M.; Eigel, W.N. (1992). Effect of feeding organic acids on selected intestinal content measurements at varying times postweaning in pigs. *Journal of Animal Science*, Vol.70, No.1, (January 1992), pp.196-206, ISSN 0021-8812

Sangild, P.T.; Cranwell, P.D.; Sorensen, H.; Mortensen, K.; Noren, O.; Wetteberg, L. & Sjostrom, H. (1991). Development of intestinal disaccharidases, intestinal peptidases and pancreatic proteases in sucking pigs. The effects of age and ACTH treatment, In: *Digestive Physiology in Pigs*, M.W.A. Verstegen; J. Huisman & L.A. den Hartog, (Eds.), 73-78, Pudoc, ISBN 978-902-2010-40-2, Wageningen, The Netherlands

Scharek, L.; Guth, J.; Reiter, K.; Weyrauch, K.D.; Tara, D.; Schwerk, P.; Schierack, P.; Schmidt, M.F.; Wieler, L.H.; Tedin, K. (2005). Influence of a probiotic *Enterococcus faecium* strain on development of the immune system of sows and piglets. *Veterinary Immunology and Immunopathology*, Vol.105, No.1-5, (May 2005), pp. 151-161, ISSN 0165-2427

Shirkey, T.W.; Siggers, R.H.; Goldade, B.G.; Marshall, J.K.; Drew, M.D.; Laarveld, B.; Van Kessel, A.G. (2006). Effects of commensal bacteria on intestinal morphology and expression of proinflammatory cytokines in the gnotobiotic pig. *Experimental Biology and Medicine*, Vol.231, No.8, (September 2006), pp.1333-1345, ISSN 1535-3702

Shulman, R.J. (1990). Oral insulin increases small intestinal mass and disaccharidase activity in the newborn miniature pig. *Pediatric Research*, Vol.28, No.2, (August 1990), pp.171-175, ISSN 0031-3998

Shurson, G.C.; Ku, P.K.; Waxler, G.L.; Yokoyama, M.T.; Miller, E.R. (1990). Physiological relationships between microbiological status and dietary copper levels in the pig. *Journal of Animal Science*, Vol.68, No.4, (April 1990), pp.1061-1071, ISSN 0021-8812

Siggers, R.H.; Thymann, T.; Siggers, J.L.; Schmidt, M.; Sangild, P.T. (2007). Bacterial colonization affects early organ and gastrointestinal growth in the neonate. *Livestock Science*, Vol.109, No.1-2, (May 2007), pp. 14-18, ISSN 1871-1413

Skrzypek, T.; Valverde Piedra, J.L.; Skrzypek, H.; Wolinski, J.; Kazimierczak, W.; Szymanczyk, S.; Pawlowska, M.; Zabielski, R. (2005). Light and scanning electron microscopy evaluation of the postnatal small intestinall mucosa development in pigs. *Journal of Physiology and Pharmacology*, Vol.56, No.3, (June 2005), pp.71-87, ISSN 0867-5910

Swords, W.E.; Wu, C.C.; Champlin, F.R.; Buddington, R.K. (1993). Postnatal changes in selected bacterial groups of the pig colonic microflora. *Biology of the Neonate*, Vol.63, No.3, (March 1993), pp. 191-200, ISSN 0006-3126

Torp, N.; Rossi, M.; Troelsen, J.T.; Olsen, J. & Danielsen, E.M. (1993). Lactase - phlorizin hydrolase and aminopeptidase N are differentially regulated in the small intestine of the pig. *Biochemical Journal*, Vol.295, No.1, (October 1993), pp.177-182, ISSN 0264-6021

Trahair, J.F. & Sanglid, P.T. (2002). Studying the development of the small intestine: Philosophical and anatomical perspectives, In: *Biology of the Intestine in Growing Animals*, R. Zabielski; P.C. Gregory & B. Westrom, (Eds.), 1-54, Elsevier, ISBN 978-044-4509-28-4, Amsterdam, The Netherlands

Walthall, K.; Cappon, G.D.; Hurt, M.E.; Zoetis, T. (2005). Postnatal development of the gastrointestinal system: a species comparison. *Birth Defects Research Part B, Developmental and Reproductive Toxicology*, Vol.74, No.2, (April 2005), pp.132-156, ISSN 1542-9733

Widdowson, E.M. & Crabb, D.E. (1976). Changes in the organs of pigs in response to feeding for the first 24 h after birth. *Biology of the Neonate*, Vol.28, No.5-6, (1976), pp.261-271, ISSN 1661-7800

Willing, B.P. & Van Kessel, A.G. (2009). Intestinal microbiota differentially affect brush border enzyme activity and gene expression in the neonatal gnotobiotic pig. *Journal of Animal Physiology and Animal Nutrition*, Vol.93, No.5, (October 2009), pp.586-595, ISSN 0931-2439

Xu, R.J. (1996). Development of the Newborn GI tract and its relation to colostrum/milk intake. A rewiev. *Reproduction, Fertility and Development*, Vol.8, No.1, (1996), pp. 35-48, ISSN 1031-3613

Zabielski, R.; Godlewski, M.M. & Guilloteau, P. (2008). Control of development of gastrointestinal system in neonates. *Journal of Physiology and Pharmacology*, Vol.59, No.1, (July 2008), pp. 35-54, ISSN 0867-5910

Zitnan, R.; Gancarcikova, S.; Nemcova, R.; Sommer, A.; Bomba, A.(2001). Some aspects of the morphological and functional development of the intestinal tract in piglets during milk feeding and weaning, *Proceedings of the Society of Nutrition Physiology*, p.116, ISBN 3-7690-4094-5, Frankfurt, Germany, May 2-3, 2001

Zoetendal, E.G.; Akkermans, A.D. & De Vos, W.M. (1998). Temperature gradient gel electrophoresis analysis of 16S rRNA from human fecal samples reveals stable and host-specific communities of active bacteria. *Applied and Environmental Microbiology*, Vol.64, No.10, (October 1998), pp.3854-3859, ISSN 0099-2240

18

Superior Mesenteric Artery Syndrome

Rani Sophia and Waseem Ahmad Bashir
Yeovil Hospital NHS Foundation Trust, Yeovil, Somerset
United Kingdom

1. Introduction

Superior mesenteric artery syndrome (SMAS) mostly occurs in adolescent or young adults and is a rare disorder. The syndrome was first described by the Von Rokitansky in 1842 and since then about 400 cases has been reported in literature but SMAS is not well recognised and often diagnosed late till the patients are far advanced with their symptoms (Geer 1990, Raissi et al1996). In general population the incidence with the help of upper gastrointestinal barium studies were reported to be around 0.013-0.3 %(Ylinen et al 1989). However after the scoliosis surgery the prevalence was reported to be in range of 0.5-4.7 %(Tsirikos, Jeans 2005). Geer (1990) reported that 75% of the cases occurred in patients aged between 10-30 years. In a large series of 75 patients it was reported that two third of the cases were women and one third men and the average age was around 40 years (Wilkie 1927). The morbidity caused by this syndrome and the difficulty in diagnosing it prompted this review, and at the same time it will also act as a fresh reminder for the clinicians.

2. Anatomy and pathology

The superior mesenteric artery (SMA) originates behind the neck of the pancreas at the level of the first lumbar vertebra and leaves the aorta at an acute angle. It forms an angle of approximately 45° with the abdominal aorta. The third part duodenum crosses caudal to the origin of superior mesenteric artery (SMA), coursing between SMA and aorta just inferior to the left renal vein from right to left (Fig 1). Any factor that sharply narrows the aortomesenteric angle from approximately 45° (range between 38-56°) to 6-25° will thus reduce the aortomesenteric distance to about 2-8mm (Hines et al 1984, Neri et al 2005). The mean radiographic aortomesenteric distance is 10–28 mm (Neri et al 2005).This can cause entrapment and compression of the third part of duodenum. Thus conditions such as loss of mesenteric and retroperitoneal fat and subsequent decrease of the aortomesenteric distance can cause SMAS.

3. Causes

- In elderly patients heavily calcified or tortuous aorta can cause SMAS.
- Other causes reducing the aortomesenteric angle are:
- Severe cachexia or catabolic states such as weight loss due to neoplasia, anorexia nervosa
- Severe head injuries or prolonged bed rest or severe burns
- Bariatric surgery or Nissan fundoplication, spinal scoliosis surgery
- Spinal deformities or trauma

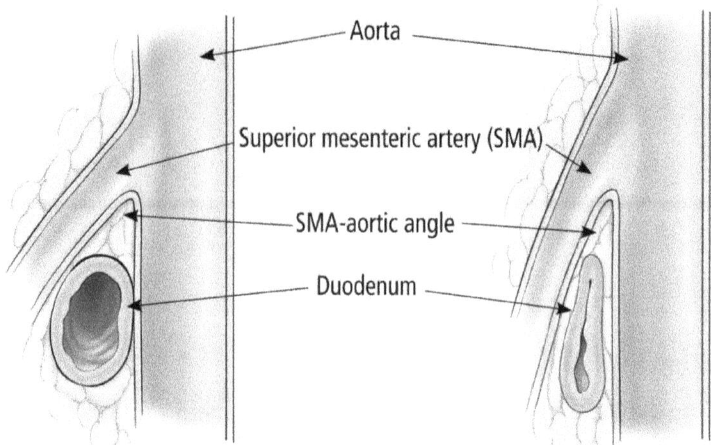

Fig. 1. Left, the normal angle between the superior mesenteric artery (SMA) and the aorta is 25 to 60 degrees. Right, in SMA syndrome, the SMA-aortic angle is more acute, and the duodenum is compressed between the aorta and the SMA (Reproduced with permission from Pasumarthy et al (2010) Cleveland Clinic Journal of Medicine. 77:45-50)

- Anatomic or congenital anomalies as high insertion of the ligament of Treitz, Intestinal malrotation, peritoneal adhesions and low origin of the superior mesenteric artery

4. Symptoms and signs

The most common symptom in these patients is intermittent abdominal pain and copious vomiting. The abdominal pain can be postprandial and the nausea, vomiting can lead to anorexia and weight loss. Early satiety, eructations, and at times sub-acute small bowel obstruction can develop. The symptoms are relieved when patient lies in left lateral decubitus, prone or knee-to-chest position (Geer 1990, Wilkie 1927, Raissi et al 1996). They are often aggravated by in an asthenic patient in supine position. Examination of the abdomen may reveal a succussion splash. Peptic ulcer disease is found in 25-45% of the patients and hyperchlohydria in 50 %(Geer 1990, Ylinen et al 1989). Dilated duodenum and stomach could predispose a patient to aspiration pneumonia and acute gastric rupture.

5. Diagnosis

To diagnose a patient with SMAS traditionally barium meal studies with hypotonic duodenography is being used. A positive diagnosis will include duodenal dilatation, retention of barium with in duodenum, the classical vertical linear impression caused by extrinsic pressure in the third part of duodenum and frequent relief of obstruction in left lateral or decubitus position (Tsirikos , Jeans 2005, Raissi et al 1996). In the past angiographic measurement of the aortomesenteric angle was thought to be a gold standard. An aortomesenteric angle of < 22–25° and a distance of <8 mm correlated well with symptoms of SMAS (Hines et al 1984). Because of its invasive nature, Computed tomography (CT) scan or CT angiogram/MR angiogram have taken over as a gold standard (Tsirikos , Jeans 2005,

Lee, Mangla 1978). CT or CT angiogram is also superior to ultrasound because it can measure the reduced aortomesenteric angle and show the gastric and duodenal dilatation at the same time. CT scan will also be helpful in finding the cause of SMAS e.g high insertion of ligament of Trietz or a neoplasia in that region. Upper gastrointestinal endoscopy is essential to rule out mechanical outlet obstruction of stomach or an ulcer (Ylinen et al 1989, Raissi et al 1996).

6. Treatment

If there is a neoplasm causing SMAS, anatomic or congenital abnormality then the treatment is surgical, otherwise this condition is treated conservatively. Patients are fed frequent small meals orally or if it is not possible then through enteral jejunal tube. After feeding the patient, he/she should be placed in either prone or lateral decubitus position. If patient cannot tolerate tube feeding because of excessive vomiting then he/she needs to be fed parentally. Both ways of feeding have shown to be effective (Barnes, Lee 1996).This conservative treatment should aim to correct the fluid and electrolyte balance and increase the body weight in an attempt to increase the retroperitoneal fat so that the aortomesenteric angle is corrected.

Surgical treatment is indicated if conservative treatment fails or if there is severe progressive weight loss, pronounced duodenal dilatation with stasis and complicating peptic ulcer disease. Several surgical procedures have been tried and tested in the management of SMAS. Gastrojejunostomy, dudenojejunostomy, Strong's operation (duodenal mobilisation for lowering the duodenojejunal flexure) have been performed to treat this condition. Gastrojejunostomy and lysis of the ligament of Treitz provided adequate decompression of the stomach but was not helpful in overcoming the duodenal obstruction and at times leading to blind loop syndrome with reflux of bile necessitating duodenojejunostomy (Lee, Mangla 1978). A review of 146 cases showed that duodenojejunostomy was the treatment of the choice (Lee, Mangla 1978) and success rate was 90 %(Raissi et al 1996). Recently laparoscopic dudenojejunostomy has become treatment of choice. Massoud (1995) reported his experience of laparoscopic division of the ligament of Treitz in 4 cases. It was successful in 3 cases. Gerson and Heniford (1998) reported first laparoscopic duodenojejunostomy and then further cases were reported in the literature (Richardson, Surowiec 2001). Minimally invasive surgery with less operative time, quick post operative recovery and relief of the symptoms were the advantages over traditional duodenojejunostomy.

7. Conclusion

SMAS is a rare disorder and is under-diagnosed in our practice of medicine. It should be ruled out in the patients with postprandial abdominal pain, vomiting and weight loss. It is caused by compression of the third part of duodenum by the narrowed aortomesenteric angle. There are different predisposing factors but severe weight loss and cachexia, spinal deformities and congenital anomalies are some of them. SMAS is treated initially conservatively but laparoscopic duodenojejunostomy has high success rate as well.

8. References

Barnes JB, Lee M (1996) Superior mesenteric artery syndrome in an intravenous drug abuser after rapid weight loss. *South Med J.* 89: 331–334.

Geer D (1990) Superior mesenteric artery syndrome. *Mil Med*. 155:321-3

Gersin KS, Heniford BT (1998) Laparoscopic duodenojejunostomy for treatment of superior mesenteric artery syndrome. *JSLS*. 2: 281–284.

Hines JR, Gore RM, Ballantyne GH (1984) Superior mesenteric artery syndrome. Diagnostic criteria and therapeutic approaches. *Am J Surg*. 148: 630–632.

Lee CS, Mangla JC (1978) Superior mesenteric artery compression syndrome. *Am J Gastroenterol* .70: 141–150.

Massoud WZ (1995) Laparoscopic management of superior mesenteric artery syndrome. *Int Surg*. 80: 322– 27.

Neri S, Signorelli SS, Mondati E, Pulvirenti D, Campanile E, Di Pino L, Scuderi M, Giustolisi N, Di Prima P, Mauceri B, Abate G,Cilio D, Misseri M, Scuderi R: (2005) Ultrasound imaging in diagnosis of superior mesenteric artery syndrome. *J intern Med*. 257: 346–351.

Raissi B, Taylor B, Traves D (1996) Recurrent mesenteric artery (Wilkie's) syndrome: a case report. *Can J Surg*. 39: 410-6.

Richardson WS, Surowiec WJ (2001) Laparoscopic repair of superior mesenteric artery syndrome. *Am J Surg*. 181: 377–78.

Tsirikos AI, Jeans LA (2005) Superior mesenteric artery syndrome in children and adolescents with spine deformities undergoing corrective surgery. *J Spinal Disord Tec*. 18:263–271.

Wilkie DPD (1927) Chronic duodenal ileus. *Am J Med Sci*. 173: 643-9

Ylinen P, Kinnunen J, Hockerstedt K (1989) Superior mesenteric artery syndrome. *J Clinn Gastroenterol*. 11: 386-91

19

Appendiceal MALT Lymphoma in Childhood – Presentation and Evolution

Antonio Marte[1,*], Gianpaolo Marte[2], Lucia Pintozzi[1] and Pio Parmeggiani[1]
1Pediatric Surgery, 2nd University of Naples, Naples
2General Surgery, 2nd University of Naples, Naples
Italy

1. Introduction

Lymphoma of mucosa-associated lymphoid tissue (MALT lymphoma) was first described by Isaacson et al. in 1983 (Isaacson & Wright, 1984). According to the WHO lymphoma classification, the indolent B cell lymphoma of MALT type is classified as a marginal zone lymphoma, thus called because it originates from the B lymphocytes normally present in a distinct anatomical location (marginal zone) of the secondary lymphoid follicles (Harris et al., 2001). MALT lymphomas comprise up to 40% of adult non-Hodgkin lymphomas (NHL); the median age at occurrence is 60 years, with a female predominance (Anonymous, 1997). In paediatric age MALT lymphomas are very rare. We report on a case of MALT lymphoma involving the appendix in a 6-year-old immunocompetent girl and its evolution toward an inflammatory bowel disease (IBD) at a middle-term follow-up.

2. Case report

P.A., a 6-year-old girl, was referred to our institution in May 2005 with a diagnosis of appendicitis. The girl had been complaining of right lower abdominal pain for 6 months. More recently, the pain was exacerbated by walking and coughing. Abdominal ultrasound showed a slight effusion of the pelvic fossa. Her postnatal history showed some period of constipation spaced by regular daily evacuations. Blood examinations showed neutrophil leucocytosis. The patient underwent laparoscopic appendectomy using the three-trocar technique, three endo-loops and the Liga-Sure for the hemostasis. During the laparoscopic exploration no hyperplastic mesenteric lymphnode was found. The appendix appeared moderately hyperemic with a slight enlargement of two-thirds of its distal portion (Fig. 1).

The postoperative course was uneventful and the girl was discharged on day 1, without any complications. The appendix underwent a routine histological examination. The morphological appearance showed thickened lamina propria and submucosa, which were occupied by pseudonodules of immunocompetent cells (Fig. 2), characterized by lymphocytes with small nuclei with a narrow cytoplasmic rim and plasma cell (Fig. 3). Immunohistochemical studies revealed positivity for CD20 (CD20, pan B cell), and

---

* Corresponding Author

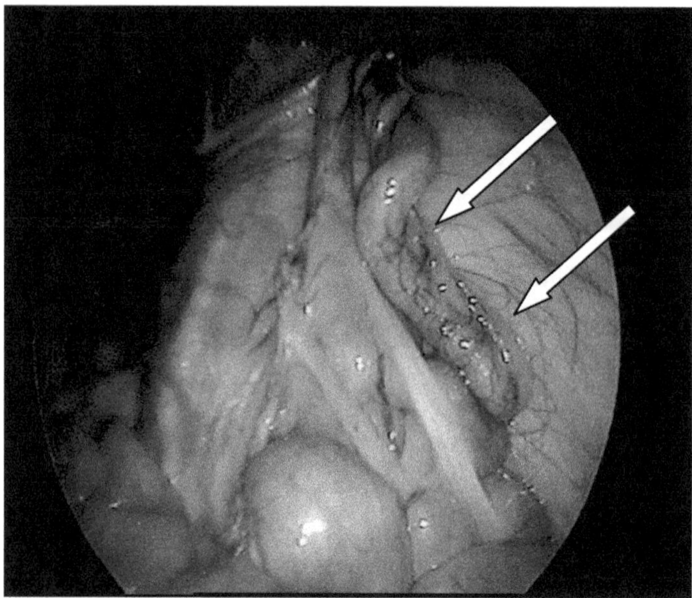

Fig. 1.

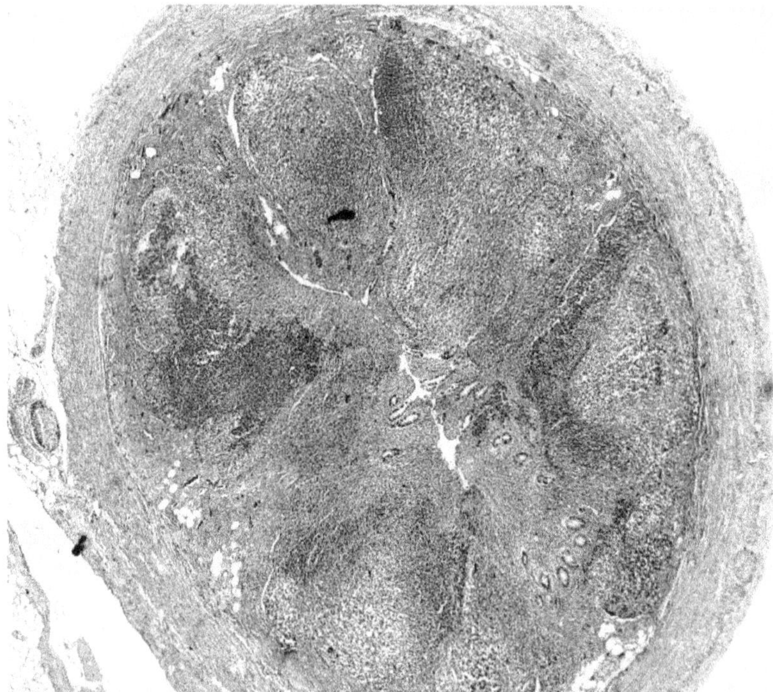

Fig. 2. Hematoxylin–eosin staining. The wall of appendix is thickened, and occupied by a compact nodular formation. The serous and muscular tunic appear thin.

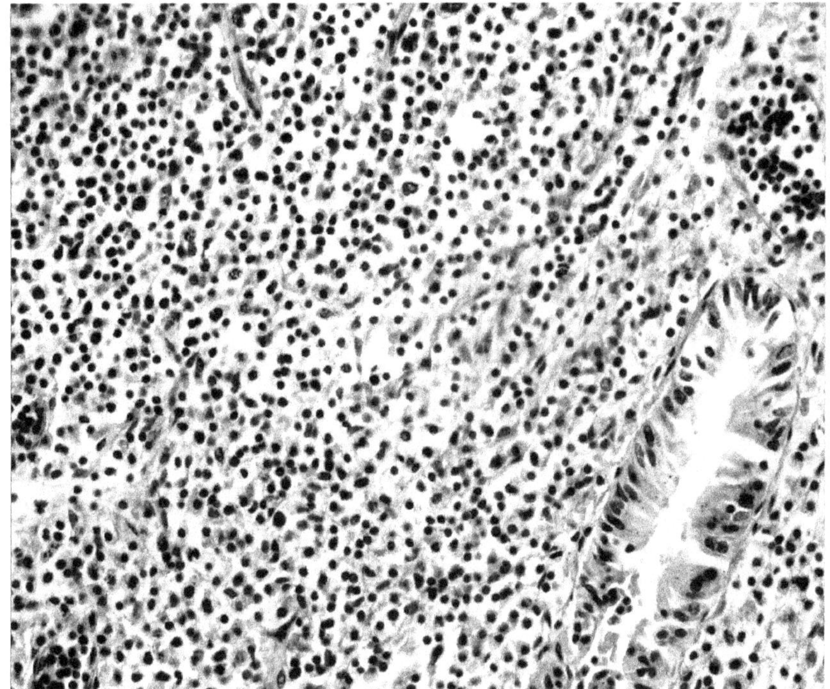

Fig. 3. Hematoxylin–eosin staining. Hyperdense lymphocytic population with small nuclei and narrow cytoplasmic rim and some plasmacytoid and monocytoid elements with great and hyperchromatic nuclei.

negativity for CD5 (CD5, Pan T cell, and B cell subsets) and CD10 using monoclonal antibodies, and positivity for anti-k (immunoglobulin light chain) using polyclonal antibodies, in addition to a low positivity to Ki-67 (proliferation-associated marker). Extensive further examination revealed that the lymphoma was restricted to the distal portion of the appendix (stage IA) and was not associated with any specific infection.

Abdominal MRI, OGDS, and capsule endoscopy of the ileum were all negative; the search for *H. pylori* was also negative. No chemotherapy was performed. After a 15-months follow-up, the patient was doing well (Marte et al., 2008). Calprotectin and clinical evaluation were repeated yearly showing no problem and the patient was asymptomatic. 3 year after, the yearly follow-up showed a slight increase of fecal calprotectin values (40µg/g) with recurrent abdominal pain and occasional episodes of diarrhea. The girl underwent a new clinical evaluation, small bowel radiological contrast study, videocapsule, OGDS, and colonoscopic examination. No fever or weight loss was present; erythrocyte sedimentation rate, C-reactive protein level were slightly higher. Perinuclear antineutrophil cytoplasmatic antibodies (pANCA) and Anti-Saccharomyces cerevisiae (ASCA) antibodies are not increased too.

The small bowel x-ray contrast, OGDS and videocapsule study demonstrated no abnormalities. Colon biopsies revealed a mild nonspecific IBD extending till 90 cm from the anal verge. (Fig.4,5,6,7)

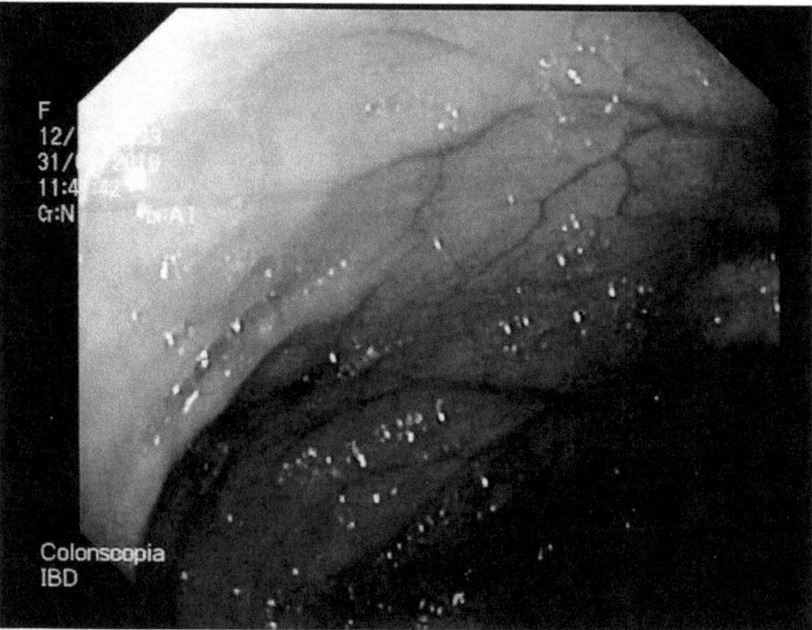

Fig. 4. Colonoscopy. Rectum and sigmoid colon: mucosal redness, nonspecific inflammatory pattern.

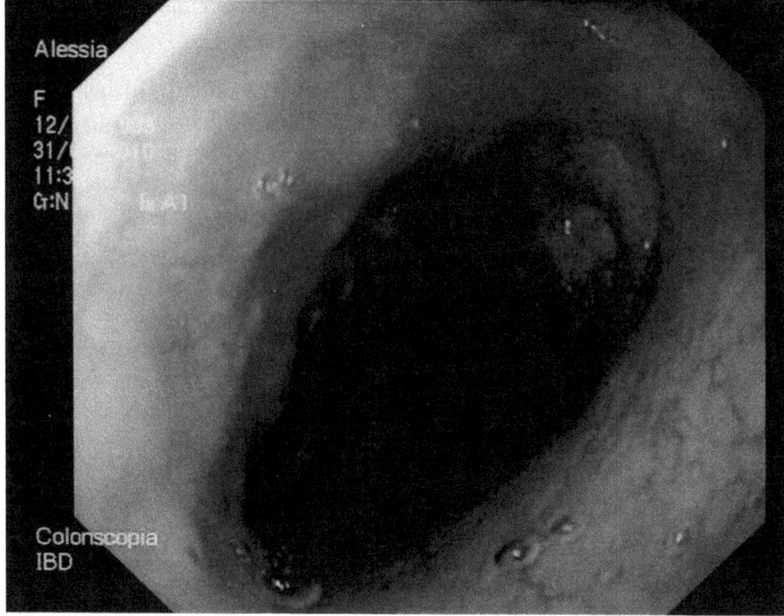

Fig. 5. Colonoscopy. Rectum and sigmoid colon: mucosal redness, nonspecific inflammatory pattern.

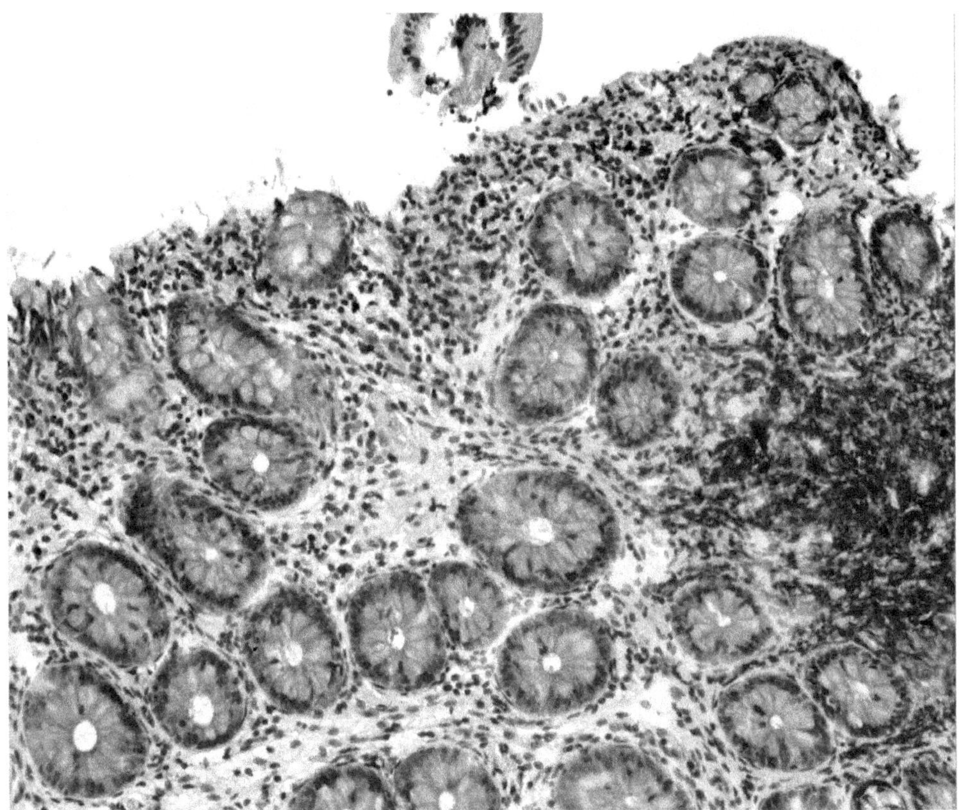

Fig. 6. Absent mucosal surface epithelium with focal reduction of the glands. The lamina propria is edematous, site of microbleeds and is infiltrated by elements of immunocompetent and heaps of eosinophils. (20 X). 90 cm from the anal verge.

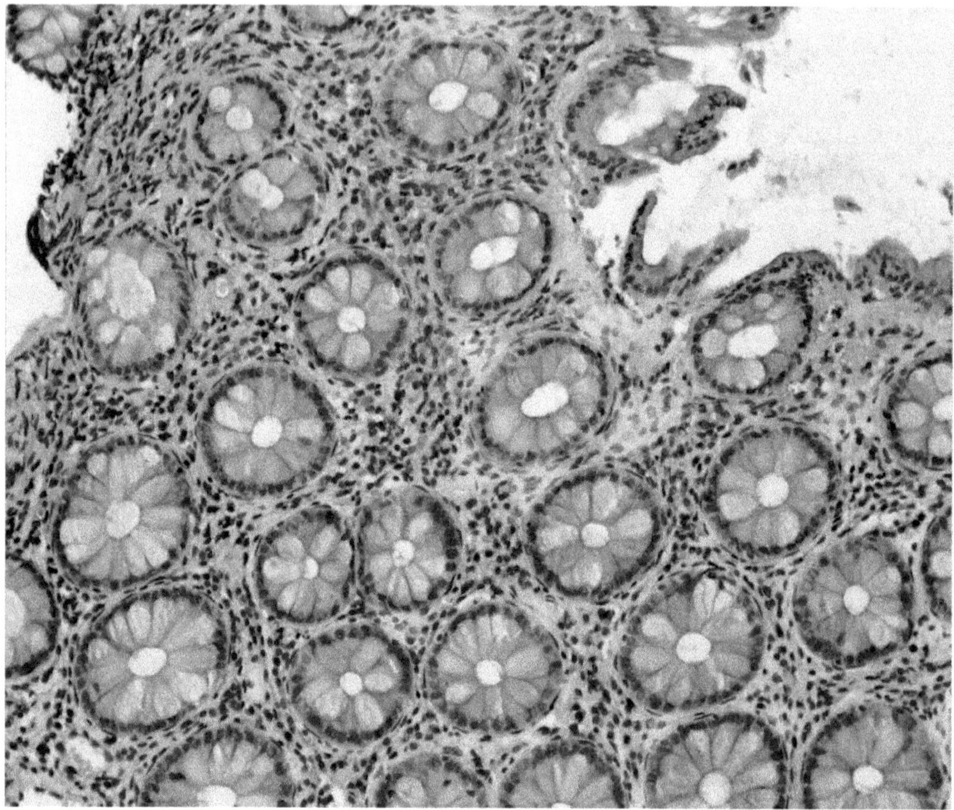

Fig. 7. Rectum (20X): 2 small erosions of the mucosa, glandular patrimony preserved, but low in mucus cells. The lamina propria is diffusely infiltrated by immunocompetent cells (lymphocytes and plasma cells).

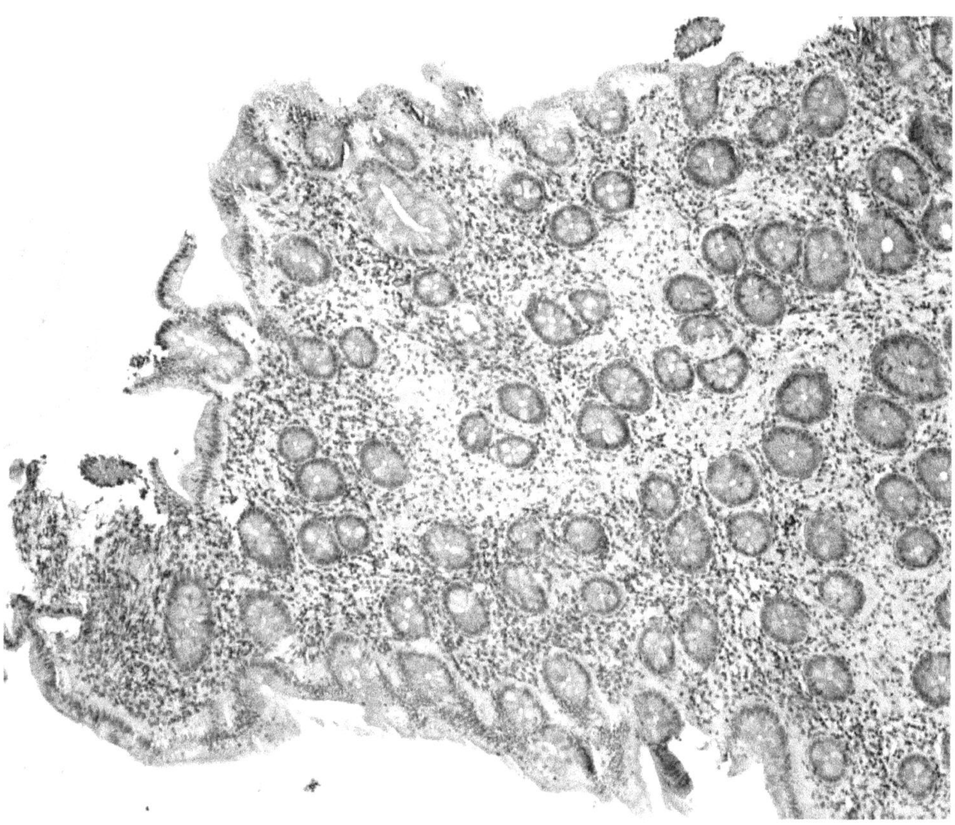

Fig. 8. Recto-sigmoid junction (10X). Mucosal home-based micro-inflammatory polyps. The glandular portion is moderately reduced. The lamina propria is edematous and infiltrated by immunocompetent elements.

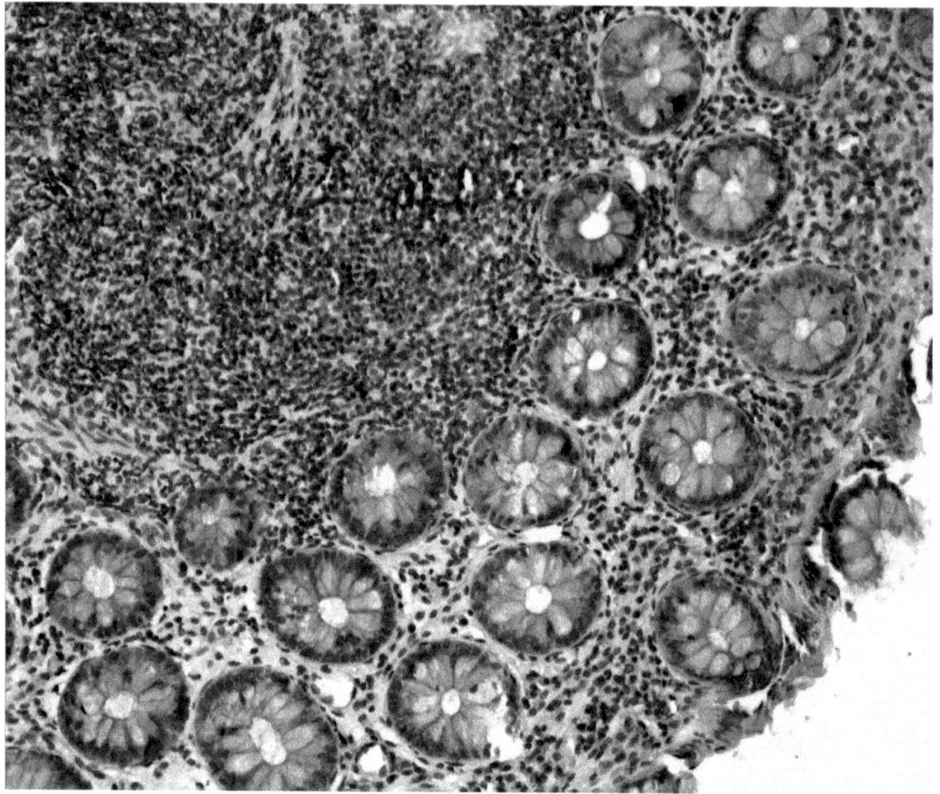

Fig. 9. Mucosal lymphocytes nodule. Glands, well structured, present a reduction of mucus cells. The lamina propria is infiltrated by immunocompetent elements. (20x). 15 cm from the anal verge.

A 6 weeks cycle of Mesalazine (5ASA), 2gr/day was administered to the patient obtaining the induction of remission and then repeated every 2 months for the prevention of recurrences. At present the patient is doing well and a strict clinical serologic follow-up with calprotectin, P-Anca and ASCA is scheduled every 6 months and, yearly, colonoscopy.

3. Discussion

Current knowledge of MALT lymphoma is largely based upon studies in adults. MALT lymphoma is rare in children; the available evidence consists mostly of isolated case reports, except for one series of ten cases (Corr et al., 1997), and another including a total of 48 cases (children and young adults) (Taddesse-Heath et al., 1997) and a pediatric NHL trial recruiting children and adolescents from Germany, Austria and Switzerland (Kaatsch et al., 2004). MALT often develops within the context of a pre-existing inflammatory response due to infection or to autoimmune disorder. Many studies show the relationship between *H. pylori* infection and gastric MALT lymphoma (Isaacson & Whright, 1984; Kurugoglu et al., 2002); some authors have reported a regression of MALT lymphoma in parotid gland (Alkan et al., 1996), lip gland (Berrebi et al., 1998), small intestine (Fischbach et al., 1997) and rectum (Matsudo et al., 1997) following *H. pylori* eradication. Other risk factors for MALT lymphoma include autoimmune diseases like Hashimoto thyroiditis or Sjogren syndrome, and Borrelia burgdorferi for skin lymphoma. A further prerequisite for the development of MALT lymphoma in children may be the presence of HIV infection (Teruya-Feldestein et al., 1995; Mo et al., 2004). In some patients no risk factors can be identified. The most common sites are the stomach and salivary glands. Others sites are: ocular adnexa, the lungs, thyroid and the skin (Zucca et al., 2000). Some retrospective analyses of histopathological results of appendectomy specimens performed for acute appendicitis in a large sample of patients, including children, report a prevalence of appendiceal malignant tumors ranging from 0.4 (Tchana et al., 2006) to 1.5% (Ravi et al., 2006). Among the malignant tumors, carcinoids have the highest incidence (Tchana et al., 2006; Ravi et al., 2006) and 70–90% of these tumors are discovered incidentally because they are usually restricted to the distal appendix (Akerstrom, 1989; Aranha & Greenle, 1980). From a review of the literature we found only one case of appendix lymphoma in paediatric age presenting with intussusception symptoms (Karabulut et al., 2005). Our report probably represents the first case of MALT lymphoma of the appendix found accidentally in a child during an appendectomy. MALT lymphomas manifest with aspecific symptoms. In our case, the clinical presentation was characterized by recurrent abdominal pain, and the only element of suspicion was the enlargement of the distal portion of the appendix. The subsequent evolution to a mild form of IBD could be considered as an evolution of the appendiceal malt-limphoma for which the phenomenon should be considered a prodromal presentation of a more extensive bowel disease which require a close follow-up and specific therapy (Aomatsu et al., 2011). Otherwise we can't exclude that the subsequent IBD could be an autonomous, subsequent disease considered that, also in this case, there are no data in the Literature. Furthermore, given the previous appendiceal malt-lymphoma, the efficacy of mesalazine alone, without the use of immunosuppressive drugs, can be considered a very favorable factor in our case. In conclusion, even if the occurrence of malignant appendiceal pathology in children is rare (Setty & Termuhlen, 2010), the probability that it is asymptomatic is very high. According to our experience, our case suggests that histological examination should always be performed following appendectomy in children and that if a MALT lymphoma were discovered, a close follow-up is strongly recommended, not only for the MALT lymphoma recurrence but also for its possible evolution towards an inflammatory bowel disease.

4. References

Akerstrom G (1989). Surgical treatment of patients with the carcinoid syndrome, *Acta Oncol* 28(3):409–414.

Alkan S, Karcher DS, Newman MA, Cohen P (1996). Regression of salivary gland MALT lymphoma after treatment for *H. pylori*, *Lancet* 348:268–269.

Anonymous (1997). A clinical evaluation of the international lymphoma study group classification of non Hodgkin's lymphoma. The non Hodgkin's lymphoma classification project, *Blood* 89:3909–3918.

Aomatsu T, Yoden A, Matsumoto K, Kimura E, Inoue K, Andoh A, Tamai H (2011). Fecal calprotectin is a useful marker for disease activity in pediatric patients with inflammatory bowel disease, *Dig Dis Sci*. Aug;56(8):2372-7.

Aranha GV, Greenle HB (1980). Surgical management of carcinoid tumors of the gastrointestinal tract, *Am Surg* 46(8):429–435.

Berrebi D, Lescoeue B, Faye A et al (1998). MALT lymphoma of labial minor salivary gland in an immunocompetent child with a gastric Helicobacter pylori infection, *J Pediatr* 133:290–292.

Corr P, Vaithilingum M, Thejpal R, Jeena P (1997). Paroid MALT lymphoma in HIV infected children, *J Ultrasound Med* 16:615–617.

Fischbach W, Tacke W, Greiner A et al (1997). Regression of immunoproliferative small intestinal disease after eradication of *H. pylori*, *Lancet* 349:31–32.

Harris NL, Jaffe ES, Stein H, Vardiman JW (2001). Pathology and genetics of tumors of the haemopoeitic and lymphoid tissues, WHO classification of tumors, *International Agency For Research On Cancer Press*, Lyon, pp 157–160.

Isaacson P, Wright DH (1984). Extranodal malignant lymphoma arising from mucosa associated lymphoid tissue, *Cancer* 53:2515–2524.

Kaatsch P, Spix C (2004). *Annual report 2004 (1980–2003)*. German childhood Cancer Registry.

Karabulut R, Sonmez K, Turkyilmaz Z, Yilmaz Y, Akyurek N, Basaklar AC, Kale N (2005). Mucosa associated lymphoma tissue lymphoma in the appendix, a lead point for intussusceptions, *J Pediatr Surg* 40(5):872–874.

Kurugoglu S, Mihmanli I, Celkan T, AkiH, Aksoy H, Korman U (2002). Radiological features in paediatric primary gastric MALT lymphoma and association with *H pylori*, *Pediatr Radiol* 32:82–87.

Marte A, Sabatino MD, Cautiero P, Accardo M, Romano M, Parmeggiani P (2008). Unexpected finding of laparoscopic appendectomy: appendix MALT lymphoma in children, *Pediatr Surg Int*. Apr;24(4):471-3.

Matsumoto T, Lida M, Shimizu M (1997). Regression of mucosa associated lymphoid tissue lymphoma of rectum after eradication of *H. pylori*, *Lancet* 350:115–116.

Mo JQ, Dimashkieh H, Mallery SR et al (2004) MALT lymphoma in children: case report and review of the literature, *Pediatr Dev Pathol* 7:407–413.

Ravi Marudanayagam, Geraint T Williams, Brian I Rees (2006). Review of the pathologiacal results of 2660 appendicectomy specimens, *J Gastroenterol* 41:745–749.

Setty BA, Termuhlen AM (2010). Rare pediatric non-Hodgkin lymphoma, *Curr Hematol Malig Rep*. Jul;5(3):163-8.

Taddesse-Heath L, Pittalunga S, Sorbara L et al (2003). Marginal zone B-cell lymphoma in children and young adults, *Am J Surg Pathol* 27:522–531.

Tchana SV, Detry O, Polus M, Thiry A, Detroz B, Maweja S, Hamoir E, Defechereux T, Cimbra C, De Roover A, Meurisse M, Honore P (2006). Carcinoid tumor of the appendix: a consecutive serie from 1237 appendectomies, *World J Gastroenterol* 7;12(41):6699–701.

Teruya-Feldstein J, Temeck BK, Sloas MM et al (1995). Pulmonary malignant lymphoma of mucosa associated lymphoid tissue (MALT) arising in a pediatric HIV-positive patient, *Am J Surg Pathol* 19:357–363.

Zucca E, Conconi A, Roggero E et al (2000). Non gastric MALT lymphomas: a survey of 369 european patients. The international extranodal lymphoma study group, *Ann Oncol* 11:99.

20

The Surgical Management
of Chronic Pancreatitis

S. Burmeister, P.C. Bornman, J.E.J. Krige and S.R. Thomson
University of Cape Town
South Africa

1. Introduction

Chronic pancreatitis (CP) has been defined as a continuing inflammatory disease of the pancreas characterized by irreversible morphological changes, often associated with pain and with the loss of exocrine and endocrine function which may be clinically relevant (Clain JE Surg Clin North Am 1999). Pain is the principal cause of intractability and together with pancreatic insufficiency may have a significantly deleterious effect on a patient's quality of life as well as their ability to work and contribute to society, often leading to loss of their' social support network (Lankisch PG Digestion 1993). Progressive disease may culminate in severe and disabling symptoms requiring narcotic analgesia and frequent hospital admission with a consequent impact on health resources (Bornman PC W J Surg 2003; Braganza JM The Lancet 2011). The incidence and prevalence of disease has not been well documented however it is considered uncommon in Europe and the USA. This is in contrast to data available from South India where a prevalence of 114-200/100 000 people has been documented. Alcohol is the leading cause in western developed countries and some developing countries such as Brazil, Mexico and South Africa while idiopathic disease predominates in Asia and the subcontinent (Braganza JM The Lancet 2011; Garg PK J Gastroenterol Hepatol 2004).

Despite extensive study, the pathogenesis of chronic pancreatitis and the mechanisms which result in the development of pain remain poorly understood. As a result, treatment strategies have been largely empirical and based on symptoms, management of clinically evident exocrine and endocrine dysfunction and gross morphological abnormalities. Modalities employed have included medical support (with analgesics, anti-diabetic medication, pancreatic enzyme replacement, nutrient support and steroids in autoimmune disease), interventional endoscopy and surgery. The role of surgery has been primarily to relieve pain refractory to medical therapy, to address complications and to resect suspected or confirmed neoplastic disease (Bornman PC S Afr Med J 2010). The causes of pain in CP are likely multifactorial and proposed factors include excessive oxygen-derived free radicals, tissue hypoxia and acidosis, inflammatory infiltration accompanied by an influx of pain transmitted substances into damaged nerve ends and the development of pancreatic ductal and tissue fluid hypertension (Bornman PC W J Surg 2003). Surgical intervention for the relief of pain focuses primarily on the latter two proposed mechanisms. Two distinct principles have been applied in the development of procedures to address these mechanisms. Resection of diseased pancreatic tissue, in particular inflamed tissue within the head of the pancreas containing altered neural tissue and diseased ducts, considered the "pacemaker of disease" (Beger HG World J Surg 1990) and drainage of the pancreatic ductal system, in order to relieve ductal and parenchymal tissue hypertension. Removal of sufficient pancreatic tissue as to result in effective and durable relief of symptoms must however be balanced against the desire to avoid surgically related morbidity and mortality as well as to prevent post-operative pancreatic functional insufficiency. This has led to the development of less extensive resections and hybrid procedures which attempt to combine the advantages while avoiding the disadvantages of each approach.

This chapter will describe the theories around the pathophysiology of pain in chronic pancreatitis, discuss the rationale and indications for surgical intervention and detail the procedures currently available. It will also review the literature guiding the choice of these procedures for the relief of pain.

2. Pathophysiology of pain in chronic pancreatitis

The pathophysiology of CP is complex and remains poorly understood, with a number of theories having been put forward. Together with this, understanding of the mechanisms leading to the development of pain has also remained largely theoretical, confounded to a large extent by small and to some degree poorly designed studies, which have at times been contradictory. Furthermore, it is likely that the cause of pain is multi-factorial and may vary during the course of the disease (Bornman PC W J Surg 2003). To date, the most predominant theories regarding genesis of pain in CP have included:

2.1 Morphological pancreatic ductal changes resulting in obstruction and pancreatic ductal and tissue hypertension

In large duct chronic pancreatitis, changes in the composition of pancreatic fluid occur including an increase in free oxygen radicals and secretion of enzymes and calcium but a concomitant decrease in serine protease inhibitor Kazal type 1 (SPINK1), bicarbonate and citrate. (Sarles H Dig Dis Sci 1986). These changes are followed by precipitation of proteins such as lactoferrin and altered levels of pancreas related secretory stress proteins (including pancreatitis associated protein and pancreatic stone protein) (Singh SM W J Surg 1990; Graf R J Surg Res 2006). Glycoprotein plugs are formed which later become calcified leading to calcific disease with associated parenchymal fibrosis. Calcified protein plugs or calculi damage the ductal epithelium further and contribute to stasis thereby facilitating further stone formation. These changes are believed to begin in the side ducts but progress to involve the main pancreatic duct (PD) with the development of pancreatic duct strictures and obstruction (PDSO) as a consequence of fibrosis or calculi. Ductal hypertension follows with associated dilatation (Nagata A Gatroenteology 1981). Together with ductal hypertension, pancreatic tissue pressure may become elevated, particularly in areas of calcification (Okazaki K Gastroenterology 1986; Manes G Int J Pancreatol 1994; Jalleh RPBr J Surg 1991). The exact mechanism of elevated PTP in CP has not been proven, however it has been speculated that it may be a reflection of obstructed pancreatic side ducts rather than main PD obstruction. This situation may be aggravated by the development of perilobular fibrosis and a fibrotic peripancreatic capsule, resulting in a compartment syndrome like scenario with consequent tissue ischaemia and acidosis. (Karanjia ND Br J Surg 1994). While PDSO with ductal and tissue hypertension have not been consistently demonstrated in CP, nor a definite correlation shown with the development of pain (Novis BH Dig Dis Sc 1985; Manes G Int J Pancreatol 1994; Ugljesic M Int J Pancreatol. 1996; Bornman PC W J Surg 2003), surgical drainage procedures have been documented to reduce pancreatic tissue pressures (PTP), while a significant association between recurrence of pain and subsequent elevation of PTP has been shown. (Ebbehøj N Scand J Gastroenterol. 1990). On the other hand, ductal dilatation has been observed in the absence of ductal obstruction giving rise to the suggestion that dilatation may also be related to parenchymal destruction; this is supported by the association between duct dilatation and pancreatic insufficiency (Jensen AR Scand J Gastroent 1984). Thus, while PDSO is likely an important factor in generating pain, there are likely factors other than main pancreatic duct abnormalities that can also be implicated (Bornman PC W J Surg 2003). Furthermore, the role of side duct obstruction in the genesis of pain has not yet been clearly defined; it may be that side branch disease contributes to the development of an inflammatory mass in the pancreatic head which is recognised as important in driving the disease process (the so called "pacemaker" of disease) (Beger HG World J Surg 1990).

2.2 Interaction between the processes of inflammation and damaged neural structures

Histological studies have shown that there is invasion of neural tissue by inflammatory cells associated with chronic pancreatitis. This is accompanied by disruptions in the perineural sheaths which expose the internal neural compartments to the inflammatory response (Bockman DE Gastroenterol 1988). In addition, there are increased amounts of pain transmitted substances, pain modulators and nerve growth factors and receptors in enlarged / damaged pancreatic nerve structures, which appear to correlate with the intensity and frequency of pain (Büchler M Pancreas 1992, Zhu ZW Dig Dis Sci 2001,McMahon SP Nat Med 1995,Friess H Ann Surg 1999). Surgical resection of a pancreatic inflammatory mass effectively removes the pain stimulus together with the altered / damaged neural structures.

2.3 Toxin metabolism and generation of excessive oxygen derived free radicals resulting in electrophilic stress and inflammation

Acinar cells and proliferated islets of Langerhans are known to express cytochrome P450 (CYP) mono-oxygenases which metabolise xenobiotics (substances foreign to a living organism), often utilizing glutathione & catalysed by glutathione transferases. (Foster JR J Pathol 1993). There may however be adverse consequences to these metabolic reactions with the generation of reactive oxygen species (ROS) and toxic xenobiotic metabolites. Prevention of cellular injury relies on defences against ROS and xenobiotic metabolites; these defences include: selenium dependant glutathione peroxidase, glutathione transferases, glutathione and ascorbic acid. These varied properties make the pancreas a versatile yet vulnerable xenobiotic metabolizing organ (Braganza JM JOP 2010; Foster JR. Toxicology of the exocrine pancreas. In: General and applied toxicology 2009). Inhaled xenobiotics (such as cigarette smoke, occupational volatile hydrocarbons and petrochemicals) that pass through the pulmonary circulation represent the biggest threat by striking the pancreas through its rich arterial supply (Braganza JM Lancet 2011). When the acinar cell's defence mechanisms are insufficient to meet the increased oxidant load from ROS and xenobiotic metabolites, eletrophilic stress results (Braganza JM Digestion 1998; Braganza JM JOP 2010; Foster JR. Toxicology of the exocrine pancreas. In: General and applied toxicology 2009). Dietary insufficiency of micronutrients and ascorbic acid may predispose to this (Braganza JM Digestion 1998). Electrophilic stress in turn results in pancreastasis, the failure of apical exocytosis in the acinar cell (Sanfey H Ann Surg 1984; Leung P Antioxid Redox Signal 2009). Enzymes (both newly synthesised & those stored in zymogen granules) not able to be released apically, are released via the basolateral memebrane into the interstitium, lymphatics and bloodstream (Cook LJ Scand J Gastroenterol 1996). Entrance of enzymes and free radical oxidation products into the interstitium causes mast cell degranulation, resulting in local inflammation, activation of nociceptive axon reflexes and fibrosis. (Cook LJ Scand J Gastroenterol 1996; Braganza JM Digestion 1998). This inflammatory response is potentiated by cytokines produced by the damaged acinar cell as a result of activated signaling cascades caused by the release of ROS. (Leung P Antioxid Redox Signal 2009).

2.4 Fibrosis as a result of pancreatic stellate cell activation in the necrosis-inflammation-fibrosis sequence and sentinel acute pancreatitis events

Pancreatic stellate cells play a central role in the fibrotic process associated with chronic pancreatitis (Stevens T Am J Gastroenterol 2004). This is particularly relevant in the necrosis-inflammation-fibrosis sequence, the most widely accepted hypothesis in the pathogenesis of chronic pancreatitis (Bornman PC in Chronic pancreatitis. Hepatobiliary and pancreatic surgery – a companion to specialist surgical practice. 2009). Initially this hypothesis held that fibrosis developed as a stepwise progressive process from recurrent bouts of acute pancreatitis (Comfort MW Gastroenterology 1946; Kloppel G Hepatogastroenterol 1991). An alternative theory suggested that alcohol might be directly toxic to the acinar cell through a change in cellular metabolism (toxic-metabolic theory). Alcohol was purported to produce cytoplasmic lipid accumulation within the acinar cell, leading to fatty degeneration, cellular necrosis and eventual fibrosis (Bordalo O Am J Gastroenterol 1977). More recently the theory of a sentinel acute pancreatitis event (SAPE) has been proposed. This theory hypothesizes that stimulation of the pancreatic acinar cell by alcohol or oxidative stress activates trypsin which results in a sentinel acute pancreatitis event. This is followed by a dual phase chronic inflammatory response, with the early phase characterised by a pro-inflammatory cell infiltrate including macrophages and lymphocytes. Cytokines released during the early phase also attract a later anti-inflammatory cellular infiltrate comprising pro-fibrotic cells, including stellate cells. These cells, once attracted, are activated by lipid peroxidation products (caused by excess ROS) and mast cell degranulation products, and are considered "primed"; continued stimulation by cytokines (in particular TGF-β1) produced by acinar cells, inflammatory cells or the stellate cells themselves as a result of oxidative stress, alcohol or recurrent acute pancreatitis, cause these activated stellate cells to deposit collagen, resulting in fibrosis and the features of chronic pancreatitis (Whitcomb DC Best Pract Res Clin Gastroenterol 2002). The transient formation of fatty acid ethanol esters and the role of macrophages and lymphocytes in pancreatic tissue destruction are also thought to be integral to this process (Pandol SJ Pancreatology 2007). It is suggested that the contractive potential and perivascular location of the stellate cells results in fibrosis that leads to microvascular ischaemia and pain (Wells RG Gastroenterol 1998).

2.5 Primary duct hypothesis

This theory suggests a primary immunological attack on ductal epithelium leading to inflammation and scarring of ductal architecture. This may have specific relevance in autoimmune pancreatitis. (Cavallini G. Ital J Gastroenterol 1993).

Once inflammation becomes established in CP, patients may enter a phase of stable disease with the histological features of acinar loss, mononuclear cell infiltrate and fibrosis (Shrikhande SV Br J Surg 2003). Subsequent progression to end stage disease is characterised by loss of all secretory tissue, disappearance of inflammatory cells and intense fibrosis. This may be accompanied by loss of pancreatic function together with diminished pain, the so-called "pancreatic burn-out syndrome"; this phenomenon is however not a universal outcome in patients with CP, thereby confounding potential treatment strategies (Girdwood AH J Clin Gastroenterol 1981; Amman RW Gastroenterol 1984; Lankisch PG Digestion 1993).

Complications of CP related to inflammation and fibrosis may develop which can alter the course of disease as well as clinical presentation. These include

1.   Biliary obstruction

This is common in advanced disease, particularly when there calcification and an inflammatory mass in the head. Obstruction may be transient when related to oedema during acute flaring of disease or more permanent when occurring as a result of a fibrotic stricture or mass effect from an adjacent pseudocyst. .

2.   Duodenal obstruction

This may be the result of peri-duodenal fibrosis or from the mass effect provided by a pseudocyst.

3.   Development of a pseudocyst / pancreatic ascites

Pancreas related fluid collections or pseudocysts occur in 30-40% of patients with CP and are thought to be the consequence of either ductal obstruction or pancreatic necrosis with ductal disruption (D'Egidio A BJS 1991). Typically cysts communicate with the pancreatic ductal system which shows gross morphological abnormalities. Postnecrotic peripancreatic collections occur only rarely, usually as a consequence of an acute on chronic attack of pancreatitis. Pseudocysts in CP are usually located either near the head when they are mostly intra-pancreatic or in the lesser sac. Pseudocysts in CP are less likely to spontaneously resolve than those associated with acute disease as they have usually matured by the time of presentation and typically communicate with the pancreatic ductal system. Pancreatic ascites occurs when there is rupture of a pseudocyst or duct into the peritoneal cavity (Bornman PC in Hepatobiliary and pancreatic surgery – a companion to specialist surgical practice. 2009).

4.   Gastro-intestinal bleeding, related to
a.   Portal hypertension

Portal hypertension may develop in up to 10% of patients as a result of venous compression or thrombosis. Splenic vein thrombosis may result in segmental portal hypertension giving rise to gastric and oesophageal varices, although frank variceal bleeding in this setting is uncommon (Bornman PC in Hepatobiliary and pancreatic surgery – a companion to specialist surgical practice. 2009).

b. Pseudoaneurysms

Enzyme rich fluid collections may erode into vascular structures resulting in false aneurysms with bleeding into the cyst and pancreatic duct, peritoneum or retroperitoneum.

3. Rationale and indications for surgical intervention

Surgery is indicated in chronic pancreatitis for the relief of pain, to manage complications and to resect confirmed or suspected neoplastic disease (Bornman PC S Afr Med J 2010). Two theoretical principles underlie the rationale for surgery to alleviate pain in CP. The first utilises the ductal / parenchymal tissue hypertension and inflammatory-neural theories on the pathogenesis of pain in CP. It postulates that surgical decompression of the main pancreatic duct will alleviate interstitial hypertension thereby improving parenchymal perfusion and acidosis (Patel AG Gastroent 1995) with consequent reduction of inflammatory stimulation and influx of mediators into damaged nerves (Salim AS HPB Surg 1997). The second principle focuses on removal of pathologically inflamed parenchyma together with altered neural tissue in particular that within the head, which is considered the "pacemaker" of disease. Emphasis has also been placed on the importance of addressing diseased side ducts, thereby limiting the possibility of recurrence (Beger HG World J Surg 1990).

The objectives of surgery for pain in CP are effective and durable relief of symptoms while preserving endocrine and exocrine function, thereby restoring the patient's quality of life. The potential for morbidity and mortality as well as recurrence should be low. Based on these objectives and the principles outlined above, a number of procedures have been developed. Essentially, these procedures fall into a spectrum covering three broad categories. At one end of the spectrum are drainage procedures which focus on decompressing the main pancreatic duct by establishing a new pancreatic-enteric communication which bypasses any native obstruction to pancreatic outflow. At the other end of the spectrum are resectional procedures which aim to remove diseased ductal and neural tissue within chronically inflamed parenchyma. Over time, a number of modified and hybrid procedures have evolved which attempt to retain the advantages while limiting the disadvantages of both the former 2 categories.

Little data exists to guide decision making regarding the optimal timing of surgery to alleviate pain in CP. There are two schools of thought. The first suggests that conservative non-surgical management should be pursued for as long as possible in order to avoid morbidity and side effects that may be associated with surgical intervention, in particular pancreatic insufficiency. They argue that the long term outcome of surgery is no different from medical management, and that the "pancreatic burn-out syndrome" is likely responsible for pain relief observed after surgery (Amman RW gastroenterol 1984). In contrast to this, others have argued that pain relief is better when surgical drainage is carried out earlier rather than later (Nealon WH Ann Surg 1993). It also remains controversial whether surgery can delay the natural course of the disease in terms of deterioration in pancreatic function (Warshaw AL Gastroenterol 1980; Nealon WH Ann Surg 1993; Jalleh RP Ann Surg 1992). Both arguments appear to have merit. While it seems foolhardy to offer surgical intervention with it's attached risk of morbidity and even mortality in patients whose symptoms might be controlled by medical means, it seems equally unreasonable to persist with a conservative approach in anticipation of pain relief, delaying surgery until narcotic addiction has developed and the outcomes from surgery may be worse (Warshaw AL gastroenterol 1984). In the absence of good evidence to guide decision making, it seems most appropriate that the decision regarding timing of surgery be individualized on a patient to patient basis. Surgical intervention should be performed only once an adequate trial of medical therapy has failed to control symptoms and the patient has been counseled regarding the risks and benefits of both modalities.

Patients referred for surgery for relief of intractable symptoms of CP should be evaluated by experienced clinicians working in a high volume, multi-disciplinary environment. All other treatment options should have been exhausted or considered not appropriate. Cross sectional imaging should be conducted to clearly delineate pancreatic morphology and detect local complications or features suggestive of neoplastic disease. The presence of portal hypertension, particularly as a result of portal or superior mesenteric vein thrombosis should be noted, as this may preclude surgical intervention (Bornman PC S Afr Med J 2010). With careful patient selection and modern surgical strategies, surgery may offer effective pain relief in over 90% of patients at 5 year follow up (Beger HG Ann Surg 1989).

In considering intervention for complications of CP, the clinical picture is paramount in decision making. Biliary obstruction may be asymptomatic, detected only biochemically or during imaging for other indications. In addition, there may be transient jaundice as a result of oedema during acute flares of the disease. The above are not indications for intervention. It must be remembered that once the biliary system has been entered, either percutaneously, endoscopically or surgically, this once sterile system should be considered contaminated with the risk of sepsis developing should obstruction recur in the future. On the other hand, persistent biliary obstruction of sufficient duration may result in secondary biliary cirrhosis, atrophy and deterioration in hepatic function. (Abdallah A HPB 2007). Obstruction longer than 4 weeks should arouse concern and warrants intervention. Decompression by means of endoscopic stenting should only be considered as a temporary bridge to surgery, in acute cholangitis or where patient factors preclude surgery (Bornman PC S Afr Med J 2010). Duodenal obstruction on the other hand typically represents either advanced fibrosis or a clinically significant pseudocyst, neither of which are likely to resolve before progression or further complications develop. Intervention is therefore indicated. Pseudocysts in CP are less likely to resolve than their acute counterparts and thus more often require drainage. The indications for drainage are the presence of symptoms or complications. Although size alone is not a criterion for intervention, cysts larger than 6cm are more likely to be symptomatic and require treatment (Bornman PC S Afr Med J 2010). Percutaneous procedures are generally not favoured for these lesions due to an increased risk of failure, introducing sepsis or creating an external fistula. Endoscopic drainage is associated with a success rate of 65-95% and a low complication rate and is preferred to surgery due to its less invasive nature. (Beckingham IJ Br J Surg 1997). Strict morphological criteria are required however, relating to cyst maturity, intra-luminal bulging, wall thickness (less than 10mm) and vascularity, particularly in the presence of portal hypertension. To this end, careful cross sectional imaging and endoscopic ultrasound are important adjuncts in assessing patients for this modality of treatment. Transmural drainage may be transduodenal or transgastric depending on the best route into the cyst while transpapillary drainage is an alternative option when communication with the pancreatic duct can be demonstrated. Surgery is indicated when endoscopic intervention fails or is not appropriate due to cyst morphology or patient factors. Surgical drainage of a pseudocyst may also be employed as part of an intervention planned for treatment of pain or additional complications. Pancreatic ascites is an uncommon but serious complication of CP which is managed in the first instance with paracentesis, nutritional support and endoscopic stenting of the pancreatic duct (Kozarek RA Gastrointest Endosc Clin North Am 1998; Bornman PC in Hepatobiliary and pancreatic surgery – a companion to specialist surgical practice 2009). Use of a somatostatin analogue remains controversial. Surgery is reserved for failures of conservative treatment. Bleeding from gastric varices related to segmental portal vein thrombosis is uncommon, thus the authors recommend intervention only once there is proven bleeding from gastric varices. Haemorrhage related to a pseudoaneurysm is best dealt with via selective angiography and embolisation due to the hazards of surgery in this setting. Surgery is reserved for failure of angiographic treatment.

4. Surgery for chronic pancreatitis – Drainage procedures

For many years longitudinal pancreaticojejunostomy (LPJ) as described by Partington and Rochelle in 1960 was the favoured surgical option in the treatment of chronic pancreatitis. This involves entering and laying open of the pancreatic duct followed by a splenic preserving pancreaticojejunostomy without resection of the pancreatic tail (Partington PF, Rochelle REL. Ann Surg 1960). This procedure is relatively simple in comparison to many of the other available operations and has a low mortality and morbidity with maximal pancreatic tissue preserved. Pain relief in the short term approximates 75% but there is frequently recurrence in the long term (Bachmann K Best Pract and res Clin Gastro 2010). This is thought to be due to incomplete decompression of the main pancreatic duct, particularly in the head. There remains a residual inflammatory mass containing altered nerve fibres (Pessaux P Pancreas 2006) as well as obstructed second and third order ducts causing ongoing intraductal hypertension (Markowitz JS Arch Surg 1994). Current indications for this procedure are isolated dilatation of the pancreatic duct greater than 7mm or where the duct has a "chain of lakes" appearance without an inflammatory mass in the head (Yekebas EF Ann Surg 2006). Where the duct is undilated (less than 3mm) a longitudinal V-shaped excision of the ventral pancreas combined with a longitudinal pancreatico-jejunostomy has been described (Izbicki JR Ann Surg 1998, 227). This may be particularly useful when a sclerosing form of chronic pancreatitis results in so called small duct disease (Bachmann K Best Pract and res Clin Gastro 2010). Good results with pain relief in 89% of patients and comparable morbidity of 19.6% have been reported (Yekebas EF Ann Surg 2006).

5. Surgery for chronic pancreatitis – Resectional procedures

With recognition that inflamed, fibrotic tissue containing damaged neural structures within the pancreatic head is critical in the generation of symptoms, pancreaticoduodenectomy became the gold standard in surgical treatment against which other procedures were measured. It has been assumed that outcomes concerning pain and quality of life are better than simple drainage procedures performed in isolation, however clear evidence of this is in randomized trials is lacking.

In the modern era, pylorus preservation as in a Pylorus Preserving Pancreaticoduodenectomy (PPPD) has been shown to result in less pain and nausea and improved quality of life when compared with the traditional Whipples pancreaticoduodenectomy (Mobius C Langenbecks Arch Surg 2007). This procedure can be performed with a mortality of 5-10% and morbidity of 20-40% and improves pain and quality of life in both the short and long term in up to 90% of patients (Bachmann K Best Pract and res Clin Gastro 2010). There are however a number of disadvantages relating to the sacrifice of functional pancreatic parenchyma and the non-diseased duodenum and common bile duct. The loss of natural bowel continuity and reduced endocrine and exocrine function result in side effects and reduced quality of life (Izbicki JR Ann Surg 1998 (228); Koninger J Surgery 2008). In order to allow organ preservation and reduce adverse effects, duodenum preserving resections of the pancreatic head (DPPHR) were developed. The Beger procedure was introduced in 1980 and was the first to include these principles (Beger HG Chirurg 1980). It consists of a subtotal resection of the head following transection of the pancreas above the portal vein. The Pancreas is then drained by an end-to-side or end-to-end pancreaticojejunostomy using a Roux-en-Y loop. Physiological gastroduodenal passage and CBD continuity are therefore preserved. This procedure could be performed with low mortality (0-3%) and morbidity (15-32%) and long term pain relief in 75-95% of patients (Izbicki JR Ann Surg 1995, Buechler MW J Gastrointest Surg 1997Frey CF Ann Surg 1994). The Frey procedure (Frey CF Pancreas 1987) subsequently combined an LPJ (as described by Partington and Rochelle) with a limited duodenum preserving excision of the head. Following exploration of the main pancreatic duct well into both the head and the tail, the head is cored out leaving a small cuff of parenchyma along the duodenal wall. This results in a lesser resection of the head than that described by Beger. In further contrast to the Beger operation, the pancreas is not divided over the SMV/portal vein complex making it an easier operation to perform. Care is taken not to enter the CBD. Drainage of the resection cavity within the head and from the opened main pancreatic duct within the body and tail is obtained with an LPJ using a Roux-en-Y loop (Frey CF Pancreas 1987). Good results have been obtained with substantial pain relief in more than 85% of patients while mortality is less than 1% and morbidity 9-39% (Izbicki JR Ann Surg 1995, Izbicki JR Ann Surg 1998, Beger HG Ann Surg 1989). Endocrine & exocrine function are well preserved and the operation may control complications such as CBD stenosis, duodenal stenosis and internal pancreatic fistulas. The Frey operation is currently the most widely performed operation for patients with an inflammatory mass in the head together with pancreatic duct dilatation while the Beger procedure is reserved for patients where the main pancreatic duct is not dilated (Bornman PC S Afr Med J 2010).

Two further modifications of the above procedures have been described. The Hamburg operation employs subtotal excision of the pancreatic head including the uncinate process(a more extensive resection than the Frey operation but comparable to Beger's procedure) together with a V-shaped excision of the ventral aspect of pancreas into the pancreatic duct. Pancreatic-enteric continuity is re-established with an LPJ using a Roux-en-Y loop (comparable to the Partington-Rochelle and Frey reconstructions).This operation combines aspects of the Frey and Beger procedures, without transection of gland over SMV/portal vein. The extent of resection is customized to pancreatic morphology while the V-shaped excicion creates a trough-like new ductal system allowing better drainage of ductal side branches (Izbicki JR Ann Surg 1998, 227, Bachmann K Med Sci Monit 2008). In the Berne operation, an extensive duodenum-preserving resection of the head is performed (as in the

Beger procedure), but without division of pancreas anterior to superior mesenteric / portal vein complex and without laying open the pancreatic duct in the body and tail. In biliary obstruction a longitudinal opening may be made in the CBD within the cavity created in the pancreatic head. Drainage of the cavity is achieved with a pancreatic-enteric anastamosis to small bowel in a Roux-en-Y reconstruction similar to the reconstructions described above. Results of the Berne procedure are comparable to the other duodenum preserving resections (Gloor B Dig Surg 2001).

Little comparative data is available to guide choice between the various available procedures in CP. Four randomized controlled trials have been conducted comparing PPPD with DPPHR, with 2 providing long term follow up (table 1). In the short to medium term,

	Follow up	Procedure	Mortality	Morbidity	Pain free	Pain relief	Better QOL	Endocrine function	Exocrine function	Weight gain
Buchler 1995	6 months							Glucose tolerance at 150min	Pancreolauryl test: pre- vs post-op	
		PPPD (n=20; FU 15)	0	4	6	4	8	130mg/dL	2.05µg/mL (0.48-6.6) vs 1.13µg/mL (0-4.87)	1.9+/- 1.2kg
		Beger (n=20; FU 16)	0	3	12	3	12	88mg/dL	2.7µg/mL (0-8.25) vs 1.4µg/mL (0-4.41)	4.1+/- 10.9kg
		P value	NS	NS	<0.05	Not stated	NS	<0.01	NS	<0.05
Klempa 1995	36 to 60 months							New onset IDDM	Steatorrhea; enzyme substitution	
		PPPD (n=21; FU 20)	1	5		14		6	20;20	Mean 4.9kg
		Beger (n=22; FU 20)	0	4		20		2	3;4	Mean 6,4Kg
		P value	NS	NS		<0.05		Not stated	<0.05	not stated
Izbicki 1998	12 - 36 months					Pan relief; median pain score (range)	Median post-op global QOL score; prof rehab	Insulin dose or Glucose tolerance: improved vs worsened	Abnormal faecal chymotrpsin, pancreolauryl test	Median (range)
		PPPD (n=30; FU 30)	0	16 (53%)		28; 18.1 (0-37.5)	85.7 (71.4-100); 13	0 vs 6	7	6.7kg (3.1-9.2)
		Frey (n=31; FU 31)	1	6 (19%)		26; 6.1 (0-40)	57.1 (33.3-100); 21	3 vs 2	1	1.9kg (0-6.3)
		P value	NS	<0.05		NS; not stated	<0.05; <0.05	Not stated	Not stated	Not stated
Farkas 2006	12 months						Prof rehab	New onset DM	Stool elastase: pre- vs post op	

	Follow up	Procedure	Mortality	Morbidity	Pain free	Pain relief	Better QOL	Endocrine function	Exocrine function	Weight gain
		PPPD (n=20; FU 20)	0	8	18	2	11/17	3	128 +/- 29µg/g vs 122.2 +/- 23 µg/g	7.8+/- 0.9kg
		Berne (n=20; FU 20)	0	0	17	3	14/18	0	124.3 +/- 33µg/g vs 132.7 +/- 39µg/g	3.2+/- 0.3kg
		P value	NS	<0.05	NS	NS	NS	NS	NS	<0.05
Muller 2008 (FU of Buchler 1995)	14 years					Median pain score	EORTC QLQ 30 – global health status (s.d.)	Presence of IDDM; new onset DM	Enzyme substitution	
		PPPD (n=20; FU=14)	5			0	58.3 (34.2)	11; 6/9	8/14	
		Beger (n=20; FU= 15)	5			0	65.0 (22.3)	7; 4/11	8/15	
		P value	NS - Mortality unrelated to surgery	N		S N	S , apart from greater appetite loss in PPPD group	0.128; 0.327	NS	
Strate 2008 (FU of Izbicki 1998)	median of 7 years					Pain score	EORTC Global quality of life	Presence of DM or abnormal glucose tolerance test	Abnormal faecal chymotrpsin	
		PPPD (n=30; FU 23)	4			18.75 (0-75)	50 (0-100)	15/23	22/23	
		Frey (n=30; FU 24)	6			17.5 (0-100)	58.35 (0-83.4)	13/23	18/21	
		P value				0.821	0.974	0.672	0.335	
		3 patients lost to FU							3 patients did not attend for assessment	

QOL= quality of life; pre-op= pre-operative; post-op= post-operative; FU= follow up; PPPD= pylorus preserving pancreatico-duodenectomy; NS= not significant; IDDM= insulin dependant diabetes mellitus; DM= diabetes mellitus: Prof rehab= professional rehabilitation; EORTC= European Organisation for Research and Treatment of Cancer; QLQ= Quality of Life Questionnaire; s.d= standard deviation
Buchler MW Am J Surg 1995
Klempa I Chirurg 1995
Izbicki JR Ann Surg 1998; 228
Farkas G Langenbecks Arch Surg 2006
Muller MW Br J Surg 2008
Strate T Gastroenterology 2008

Table 1. Outcomes of Pylorus preserving pancreaticoduodenectomy (PPPD) vs duodenum preserving pancreatic head resection (DPPHR)

	Follow up	Procedure	Mortality	morbidity	Pain relief	QOL	Endocrine function	Exocrine function	Weight gain
Izbicki 1995	Mean 1.5 yrs (6-24 months)				Pre-op vs post-op pain score	Prof rehab; post-op global QOL score	worsened DM control; new onset DM; newly abnormal Oral GTT	New faecal chymotrypsin/ Pancreolauryl test abnormality on post-operative FU	
		Beger (n=20)	0	6	62.25; 3	14; 28.6	2; 0; 1	2	6.7 +/- 2.1kg
		Frey (n=22)	0	2	61.50; 4	15; 28.6	0; 0; 1	2	6.4 +/- 2.5kg
		P value	NS	<0.05	NS	NS; NS	Not stated	NS	Not stated
						Less fatigue with Beger			
Strate 2005 (FU of Izbicki 1995)	Median 8.5 yrs (72-144 months)			Pancreas related repeat surgery	Pain score	global QOL score; Prof rehab	Presence of DM	Abnormal faecal pancreatic elastase	
		Beger (n=38; FU= 26)	8	3	11.25 (0 - 75)	66.7 (0-100); 16	14/25	22/25	
		Frey (n=36; FU=25)	8	0	11.25 (0 - 99.75)	58.35 (0-83.4); 11	15/25	18/23	
		P value	NS	0.08	0.679	0.476; NS	0.774	0.157	
		7 patients lost to FU (Beger 4, Frey 3)					1 patient declined testing	3 patients declined testing	
Köninger 2008	6 months and 2 years					EORTC QLQ-C30, QLQ-PAN26 scores			

	Follow up	Procedure	Mortality	morbidity	Pain relief	QOL	Endocrine function	Exocrine function	Weight gain
		Beger (n=32; FU=30 and 26)		6		65.6 +/- 24.8, 63.9 +/- 23.7			
		Berne (n=33; FU=32 and 29)		7		71.3 +/- 21.6, 75.8 +/- 15.7			
		P value		>9.9		0.371, 0.037			
		Patients analysed on intention to treat; but 8 in Beger and 6 in Berne groups had technique converted							

QOL= quality of life; pre-op= pre-operative; post-op= post-operative; GTT= glucose tolerance test; FU= follow up; NS= not significant; DM= diabetes mellitus: Prof rehab= professional rehabilitation; EORTC= European Organisation for Research and Treatment of Cancer; QLQ= Quality of Life Questionnaire

Izbicki JR Ann Surg 1995

Strate T Ann Surg 2005

Koninger J Surgery 2008

Table 2. Comparisons of duodenum preserving resections of the pancreatic head.

there was evidence for significant benefit of DPPHR over PPPD in terms of morbidity (2 trials), pain relief (2 trials), quality of life (1 trial), endocrine function (1 trial), exocrine function (1 trial) and weight gain (2 trials). In addition, 2 trials showed a benefit for DPPHR in terms of operating time while hospital stay and requirement for blood transfusion were improved in 1 trial each. A Cochrane review on short term outcomes concluded that there was benefit for DPPHR in respect of quality of life and professional rehabilitation, exocrine insufficiency, weight gain, hospital stay and intra-operative blood replacement. There was also a trend towards reduced post-operative diabetes (Diener MK Ann Surg 2008). However, in the 2 studies examining long term outcomes, it was seen that many of the short term clinical benefits described above were not maintained. Proposed reasons for this were study error related to the small population sizes studied and that pancreatic gland burn-out might be delayed by DPPHR (Muller MW Br J Surg 2008). Nevertheless, at 14 year follow up there remained a trend towards better endocrine function, while there was significant benefit in terms of appetite, subjective feeling of well being and mean period of employment after surgery for patients undergoing DPPHR(Muller MW Br J Surg 2008). Thus, while short term results favour DPPHR over PPPD in CP, long term results appear equivalent and probably reflect the natural course of the disease.

Only 2 randomized trials have compared different DPPHR procedures, with 1 trial undergoing long term follow up (table 2). The first trial compared the Beger and Frey procedures with no significant differences being found in the short term apart from a benefit for the Frey operation in terms of morbidity. After a median of 8.5 years, all variables had comparable outcomes while almost all patients were noted to be exocrine insufficient (Izbicki JR Ann Surg 1995; Strate T Ann Surg 2005). The second study compared the Beger and Berne procedures, suggesting a benefit for the Berne operation in terms of operation time and hospital stay. Results were analysed on intention to treat basis however, including 8 out of 32 (Beger procedure) and 6 out of 33 (Berne procedure) patients who had their operations altered for technical reasons. When patients were analysed per protocol ie only those who underwent their assigned procedure, only the difference in operating times remained significant.

More extensive pancreatic resections such as total or near total distal pancreatectomy offer only short term relief and are associated with significant mortality and morbidity, often as a result of markedly reduced pancreatic function. They have largely been abandoned with their main role being as salvage procedures for complications relating to previous surgical interventions (including anastamotic leakage, pancreatic fistula and intractable pain following previous adequate resection or drainage surgery).

6. Surgery for the complications of chronic pancreatitis

Surgery for the complications of CP should be individualized to cater to a patient's specific morphology and clinical presentation.

6.1 Biliary obstruction

Choledocho-duodenostomy or hepatico-jejunostomy using a Roux-en-Y loop are the preferred procedures to resolve isolated biliary obstruction although the former may result in enteric refux and a sump-like syndrome. Cholecysto-enterostomy has been associated with poor results and has fallen into disfavour. A Hepatico-jejunostomy may be included in the Roux loop used to drain the pancreatic duct in dedicated drainage, resection or hybrid procedures performed to relieve pain. Alternatively, the CBD may opened within the surgically created cavity in the pancreatic head during the Berne procedure.

6.2 Duodenal obstruction

Surgical relief of obstruction related to a fibrotic stricture involves duodenal mobilization by Kocher's maneouvre with division of all fibrotic tissue. Should this be insufficient to restore patency, duodeno-duodenostomy or a gastro-jejunostomy may be considered, although the latter may be associated with biliary reflux. Where biliary obstruction co-exists in the presence of duodenal obstruction together with an inflammatory mass in the head, two options exist: PPPD or gastric bypass with a gastro-jejunostomy as part of the Roux drainage limb in a DPPHR.

6.3 Development of a pseudocyst

The choice of surgical procedure is dictated by the location of the pseudocyst and its proximity to a section of bowel suitable for drainage. Cyst-gastrostomy, cyst-duodenostomy and cyst-jejunostomy may all be employed depending on individual patient characteristics. Distal pancreatectomy may be employed for segmental disease within the body/tail together with an associated pseudocyst (Bornman PC S Afr Med J 2010). Surgery for pancreatic fistulae / ascites entails either a roux-en-Y jejunostomy to the fistula tract or an appropriate resection.

6.4 Gastro-intestinal bleeding, related to

a. Portal hypertension

Patients who have bled from gastric varices related to segmental portal hypertension as a consequence of splenic vein thrombosis can usually be managed with distal pancreatectomy.

b. Pseudoaneurysms

Where angiographic embolisation has failed to control a bleeding pseudoaneurysm vascular control may be achieved using a Frey-type procedure in preference to a more extensive resection which may be hazardous under these circumstances, while bleeding from the tail can usually be dealt with safely by means of a distal pancreatectomy (Bornman PC S Afr Med J 2010).

Surgery for suspected malignancy should utilize either a pancreatico-duodenectomy or distal pancreatectomy depending on tumour location and should be performed in keeping with the oncological principle of clear resection margins.

7. Conclusion

The pathophysiology of chronic pancreatitis is complex and as yet incompletely understood, confounding attempts at effective management strategies. The clinical picture is dominated by progressive pain which may become intractable and pancreatic endocrine and exocrine dysfunction which may severely impact on a patient's quality of life. Surgery aims to relieve ductal and tissue hypertension related to obstruction in the main and side branch ducts while also removing inflamed and fibrotic parenchymal tissue containing diseased nerve fibres. Duodenal preserving pancreatic head resections, usually combined with drainage of the main pancreatic duct, achieve both objectives with short and long term relief of pain in approximately 90% of patients at 5 year follow up. By preserving some parenchymal tissue these procedures attempt to limit pancreatic functional insufficiency. With acceptable morbidity and mortality figures, they have evolved as the surgical procedure of choice for the majority of patients with pain refractory to medical treatment. Surgery for complications of CP should be individualized while resection for neoplastic disease should be performed according to oncological principles, ensuring a clear margin of resection. More extensive resections should generally only be performed as salvage procedures for complications of previous surgery. Patients requiring surgery for chronic pancreatitis should be evaluated and treated by experienced surgeons in high volume centres utilizing a multi-disciplinary approach. Prior to undergoing surgery for pain, patients should have completed an adequate trial of medical therapy and been thoroughly counseled regarding the risks of surgery and its likely outcomes.

8. References

[1] Abdallah AA, Krige JEJ, Bornman PC. Biliary tract obstruction in chronic pancreatitis. HPB 2007; 9: 421-428

[2] Amman RW, Akovbiantz A, Largiader F et al. Course and outcome of chronic pancreatitis. Longitudinal study of a mixed medical-surgical series of 245 patients. Gastroenterol 1984; 86: 820-828

[3] Bachmann K, Izbicki JR, Yekebas EF. Chronic pancreatitis: modern surgical management Langenbecks Arch Surg. 2011 Feb; 396(2):139-49.

[4] Bachmann K, Kutup A, Mann O et al. Surgical treatment in chronic pancreatitis timing and type of procedure. Best Pract and res Clin Gastro 2010; 24: 299-310

[5] Bachmann K, Mann O, Izbicki JR et al. Chronic pancreatitis – a surgeons' view. Med Sci Monit 2008; 14:RA 198-205

[6] Beckingham IJ, Krige JEJ, Bornman PC et al. Endoscopic management of pancreatic pseudocysts. Br J Surg 1997; 84: 1638-1645

[7] Beger HG, Büchler M. Duodenum preserving resection of the head of the pancreas in chronic pancreatitis with inflammatory mass in the head. World J Surg 1990; 14: 83-87

[8] Beger HG, Buechler M, Bittner R et al: Duodenum preserving resection of the head of the pancreas in severe chronic pancreatitis. Ann Surg 1989: 209: 273-278

[9] Beger HG, Witte C, Krautzberger W et al. [Experiences with duodenum-sparing pancreas head resection in chronic pancreatitis]. Chirurg 1980; 51: 303-307

[10] Bockman DE, Büchler M, Malfertheiner P et al. Analysis of nerves in chronic pancreatitis. Gastroenterol 1988; 94: 1459-146

[11] Bordalo O, Goncalves D, Noronha M et al. Newer concept for the pathogenesis of chronic alcoholic pancreatitis. Am J Gastroenterol 1977; 68:278-285

[12] Bornman PC (Eds) O James Garden 4th edition. Chronic pancreatitis. Hepatobiliary and pancreatic surgery – a companion to specialist surgical practice. WB Saunders Co Ltd, London, Edinburgh, New York 2009: 259-283

[13] Bornman PC, Botha JF, Ramos JM et al. Guidelines for the diagnosis and treatment of chronic pancreatitis. S Afr Med J 2010; 100(12): 845-860

[14] Bornman PC, Marks IN, Girdwood AW et al. Pathogenesis of Pain in Chronic Pancreatitis: Ongoing Enigma. W J Surg 2003; 27: 1175-1182

[15] Bornman PC, Marks IN, Girdwood AW et al. Is pancreatic duct obstruction or stricture a major cause of pain in calcific pancreatitis. Br J Surg 1980; 67: 425-428

[16] Braganza JM. A framework for the aetiogenesis of chronic pancreatitis Digestion 1998; 58(suppl 4): 1-12

[17] Braganza JM, Dormandy TL. Micronutrient therapy for chronic pancreatitis: rationale and impact. JOP 2010; 11: 99-112

[18] Braganza JM, Lee SH, McCloy RF et al. Chronic pancreatitis. The Lancet 2011; 377, April 2: 1184 – 1197

[19] Buchler MW, Friess H, Muller MW et al. Randomised trial of duodenum-preserving pancreatic head resection versus pylorus-preserving Whipple in chronic pancreatitis. Am J Surg 1995; 169: 65-69

[20] Büchler M, Weihe E, Friess H et al. Changes in peptidergic innervations in chronic pancreatitis. Pancreas 1992; 7: 182-192

[21] Buechler MW, Friess H, Bittner R et al. Duodenum-preserving pancreatic head resection: long term results. J Gastrointest Surg 1997; 1: 13-19

[22] Cavallini G. Is chronic pancreatitis a primary disease of the pancreatic ducts. A new pathogenetic hypothesis. Ital J Gastroenterol 1993; 25:400-407

[23] Clain JE, Pearson RK. Diagnosis of chronic pancreatitis: is a gold standard necessary? Surg Clin North Am 1999; 79: 829-845

[24] Comfort MW, Gaubill EE, Baggenstos AM. Chronic pancreatitis: a study of 29 cases without associated disease of the biliary or gastro-intestinal tract. Gastroenterology 1946; 6:239

[25] Cook LJ, Musa OA, Case RM. Intracellular transport of pancreatic enzymes. Scand J Gastroenterol 1996; 219(suppl): 1-5

[26] D'Egidio A, Schein M. Pancreatic pseudocysts: a proposed classification and its management implications. BJS 1991; 78(8): 981-984

[27] Diener MK, Rahbari NN, Fisher L et al. Duodenum-preserving pancreatic head resection versus pancreaticoduodenectomy for surgical treatment of chronic pancreatitis: a systemic review and meta-analysis. Ann Surg 2008; 247: 950-961

[28] Ebbehøj N, Borly L, Bülow J et al. Evaluation of pancreatic tissue fluidpressure and pain in chronic pancreatitis. A longitudinal study. Scand J Gastroenterol. 1990; 25: 462-466

[29] Farkas G, Leindler L, Daroczi M et al. Long term follow-up after organ preserving pancreatic head resection in patients with chronic pancreatitis. J Gastrointest Surg 2008; 12: 308-312

[30] Farkas G, Leindler L, Daroczi M et al. Prospective randomised comparison of organ preserving pancreatic head resection with pylorus-preserving pancreaticoduodenectomy. Langenbecks Arch Surg 2006; 391: 338-342

[31] Foster JR. Toxicology of the exocrine pancreas. In: Ballantyne B, Marrs T, Syversen T eds. General and applied toxicology, 3rd edition. Chichester: John Wiley and sons, 2009: 1411-1455

[32] Foster JR, Idle JR, Hardwick JP et al. Induction of drug metabolisingenzymes in in human pancreatic cancer and chronic pancreatitis. J Pathol 1993; 169: 457-463

[33] Friess H, Zhu ZW, di Mola FF et al. Nerve growth factor and its high affinity receptor in chronic pancreatitis. Ann Surg 1999; 230: 615-624

[34] Frey CF, Amikura K. Local resection of the head of the pancreas combined with longitudinal pancreaticojejunostomy in the management of patients with chronic pancreatitis. Ann Surg 1994; 220: 492-507

[35] Frey CF, Smith GJ. Description and rationale of a new operation for chronic pancreatitis. Pancreas 1987; 2: 701-707

[36] Garg PK, Tandon RK. Survey on chronic pancreatitis in the Asia-Pacific region. J Gastroenterol Hepatol 2004; 19: 998-1004

[37] Graf R, Scheisser M, Reding T. Exocrine meets endocrine: pancreatic stone protein and regenerating protein – two sides of the same coin. J Surg Res 2006; 133: 113-120

[38] Girdwood AH, Marks IN, Bornman PC et al. Does progressive pancreatic insufficiency limit pain in calcific pancreatitis with duct stricture or continued alcohol insult. J Clin Gastroenterol 1981; 3:241-245

[39] Gloor B, Friess H, Uhl W et al. A modified technique of the Beger and Frey procedure in patients with chronic pancreatitis. Dig Surg 2001; 18: 21-25

[40] Izbicki JR, Bloechle C, Broering DC et al. Extended drainage versus resection in surgery for chronic pancreatitis – prospective randomized trial comparing the longitudinal pancreaticojejunostomy combined with local pancreatic head excision with the pylorus preserving pancreaticoduodenectomy. Ann Surg 1998; 228: 771-779

[41] Izbicki JR, Bloechle C, Broering DC et al. Longitudinal V-shaped excision of the ventral pancreas for small duct disease in severe chronic pancreatitis. Ann Surg 1998; 227: 213-219

[42] Izbicki JR, Bloechle C, Knoefel WT et al. Complications of adjacent organs in chronic pancreatitis managed by duodenum preserving resection of the head of the pancreas. Br J Surg 1994; 81: 1351-1355

[43] Izbicki JR, Bloechle C, Knoefel WT et al. Duodenum preserving resections of the head of the pancreas in chronic pancreatitis – a prospective randomized trial. Ann Surg 1995; 221: 350-358

[44] Jalleh RP, Aslam M, Williamson RCN. Pancreatic tissue and ductal pressures in chronic pancreatitis. Br J Surg 1991; 78: 1235-1237

[45] Jensen AR, Matzen P, Malchow-Møller A et al. Pattern of pain, duct morphology and pancreatic function in chronic pancreatitis. A comparative study. Scand J Gastroent 1984; 9: 334-338

[46] Karanjia ND, Widdison AL, Leung F et al. Compartment syndrome in experimental chronic obstructive pancreatitis: effects of decompressing the main pancreatic duct. Br J Surg 1994; 81: 259-264

[47] Klempa I, Spatny M, Menzel J et al. Pankreasfunktion und lebensqualität nach pankreaskopfresektion bei der chronischen pankreatitis. Chirurg 1995; 66: 350-359

[48] Kloppel G, Maillet B. Chronic pancreatitis: evolution of the disease. Hepatogastroenterol 1991; 38: 408-412

[49] Koninger J, Seiler CM, Sauerland S et al. Duodenum-preserving pancreatic head resection – a randomised controlled trial comparing the original Beger procedure with the Berne modification. Surgery 2008; 143: 490-498

[50] Kozarek RA. Endoscopic therapy of complete and partial pancreatic duct disruption. Gastrointest Endosc Clin North Am 1998; 8: 39-53

[51] Lankisch PG, Löhr-Happe A, Otto J et al. Natural course in chronic pancreatitis. Pain, exocrine and endocrine pancreatic insufficiency and prognosis of the disease. Digestion 1993; 54: 148-155

[52] Leung P, Chan YC. Role of oxidative stress in pancreatic inflammation. Antioxid Redox Signal 2009; 11: 135-165

[53] McMahon SP, Bennett DL, Priestly JV et al. The biological effects of endogenous nerve growth factor on adult sensory nerves revealed by a tryA-IgG fusion molecule. Nat Med 1995; 1: 774-780

[54] Manes G, Büchler M, Pieramico O et al. Is increased pancreatic pressure related to pain in chronic pancreatitis? Int J Pancreatol 1994; 15: 113-117

[55] Markowitz JS, Rattner DW, Warshaw AL. Failure of symptomatic relief after pancreaticojejunal decompression for chronic pancreatitis. Strategies for salvage. Arch Surg 1994; 129: 374-379

[56] Mobius C, Max D, Uhlmann D et al. Five-year follow -up of a prospective non-randomized study comparing duodenum-preserving pancreatic head resection with classic Whipple procedure in the treatment of chronic pancreatitis. Langenbecks Arch Surg 2007; 392: 359-364

[57] Muller MW, Friess H, Martin DJ et al. Long term follow-up of a randomized clinical trial comparing Beger with pylorus-preserving Whipple procedure for chronic pancreatitis. Br J Surg 2008; 95: 350-356

[58] Nagata A, Homma T, Tamai K et al. A study of chronic pancreatitis by serial endoscopic pancreatography. Gatroenteology 1981; 81: 884-891

[59] Nealon WH, Thompson JC. Progressive loss of pancreatic function in chronic pancreatitis is delayed by main pancreatic duct decompression – a longitudinal prospective analysis of the modified Peustow procedure. Ann Surg 1993; 217: 458-468

[60] Novis BH, Bornman PC, Girdwood AH et al. Endoscopic manometry of the pancreatic duct and sphincter zone in patients with chronic pancreatitis. Dig Dis Sc 1985; 30:225-228

[61] Okazaki K, Yamamoto Y, Ito K et al. Endoscopic measurement of papillary sphincter zone and pancreatic main ductal pressure in patients with chronic pancreatitis. Gastroenterology 1986; 91: 409-418

[62] Pandol SJ, Raraty M. Pathobiology of alcoholic pancreatitis. Pancreatology 2007; 7:105-114

[63] Partington PF, Rochelle REL. Modified Puestow procedure for retrograde drainage of the pancreatic duct. Ann Surg1960; 152: 1037-43

[64] Patel AG, Toyoma MT, Alvarez C et al. Pancreatic interstitial pH in human and feline chronic pancreatitis. Gastroenterology 1995; 109: 1639-1645

[65] Pessaux P, Kianmanesh R, Regimbeau JM et al. Frey procedure in the treatment of chronic pancreatitis: short term results. Pancreas 2006; 33: 354-358

[66] Salim AS. Perspectives in pancreatic pain. HPB Surg 1997; 10: 269-277

[67] Sanfey H, Bulkley B, Cameron JL. The role of oxygen derived free radicals in the pathogenesis of acute pancreatitis. Ann Surg 1984; 200:405-413

[68] Sarles H. Etiopathogenesis and definition of chronic pancreatitis. Dig Dis Sci 1986; 11(suppl): s91-107

[69] Shrikhande SV, Martignoni ME, Shrikhande M et al. Comparison of histological features and inflammatory cell reaction in alcoholic, idiopathic and tropical chronic pancreatitis. Br J Surg 2003; 90: 1565-1572

[70] Singh SM, Reber HA. The pathology of chronic pancreatitis. W J Surg 1990; 14: 2-10

[71] Stevens T, Conwell DL, Zuccaro G. Pathogenesis of chronic pancreatitis: an evidence-based review of past theories and recent developments. Am J Gastroenterol 2004; 99: 2256-2270

[72] Strate T, Bachman K, Busch P et al. Resection vs drainage in treatment of chronic pancreatitis: long term results of a randomized trial. Gastroenterology 2008; 134: 1406-1411

[73] Strate T, Knoefel WT, Yekebas E et al. Chronic pancreatitis: etiology, pathogenesis, diagnosis and treatment. Int J Colorectal Dis 2003; 18: 97-106

[74] Strate T, Taherpour Z, Bloechle C et al. Long-term follow-up of a randomized trial comparing the Beger and Frey procedures for patients suffering from chronic pancreatitis. Ann Surg 2005; 241: 591-598

[75] Ugljesic M, Bulajic M, Milosavljevic T et al. Endoscopic manometry of the sphincter of Oddi and pancreatic duct in patients with chronic pancreatitis. Int J Pancreatol. 1996; 19: 191-195

[76] Wells RG, Crawford JM. Pancreatic stellate cells. The new stars of chronic pancreatitis? Gastroenterol 1998; 115: 491-493

[77] Whitcomb DC, Schneider A. Hereditary pancreatitis: a model for inflammatory disease of the pancreas. Best Pract Res Clin Gastroenterol 2002; 16: 347-363

[78] Zhu ZW, Friess H, Wang L et al. Brain derived neurotrophic factor (BDNF) is upregulated and associated with pain in chronic pancreatitis. Dig Dis Sci 2001; 46: 1633-1639

[79] Warshaw AL. Pain in chronic pancreatitis: patients, patience and the impatient surgeon. Gastroenterol 1984; 86: 987-989

[80] Warshaw AL, Popp JL, Schapiro RH. Long-term patency, pancreatic function, and pain relief after lateral pancreaticojejunostomy for chronic pancreatitis. Gastroenterol 1980; 79: 289-293

[81] Yekebas EF, Bogoevski D, Honarpisheh H et al. Long-term follow-up in small duct chronic pancreatitis: a plea for extended drainage by "V-shaped excision" of the anterior aspect of the pancreas. Ann Surg 2006; 244:940-946

21

The Influence of Colonic Irrigation on Human Intestinal Microbiota

Yoko Uchiyama-Tanaka
Yoko Clinic
Japan

1. Introduction

It has been documented that the intestinal tract is inhabited by more than 10^{12} bacterial cells per gram of dry matter (Hayashi et al., 2002a; Langendijk et al., 1995; Suau et al., 1999), which is comprised of an estimated 400 to 500 bacterial species (Moor & Holdeman, 1974). The composition and activities of the indigenous intestinal microbiota are of paramount importance in human immunity, nutrition, and pathological processes, and therefore, the health of the individual (Van der Waaij et al., 1971). It is well established that the intestine is an important site of local immunity, and recent reports have suggested that it is a major site of extrathymic T cell differentiation (Cerf-Bensussan et al., 1985; Guy-Grand et al., 1991; Iiai eta al., 2002; Uchiyama-Tanaka, 2009). Numerous activated and quiescent lymphocytes are produced within gut-associated lymphatic tissues (GALT), such as Peyer's patches (Takahashi et al., 2005). Thus, it has been speculated that people who suffer from constipation and who harbor fecal residues in the intestine may have decreased local immune system function.

Colonic irrigations referred to as a colonics are a type of colonic hydrotherapy performed using an instrument in combination with abdominal massage, but without drugs or mechanical pressure. I previously reported that colonic irrigation may induce lymphocyte transmigration from GALT into the circulation, which may improve the functions of both the colon and immune system (Uchiyama-Tanaka, 2009). Colonic irrigation was developed about 40 years ago and no serious complications associated with its use have been reported. However, the impact of this method, which use a large amount of water, on the intestinal microbiota and serum electrolytes remains unknown. In this study, colonic irrigations were performed 3 times for each of the 10 subjects with no history of malignant or inflammatory disease.

2. Materials and methods

2.1 Study design and subjects

The procedures used in this study were in accordance with the guidelines of the Declaration of Helsinki for Human Experimentation, 2000 and all subjects provided informed consent. Ten outpatients from the Yoko Clinic (4 men and 6 women; mean age=38 ± 6 years; age range: 27–47 years) admitted to the hospital between April and May 2009 were enrolled in this study. None of the subjects had cancer or any active inflammatory disease.

2.2 Analysis of fecal microbiotauction

Fecal samples were collected before the first colonic irrigation and at 1 week after the third irrigation. These samples were analyzed using a kit from TechnoSuruga Laboratory Co., Ltd. (Shizuoka Japan). Fecal microbiota analysis targeted bacterial 16S rRNA genes with a terminal restriction fragment length polymorphism (T-RFLP) analysis program (Nagashima's method) (Ando et al., 2007; Nagashima et al. 2002, 2006). T-RFLP was performed as previously described by Nagashima et al. (2002, 2006). The 16S rRNA genes were amplified using a forward primaer, 516f [5′-TGCCAGCAGCCGCGGTA-3′] and a reverse primer, 1510r [5′-GGTTACCTTGTTACGACTT-3′]. The 5′ ends of the forward primer, 516f were labeled with 6′-carboxyfluorescein, which was synthesized by Applied Biosystems Japan (Tokyo, Japan). The purified PCR products (2 µL) were digested with 10 U of either BslI (New England BioLabs, Inc., Ipswich, MA, USA) at 55°C for 3 h. The lengths of terminal restriction fragments were determined with the ABI PRISM 3130xl Genetic Analyzer (Applied Biosystems, Tokyo, japan).

2.3 Laboratory determinations

Blood samples were collected from the subjects in a sitting position before the start and at 10 min after the third irrigation. Serum samples were analyzed using a commercial kit.

2.4 Colonic irrigations

Each patient underwent 3 colonic irrigations over a period 2 weeks. Same trained physician performed colonic irrigations for all subjects. Irrigations using an intestinal irrigation devide (Colon Hydromat Comfort: Herrmann Apparatebau GmbH, Kleinwallstadt, Germany) that circulated approximately 30–50 L of purified warm water (38°C) through a filter (Uchiyama-Tanaka, 2009). During an irrigation process, which lasts for approximately 1 hour, a subject is laid supine on a bed and given abdominal massage. Because colonic irrigations utilize a large amount of water introduced using a tube and abdominal massage, there are some contraindications, such as renal failure, heart failure, liver cirrhosis, severe hemorrhoids, after post-intestinal polypectomy, post-abdominal surgery and pregnacy. The principle of the Colon Hydromat Comfort's function is shown in Figure1.

Filtered hot water and ordinary water are mixed and passed into a patient's colon through the speculum. The sewage water flows out due to the pressure in the water-filled colon. Some pictures of fecal residues and intestinal epithelium during colon irrigations are shown below.

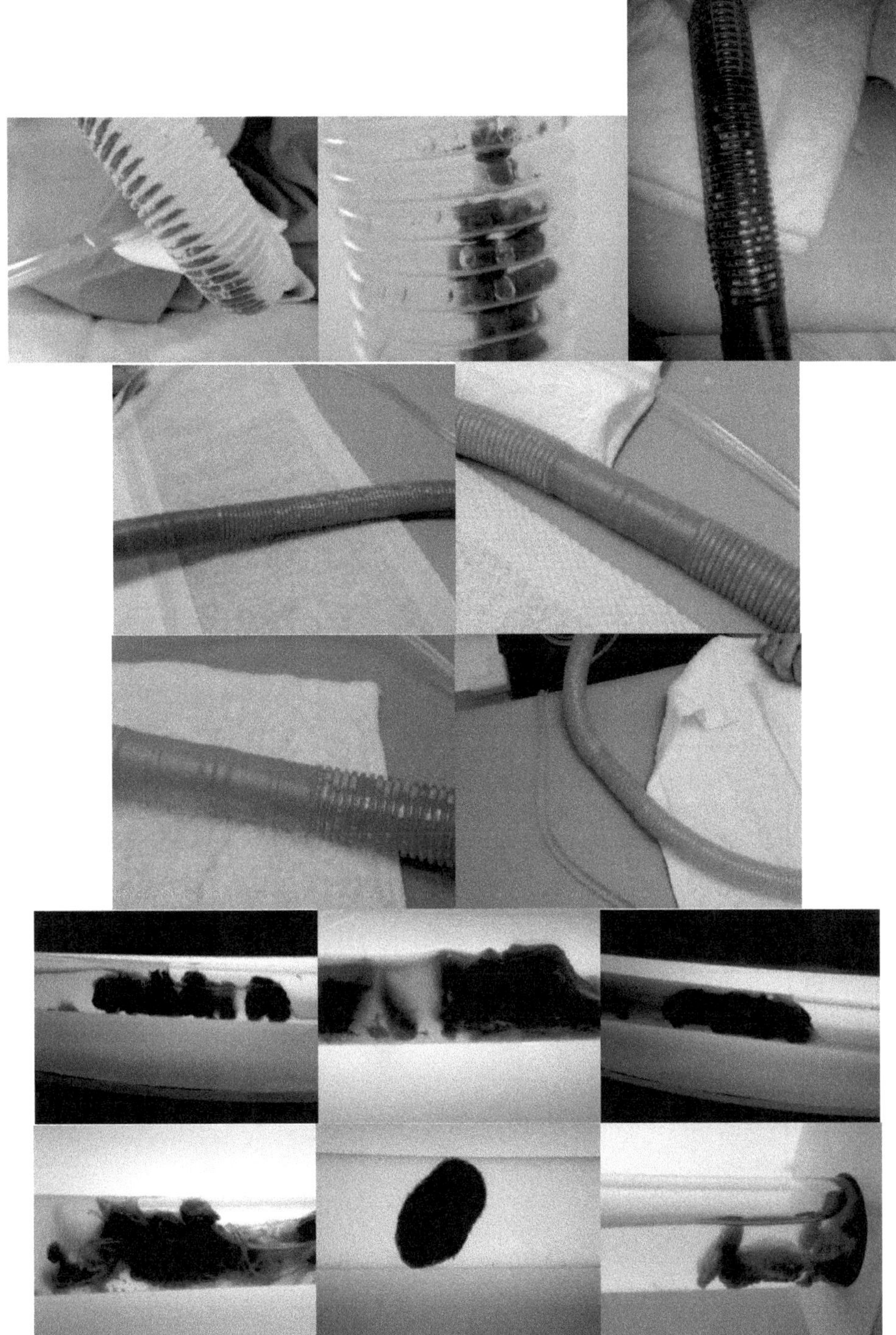

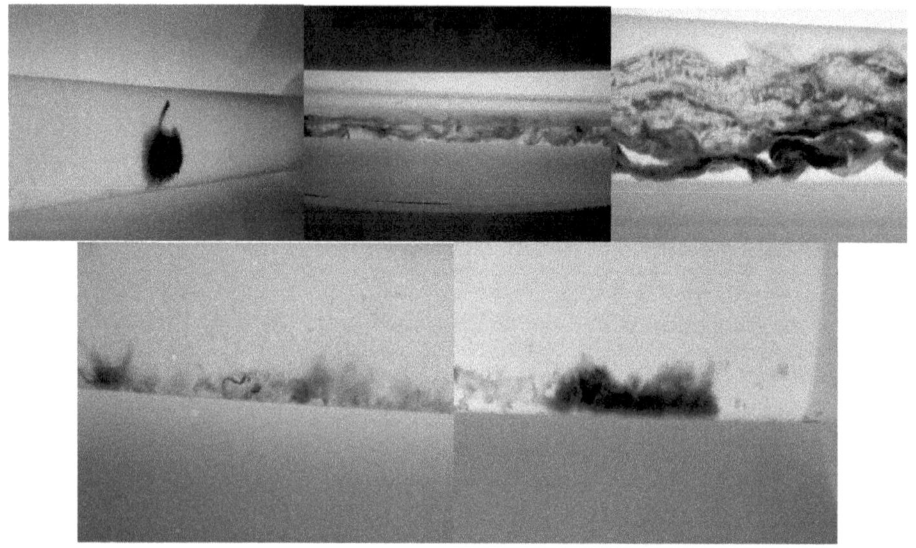

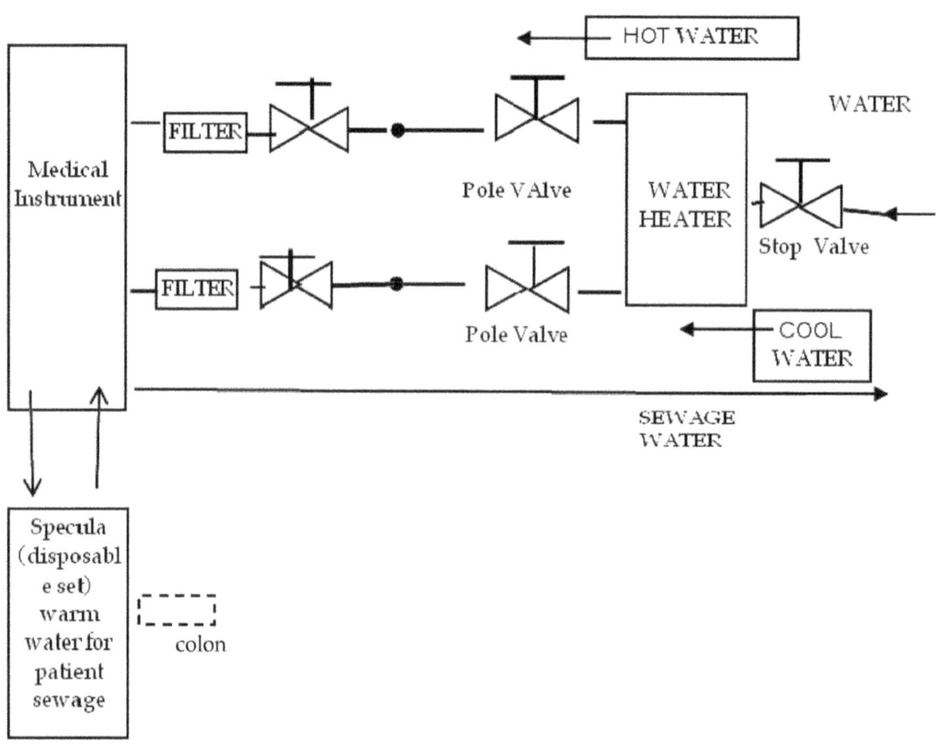

Fig. 1. Principle of the Colon Hydromat Comfort

2.5 Statistics

Results are given as means ± standard deviations (SD). Student's paired t-test was used to compare results before and after irrigations. P < 0.05 was considered statistically significant.

3. Results

Patient clinical characteristics are summarized in Table 1.

Patient	Age	Gender	Underlying disease	Symptom change
No. 1	44	Male	Pollen allergy	Symptom-free (after 7 times)
No. 2	47	Female	Constipation	Better
No. 3	45	Female	Ovarian cysts	Size Smaller (8 cm to 6 cm, after 3 times)
No. 4	47	Male	Atopic dermatitis	Decreased itching
No. 5	28	Male	Psoriasis	Better (still undergoing irrigation)
No. 6	38	Female	Constipation	Better
No. 7	38	Female	Constipation	Better
No. 8	32	Female	Face eruption	Better
No. 9	39	Female	Constipation	Better
No. 10	29	Male	Allergic Rhinitis	Decreased blowing of nose

Table 1. Subject's clinical characteristics and symptom changes after irrigations

Each patient underwent 3 colonic irrigations over a period of 2 weeks. Fecal samples were collected before the first colon irrigation and at 1 week after the third irrigation. The relative proportions of bacteria found in the fecal samples of each patient before and after colonic irrigation are shown in Table 2.

	1		2		3		4	
Presumed bacterium	b	a	b	a	b	a	b	a
Bifidobacterium	18.6	16.5	22.9	17.1	8.7	14.9	1.8	14.5
Lactobacillales	2.2	4.5	4.1	0	6.1	4	0	0
Bacteroides	23	17	21.3	20.9	31.7	31.6	44.4	38.3
Prevotella	9.1	2.8	7.8	8.9	0	0	0	0
Clostridium cluster IV	11.6	15.4	14.5	19.1	25.5	23	22.7	13.9
Clostridium subcluster XIVa	13	16.3	17.7	24.7	21.3	19.4	14.6	22.4
Clostridium cluster XI	2.6	4.2	0	0	0	0	2.4	2.3
Clostridium cluster XVIII	7	4.4	2	1.4	0	0	5.1	0
others	13	18.8	9.6	8	6.7	7.1	9.1	8.6

Table 2. Continued

5		6		7		8		9		10	
b	a	b	a	b	a	b	a	b	a	b	a
1.9	2	17.9	2.6	22.6	28.2	9.9	1	0	28.5	5.6	26.7
0	0	1.5	0	2.7	2.5	0	0	3.3	3.2	1.6	1.5
28.3	14.7	13.5	14.4	15.6	25.4	29.8	12.3	59.8	30.3	32.9	33
38.3	31.6	23.9	30.3	0	0	0	40.3	0	0	0	0
2.8	8.1	3.8	1.5	12.6	11.7	0	19.7	0	19.1	0	4.8
3.9	15.8	19	11.2	22.8	17.4	26.5	11.6	7.7	13	24.4	15.1
1.7	0	1	3.4	11.1	3	13.8	2.5	3.3	3.3	0	0
1.1	0	1.1	0.6	0	1.5	0	1.2	1.7	0	0	0
22	27.8	18.3	35.9	12.6	10.3	20	11.3	24.3	2.4	35.5	18.9

No 1-10: Patients in Table 1. b: Before colonic irrigations. a: After 3 times colonic irrigations

Table 2. The changes in the fecal microbiota between prior to and after 3 clonic irrigations

There were no significant differences in the overall quantities of fecal bacteria in samples collected before and after irrigations. There was also no tendency for changes int the proportions of Lactobacillales and *Bifidobacterium* and *Clostridium* subclusters. The proportions of these bacterial orders are shown in Table 3.

Presumed microbiota %	prior to (mean ± SD)	after	p
Bifidobacterium	10.99±8.85	15.29±10.74	p>0.05
Lactobacillales	2.15±1.99	1.57±1.84	p>0.05
Bacteroids	30.08±13.86	23.8±9.2	p>0.05
Prevotella	7.88±13.07	11.39±16.09	p>0.05
Clostridium IV	9.4±9.62	13.62±7.04	p>0.05
Clostridum XIVa	17.07±7.33	16.64±4.42	p>0.05
Clostridum XI	3.61±4.9	1.87±1.69	p>0.05
Clostridum XVIII	1.8±2.4	0.91±1.38	p>0.05
Others	17.13±8.85	14.92±10.42	p>0.05

Table 3. The mean changes in the microbiota between prior to and after 3 colonic irrigations

According to Collins et al. (1994), *Clostridium* clusters and subclusters cannot revide the unknown pole in intestine. For example, *Faecalibacterium prausnitzil* is an important bacteria as butyrate-producing bacterium in *Clostridium* cluster IV. In contrast, *Clostridium perfringens* is a well known as harmful bacterium in *Clostridium* cluster I. Lactobacillales and *Bifidobacterium* are considered to be healthy, beneficial fecal bacteria. In this study, beneficial bacteria decreased in some patients. Serum electrolytes after irrigations (sodium, potassium, and chlorine) exhibited no significant changes from their values before irrigation (data not shown). Patient symptoms were improved after irrigations (Table 1), and they did not experience any difficulties.

4. Discussion

This study showed that colonic irrigations are safe in terms of serum electrolytes for subjects with normal renal function and had a positive impact on these subjects' symptoms. However, these irrigations showed no tendency for any effects on the intestinal microbiota. Colonic irrigation was developed at the National Aeronautics and Space Administration and has been used worldwide in the care of allergic and pollen diseases, skin disorders, and constipation. I previously reported that colonic irrigation may induce lymphocyte transmigration from GALT into the circulation, which may improve the function of both the colon and the immune system functions (Uchiyama-Tanaka, 2009). The increase in the lymphocytes was suspected to be the result of lymphocytes transmigrating as intraepithelial lymphocytes from Peyer's patched and lymph nodes around the intestine as a result of irrigation and abdominal massage.

Based on my personal experience, patient symptoms can improve after colonic irrigations. However, it has been proposed that colon irrigations with large volumes of water may obliterate the microbiota and induce electrolyte abnormalities, but no studies support these claims. The results of this study suggests that after 3s colonic irrigations, the composition of the microbiota changes, but there is no tendency for the changes in the bacterial components.

Colonic irrigations are different from enemas for the following reasons: (a) they are not self-administered, but are administered by a professionally trained person; and (b) they are administered using a device that controls water flow and infuses the entire colon with water, in contrast to the more limited infusion of warm filtered water into the rectum. The water circulates throughout the colon and removes its contents while the patient lies on a bed. The temperature and pressure of water are closely monitored and regulated during a series of fills and releases to aid colonic peristalsis. Because this method involves a closed system, the waste materials are removed without any unpleasant odor or discomfort, which are usually associated with enemas.

The intestine is an important site of local immunity and nutrition (Iiai et al., 2002). It is a major site of extrathymic T cell differentiation, and numerous activated and quiescent lymphocytes are produced within GALT. The very important role of the intestine, as a part of the immune system is due to the intestinal microbiota. Thus, it has been speculated in peoplewho suffer from constipation and who harbor fecal residues, the intestine may have a diminished function in the immune system (Alveres, 2001, 1924).

The intestinal epithelium is the first line of defense system to encounter intestinal pathogens and dietary antigens. It has been speculated that when the intestine is filled with feces, there may be a reduced function of this immune system caused by toxins leaking from the gut, in addition to bacterial translocation from the gut to the systemic circulation caused by a breakdown of the intestinal wall. This breakdown can be caused by a variety of injuries to the body at further locations far from the gut.

It has been reported that increased gut permeability and bacterial translocation play a role in multiple organ failure (MOF: Swank & Deitch, 1996). Failure of the gut barrier is central to the hypothesis that toxins escaping from the gut lumen contribute to the activation of a host's immune inflammatory defense mechanisms, which subsequently leads to autointoxication and tissue destruction that are seen in the septic response characteristics of MOF (Swank & Deitch,1996; Garcia-Tsao et al., 1995; Purohit et al., 2008). Thus, colonic irrigation is useful for removing fecal residues.

Although irrigation is useful for establishing a "good" status in the intestine in terms of removing fecal residues, we should not expect too much from these irrigations. Factors like proper nutrition and food intake and a stress-free life style are also important in improving the microbiota, rather than colonic irrigations alone. One report showed that the microbiota of people on a strict vegetarian diet was very different from those on normal diets (Hayashi et al. 2002b). The removal of residual fecal matter in the colon may provide a break from a bad dietary cycle and highlight the importance of intestinal care in everyday life.

Colonic irrigation is relatively safe and is a good method for impressing upon patients the importance of intestinal care. But according to the results of this study, some patients' microbiota deteriorated. Although safe in terms of serum electrolytes, it should be noted that colonic irrigations should not be performed for patients with renal failure, heart disease, liver cirrhosis with ascites, recent abdominal surgery, pregnancy, and other conditions. In addition, excessive therapy such as everyday irrigations should be avoided. This may result in the loss of massive amount of digestive fluid. Except for the first 3 times of colonic irrigation, subsequent irrigations should be performed within a minimum 1 month interval.

This study was limited by its small study population. Some subjects showed reduced proportions in beneficial fecal bacteria, although their symptoms including allergic rhinorrhea, constipation, skin itching, and eczema, were improved. We should be careful with regard to the duration and number of irrigations administered and preferably take probiotics after colonic irrigation. If the patient is in a "good" status in terms of stool analysis, a single trial with an adequate duration would be sufficient.

Another limitation of this study was that the actual numbers of bacteria were not determined using these methods. T-RFLP is only useful for estimating the proportions of bacteria. Hence, we need a more efficient quantitative method for bacterial analysis in addition to the existing one with an advantageous cost versus performance.

In conclusion, colonic irrigation has no influence on serum electrolytes and may induce improvements in symptoms without any effects on the intestinal microbiota.

5. References

Alveres, WC. (2001). Origin of so-called autointoxication symptoms. *JAMA*.72: pp. 8-13.
Alverez, WC.; Freedlander. BL.(1924). The rate of progress of food residues through the bowel. *JAMA*. 83: pp. 576-580.
Ando, A.; Sakata, S., Koizumi, Y., Mitsuyama, K., Fujiyama, Y., Benno, Y.(2007). Terminal restriction fragment length polymorphism analysis of the diversity of fecal microbiota in patients with ulcerative colitis. *Inflamm Bowel Dis*. 13: pp. 955-962.
Cerf-Bensussan, N.; Guy-Grand, D., Griscelli, C. (1985). Intraepithelial lymphocytes of human gut: isolation, characterization and study of natural killer activity. *Gut*. 26: pp.81-88

Collins, MD.; Lawson, PA., Willems ,A., Cordoba, JJ., Fernandez-Garayzabal, J., Garcia, P., Cai, J., Hippe, H., Farrow, JAE.(1994). The Phylogeny of the Genus Clostridium: Proposal of Five New Genera and Eleven New Species Combinations. *Int J Syst Bacteriol.* 44: pp. 812-826.

Garcia-Tsao, G.; Lee, FY., Bardeb, GE., Cartun, R., West, AB. (1995) Bacterial translocation to mesenteric lymph nodes is increased in cirrhotic rats with ascites. *Gastroenterology* 108: pp. 1835-1841

Guy-Grand, D.; Cerf-Bensussan, N., Malissen, B., Malassis-Seris ,M., Briottet, C., Vassalli, P. (1991). Two gut intraepithelial CD8+ lymphocyte population with different T cell receptors. A role for the gut epithelium in T cell differentiation. *J Exp Med.* 173: pp. 471-481.

Hayashi, H.; Sakamoto, M. & Benno, Y. (2002). Phylogenetic analysis of human gut microbiota using 16S rDNA clone libraries and strictly anaerobic culture-based methods. *Microbiol Immunol,* 46: pp. 535-548

Hayashi, H.; Sakamoto, M., Bennno, Y. (2002). Fecal microbial diversity in a strict vegetarian as determined by molecular analysis and cultivation. *Microbiol Immunol* 46: pp.819-831.

Iiai, T.; Watanabe, H., Suda, T., Okamoto, H., Abo, T., Hatakeyama, K. (2002). CD161+T (NT) cells exist predominantly in human intestinal epithelium as well as in liver. *Clin Exp Immunol* 129: pp. 92-98.

Langendijk, PS.; Schut, F., Jansen, GJ., Raangs, GC., Kamphuius, GR., Wilkison ,MH., Welling, GW. (1995). Quantitative fluorescence in situ hybridization of Bifidobacterium spp. With genus-specific 16S rRNA-targeted probes and its application in fecal samples. *Appl Environ Microbiol* 61: pp. 3069-3075

Moor, WE.; Holdeman, LV.(1974). Human fecal flora: the normal flora of 20 Japanese-Hawaiians. *Appl Environ Microbiol.* 27: pp. 961-979

Nagashima, K.; Hisada ,T., Sato, M., Mochizuki, J. (2002). Application of new primer-enzyme combinations to terminal restriction fragment length polymorphism profiling of bacterial populations in human feces. *Appl Environ Microbiol* 69: pp. 1251-1262

Nagashima, K.; Mochizuki, J., Hisada, T., Suzuki, S., Shimomura, K. (2006). Phylogenetic analysis of 16S ribosomal RNA gene sequences from human fecal microbiota and improved utility of terminal restriction fragment length polymorphism profiling. *Bioscience Microflora.* 25: pp. 99-107.

Purohit, V.; Bode, JC., Bode, C., Brenner, DA., Choudhry, MA., Hamilton, F., Kang, YJ., Keshavarzin, A., Rao, R., Sartor, RB., Swanson, C., Turner, JR. (2008) Alcohol, intestinal bacterial growth, intestinal permeability to endotoxin, and medical consequences: Summary of a symposium. *Alcohol* 42: pp. 349-361

Suau, A.; Bonnet, R., Sutren, M., Godon, JJ., Gibson, G.R., Collins, MD., Dore, J. (1999). Direct analysis of genes encoding 16S rRNA from complex communities reveals many novel molecular species within the human gut. *Appl Environ Microbiol* 65: pp. 4799-4807

Swank, GM.; Deitch, EA. (1996) Role of the gut in multiple organ failure. Bacterial translocation and permeability changes. *World J Surg* 20: pp. 411-417

Takahashi, S.; Kawamura ,T., Kanda, Y., Taniguchi, T., Nishizawa, T., Iiai, T., Hatakeyama, K., Abo, T.(2005). Multipotential acceptance of Peyer's patches in the intestine for both thymus-derived T cells and extrathymic T cells in mice. *Immunol Cell Biol.* 83: pp.504-510.

Uchiyama-Tanaka, Y.; (2009). Colon irrigation and lymphocyte movement to peripheral blood. *Biochemical Research.* 30:pp. 311-314.

Van der Waaij, D.; Berghuis-de Vries, JM., Lekkerkerk van der ,Wees. (1971). Colonization resistance of digestive tract in conventional and antibiotic treated mice. *J Hyg.* 67: pp. 405-411.

Section 4

Diseases of the Liver and Biliary Tract

22

Pancreato-Biliary Cancers – Diagnosis and Management

Nam Q. Nguyen
Department of Gastroenterology, Royal Adelaide Hospital,
North Terrace, Adelaide, SA
Australia

1. Introduction

Pancreato-biliary cancers are relatively uncommon and in general, including cancers arise from the pancreas, bile duct and major ampullae. These tumours are uniformly carried a poor prognosis due to late presentation and surgical resection is only possible in less than 20% patients (David et al., 2009; Luke et al., 2009). Despites many medical advances in the imaging diagnosis, chemo-radio-therapy, surgical technique and post-operative care over the last 2 decades, the overall survival of patients with pancreato-biliary neoplasm has not improved significantly (Luke et al., 2009). The aim of the current chapter is to review and discuss current techniques and approaches to the diagnosis and management of pancreato-biliary neoplasm.

2. Clinico-pathology of pancreato-biliary tumours

2.1 Pancreatic carcinoma

In the Western world, pancreatic cancer is the fourth leading cause of cancer related mortality with the approximate incidence of 11 per 100 000, and ranks second after colorectal cancer among all gastrointestinal malignancies (Shaib et al., 2006). Men are more frequently affected than women and over 80% patients are diagnosed at the age older than 60 years. Almost 50% patients have distant metastases at the time of presentation with poor 5-year survival of 5% (Shaib et al., 2006). Recent data suggest that although the mortality rate for males has decreased by 0.4% from 1990 to 2005, the mortality rate for females has increased by 4.4% (Shaib et al., 2006; Jemal et al., 2009). The reason for this gender difference in mortality is unknown. Risk factors for pancreatic cancer include smoking, alcohol, diabetes mellitus, chronic pancreatitis, family history of pancreatic cancer. Patients with hereditary pancreatitis, Puetz-Jeghers syndrome, familial atypical multiple mole melanoma, familial breast and ovarian cancer, Li-Fraumeni syndrome, Fanconi anaemia, ataxia-telangiectasia, familial adenomatous polyposis, cystic fibrosis and possible hereditary non-polyposis colon cancer syndrome are also at higher risk of having pancreatic cancer (Shaib et al., 2006; Klapman and Malafa, 2008).

Ductal infiltrating adenocarcinoma is the most common type of pancreatic cancer with 78% located in the head, 11% in the body and 11% in the tail (Lillemoe et al., 2000; Ghaneh et al.,

2008). Less than 15% of pancreatic cancers are intraductal mucinous papillary neoplasm (IPMN), solid pseudopapillary neoplasm, pancreatoblastoma, mucinous cystadenocarcinoma, adenosquamous carcinoma and acinar cell carcinoma (Ghaneh et al., 2008). Given the preponderance pancreatic head location of the tumours, painless cholestatic symptoms are the most common presentation (Ghaneh et al., 2008). Anorexia, abdominal pain or mass and weight loss often indicate the presence of advanced disease.

2.2 Cholangiocarcinoma

This is rare malignant disease of the epithelial cells in the intra- and extrahepatic bile ducts and the incidence is increasing, especially the intra-hepatic subtype (Patel, 2001). In addition to liver flukes infestation, hepatitis B and C infections have recently been associated with rise of cholangiocarcinoma in the developing countries, and are thought to be responsible for the increasing incidence of intra-hepatic cholangiocarcinomas. In the western countries, primary sclerosing cholangitis and congenital anomalies such as Caroli's syndrome and choledochal cysts are the main predisposing risk factors for cholangiocarcinoma (Patel, 2006).

As with pancreatic cancer, most of the cholangiocarcinomas are unresectable at presentation and the prognosis for these patients is dismal. Clinical presentations of cholangiocarcinoma are dependent on tumour location (Patel, 2006). Extrahepatic tumours, including those involving the bifurcation usually show signs of biliary obstruction with jaundice and pale stools. In contrast, intra-hepatic cholangiocarcinomas more often present with late symptoms of malignancy such as weight loss, loss of appetite, and abdominal pain or mass.

2.3 Ampullary tumours

Compared to pancreatic carcinoma and cholangiocarcinoma, ampullary neoplasm is the least common and aggressive tumour. In general, ampullary tumour has better clinical outcomes even when the tumour is not resectable (Heinrich and Clavien 2010). Whilst ampullary tumours can occur sporadically, they are often seen in the context of genetic syndromes such as familial adenomatous polyposis and hereditary non-polyposis colorectal cancer, in whom the risk is 100 times more than the general population (Offerhaus et al., 1992). As endoscopic screening and surveillance program is adopted for these at-risk individuals, most tumours are adenomas at detection, though the potential of malignant transformation to carcinomas is high (Jean and Dua, 2003; Fischer and Zhou, 2004). Currently, there is no consensus on the management of ampullary tumors. Factors that impact treatment strategy include the patient's general health, tumor characteristics, and available expertise. Ampullary adenomas, especially those with high-grade dysplasia, warrant therapy because they are "time bombs" for malignancy and may already harbor malignancy missed on biopsy (Heinrich and Clavien 2010). Although endoscopic resection is widely embraced as first-line therapy in patients with benign ampullary tumors (Binmoeller et al., 1993; Beger et al., 1999; Cheng et al., 2004), the final treatment decision is based on the histological findings of the ampullectomized specimen. The presence of invasive carcinoma in the specimen indicates the need for definitive surgical resection. In patients who are poor candidates for surgery or who refuse surgery, endoscopic resection with ablative therapy can be considered despite unfavorable tumor characteristics (Nguyen et al. 2010). Endoscopic ampullectomy has also been reported to successfully eradicate large ampullary adenomas (Zadorova et al., 2001), early T1 ampullary adenocarcinoma

(Katsinelos et al., 2007), and even lesions with intraductal growth (Bohnacker et al., 2005). Given its tumour behaviour, clinical presentation and treatment modality are very different to that of pancreatic cancer and cholangiocarcinoma, ampullary tumours will not be discussed further in this chapter.

3. Investigations of pancreato-biliary cancers

The imaging modalities involve in the detection, staging and management of pancreatic cancer are computer tomography (CT), magnetic resonance imaging (MRI), endoscopic retrograde cholangiopancreatography (ERCP), endoscopic ultrasound (EUS) and positron emission tomography (PET) (Clarke et al., 2003; Chang et al., 2009; Peddu et al., 2009). The diagnosis can potentially be made by any, or a combination of the above modalities. The roles and relative importance of these imaging modalities have changed over the last few decades and continue to change with rapid technological advancement in medical imaging.

Base on current best available evidence, CT should be used as first line for diagnosis, staging and the assessment of resectability in pancreato-biliary cancer. MRI should be reserved for patients with iodine contrast allergy or who cannot be exposed to radiation or to be used as an adjunct to CT in patients with suspicious liver lesions that need to be to better characterized (Clarke et al., 2003; Peddu et al., 2009). MR cholangio-pancreatography (MRPC) is an essential part of the evaluation for cholangiocarcinoma as it can identify the luminal involvement of the cancer as well as the road map of the biliary tree (Patel, 2006). Such information is not only important in local staging but also critical in determining respectability, type of surgery and/or identifying the dominant obstructive ductal system for biliary drainage. In selected cases, cholangioscopy is helpful by providing direct endoscopic visualization of the intra-ductal lesion that responsible for the biliary stricture (Patel, 2006). The recent development of SpyGlass cholangioscopy system has also allowed tissue sample under direct vision.

EUS should be used for local staging and assessment of resectability if it remains inconclusive on non-invasive imaging modalities (Chang et al., 2009; Iglesias Garcia et al., 2009). It should also be used in patients with a high clinical suspicion of a lesion that has not been clearly demonstrated using other modalities. EUS-FNA should also be the biopsy route of choice in patients where a tissue diagnosis or tissue from regional lymph nodes may alter the course of treatment, or if neo-adjuvant treatment is contemplated. If there is disagreement between CT and EUS images, then laparotomy and trial of dissection should be considered (Chang et al., 2009). PET/CT should be used selectively such as when metastatic disease is suspected but has not been demonstrated with other imaging modalities (Nguyen and Bartholomeusz, 2011; Serrano et al. 2010). The availability and local expertise of each imaging modality will also influence their use. A suggested management algorithm for patients with suspected pancreato-biliary cancer is shown in Figure 1.

3.1 Tumour markers

The role of tumour marker in the diagnosis and management of pancreato-biliary cancers remains controversial (Balzano and Di Carlo, 2008). Carbohydrate antigen 19-9 (CA19-9), which is caused by the up-regulation of glycosyl transferase genes, is the most commonly used marker and can provide useful diagnostic and prognostic information (Duffy et al.

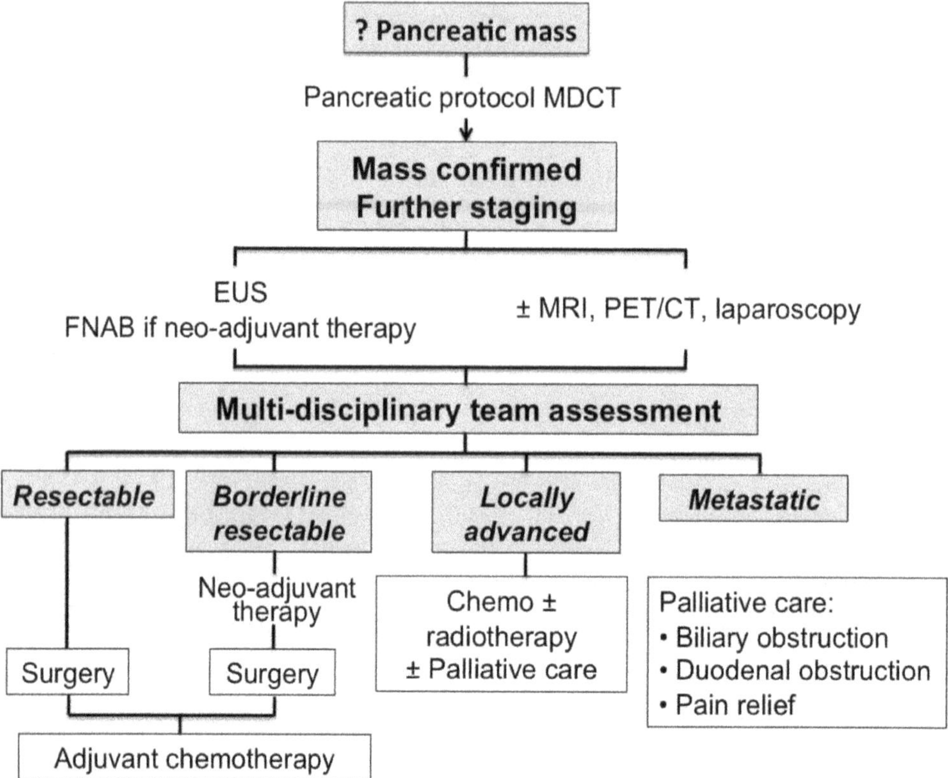

Fig. 1. Suggested algorithm for the evaluation and management of patients with suspected pancreatic.

2010). Its sensitivity (70%-90%) and specificity (43%-91%) for diagnosing pancreatic cancer are only modest and can be falsely increased by high serum bilirubin (Duffy et al. 2010). However, for those with confirmed pancreatic cancer, high serum CA19-9 is associated with a worse survival (Park et al., 2008). Similarly, in patients who undergo curative resection for pancreatic cancer, a normalizing post-operative CA19-9 level is associated with a longer median and disease-free survival compared to those with persistently high level (Duffy et al., 2008; Balzano and Di Carlo, 2008).

3.2 Tissue sampling

A distinct advantage of EUS is its ability to obtain tissue via fine needle aspiration (FNA). This approach is superior to percutaneous biopsy (via US or CT guided) in the investigation of pancreato-biliary malignancies with higher diagnostic yield (84% vs. 62%) and significantly lower risk of tumour seeding from the needle tract (<2% vs. 16%) (Paquin et al., 2005). Apart from biopsy of the primary tumour, it also has the ability to biopsy lymph nodes, liver lesions and ascitic fluid, which is critical in accurate staging and avoiding unnecessary resection (Figure 2). For pancreatic head lesions, the possibility of seeding is eliminated, as the needle track is included in the resection specimen (Yamao et al., 2005). In

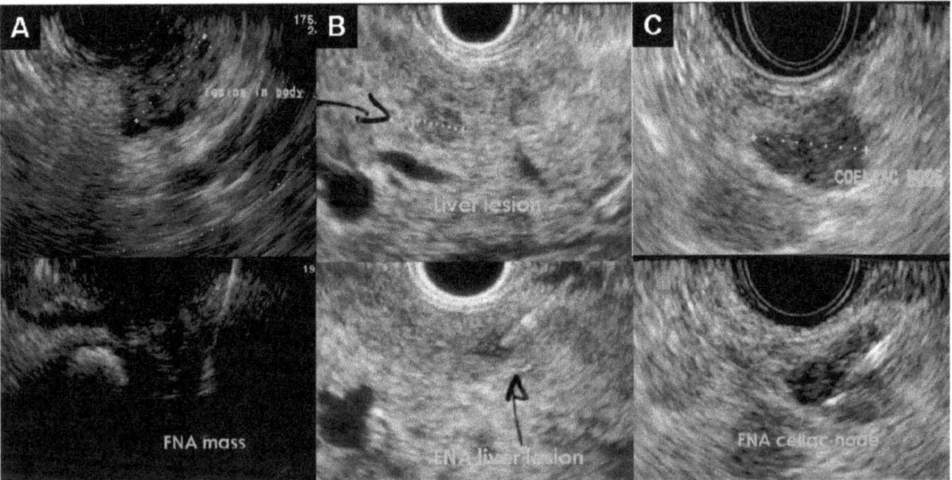

Fig. 2. Examples of EUS-guide FNA of a pancreatic mass in the body (panel A), a liver lesion (panel B) and pathological celiac node (panel C).

contrast, for lesions in the pancreatic body and tail, where the needle track is not resected, the risks and benefits of pre-operative biopsy should be carefully assessed on an individual basis. Due to its anatomical position, tissue acquisition from biliary lesion via EUS guided FNA is more difficult and in general, the diagnostic yield is lower than that for pancreatic cancer and is dependent on the location of the lesion. As it is easier to visualize and access the distal biliary lesions, the diagnostic yield is significantly higher in distal compared with proximal lesions (81% vs 59%) (Mohamadnejad et al. 2011).

3.3 Cholangioscopy

In cases where the diagnosis of the biliary stricture remains unclear after conventional MDCT, MRI and EUS evaluation, directly visualization of the appearance of the ductal strictures and biopsy can be helpful in differentiating benign from malignant disorders (Figure 3). Although video "mother-baby" cholangioscope provides high quality images, it is fragile and often lack of accessory channel for tissue sampling (Nguyen, 2009; Nguyen et al., 2009). The diagnostic yield of malignancy based on cholangioscopic appearance of the intra-ductal lesion varied from 70% to 88% (Nguyen, 2009; Nguyen et al., 2009). Currently, tissue sampling is only possible with the single-operator disposable SpyGlass system, which has a 1.2mm accessory channel. Although SpyGlass guided tissue sample is successful in up to 96% of cases, its overall accuracy in confirming a malignant stricture is only modest (49% of cases) (Nguyen, 2009; Nguyen et al., 2009). This is mainly due to the poor sensitivity of SpyGlass guided biopsy in the diagnosis of malignancy from extrinsic cancers (8%) as compared to that of intrinsic cancers (66%) (Nguyen, 2009; Nguyen et al., 2009).

4. Therapeutic approaches for pancreato-biliary cancers

Patients with suspected or confirmed diagnosis of pancreato-biliary malignancy should be assessed by a multidisciplinary team and stratified as resectable, borderline resectable,

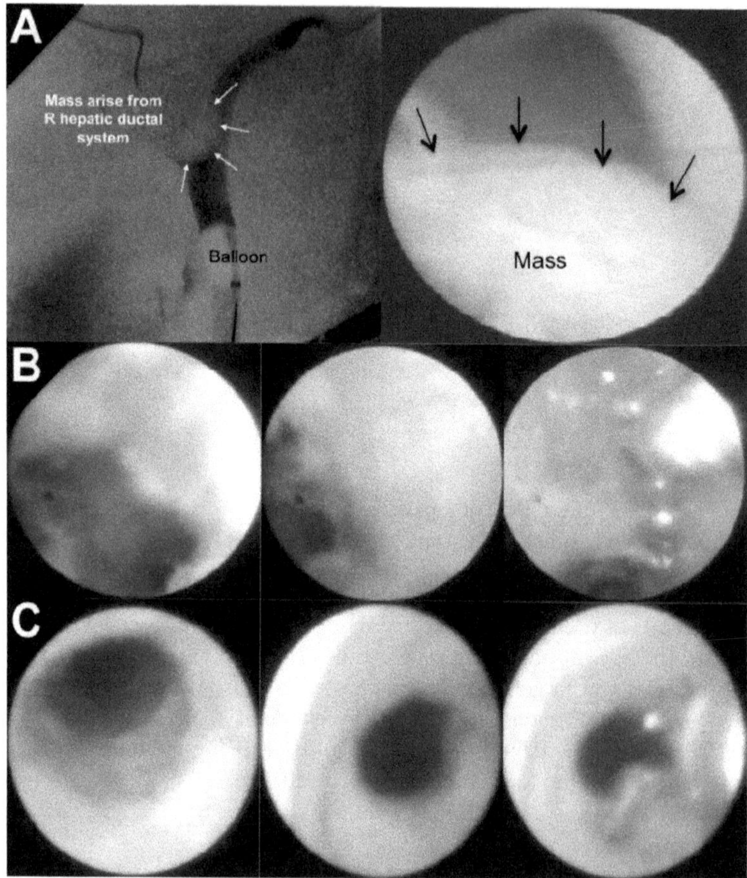

Fig. 3. Cholangioscopic images from SpyScope for investigation of suspected biliary strictures. A case of a hepatoma causing a polypoid protrusion into the right hepatic duct at the hilum, mimicking a cholangiocarcinoma on cholangiography (panel A). A case of cholangiocarcinoma in the upper common bile duct (CBD) stricture, confirmed on SpyGlass guided biopsy (panel B). A case of mid-CBD stricture in a patient with primary sclerosing cholangitis, which appeared benign on SpyScope and was confirmed on biopsy (panel C).

locally advanced unresectable or metastatic disease. Treatment should be planned according to local expertise and established guidelines, as resectable and borderline patients should be referred to surgeons, unresectable and metastatic patients should be referred to medical and radiation oncologists and palliative care teams. Endoscopic interventions to alleviate biliary or duodenal obstruction are also important in improving the performance status and quality of life in these patients. A multidisciplinary approach to pancreato-biliary malignancy is necessary to improve the overall outcome of these patients, especially for borderline resectable or unresectable disease as neo-adjuvant chemo-radiation therapy may play a role in down-staging and the conversion to potentially resectable, and in some case "curable", disease (Verslype et al., 2007; Chang et al., 2008). The therapeutic approach for pancreatic cancers is summarized in Figure 1.

4.1 Surgery

Surgical resection remains the only possibility of cure for pancreato-biliary cancers as chemotherapy and radiotherapy offering only a modest survival benefit. Patients who undergo complete surgical resection for localized, non-metastatic adenocarcinoma of the pancreas have a 5-year survival rate of approximately 20 to 25%, and a median survival of 22 months (Cameron et al., 2006). Unfortunately less than 20% of patients with pancreatic cancer have disease amendable to surgical resection at the time of presentation (Yeo et al., 1997) because patients often present at an advanced stage with widespread metastatic or locally advanced disease. The type of resection depends on the location of the tumours with Whipple's procedures are most commonly performed as most cancers locate in the head of pancreas.

Similarly, the type and extend of resection for cholangiocarcinoma depends on the location of the tumour. The indication and type of resection of intra-hepatic cholangiocarcinoma is similar to those of liver cancers. In contrast, curative surgery for extra-hepatic cholangiocarcinoma is rare and is only possible for distal ductal tumours (Witzigmann et al., 2008; Lang et al., 2009). Hilar tumours involving the bifurcation are usually contraindicated for surgery and have very poor prognosis. Even in patients whose resection is considered successful, the overall five-year survival rate in the range of 25–30% (Lang et al., 2009).

4.2 Chemo-radiotherapy

Given the high loco-regional recurrence rate and a tendency towards early liver metastasis after pancreatic resection, adjuvant chemotherapy has been employed though its benefits remain controversial with mixed results until recently (Brennan, 2004; Zuckerman and Ryan, 2008). Of the six randomized controlled trials that examined the effects of adjuvant chemotherapy after pancreatic resection (Kalser and Ellenberg, 1985; Moertel et al., 1994; Neoptolemos et al., 2001; Neoptolemos et al., 2004; Oettle et al., 2007; Regine et al., 2008), only two trials were able to demonstrate a survival benefit of adjuvant chemotherapy (Neoptolemos et al., 2001; Neoptolemos et al., 2004). In the ESPAC-1 study, the survival of patients treated with adjuvant 5-Fluorouracil (5-FU) was significantly longer than that without adjuvant chemotherapy (20.1 months vs 15.5 months) (Neoptolemos et al., 2001; Neoptolemos et al., 2004). Subsequent meta-analysis supports the results of ESPAC-1 trial and indicated that 5-FU reduced the risk of death by 25% (Stocken et al., 2005). More recently, German investigators (Oettle et al., 2007) have demonstrated a disease-free survival advantage of patients who received gemcitabine adjuvant chemotherapy (13.4 months vs 6.9 months), but not the overall survival (22.1 months vs 20.2 months). Given the encouraging data from these trials (Neoptolemos et al., 2001; Neoptolemos et al., 2004; Oettle et al., 2007), adjuvant chemotherapy with either 5-FU or gemcitabine or both is increasingly used in patients with resected pancreatic cancer (Fogelman et al., 2004; Goldstein et al., 2004). Compared with 5-FU, gemcitabine is better tolerated with lesser incidence of grade 3 and 4 haematological toxicity (Oettle et al., 2007; Palmer et al., 2007).

Similarly, in order to convert borderline resectable to resectable tumors or to increase the probability of complete microscopic tumor resection, neo-adjuvant chemo-radiotherapy has also been evaluated (Gillen et al., 2010; Heinrich et al., 2010; van Tienhoven et al., 2011;

Vinciguerra 2011). A recent systematic review evaluating retrospective and prospective studies on neo-adjuvant chemo-radiotherapy from 1966 to 2009 included a total of 111 studies and 4,394 patients suggests that up to one third of patients with previously borderline resectable cancers are eligible for resection after neoadjuvant treatment (Gillen et al. 2010). More importantly, these patients were found to have comparable median survival as those who undergoing resection followed by adjuvant therapy (20.1 vs. 23.6 months, respectively). In contrast, neoadjuvant therapy did not seem to improve overall outcome for patients with resectable cancer at presentation (Gillen et al. 2010).

In contrast to pancreatic cancer, cholangiocarcinoma has been shown to be resistant to common chemotherapy (Anderson and Kim, 2009). Numerous drugs have been tested alone and in combination, and thus far, the response rate has been unacceptably low. Although gemcitabine chemotherapy is often given to patients with unresectable cholangiocarcinoma, the survival benefit has not been proven in a randomised controlled trial (Gruenberger et al. 2010).

5. Palliative endoscopic interventions

Given that up to 80-85% of pancreato-biliary cancers are unresectable and the survival benefit of chemo-radiation therapy is very modest, palliative treatment plays a very important role in the care of these patients. Relief of symptoms secondary to gastro-duodenal obstruction, jaundice and pain are essential to improve their quality of life and overall survival. In the past, surgical palliative approaches, such as gastric bypass and hepatico-enteric decompression, are more common used as the diagnosis of unresectable disease is frequently made in the operating room. With the recent improvement in pre-operative staging, diagnostic laparotomy is rarely performed and biliary or gastro-duodenal obstruction is mostly managed by minimally invasive endoscopic interventions.

5.1 Alleviation of biliary obstruction

Currently, endoscopic biliary stenting is the treatment of choice for unresectable pancreato-biliary cancers with obstructive jaundice (Figure 4). Endoscopic placement of plastic stent(s) was equally effective as surgical technique in palliating obstructive jaundice, but endoscopic stent was associated with fewer procedural complications and death (Taylor et al., 2000). More recently, the invention of larger diameter self-expandable metallic (SEM) biliary stents provides longer stent patency for drainage. Compared to plastic stents, SEM stents are significantly less likely to be occluded and thus, minimized the number of repeated ERCP. As with plastic stents, endoscopic placement of SEM stents has been shown to provide similar overall survival to surgical decompression but is more cost-effective and better quality of life (Knyrim et al., 1993; Prat et al., 1998). The concurrent use of chemotherapeutic agents in patients palliated with SEM stents does not increase the risk for ascending cholangitis (Nakai et al., 2005).

Percutaneous trans-hepatic stenting (PTHS) is often reserved for patients in whom ERCP has failed due to a higher complication rate as well as poorer quality of life (Pinol et al., 2002). More recently, the advent of EUS assisted ductal drainage and stenting has significantly improved the success rate of endoscopic approach and thus, reduced the need for PTHS. This approach involves puncturing a dilated intra-hepatic duct, under direct EUS

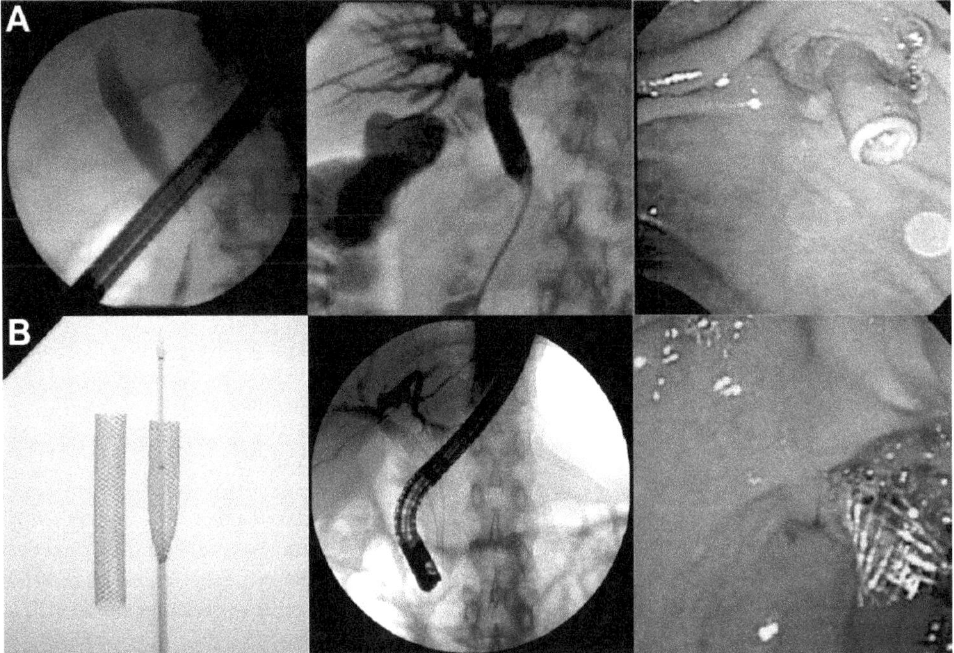

Fig. 4. Examples of biliary obstruction from pancreatic cancer requiring biliary drainage using plastic biliary stent (panel A) and SEM biliary stent (panel B).

guidance, to pass a guide wire into the duodenum, which then allows successful canulation of the biliar tree via ERCP and stenting (Shami and Kahaleh, 2007). In cases of duodenal obstruction, direct biliary drainage from a dilated intrahepatic duct into the stomach or duodenum via a SEM is an effective alternative for palliation with reasonable safety profile (Iwamuro et al., 2010; Nguyen-Tang et al. 2010). Surgical biliary bypass is only considered for patients who have relatively preserved functional status with obstructive jaundice and have failed on endoscopic stent placement.

5.2 Alleviation of gastro-duodenal obstruction

Although gastric bypass is commonly performed for unresectable patients with gastro-duodenal obstruction, the introduction of self-expanding metallic duodenal stents has changed the options for palliation (Figure 5). Current data suggest that placement of self-expandable metallic duodenal stents for malignant gastric outlet obstruction is successful in 98% of cases with a median duration of patency of 10 months (van Hooft et al., 2009). Serious complications from duodenal stenting, such as gastrointestinal bleeding or perforation, are rare with long-term stent dysfunction occurs in 14% of patients and migration in only 2% (van Hooft et al., 2009). Compared with palliative surgery, stent placement provides a shorter hospital stay, earlier resumption of oral intake, fewer complications and lower hospital costs (Maetani et al., 2004; Maetani et al., 2005). Currently, surgical palliation is often reserved for patients who are expected have a long life-expectancy and need both biliary and gastric bypass.

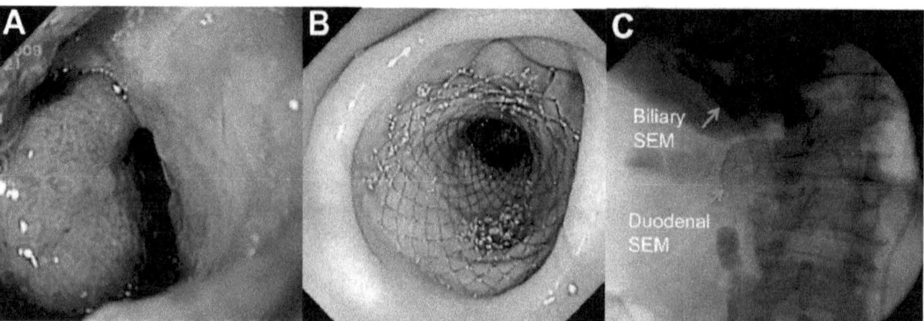

Fig. 5. A case of duodenal obstruction caused by locally advanced pancreatic cancer (A) and was successfully treated with a SEM duodenal stent (B).This patient also had a SEM biliary stent inserted for biliary drainage prior to the duodenal stent placement (C).

5.3 Alleviation of pain

Approximately 70% of patients with unresectable pancreato-biliary cancer develop clinically important pain, which can significantly reduce the quality and quantity of life of these patients (Andren-Sandberg et al., 1999). Good pain relief is, therefore, an essential part of effective palliative care. Although opioid analgesics are most commonly used as the first line pain relieved medication, one third of patients experience inadequate control of pain with significant side effects such as constipation and drowsiness (Andren-Sandberg et al., 1999). In these patients, neurolytic celiac plexus block under radiological or surgical guidance with absolute alcohol can be performed with up to 90% success rate (Mercadante et al., 2003; Wong et al., 2004; Noble and Gress, 2006). Recent studies have shown that EUS-guided neurolysis is equally effective but has significantly fewer serious complications associated with surgical or percutaneous approaches (O'Toole and Schmulewitz, 2009; Puli et al., 2009)

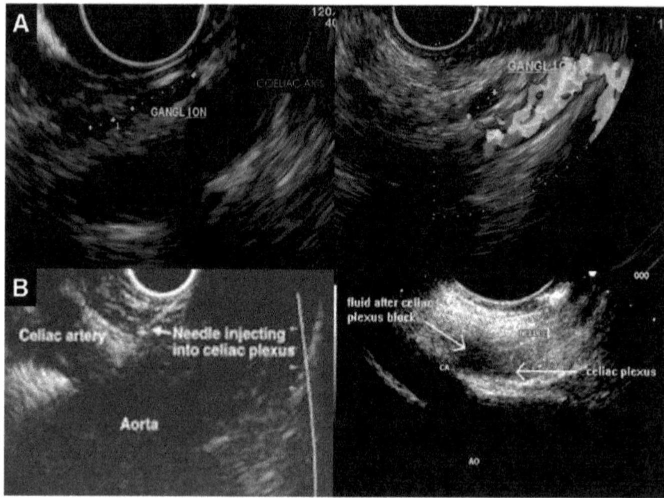

Fig. 6. Celiac ganglia can be visualized clearly on EUS imaging (panel A). Examples of EUS guided celiac ganglion blockage with alcohol injection (panel B).

(Figure 6). A recent double-blind randomized controlled study has also found that celiac plexus block is superior than systemic analgesic therapy in providing pain relief and improving quality of life (Wong et al., 2004). Thus, EUS-guided celiac neurolysis should be considered in all patients who have abdominal pain related to the pancreato-biliary cancer.

6. Conclusions

Despite the recent advances in diagnostic modalities, chemo-radiotherapy, surgical and post-operative care, the overall prognosis of pancreato-biliary malignancies has barely changed over the last few decades. The management of these patients is often complex and requires expertise in many fields. Thus, multidisciplinary teams are necessary to optimize the overall care. As the majority of these patients are diagnosed in advanced stages, good palliative care measures are essential to the management. Fortunately, a number of advances in endoscopic techniques have been made to improve the quality of life of these patients and avoid unnecessary surgery.

7. References

Anderson, C. and R. Kim (2009). "Adjuvant therapy for resected extrahepatic cholangiocarcinoma: a review of the literature and future directions." *Cancer Treat Rev* 35(4): 322-7.

Andren-Sandberg, A., A. Viste, A. Horn, D. Hoem and H. Gislason (1999). "Pain management of pancreatic cancer." *Ann Oncol* 10 Suppl 4: 265-8.

Balzano, G. and V. Di Carlo (2008). "Is CA 19-9 useful in the management of pancreatic cancer?" *Lancet Oncol* 9(2): 89-91.

Beger, H. G., F. Treitschke, F. Gansauge, N. Harada, N. Hiki and T. Mattfeldt (1999). "Tumor of the ampulla of Vater: experience with local or radical resection in 171 consecutively treated patients." *Arch Surg* 134(5): 526-32.

Binmoeller, K. F., S. Boaventura, K. Ramsperger and N. Soehendra (1993). "Endoscopic snare excision of benign adenomas of the papilla of Vater." *Gastrointest Endosc* 39(2): 127-31.

Bohnacker, S., U. Seitz, D. Nguyen, F. Thonke, S. Seewald, A. deWeerth, R. Ponnudurai, S. Omar and N. Soehendra (2005). "Endoscopic resection of benign tumors of the duodenal papilla without and with intraductal growth." *Gastrointest Endosc* 62(4): 551-60.

Brennan, M. F. (2004). "Adjuvant therapy following resection for pancreatic adenocarcinoma." *Surg Oncol Clin N Am* 13(4): 555-66, vii.

Cameron, J. L., T. S. Riall, J. Coleman and K. A. Belcher (2006). "One thousand consecutive pancreaticoduodenectomies." *Ann Surg* 244(1): 10-15.

Chang, D. K., N. D. Merrett and A. V. Biankin (2008). "Improving outcomes for operable pancreatic cancer: is access to safer surgery the problem?" *J Gastroenterol Hepatol* 23(7 Pt 1): 1036-45.

Chang, D. K., N. Q. Nguyen, N. D. Merrett, H. Dixson, R. W. Leong and A. V. Biankin (2009). "Role of endoscopic ultrasound in pancreatic cancer." *Expert Rev Gastroenterol Hepatol* 3(3): 293-303.

Cheng, C. L., S. Sherman, E. L. Fogel, L. McHenry, J. L. Watkins, T. Fukushima, T. J. Howard, L. Lazzell-Pannell and G. A. Lehman (2004). "Endoscopic snare papillectomy for tumors of the duodenal papillae." *Gastrointest Endosc* 60(5): 757-64.

Clarke, D. L., S. R. Thomson, T. E. Madiba and C. Sanyika (2003). "Preoperative imaging of pancreatic cancer: a management-oriented approach." *J Am Coll Surg* 196(1): 119-29.

David, M., C. Lepage, J. L. Jouve, V. Jooste, M. Chauvenet, J. Faivre and A. M. Bouvier (2009). "Management and prognosis of pancreatic cancer over a 30-year period." *Br J Cancer* 101(2): 215-8.

Duffy, M. J., C. Sturgeon, R. Lamerz, C. Haglund, V. L. Holubec, R. Klapdor, A. Nicolini, O. Topolcan and V. Heinemann (2010). "Tumor markers in pancreatic cancer: a European Group on Tumor Markers (EGTM) status report." *Ann Oncol* 21(3): 441-7.

Fischer, H. P. and H. Zhou (2004). "Pathogenesis of carcinoma of the papilla of Vater." *J Hepatobiliary Pancreat Surg* 11(5): 301-9.

Fogelman, D. R., J. Chen, J. A. Chabot, J. D. Allendorf, B. A. Schrope, R. D. Ennis, S. M. Schreibman and R. L. Fine (2004). "The evolution of adjuvant and neoadjuvant chemotherapy and radiation for advanced pancreatic cancer: from 5-fluorouracil to GTX." *Surg Oncol Clin N Am* 13(4): 711-35, x.

Ghaneh, P., E. Costello and J. P. Neoptolemos (2008). "Biology and management of pancreatic cancer." *Postgrad Med J* 84(995): 478-97.

Gillen, S., T. Schuster, C. Meyer Zum Buschenfelde, H. Friess and J. Kleeff (2010). "Preoperative/neoadjuvant therapy in pancreatic cancer: a systematic review and meta-analysis of response and resection percentages." *PLoS Med* 7(4): e1000267.

Goldstein, D., S. Carroll, M. Apte and G. Keogh (2004). "Modern management of pancreatic carcinoma." *Intern Med J* 34(8): 475-81.

Gruenberger, B., J. Schueller, U. Heubrandtner, F. Wrba, D. Tamandl, K. Kaczirek, R. Roka, S. Freimann-Pircher and T. Gruenberger (2010). "Cetuximab, gemcitabine, and oxaliplatin in patients with unresectable advanced or metastatic biliary tract cancer: a phase 2 study." *Lancet Oncol* 11(12): 1142-8.

Heinrich, S. and P. A. Clavien (2010). "Ampullary cancer." *Curr Opin Gastroenterol* 26(3): 280-5.

Heinrich, S., B. Pestalozzi, M. Lesurtel, F. Berrevoet, S. Laurent, J. R. Delpero, J. L. Raoul, P. Bachellier, P. Dufour, M. Moehler, A. Weber, H. Lang, X. Rogiers and P. A. Clavien (2010). "Adjuvant gemcitabine versus NEOadjuvant gemcitabine/oxaliplatin plus adjuvant gemcitabine in resectable pancreatic cancer: a randomized multicenter phase III study (NEOPAC study)." *BMC Cancer* 11: 346.

Iglesias Garcia, J., J. Larino Noia and J. E. Dominguez Munoz (2009). "Endoscopic ultrasound in the diagnosis and staging of pancreatic cancer." *Rev Esp Enferm Dig* 101(9): 631-8.

Iwamuro, M., H. Kawamoto, R. Harada, H. Kato, K. Hirao, O. Mizuno, E. Ishida, T. Ogawa, H. Okada and K. Yamamoto "Combined duodenal stent placement and endoscopic ultrasonography-guided biliary drainage for malignant duodenal obstruction with biliary stricture." *Dig Endosc* 22(3): 236-40.

Jean, M. and K. Dua (2003). "Tumors of the ampulla of Vater." *Curr Gastroenterol Rep* 5(2): 171-5.

Jemal, A., R. Siegel, E. Ward, Y. Hao, J. Xu and M. J. Thun (2009). "Cancer statistics, 2009." *CA Cancer J Clin* 59(4): 225-49.

Kalser, M. H. and S. S. Ellenberg (1985). "Pancreatic cancer. Adjuvant combined radiation and chemotherapy following curative resection." *Arch Surg* 120(8): 899-903.

Katsinelos, P., J. Kountouras, G. Chatzimavroudis, C. Zavos, G. Paroutoglou, R. Kotakidou, K. Panagiotopoulou and B. Papaziogas (2007). "A case of early depressed-type ampullary carcinoma treated by wire-guided endoscopic resection." *Surg Laparosc Endosc Percutan Tech* 17(6): 533-7.

Klapman, J. and M. P. Malafa (2008). "Early detection of pancreatic cancer: why, who, and how to screen." *Cancer Control* 15(4): 280-7.

Knyrim, K., H. J. Wagner, J. Pausch and N. Vakil (1993). "A prospective, randomized, controlled trial of metal stents for malignant obstruction of the common bile duct." *Endoscopy* 25(3): 207-12.

Lang, H., G. C. Sotiropoulos, G. Sgourakis, K. J. Schmitz, A. Paul, P. Hilgard, T. Zopf, T. Trarbach, M. Malago, H. A. Baba and C. E. Broelsch (2009). "Operations for intrahepatic cholangiocarcinoma: single-institution experience of 158 patients." *J Am Coll Surg* 208(2): 218-28.

Lillemoe, K. D., C. J. Yeo and J. L. Cameron (2000). "Pancreatic cancer: state-of-the-art care." *CA Cancer J Clin* 50(4): 241-68.

Luke, C., T. Price, C. Karapetis, N. Singhal and D. Roder (2009). "Pancreatic cancer epidemiology and survival in an Australian population." *Asian Pac J Cancer Prev* 10(3): 369-74.

Maetani, I., S. Akatsuka, M. Ikeda, T. Tada, T. Ukita, Y. Nakamura, J. Nagao and Y. Sakai (2005). "Self-expandable metallic stent placement for palliation in gastric outlet obstructions caused by gastric cancer: a comparison with surgical gastrojejunostomy." *J Gastroenterol* 40(10): 932-7.

Maetani, I., T. Tada, T. Ukita, H. Inoue, Y. Sakai and J. Nagao (2004). "Comparison of duodenal stent placement with surgical gastrojejunostomy for palliation in patients with duodenal obstructions caused by pancreaticobiliary malignancies." *Endoscopy* 36(1): 73-8.

Mercadante, S., E. Catala, E. Arcuri and A. Casuccio (2003). "Celiac plexus block for pancreatic cancer pain: factors influencing pain, symptoms and quality of life." *J Pain Symptom Manage* 26(6): 1140-7.

Moertel, C. G., L. L. Gunderson, J. A. Mailliard, P. J. McKenna, J. A. Martenson, Jr., P. A. Burch and S. S. Cha (1994). "Early evaluation of combined fluorouracil and leucovorin as a radiation enhancer for locally unresectable, residual, or recurrent gastrointestinal carcinoma. The North Central Cancer Treatment Group." *J Clin Oncol* 12(1): 21-7.

Mohamadnejad, M., J. M. DeWitt, S. Sherman, J. K. LeBlanc, H. A. Pitt, M. G. House, K. J. Jones, E. L. Fogel, L. McHenry, J. L. Watkins, G. A. Cote, G. A. Lehman and M. A. Al-Haddad "Role of EUS for preoperative evaluation of cholangiocarcinoma: a large single-center experience." *Gastrointest Endosc* 73(1): 71-8.

Nakai, Y., H. Isayama, Y. Komatsu, T. Tsujino, N. Toda, N. Sasahira, N. Yamamoto, K. Hirano, M. Tada, H. Yoshida, T. Kawabe and M. Omata (2005). "Efficacy and safety of the covered Wallstent in patients with distal malignant biliary obstruction." *Gastrointest Endosc* 62(5): 742-8.

Neoptolemos, J. P., J. A. Dunn, D. D. Stocken, J. Almond, K. Link, H. Beger, C. Bassi, M. Falconi, P. Pederzoli, C. Dervenis, L. Fernandez-Cruz, F. Lacaine, A. Pap, D.

Spooner, D. J. Kerr, H. Friess and M. W. Buchler (2001). "Adjuvant chemoradiotherapy and chemotherapy in resectable pancreatic cancer: a randomised controlled trial." *Lancet* 358(9293): 1576-85.

Neoptolemos, J. P., D. D. Stocken, H. Friess, C. Bassi, J. A. Dunn, H. Hickey, H. Beger, L. Fernandez-Cruz, C. Dervenis, F. Lacaine, M. Falconi, P. Pederzoli, A. Pap, D. Spooner, D. J. Kerr and M. W. Buchler (2004). "A randomized trial of chemoradiotherapy and chemotherapy after resection of pancreatic cancer." *N Engl J Med* 350(12): 1200-10.

Nguyen-Tang, T., K. F. Binmoeller, A. Sanchez-Yague and J. N. Shah (2010). "Endoscopic ultrasound (EUS)-guided transhepatic anterograde self-expandable metal stent (SEMS) placement across malignant biliary obstruction." *Endoscopy* 42(3): 232-6.

Nguyen, N. Q. (2009). "Application of per oral cholangiopancreatoscopy in pancreatobiliary diseases." *J Gastroenterol Hepatol* 24(6): 962-9.

Nguyen, N. Q. and D. F. Bartholomeusz "18F-FDG-PET/CT in the assessment of pancreatic cancer: is the contrast or a better-designed trial needed?" *J Gastroenterol Hepatol* 26(4): 613-5.

Nguyen, N. Q., K. F. Binmoeller and J. N. Shah (2009). "Cholangioscopy and pancreatoscopy (with videos)." *Gastrointest Endosc* 70(6): 1200-10.

Nguyen, N. Q., J. N. Shah and K. F. Binmoeller "Outcomes of endoscopic papillectomy in elderly patients with ampullary adenoma or early carcinoma." *Endoscopy* 42(11): 975-7.

Noble, M. and F. G. Gress (2006). "Techniques and results of neurolysis for chronic pancreatitis and pancreatic cancer pain." *Curr Gastroenterol Rep* 8(2): 99-103.

O'Toole, T. M. and N. Schmulewitz (2009). "Complication rates of EUS-guided celiac plexus blockade and neurolysis: results of a large case series." *Endoscopy* 41(7): 593-7.

Oettle, H., S. Post, P. Neuhaus, K. Gellert, J. Langrehr, K. Ridwelski, H. Schramm, J. Fahlke, C. Zuelke, C. Burkart, K. Gutberlet, E. Kettner, H. Schmalenberg, K. Weigang-Koehler, W. O. Bechstein, M. Niedergethmann, I. Schmidt-Wolf, L. Roll, B. Doerken and H. Riess (2007). "Adjuvant chemotherapy with gemcitabine vs observation in patients undergoing curative-intent resection of pancreatic cancer: a randomized controlled trial." *Jama* 297(3): 267-77.

Offerhaus, G. J., F. M. Giardiello, A. J. Krush, S. V. Booker, A. C. Tersmette, N. C. Kelley and S. R. Hamilton (1992). "The risk of upper gastrointestinal cancer in familial adenomatous polyposis." *Gastroenterology* 102(6): 1980-2.

Palmer, D. H., D. D. Stocken, H. Hewitt, C. E. Markham, A. B. Hassan, P. J. Johnson, J. A. Buckels and S. R. Bramhall (2007). "A randomized phase 2 trial of neoadjuvant chemotherapy in resectable pancreatic cancer: gemcitabine alone versus gemcitabine combined with cisplatin." *Ann Surg Oncol* 14(7): 2088-96.

Paquin, S. C., G. Gariepy, L. Lepanto, R. Bourdages, G. Raymond and A. V. Sahai (2005). "A first report of tumor seeding because of EUS-guided FNA of a pancreatic adenocarcinoma." *Gastrointest Endosc* 61(4): 610-1.

Park, J. K., Y. B. Yoon, Y. T. Kim, J. K. Ryu, W. J. Yoon and S. H. Lee (2008). "Survival and prognostic factors of unresectable pancreatic cancer." *J Clin Gastroenterol* 42(1): 86-91.

Patel, T. (2001). "Increasing incidence and mortality of primary intrahepatic cholangiocarcinoma in the United States." *Hepatology* 33(6): 1353-7.

Patel, T. (2006). "Cholangiocarcinoma." *Nat Clin Pract Gastroenterol Hepatol* 3(1): 33-42.

Peddu, P., A. Quaglia, P. A. Kane and J. B. Karani (2009). "Role of imaging in the management of pancreatic mass." *Crit Rev Oncol Hematol* 70(1): 12-23.

Pinol, V., A. Castells, J. M. Bordas, M. I. Real, J. Llach, X. Montana, F. Feu and S. Navarro (2002). "Percutaneous self-expanding metal stents versus endoscopic polyethylene endoprostheses for treating malignant biliary obstruction: randomized clinical trial." *Radiology* 225(1): 27-34.

Prat, F., O. Chapat, B. Ducot, T. Ponchon, G. Pelletier, J. Fritsch, A. D. Choury and C. Buffet (1998). "A randomized trial of endoscopic drainage methods for inoperable malignant strictures of the common bile duct." *Gastrointest Endosc* 47(1): 1-7.

Puli, S. R., J. B. Reddy, M. L. Bechtold, M. R. Antillon and W. R. Brugge (2009). "EUS-guided celiac plexus neurolysis for pain due to chronic pancreatitis or pancreatic cancer pain: a meta-analysis and systematic review." *Dig Dis Sci* 54(11): 2330-7.

Regine, W. F., K. A. Winter, R. A. Abrams, H. Safran, J. P. Hoffman, A. Konski, A. B. Benson, J. S. Macdonald, M. R. Kudrimoti, M. L. Fromm, M. G. Haddock, P. Schaefer, C. G. Willett and T. A. Rich (2008). "Fluorouracil vs gemcitabine chemotherapy before and after fluorouracil-based chemoradiation following resection of pancreatic adenocarcinoma: a randomized controlled trial." *Jama* 299(9): 1019-26.

Serrano, O. K., M. A. Chaudhry and S. D. Leach "The role of PET scanning in pancreatic cancer." *Adv Surg* 44: 313-25.

Shaib, Y. H., J. A. Davila and H. B. El-Serag (2006). "The epidemiology of pancreatic cancer in the United States: changes below the surface." *Aliment Pharmacol Ther* 24(1): 87-94.

Shami, V. M. and M. Kahaleh (2007). "Endoscopic ultrasonography (EUS)-guided access and therapy of pancreatico-biliary disorders: EUS-guided cholangio and pancreatic drainage." *Gastrointest Endosc Clin N Am* 17(3): 581-93, vii-viii.

Stocken, D. D., M. W. Buchler, C. Dervenis, C. Bassi, H. Jeekel, J. H. Klinkenbijl, K. E. Bakkevold, T. Takada, H. Amano and J. P. Neoptolemos (2005). "Meta-analysis of randomised adjuvant therapy trials for pancreatic cancer." *Br J Cancer* 92(8): 1372-81.

Taylor, M. C., R. S. McLeod and B. Langer (2000). "Biliary stenting versus bypass surgery for the palliation of malignant distal bile duct obstruction: a meta-analysis." *Liver Transpl* 6(3): 302-8.

van Hooft, J. E., M. J. Uitdehaag, M. J. Bruno, R. Timmer, P. D. Siersema, M. G. Dijkgraaf and P. Fockens (2009). "Efficacy and safety of the new WallFlex enteral stent in palliative treatment of malignant gastric outlet obstruction (DUOFLEX study): a prospective multicenter study." *Gastrointest Endosc* 69(6): 1059-66.

van Tienhoven, G., D. J. Gouma and D. J. Richel (2011). "Neoadjuvant chemoradiotherapy has a potential role in pancreatic carcinoma." *Ther Adv Med Oncol* 3(1): 27-33.

Verslype, C., E. Van Cutsem, M. Dicato, S. Cascinu, D. Cunningham, E. Diaz-Rubio, B. Glimelius, D. Haller, K. Haustermans, V. Heinemann, P. Hoff, P. G. Johnston, D. Kerr, R. Labianca, C. Louvet, B. Minsky, M. Moore, B. Nordlinger, S. Pedrazzoli, A. Roth, M. Rothenberg, P. Rougier, H. J. Schmoll, J. Tabernero, M. Tempero, C. van de Velde, J. L. Van Laethem and J. Zalcberg (2007). "The management of pancreatic cancer. Current expert opinion and recommendations derived from the 8th World

Congress on Gastrointestinal Cancer, Barcelona, 2006." *Ann Oncol* 18 Suppl 7: vii1-vii10.

Vinciguerra, V. (2011). "Adjuvant and neoadjuvant therapy for pancreatic cancer." *Oncology (Williston Park)* 25(2): 192-3.

Witzigmann, H., H. Lang and H. Lauer (2008). "Guidelines for palliative surgery of cholangiocarcinoma." *HPB (Oxford)* 10(3): 154-60.

Wong, G. Y., D. R. Schroeder, P. E. Carns, J. L. Wilson, D. P. Martin, M. O. Kinney, C. B. Mantilla and D. O. Warner (2004). "Effect of neurolytic celiac plexus block on pain relief, quality of life, and survival in patients with unresectable pancreatic cancer: a randomized controlled trial." *Jama* 291(9): 1092-9.

Yamao, K., A. Sawaki, N. Mizuno, Y. Shimizu, Y. Yatabe and T. Koshikawa (2005). "Endoscopic ultrasound-guided fine-needle aspiration biopsy (EUS-FNAB): past, present, and future." *Journal of Gastroenterology* 40(11): 1013-1023.

Yeo, C. J., J. L. Cameron, T. A. Sohn, K. D. Lillemoe, H. A. Pitt, M. A. Talamini, R. H. Hruban, S. E. Ord, P. K. Sauter and J. Coleman (1997). "Six hundred fifty consecutive pancreaticoduodenectomies in the 1990s: pathology, complications, and outcomes." *Ann Surg* 226(3): 248-257.

Zadorova, Z., M. Dvofak and J. Hajer (2001). "Endoscopic therapy of benign tumors of the papilla of Vater." *Endoscopy* 33(4): 345-7.

Zuckerman, D. S. and D. P. Ryan (2008). "Adjuvant therapy for pancreatic cancer: a review." *Cancer* 112(2): 243-9.

23

Recontructive Biliary Surgery in the Treatment of Iatrogenic Bile Duct Injuries

Beata Jabłońska and Paweł Lampe
Medical University of Silesia in Katowice,
Department of Digestive Tract Surgery
Poland

1. Introduction

The aim of this chapter is to present different types of biliary reconstructions used in the surgical treatment of iatrogenic bile duct injuries (IBDI).

IBDI remain an important problem in gastrointestinal surgery. The most frequently, they are caused by laparoscopic cholecystectomy which is one of the commonest surgical procedure in the world. The early and proper diagnostics of IBDI is very important for surgeons and gastroenterologists, because unrecognized IBDI lead to serious complications such as biliary cirrhosis, hepatic failure and death. Choice of the proper treatment of IBDI is very important, because it may avoid these serious complications and improve quality of life in patients. Non-invasive, percutaneous radiological and endoscopic techniques are recommended as initial treatment of IBDI. When endoscopic treatment is not effective, surgical management is considered. The goal of surgical treatment is to reconstruct the proper bile flow to the alimentary tract. In order to achieve this goal, many techniques are used. There are contradictory reports on the effectiveness of bile duct reconstruction methods in the literature.

2. Historical perspectives of reconstructive biliary surgery

The first descriptions of the anatomy of the liver and bile ducts originate 2000 years BC in Babylon. The presence of gallbladder stones were found in mummy priestess who lived in the eleventh century BC. Historical records derived from ancient Mesopotamia, Greece, Egypt and Rome, also demonstrate the presence of biliary tract diseases in those days. The first surgical procedures within the bile ducts were simple and uncomplicated. In 1618, Fabricus removed gallstones from the gallbladder. In 1867, Bobbs performed cholecystostomy. Cholecystostomy procedures were also performed by: Sims in 1878, Kocher in 1878 and Tait in 1879. The first planned cholecystectomy, performed on July 15, 1882, by the Berlin surgeon Langenbuch (1846-1901), was a breakthrough in the development of biliary surgery. In 1890, Couvoissier the performed the first choledochotomy. Development of operations performed on the bile ducts caused the the problem of iatrogenic bile duct injuries. In 1891, Sprengel, first described the case of bile duct injury. With the rise of this problem, the first reports of surgical reconstruction of the injuried bile ducts have appeared. In 1892, Doyen, as first, described the biliary ductal end-to-end anastomosis. The idea of biliary-alimentary anastomoses appeared as early as the nineteenth century. Cholecystoenterostomy (anastomosis between the gallbladder and colon), made by Winiwater in 1881, was the he first recorded biliary-alimentary anastomosis. In 1905, Mayo made the first biliary reconstruction as the end-to-side anastomosis between the common bile duct anastomosis (CBD) and the duodenum called choledochoduodenostomy. In 1908, Monprofit described biliary-alimentary anastomosis with a loop of small intestine Roux-Y as a way to repair the biliary tract. In 1909, Dahl reported a similar case. In 1944, Manteuffel performed hepaticojejunostomy conncting intrahepatic biliary ducts with a small intestine. In 1948, Cole attempted to produce mucosal-intestinal anastomosis by moving a segment of small intestine mucosa by incision the proximal hepatic duct. However, in this method, the mucosal fragment had not got sufficient blood supply. This technique was modified in 1969 by Smith, who described it as a mucosal graft. In 1964, Gilbert and in 1969, Grassi used in the insertion of the small intestine pedunculated on biliary vessels in the biliary reconstruction. The role of the Berlin surgeon Kehr (1862-1916), as the creator of the most widely used today T biliary drain, should be also emphasized. The French surgeons, Couinaud in 1954 and in 1956, Hepp and Couinaud, described the hepatic hilum of the liver and long extrahepatic left hepatic duct, using it to perform a wide biliary-alimentary anastomosis, after the dissection of tissue within the hilum the liver to perform, in cases of intrahepatic bile duct injuries. In 1948, Longmire and Sanford also described a technique of isolating the left hepatic duct to use it for a biliary-intestinal anastomosis, consisting of partial resection of the left lobe of the liver. In 1957, this technique has been modified and used by Soupault and Couinaud to isolate the hepatic segment of the third hepatic segment in order to perform the biliary-intestinal anastomosis in the case of atypical sectoral biliary system. In 1994, Blumgart described the technique of the hilar and intrahepatic biliary-enteric anastomosis. In 1965, Thomford and Hallenbeck described the modification of an animal model of biliary-enteric anastomosis using Roux-Y loop, consisting of the jejunostomy (intestinal loop sutured into the abdominal shell) which allowed postoperative endoscopic control and dilatation of the anastomosis. In 1984, Hutson described the application of this technique in patients with postoperative stenosis within the biliary anastomosis. This method of reconstruction has not been widely accepted and incorporated into the standard surgical treatment of iatrogenic bile duct injuries (IBDI). In Poland, the modified biliary-enteric anastomosis with using Roux-Y loop sutured into the hole in the layer of musculo-fascial, was first described in 1997 by Jędrzejczyk et al. [8]. The increase in the IBDI incidence has been reported in the early 90's, which was connected with the introduction of laparoscopic cholecystectomy. The first laparoscopic cholecystectomy was performed in 1986 by Muhe.

3. Pathogenesis of bile duct injuries

Iatrogenic bile duct injury account for about 95% of all benign biliary strictures (BBS). "Benign biliary strictures" is a broad concept encompassing not only strictures caused by injuries, but also as a result of other causal factors [1, 11 12]. Causes of BBS can be divided into several groups and they are summarized in table 1.

There are two basic groups of surgical procedures, which may lead to IBDI. The first group are the operations performed on the bile ducts: an open cholecystectomy (OC) and

Congenital strictures: Biliary atresia and congenital cysts
Bile duct injuries:
Iatrogenic: postoperative, following endoscopic and percutaneous procedures
Following blunt or penetrating trauma of the abdomen
Inflammatory strictures:
Cholelithiasis and choledocholithiasis
Mirizzi's syndrome
Chronic pancretitis
Chronic ulcer or diverticulum of duodenum
Abscess or inflammation of liver or subhepatic region
Parasitic, viral infection
Toxic drugs
Recurrent pyogenic cholangitis
Primary sclerosing cholangitis
Radiation-induced strictures
Papillary stenosis

Table 1. Main causes of benign biliary strictures.

laparoscopic cholecystectomy (LC), choledochotomy, and previous biliary reconstruction. The second group includes the operations performed on other abdominal organs, such as gastric resection (Bilroth II partial resection), liver resection, liver transplantation, pancreatic resection (pancreatoduodenectomy, extended distal pancreatic resection and pancreatic cyst drainage), biliary-enteric and porto-caval anastomoses, and lymphadenectomy or other procedures within the hepatoduodenal ligament.Cholecystectomy is the most common cause of IBDI. Injuries caused during cholecystectomy represent 92.5% of IBDI.

Data regarding the exact prevalence of IBDI after OC and laparoscopic LC vary depending on the literature source. However, according to most authors IBDI occur 2-4 times more likely after laparoscopic cholecystectomy than after open cholecystectomy. IBDI number has increased in recent years, twice in connection with the introduction of laparoscopic cholecystectomy. Table 2 summarizes IBDI incidence following OC and LC.

Author	IBDI incidence following OC	IBDI incidence following LC
Mc Mahon 1995	0.2%	0.81%
Strasberg 1995	0.7%	0.5%
Shea 1996	0.19-0.29%	0.36-0.47%
Targarona 1998	0.6%	0.95%
Lillemoe 2000	0.3%	0.4-0.6%
Gazzaniga 2001	0.0-0.5%	0.07-0.95%
Savar 2004	0.18%	0.21%
Moore 2004	0.2%	0.4%
Misra 2004	0.1-0.3%	0.4-0.6%
Gentileschi 2004	0.0-0.7%	0.1-1.1%
Kaman 2006	0.3%	0.6%

BDI iatrogenic bile duct injuries; OC open cholecystectomy; LC laparoscopic cholecystectomy.

Table 2. Incidence of IBDI following cholecystectomy.

There are many factors that increase the IBDI risk during surgery. Coexisting chronic or exacerbated inflammation of the operated area, obese patient, the presence of abundant adipose tissue around the hepatoduodenal ligament, not sufficiently broad insight into the operative field, and bleeding increases the difficulty of surgery and promote bile duct injuries. The conditions in which laparoscopic cholecystectomy is performed, also affect the rate of IBDI formation. Adverse factors include older age, male gender and long duration of symptoms prior to surgery. Biliary anomalies and variability of the arteries are also the factors associated with increased IBDI risk. Unusually reputed hepatic duct may be mistakenly regarded as the cystic duct and ligated or cut. Excessive, more than is necessary, dissection around the hepatoduodenal ligament during cholecystectomy may lead to damage to the axial arteries running along the CBD. Vascular damage is the cause of postoperative biliary strictures due to ischemia . According to the literature, during the distal bile duct injury the axial artery damage usually occurs (incidence 10-15% of cases), while during high biliary injuries of the proximal bile duct damage to the branches of the proper hepatic artery occurs (incidence 40-60% of cases).

4. Clinical presentation of iatrogenic bile duct injuries

The most frequently observed clinical symptoms include jaundice, fever, chills, abdominal pain, pruritus. Clinical symptoms can be divided into two main groups. The first group are patients with the bile leakage in the early postoperative period due to the bile duct injury. In the presence of a drain in the peritoneal cavity, the injury indicates the appearance of bile in the drain. In patients without a catheter in the peritoneal cavity, bile leak into the abdominal cavity, leading to biloma or bile peritonitis. In these patients, jaundice is not observed because there is no cholestasis. In the second group of patients, usually in a remote time after surgery, there are primarily clinical symptoms resulting from cholestasis due to biliary obstruction. This is most commonly jaundice,

5. Diagnosis of iatrogenic bile duct injuries

5.1 Laboratory diagnosis

Laboratory tests and imaging are used in IBDI diagnostics. In the laboratory tests, cholestasis and liver function indicators, such as bilirubin, alkaline phosphatase (FA), gamma-glutamyl-transpeptidase (GGT), alanine transaminase (ALT) and aspartate transaminase (AST), are the most useful. In patients with biliary stenosis cholestasis parameters are increased: serum bilirubin, FA, GGT and 5'-nucleotidase and leucine aminoptidase (LAP) (less marked in the laboratory), and transaminase values usually remain normal (the liver is not damaged). Elevated transaminase levels indicate damage to liver parenchyma and the development of secondary biliary cirrhosis hypoalbuminemia and prolonged prothrombin time occur due to damaged liver synthetic function.

5.2 Radiological diagnosis

In IBDI diagnostics, imaging ultrasound (USG), abdominal computed tomography (CT) scan of the abdominal cavity, percutaneous cholangiography, endoscopic cholangiography and magnetic resonance imaging are performed. Abdominal ultrasound allows the visualization of intra-and extrahepatic bile ducts with the measurement of width and visibility of the biloma within the peritoneal cavity in the case of bile leakage. In doubtful cases, you can perform abdominal CT to accurately depict the reservoir of bile. Accurate assessment of biliary tree can be made using cholangiography. Percutaneous cholangiography (percutaneous transhepatic cholangiography, PTC) is useful to evaluate the bile ducts proximal to the injury. Endoscopic cholangiography (endoscopic retrograde cholangiopancreatography, ERCP) plays a very important role in the imaging of biliary tract injuries. During ERCP it is possible to supply minor injuries through the establishment of the prosthesis into the lumen of the damaged bile ducts. The advantage of magnetic resonance cholangiography (cholangio-MR) imaging is the high accuracy of the biliary tree and it is non-invasive. This investigation is primarily used to assess the biliary tract before the reconstructive surgery.

6. Classification of iatrogenic bile duct injuries

Different IBDI classifications are described in the literature. In our opinion, the Bismuth classification is the most useful in a clinical practice (described in figure 1). It is based on location of the injury in the biliary tract. This classification is very helpful in prognosis after repair, but does not involve the wide spectrum of possible biliary injuries. The another classification is the Strasberg scale which, in difference from the Bismuth scale, allows to distinguish small (bile leakage from the cystic duct) and serious injuries performed during laparoscopic cholecystectomy, but it does not play an important role in choice of surgical treatment method. The Mattox classification of IBDI takes into consideration a kind of injuring factor (contusion, laceration, perforation, transsection, distraction or interruption of the bile duct or the gallbladder). There are several classifications of IBDI performed during laparoscopic cholecystectomy (Steward and Way, Schmidt, Hannover) in the literature.

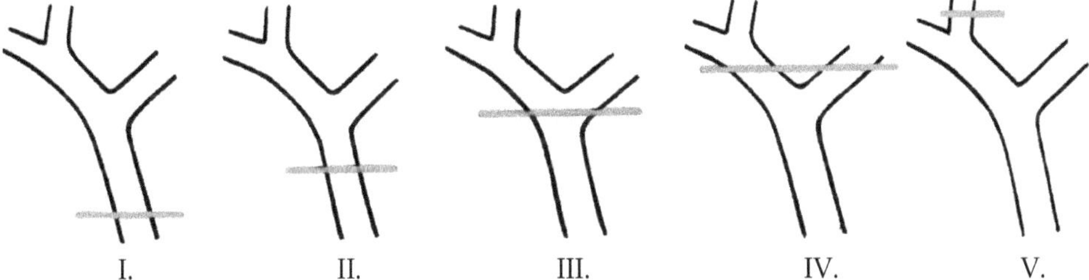

I. Common bile duct (CBD) and low common hepatic duct (CHD) > 2cm. from hepatic duct confluence. II. Proximal CHD < 2cm from confluence. III. Hilar injury with no residual CHD – confluence intact. IV. Destruction of confluence – right and left hepatic ducts separated. V. Involvement of aberrant right sectoral hepatic duct alone or with concomitant injury of CHD.

Fig. 1. Bismuth classification of IBDI.

7. Treatment of iatrogenic bile duct injuries

7.1 Non-invasive treatment of iatrogenic bile duct injuries

Non-invasive, percutaneous radiological end endoscopic techniques are recommended as initial treatment of IBDI. When these techniques are not effective, surgical management is considered.

Type	Injury type
A	Injury of small bile ducts in communication with the main biliary system, with leakage of bile from the Luschka's or cystic ducts.
B	Injury of the sectoral bile duct, with subsequent obstruction of the main biliary system.
C	Injury of the sectoral bile duct with bile leakage of bile from bile duct, without communication with the main biliary system.
D	Side extrahepatic bile duct injury.
E1	CBD or CHD stricture at a distance> 2 cm from the hepatic duct confluence.
E2	CHD stricture at a distance< 2 cm from the hepatic duct confluence.
E3	CHD stricture within the hepatic duct confluence.
E4	Stricture involving the right and left hepatic ducts separately.
E5	Complete closure of all the bile ducts, including sectoral bile ducts.

Table 3. Strasberg classification of IBDI.

Type	Injury type
I	Contusion of the gallbladder or hepatic triad.
II	Jagged or perforation of the gallbladder.
III	The total separation of the gallbladder from the liver.
IV	CBD or CHD partial <50% CBD or CHD laceration or CSF.
V	CBD or CHD transsection> 50% and injury of intrapancreatic or intraduodenal part of bile ducts.

Table 4. Mattox classification of IBDI.

Type	Injury type
I	Small incisions or incomplete intersections of CBD.
II	Stricture caused by thermal injury or clips.
III	Total transsection or excision of the or CBD, CHD or the right or left hepatic ducts.
IV	Resection of the right hepatic cord erroneously recognized as the cystic duct.

Table 5. Steward i Way classification of IBDI.

Type	Injury type
A	Leak from the cystic duct (A1) or an accessory hepatic duct within gallbladder fossa (A2).
B	Clip closure of CBD or CHD incomplete (B1) or complete (B2).
C	Side injury of CBD or CHD over a distance of up to 5 mm (C1) or more than 5 mm (C2).
D	Transsection of CBD or CHD without loss (D1) or loss (D2) of bile duct.
E	Stricture of CBD or CHD over a distance of up to 5 mm (E1),> 5 mm (E2) or the hepatic ducts confluence (E3) or only the right hepatic duct (E4).

Table 6. Schmidt classification of IBDI.

Type	Injury type
A	Peripheal bile leakage (in communication with main biliary system).
A1	Bile leakage from the cystic duct.
A2	Bile leakage from the gallbalder fossa.
B	CHD or CBD stricture without damage (eg caused by a clip).
B1	Incomplete.
B2	Complete.
C	Lateral CHD or CBD injury.
C1	Small spot injury (< 5 mm).
C2	Large injury (> 5 mm) below the hepatic ducts confluence.
C3	Large injury at the level of the hepatic ducts confluence.
C4	Large injury above the hepatic ducts confluence.
D	Total transsection of CHD Or CBD.
D1	Without ductal loss below the hepatic ducts confluence.
D2	With ductal loss below the hepatic ducts confluence.
D3	At the level of the hepatic ducts confluence.
D4	Above the hepatic ducts confluence. (with or without ductal loss).
E	CHD or CBD stricture.
E1	Short, circular (< 5 mm) CHD or CBD stricture.
E2	Longitudinal CBD stricture (>5 mm).
E3	Stricture at the level of the hepatic ducts confluence
E4	Stricture of the right hepatic duct / sectorral hepatic duct.
E5	The complete closure of all the bile ducts, including sectoral bile ducts.

Table 7. Hannover classification of IBDI.

7.1.1 Percutaneous dilatation under radiological control

The effectiveness of percutaneous diltatation of biliary strictures with transhepatic insertion of the stent under radiological control is 40-85%. The main treatment-related complications associated with the liver puncture include haemorrhage, bile leakage and cholangitis. The other less common complications include pneumothorax which is the result of damage to the pleura, biliary-pleural fistula and perforation of adjacent organs, including the colon. Percutaneous technique is less effective (52%) than surgical therapy (89%). Also frequently than post-surgical complications observed (35% and 25% of complications). It is also associated with the higher number of complications (35%) than surgery (25%). The most frequently, it is recommended in very difficult cases of very high, hilar biliary strictures or in the treatment of very small bile ducts in the diameter.

7.1.2 Endoscopic dilatation during ERCP

Endoscopic dilatation associated with insertion of biliary prosthesis during ERCP investigation is the most frequently used non-surgical method in the treatment of IBDI. The effectiveness of endoscopic (72%) and surgical (83%) treatment is comparable. Incidence of complications in both methods of treatment is also comparable (35% vs. 26%). The common complications of endoscopic techniques regarding placement of biliary prosthesis include cholangitis, pancreatitis, prosthesis occlusion, migration, dislodgement and perforation of the bile duct.

Endoscopic treatment is recommended as initial treatment of benign biliary strictures, biliary fistula in the presence and in patients not not qualified to surgical treatment.

7.2 Surgical treatment of iatrogenic bile duct injuries

7.2.1 Immediate repair of IBDI

In the case of intraoperative recognition of bile duct injury, it is recommended that intraoperative cholangiography or conversion from laparoscopic cholecystectomy to open, allowing a better insight into the operative field and immediate repair. The injury should be repaired by an experienced hepatobiliary surgeon. If it is impossible, a patient should be transferred to a referral hepatobiliary surgery center, after adequate drainage of a subhepatic region. If the cut bile duct is less than 2-3 mm in diameter, without communication with the main biliary system, it should be ligated in order to avoid postoperative bile leak leading to development of the biloma and abscess in the subhepatic region. Bile ducts with a diameter of 3-4 mm or more should be surgically repaired because they drain the larger area of the liver. Interruption of CHD or CBD continuity can be repaired by immediate tension-free end-to-end ductal anastomosis with or without a T tube, using absorbable sutures. Security of the immediately repaired bile duct with a T tube is controversial. If the bile duct loss is too long and immediate end-to-end biliary anastomosis is not possible without tension, hepaticojejunostomy Roux-Y is recommended.

7.2.2 Surgical reconstructions of iatrogenic bile duct injuries

Over 2/3 bile duct injuries are recognized at least a few days after surgery, during which the injury occurred. The surgical treatment of elective IBDI is made using different methods of biliary reconstructions. The main aim of surgical treatment is the reconstruction of proper flow of bile to the alimentary tract. The following operations are performed in biliary injuries surgical treatment: Roux-Y hepaticojejunostomy, end-to-end ductal biliary anastomosis with T drainage or endoprothesis conducted into the duodenum according to Górka, choledochoduodenostomy, Lahey hepaticojejunostomy, jejunal interposition hepaticoduodenostomy, Blumgart (Hepp) anastomosis, Heinecke-Mikulicz biliary plastic reconstruction and Smith mucosal graft.

Conditions of proper healing of each biliary anastomosis

- The anastomosed edges should be healthy, without inflammation, ischemia and fibrosis.
- The anastomosis should be tension-free and properly vascularized.
- It should be performed in a single layer with absorbable sutures.

7.2.2.1 Types of surgical reconstructions performed in IBDI

7.2.2.1.1 End-to-end ductal anastomosis (EE)

We recommend this method as the first, because end-to-end ductal anastomosis (EE) is the most physiological biliary reconstruction [1, 46, 48, 49]. In this type of reconstruction, extensive mobilization of the duodenum with the pancreatic head through the Kocher maneuver, excision of the bile duct stricture, and refreshment of the proximal and distal stumps should be performed. Anastomosis is performed in a single layer with interrupted absorbable PDS 4-0 or 5-0 sutures. This reconstruction is not recommended by most authors due to the higher number of anastomosis strictures in comparison with Roux-y hepaticojejunostomy (HJ). We recommend EE first, because in some patients, extensive mobilization of the duodenum with the pancreatic head by the Kocher maneuver allows to perform the tension-free anastomosis after the extensive length-loss of the bile duct. Excision of the bile duct stricture, dissection and refreshing of the proximal and distal stumps as far as the tissues are healthy and without inflammation, and the use of non-traumatic, monofilament-interrupted sutures 5-0 allows the achievement of good long-term results. Using of an internal Y tube conducting from the right and left hepatic ducts into the duodenum through EE and the papilla of Vater also allows the proper healing of this anastomosis. This reconstruction can be performed when the bile duct loss is from 0.5 to 4 cm. It allows the achievement of very good long-term results with effectiveness comparable with HJ. It is important that establishing a physiological bile pathway allows proper digestion and absorption, which causes a higher gain weight in patients following EE, which was noted in study performed in our department. Another essential advantage of EE is possibility of of endoscopic control after surgery.The lower number of early complications is observed after EE than HJ, which is associated with opening of the alimentary tract and the higher number of performed anastomoses (biliary-enteric and entero-enteric) in patients with HJ. The disadvantage is the higher incidence of recorded postoperative stenosis at the anastomosis due to poorer blood supply of the operated area. It can't be performed in patients with bile duct loss more than 4 cm. The diameter of both anastomosed ends should be comparable. If there is a difference between a diameter of anastomosed ends, the thinner end should be incised longitudinally in the anterior surface in order to extend it before creation of anastomosis. This repair should not be carried out in bile ducts that are too thin (diameter less than 4 mm). In our opinion a patient, whom we perform first or exceptionally second bile ducts repair, is a candidate for EE. Because of a number of advantages, EE is recommended as the first method of choice for patients with IBDI.

7.2.2.1.2 Roux-Y hepaticojejunostomy

Roux-Y hepaticojejunostomy (HJ) is the most frequently performed surgical reconstruction of IBDI. In this surgical technique, a proximal common hepatic duct is identified and prepared and the distal common bile duct is sutured. End-to-side or end-to-end HJ is performed in a single layer using interrupted absorbable polydioxanone (PDS 4-0 or 5-0) sutures. Most authors prefer HJ due to the lower number of postoperative anastomosis strictures. According to Terblanche et al, HJ is effective in 90% of cases [50]. However, after this reconstruction, bile flow into the alimentary tract is not physiological, because the duodenum and upper part of the jejunum are excluded from bile passage. Physiological conditions within the proximal gastrointestinal tract are changed as a result of duodenal exclusion from bile passage. An altered bile pathway is a cause of disturbances in the release of gastrointestinal hormones. There is a hypothesis that in patients with HJ, the bile bypass induces gastric hypersecretion leading to a pH change secondary to altered bile synthesis and release of gastrin. A higher number of duodenal ulcers is observed in patients with HJ, which may be associated with a loss of the neutralizing effect of the bile, including bicarbonates and the secondary gastric hypersecretion. Laboratory investigations revealed increased gastrin and glucagon-like immunoreactivity (GLI) plasma levels and decreased triglycerides, gastric inhibitory polypeptide (GIP), and insulin plasma levels in patients with HJ. An altered pathway of bile flow is also a cause of disturbance in fat metabolism in patients undergoing HJ. Moreover, the total surface of absorption in these patients is also decreased due to exclusion of the duodenum and upper jejunum from the food passage. In our department a significantly lower weight gain in patients undergoing HJ in comparison to patients following physiological end-to-end ductal anastomosis was reported [1, 49]. The another disadvantage of HJ is a lack of capability of control endoscopic examination and endoscopic dilatation of strictured biliary anastomosis. In order to resolve this problem, a longer jejunal loop (jejunostomy) is prepared and sutured to the abdominal subcutaneous tissue in the right subcostal region. Jejunostomy can be open or closed with possibility of opening in a case of biliary anastomosis stricture, which should be endoscopically dilated. Jejunostomy is asscociated with bile loss of about 40 ml/day in patients.

7.2.2.1.3 Choledochoduodenostomy (ChD)

Choledochoduodenostomy (ChD) is actually rarely performed operation recommended by some authors only in cases of injury within the distal portion of the common bile duct. It guarantees physiological bile flow into duodenum and anastomosis endoscopic control, and it is easier technically. It is recommended in some cases of distal strictures, when use of the jejunal loop due to numerous adhesions is impossible. It should be performed on the large common bile duct (>15 mm diameter) because the postoperative strictures are more frequent within the narrow duct. ChD should be created between the duodenum and the distal CBD in order to decrease a risk of so-called sump syndrome noted in 0.14-3.3% of cases in the literature. In patients following ChD, recurrent ascending cholangitis due to bile reflux is noted in 0-4%. A higher rate of bile duct cancer in patients with ChD in comparison of HJ (7.6 vs. 1.9%) was reported in the literature .

7.2.2.1.4 Jejunal interposition hepaticoduodenostomy (JIHD)

Jejunal interposition hepaticoduodenostomy, using 25-35 cm of the jejunal loop, is performed in some surgical centers including our department. This reconstruction includes three (biliary-enteric, enteric-duodenal and entero-enteric) anastomoses. Biliary-enteric anastomosis is performed in a single layer with interrupted absorbable sutures 5-0 and enteric-duodenal in a single layer with interrupted or continuous absorbable sutures 4-0. In our opinion, JIHD should be used only in patients in good general condition, without active inflammation within the peritoneal cavity, with protein level more than 6 g/dl and serum bilirubin level less than 20 mg/dl. Good condition of the duodenal wall is important factor for proper healing of hepaticoduodenostomy with jejunal interposition. The advantage of this reconstruction is physiological bile flow into the duodenum, which prevents duodenal ulcer caused by changes in the neurohormonal axis within the upper alimentary tract. This method of reconstruction is recommended mainly in patients with concomitant duodenal ulcer The disadvantage is a higher number of early complications due to presence of three anastomoses.

7.2.2.1.5 Reconstructions of hilar bile duct injuries

The repair of hilar IBDI requires special surgical techniques. In the past, so-called "mucosal graft technique" described by Smith in the 1960s was performed. This reconstruction involves creating a mucosal dome of jejunum (by removing a seromuscular patch) near the end of Roux-Y loop through which a straight rubber tube is brought via hepatic ducts and through liver parenchyma. This technique is based on the hypothesis that jejunal mucosa grafts to the biliary epithelium and mucosa-to-mucosa anastomosis is created. Short-term results were good, but in long-term results a high number of anastomosis strictures was observed. Therefore, currently, not Smith but Blumgart-Hepp technique is used in reconstruction of hilar IBDI. In this technique, dorsal surface of the left hepatic duct parallel to the quadrate hepatic lobe. Dissection and opening of the left hepatic duct longitudinally allows to create a wide anastomosis of 1-3 cm in diameter.

Other methods of IBDI reconstruction, such as Lahey hepaticojejunostomy, jejunal Heinecke-Mikulicz biliary plastic operation Kirtley operation and others are performed sporadically.

7.2.2.2 Types of surgical biliary drainage used in IBDI reconstructions

7.2.2.2.1 External T-drainage

External T-drainage - using a typical Kehr tube with insertion of its short branches into the bile duct and conducting of its long branch through the abdominal wall outside.

7.2.2.2.2 External Y-drainage

External Y-drainage - insertion of short branches of the Kehr tube into both right and left hepatic ducts, splinting of the anastomosis and conducting of its long branch through the jejunal loop and abdominal wall outside.

7.2.2.3 Internal Y-drainage

Internal Y-drainage - insertion of short branches of the Kehr tube into both right and left hepatic ducts, splinting of the anastomosis and conducting of its long branch into the duodenum by the papilla of Vater.

7.2.2.4 Rodney-Smith drainage

Rodney Smith drainage - using two straight rubber tubes splinting the biliary-enteric anastomosis that are brought via hepatic ducts and through liver parenchyma and conducted through the abdominal wall outside. This drainage type is used in high intrahilar biliary-enteric anastomosis. In the past, it was used in Smith "mucosal graft technique".

7.2.2.5 No drainage

Drainage using is still controversial. The advantage of biliary drainage is limitation of the inflammation and fibrosis occurring after the surgical procedure. In some authors' opinion, the presence of the biliary tube prevents anastomosis stricture. The disadvantage of biliary drainage is a higher risk of postoperative complications. There are recommendations (according to Mercado et al) to use transanastomotic stents when there is a thin bile duct less than 4 mm in diameter, and when there is inflammation within the ductal anastomosed edges that makes proper healing of the anastomosis questionable.

8. Treatment of iatrogenic bile duct injuries – Assesment of results in the surgical treatment of iatrogenic bile duct injuries

8.1 Short-term results and early complications

The early postoperative morbidity rate is 20-30% and mortality rate 0-2%. The most frequent early complication is wound infection (8-17.7%). Other complications are the following: bile collection, intra-abdominal abscess, biliary-enteric anastomosis dehiscence, biliary fistula, cholangitis, peritonitis, eventration, pneumonia, circulatory insufficiency, intra-abdominal bleeding, sepsis, infection of the urinary tract, pneumothorax, acute pancreatitis, thrombosis and embolic complications, diarrhea, ileus and multi-organ insufficiency.

8.2 Long-term results and quality of life

8.2.1 Follow-up after surgical reconstructions

8.2.1.1 Duration of follow-up

IBDI remain a serious clinical problem and a challenge for even the most experienced surgical centers of reference. According to literature, the effectiveness of surgical treatment of IBDI is 70-90%. The recurrent strictures after biliary reconstruction occur in 10-30% of cases. About 80% of postoperative recurrence of biliary strictures are observed during the first five years following reconstruction. Two-thirds (65%) of recurrent biliary strictures develop within 2-3 years after the reconstruction, 80% within 5 years, and 90% within 7 years. Recurrent strictures 10 years after the surgical procedure are also described in the literature. Therefore, the objective assessment of long-term results of surgical treatment plays an important role in the observation period (follow-up) (FU). According to most authors, patients following biliary reconstruction should be observed at least 3 years; according to some authors even 5 to 10 years. Satisfactory length of follow-up, which is necessary in order to assess the long-term results of the repair procedure, is 2 to 5 years. Some authors recommend 10 or 20 years of observation. The criteria of success of surgery include: the absence of clinical symptoms such as biliary jaundice or cholangitis and absence of recurrent stenosis after surgery requiring endoscopic or surgical correction.

The early proper biliary reconstruction is very important, because duration of biliary obstruction is the most important risk factor of biliary cirrhosis. According to literature, prolonged time from injury to repair and portal hypertension are important parameters correlating with secondary biliary cirrhosis. So, early biliary repair can prevent liver fibrosis. According to the literature, biliary cirrhosis occurs in two thirds of patients without effective biliary repair. Portal hypertension is noted in 15-25% of patients with biliary cirrhosis due to IBDI. Reoperations within inflammation, fibrosis and a higher risk of intra-operative bleeding due to portal hypertension with collateral circulation and intraperitoneal adhesions are very difficult and associated with increased mortality rate. Therefore, early and proper biliary reconstruction increases survival rate and decreases morbidity and mortality rates in patients with IBDI.

8.2.1.2 Follow-up classifications

Different classifications are used for an objective assessment of the effectiveness of biliary repair. The Terblanche scale taking into account clinical parameters is the most frequently used classification [50, 72]. Other less frequently used classifications are the following: the McDonald, Brummelkamp Lygidakis, Cardenas and Munoz, and Nielubowicz scales.

I	**Excellent result.** No biliary symptoms with normal liver function.
II	**Good result.** Transitory symptoms, currently no symptoms and normal liver function.
III	**Fair result.** Clearly related symptoms requiring medical therapy and/or deteriorating liver function.
IV	**Poor result.** Recurrent stricture requiring correction or related death.

Table 8. Terblanche classification.

A	No clinical symptoms from the biliary tract, proper laboratory liver funtion parameters tests.
B	No clinical signs, laboratory liver function parameters tests slightly elevated liver function parameters, or periodically occurring episodes of pain or fever.
C	Pain, cholangitis with the presence of fever with jaundice and abnormalities in laboratory tests.
D	Condition requiring surgical or endoscopic correction.

Table 9. McDonald classification.

I	Without pain, normal liver function tests.
II	Minor clinical symptoms due to periodic cholangitis resolved after antibiotic therapy, occurring 2-3 times a year, not requiring hospitalization. Proper liver function tests, except of increased serum bilirubin and alkaline phosphatase, with rapid normalization after symptoms resolution.
III	Severe recurrent cholangitis, occuring in more 3 times a year,, lasting over a week and requiring hospitalization. Laboratory tests showing a tendency do increased ALT and AST and transit but rapid increased serum bilirubin and alkaline phosphatase.

Table 10. Lygidakis i Brummelkamp classification.

I	Asymtomatic course.
II	Minor clinical symtoms.
III	Recurrent cholangitis.

Table 11. Muňoz-Cardenas classification.

Very good result	Without clinical symptoms.
Good result	Cholangitis 1-2 a year without jaundice, and without debilitating normal life and work of the patient.
Poor result	Often repeated bouts of cholangitis with jaundice, showing recurrence of stenosis.

Table 12. Nielubowicz classification.

9. Conclusion

The early and proper treatment of IBDI is very important, because it can prevent serious complications and improve quality of life in patients. Non-invasive methods are used as initial treatment. When it is not effective, surgical management should be considered. Surgical treatement includes different types of reconstructions.

10. References

[1] Ahrendt S.; & Pitt H. (2001). Surgical Therapy of Iatrogenic Lesions of Biliary Tract. Word J Surg, Vol. 25, pp. 1360-1365.

[2] Barker E.M.; & Winkler M. (1984). Permanent-access hepaticojejunostomy. Br J Surg, Vol. 71, pp. 188-191.

[3] Beal J.M. (1984). Historical perspective of gallstone disease. Surg Gynecol Obstet, Vol. 158, pp. 181-189.

[4] Bektas H.; Schrem H.; Winny M.; & Klempnauer J. (2007). Surgical treatment and outcome of iatrogenic bile duct lesions after cholecystectomy and the impact od different clinical classification systems. Br J Surg 2007, Vol. 94, No. 9, pp. 1119-1127.

[5] Bismuth H.; & Franco D. (1978). Long term results of Roux-en-Y hepaticojejunostomy. Surg Gyn Obstet, Vol. 146, No. 2, pp. 161-167.

[6] Bismuth H.; & Majno P.E. (2001). Biliary strictures: classification based on the principles of surgical treatment. Word J Surg, Vol. 25, pp. 1241-1244.

[7] Blumgart L.H. (1994). Hilar and intrahepatic biliary enteric anastomosis. Surg Clin North Am;, Vol. 74, pp. 731-740

[8] Bolton J.S.; Braasch J.W.; & Rossi R.L. (1980). Management of benign biliary stricture. Surg Clin North Am, Vol. 60, pp. 313-332.

[9] Braasch J.W. (1994). Historical perspectives of biliary tract injuries . Surg Clin North Am, Vol 74, No. 4 pp. 731-740.

[10] Buell J.F.; Cronin D.C.; Funaki B.; & al. (2002). Devastating and Fatal Compilactions Associated With Combined Vascular and Bile Injuries During Cholecystectomy. Ann Surg, Vol. 137, pp. 703-710.

[11] Chaudhary A.; Chandra A.; Negi S.; & Sachdev A. (2002). Reoperative Surgery for Postcholecystectomy Bile Duct Injuries. Dig Surg, Vol. 19, pp. 22-27.

[12] Coleman J.A.; & Yeo Ch.J. (2000). Postoperative Bile Duct Strictures: Management and Outcome In the 1990s. Ann Surg, Vol. 232, No. 3, pp. 430-441.

[13] Connor S.; & Garden O.J. (2006). Bile duct injury in the era of laparoscopic cholecystectomy. Br J Surg, Vol. 93, pp. 158-168.

[14] Davids P.; Tanka A.; Rauws E, Gulik T.; Leeuwen D.; Wit L.; Verbeek P,.; Huibregtse K.; Heyde N.; & Tytgat G. (1993). Benign Biliary Strictures. Surgery or Endoscopy? Ann Surg, Vol. 217, No. 3, pp. 237-243.

[15] Flum D.R.; Cheadle A.; Prela C.; Dellinger E.P.; & Chan L. (2003). Bile Duct Injury During Cholecystectomy and Survival in Medicare Beneficiares. JAMA 2003, Vol. 290, No. 16, pp. 2168-2173.

[16] Gazzaniga G.M.; Filauro M.; & Mori L. (2001). Surgical treatment of Iatrogenic Lesions of the Proximal Common Bile Duct. Word J Surg, Vol. 25, pp. 1254-1259.

[17] Gentileschi P.; Di Paola M.; Catarci M.; & al. (2004). Bile duct injuries during laparoscopic cholecystectomy. A 1994-2001 audit on 13,718 operations in the area of Rome. Surg Endosc, Vol. 18, pp. 232-236.

[18] Górka Z.; & Rudnicki M. (1991). Zespolenie przewodowo-czczo-dwunastnicze w operacjach odtwórczych dróg żółciowych. Pol Przegl Chir, Vol. 63, pp. 1003-1008.

[19] Górka Z.; Ziaja K.; Nowak J.; Lampe P.; & Wojtyczka A. (1992). 195 operacji kalectwa żółciowego. Pol Przegl Chir, Vol. 64:, pp. 969-976.

[20] Górka Z.; Ziaja K.; Wojtyczka A.; Kabat J.; & Nowak J. (1992). End-to-end anastomosis as a method of choice in surgical treatment of selected cases of biliary handicap. Pol J Surg, Vol. 64, pp. 977-979

[21] Gouma D.J.; & Obertop H. (2002). Management of Bile Duct Injuries: Treatment and Long-Term Results. Dig Surg; Vol. 19, pp. 117-122.

[22] Hall J.G.; & Pappas TN. (2004). Current Management of Biliary Strictures. J Gastrointest Surg, Vol. 8, No. 8, pp. 1098-1110.

[23] Hardy K.J. (1993). Carl Langenbuch and the lasarus Hospital: events and circumstanses surrounding the first cholecystectomyAust N Z J Surg, Vol. 63, No. 1, pp. 56-64.

[24] Imamura M.; Takahashi M.; Sasaki I.; Yamauchi H.; & Sato T. (1988). Effects of the Pathway of Bile Flow on the Digestion of FAT and the Release of Gastrointestinal Hormones. Am J Gastroenterol, Vol. 83, pp. 386-392.

[25] Jabłońska B.; Lampe P.; Olakowski M.; Lekstan A.; & Górka Z. (2008). Surgical treatment of iatrogenic biliary injuries – early complications. Przegl Chir, Vol. 80, No. 6, pp. 299-305.

[26] Jabłońska B.; Lampe P.; Olakowski M.; Górka Z.; Lekstan A.; & Gruszka T. (2009). Hepaticojejunostomy vs. end-to-end biliary reconstructions in the treatment of iatrogenic bile duct injuries. J Gastrointest Surg, Vol. 13, No.6, pp. 1084-1093.

[27] Jabłońska B.; & Lampe P. (2009). Iatrogenic bile duct injuries – etiology, diagnosis and management. WorldJ Gastroenterol, Vol. 15, No. 33, pp. 4097-4104.

[28] Jabłońska B.; Lampe P.; Olakowski M.; Lekstan A.; & Górka Z. (2010). Long-term Results in the Surgical Treatment of Iatrogenic Bile Duct Injuries. Pol J Surg, Vol. 82, No. 6, pp. 354-361.

[29] Jarnagin W.R,.; & Blumgart LH (1999). Operative Repair of Bile Duct Injuries Involving the Hepatic Duct Confluence. Arch Sur, Vol. 134, pp. 769-775.

[30] Jarnagin W.R.; & Blumgart L.H. (2002). Benign biliary strictures. [In:] Blumgart LH, Fong Y, ed. Surgery of the liver and biliary tract. WB Saunders Company, Philadelphia 2002: pp. 895-929.

[31] Jędrzejczyk W.; Juźków H.; & Jackowski M. (1997). Modyfikacja techniki operacyjnej w kalectwie dróg żółciowych – nadzieje i obawy. Pol Przegl Chir, Vol. 69, No. 3, pp. 297-300.

[32] Kaman L.; Sanyal S.; Behera A.; Singh R.; & Katariya R.N. (2006). Comparision of major bile duct injuries following laparoscopic cholecystectomy and open cholecystectomy. ANZ J Surg, Vol. 76, pp. 788-791.

[33] Koffron A.; Ferrario M.; Parsons W.; Nemcek A.; Saker M.; & Abecassis M. (2001). Failed primary management of iatrogenic biliary injury: Incidence and significance of concomitant hepatic arterial disruption. Surgery, Vol. 130, pp. 722-731.

[34] Kosiński B.; Umiński M.; J& agielski G. (1995). Kalectwo dróg żółciowych. Pol Przegl Chir, Vol. 67, No. 2, pp. 141-144.

[35] Kozicki I.; & Bielecki K. (1997). Hepaticojejunostomy in Benign Biliary Stricture – Influence of Careful Postoperative Observations on Long-Term Results. Dig Surg, Vol. 14, pp. 527-533.

[36] Kozicki I.; & Bielecki K.; the late Kowalski A.; & Krolicki L. (1994). Repeated reconstruction for recurrent benign bile duct stricture. Br J Surg, Vol. 81, pp. 677-679.

[37] Kozicki I.; Bielecki K.; & Lembas L. (2000). Leczenie śródwnękowych urazów dróg żółciowych po cholecystektomii laparoskopowej. Pol Przegl Chir, Vol. 72, No. 11, pp. 1049-1060.

[38] Krawczyk M.; & Patkowski W. (2001). Taktyka postępowania w jatrogennym uszkodzeniu dróg żółciowych. Pol Przegl Chir, Vol. 73, No. 1, pp. 4-16.

[39] Lillemoe K.D.; Melton G.B.; Cameron J.L.; Pitt H.A.; Campbell K.A.; Talamini M.A.; Sauter P.A.; Coleman J.; & Yeo C.J. (2000). Postoperative Bile Duct Strictures: Management and Outcome in the 1990s. Ann Surg, Vol.232, No. 3, pp. 430-441.

[40] Lygidakis N.J.; & Brummelkamp W.H. (1986). Surgical management of proximal benign biliary strictures. Acta Chir Scand, Vol. 152, pp. 367-371.

[41] Mattox K.L.; Feliciano D.V.; & Moore E.E.(1996). Trauma. 3rd Ed. Stamford, CT: Applenton&Lange, 1996: 515-519.

[42] Mc Mahon A.J.; Fullarton G.; Barter J.N.; & O'Dwyer P.J. (1995). Bile duct injury and bile leakage In laparosopic cholecystectomy. Br J Surg; Vol. 82, pp. 307-313.

[43] McDonald M.L.; Farnell M.B.; Nagorney D.M.; Ilstrup D.M.; & Kutch J.M. (1995). Benign biliary strictures: repair and outcome with contemporary approach. Surgery, Vol. 118, pp. 582-591.

[44] Mercado M.A.; Chan C.; Orozco H.; Cano-Gutiérrez G.; Chaparro J.M.; Galindo E.; Vilatobá M..; & Samaniego-Arvizu G. (2002) To stent or not to stent bilioenteric anastomosis after iatrogenic injury: A Dilemma not answered? Surgery, Vol. 137:, pp. 60-63.

[45] Mercado M.A.; Chan C.; Orozco H.; Tielve M.; & Hinojosa C.A. (2003). Acute bile duct injury. The need for a high repair. Surg Endosc, Vol. 17, pp. 1351-1355.

[46] Misra S.; Melton G.B.; Geschwind J.F.; Venbrux A.C.; Cameron J.L.; & Lillemoe K.D. (2004). Percutaneous Management of Bile Duct Strictures and Injuries Associated with Laparoscopic Cholecystectomy: A Decade of Experience. J Am Coll Surg, Vol. 198, pp. 218-226.

[47] Moore D.F.; Feurer I..D.; Holzman M.D.; & al. (2004). Long-term Detrimental Effect of Bile Injury on Health-Related Quality of Life. Arch Surg, Vol. 139, pp. 476-482.

[48] Muñoz R.; & Cardenas S. (1990). Thirty Years' Experience with Biliary Tract Reconstruction by Hepaticoenterostomy and Transhepatic T Tube. Am J Surg, Vol. 159, pp. 405-410.

[49] Murr M.M.; Gigot J.F.; Nagorney D.M.; Harmsen W.S.; Ilstrup D.M.; & Farnell MB. (1999). Long-term Results of Biliary Reconstruction After Laparoscopic Bile Duct injuries. Arch Surg, Vol. 134, No. 6, pp. 604-610

[50] Negi S.S,.; Sakhuja P.; Malhotra V.; & al. (2004). Factors Predicting Advanced Hepatic Fibrosis in Patients With Postcholecystectomy Bile Duct Strictures. Arch Surg, Vol. 139, pp. 299-303.

[51] Nielsen M.K.; Jensen S.L.; Malstrom J.; & Niwlsen O.V. (1980). Gastryn and gastric acid secretion in hepaticojejunostomy Roux-en-Y. Surg Gyn Obstet, Vol. 150, pp. 61-64.

[52] Nielubowicz J.; Olszewski K.; & Szostek M. (1973). Operacje odtwórcze w kalctwie dróg żółciowych. Pol Przegl Chir, Vol. XLV, No. 12, pp. 1389-1395.

[53] Pellegrini C.A.; Thomas M.J.; & Way L.W. (1984). Recurrent biliary stricture: patterns of recurrence and outcome of surgical therapy. Am J Surg, No. 147, pp. 175-180.

[54] Perakath B.; Sitaram V.; Mathew G.; & al.(2003). Postcholecystectomy benign biliary stricture with portal hypertension: is a portosystemic shunt before hepaticojejunostomy necessary? Ann R Coll Surg Engl, Vol. 85, pp. 317-320.

[55] Pitt H.A.; Kaufman H.S.; Coleman J.; White R.I.; & Cameron JL. (1989). Benign postoperative biliare strictures. Operate or dilate? Ann Surg, Vol. 210, pp. 417-425.

[56] Pitt H.A.; Miyamoto T.; Parapatis S.K.; Tompkins R.K.; & Longmire W.P .Jr. (1982). Factors influencing outcome in patients with postoperative biliary strictures. Am J Surg, Vol. 144, pp. 14-21.

[57] Reynolds W. Jr. 2001The first laparoscopic cholecystectomy. JSLS. Jan-Mar;5(1):89-94.

[58] Robinson T.N,.; Stiegmann G.V.; Durham J.D.; Johnson S.I.; Wachs M.E.; Serra A.D.; & Kumpe D.A. (2001). Management of major bile duct injury associated with laparoscopic cholecystectomy. Surg Endosc, Vol. 15, pp. 1381-1385.

[59] Rossi R.L.; & Tsao J.I. (1994). Biliary reconstruction. Surg Clin North Am, Vol. 74, No. 4, pp. 825-841.

[60] Rudnicki M.; McFadden D.W.; Sheriff S. & Ischer J.E. (1992). Roux-en-Y jejunal Bypass abolishes postprandial neuropeptide Y release. J Surg Res, Vol. 53, pp. 7-11.

[61] Savar A.; Carmody I.; Hiatt J.R.; & Busuttil R.W. (2004). Laparoscopic Bile Duct Injuries: Management at a Tertiary Liver Center. Am Surg, Vol. 70, pp. 906-909.

[62] Schmidt S.C.; Langrehr J.M.; Hintze R.E.; & Neuhaus P. (2005). Long-term results and risk factors influencing outcome of major bile duct injuries following cholecystectomy. Br J Surg, Vol. 92, pp. 76-82.

[63] Schmidt S.C.; Settmacher U.; Langrehr J.M.; & Neuhaus P. (2004). Management and outcome of patients with combined bile duct and hepatic arterial injuries after laparoscopic cholecystectomy. Surgery, No. 135, pp. 613-618.

[64] Shamiyeh A.; & Wayand W. (2004). Laparoscopic cholecystectomy: early and late complications and their treatment. Langenbecks Arch Surg, No. 389, Vo.3, pp. 164-171.

[65] Shea J.A.; Healey M.J.; Jesse A.; & al. (1996). Mortality and Complications Associated with Laparoscopic Cholecystectomy: A Meta-Analysis. Ann Surg, Vo. 224, No. 5, pp. 609-620.

[66] Sicklick J.K.; Camp M.S.; Lillemoe K.D.; & al. (2005). Surgical Management of Bile Duct Injuries Sustained During Laparoscopic Cholecystectomy. Perioperative Results in 200 Patients. Ann Surg, Vol. 241, No. 5, pp. 786-795.

[67] Sicklick J.K.; Camp M.S.; Lillemoe K.D.; Melton G.B.; Yeo C.J.; Campbell K.A.; Talamini M.A.; Pitt H.A.; Coleman J.; Sauter P.A,.; & Cameron J.L. (2005). Surgical Management of Bile Duct Injuries Sustained During Laparoscopic Cholecystectomy. Perioperative Results in 200 Patients. Ann Surg, Vol. 241, pp. 786-795.

[68] Sikora S.S.; Pottakkat B.; Srikanth G.; Kumar A.; Saxena R.; & Kapoor V.K. (2006). Postcholecystectomy Benign Biliary Strictures – Long-Term Results. Dig Surg, Vol. 23, pp. 304-312.

[69] Sikora S.S.; Srikanth G.; Agrawal V.; & al. (2008). Liver histology in benign biliary stricture: fibrosis to cirrhosis... and reversal? J Gastroenterol Hepatol, Vol. 23, No. 12, pp. 1879-84.

[70] Smith R. (1964). Hepaticojejunostomy with transhepatic intubation: a technique for very high strictures of the hepatic ducts. Br J Surg, Vol. 51, pp. 186-194.

[71] Steward L.; & Way L.W. (1995). Bile Duct Injuries During Laparoscopic Cholecystectomy. Factors That Influence the Results of Treatment. Arch Surg, Vol. 130, pp. 1123-1128.

[72] Strasberg S.M.; Hertz M.; & Soper N.J. (1995). An analysis of the problem of biliary injury during laparoscopic cholecystectomy. J Am Coll Surg, Vol. 189, pp. 101-125.

[73] Targarona E.M.; Marco C.; Balague C.; & al. (1998). How, when and why bile duct injury occurs. A comparision between open and laparoscopic cholecystectomy. Surg Endosc, Vol. 12, No. 4, pp. 322-326.

[74] Terblanche J.; Worthley C.; & Krige J. (1990). High or low hepaticojejunostomy for bile duct strictures? Surgery, Vol. 108, pp. 828-834.

[75] Tocchi A.; Costa G.; Lepre L.; Lotta G.; Mazzoni G.; & Sita A. (1996). The Long-Term Outcome of Hepaticojejunostomy In the Treatment of Benign Bile Duct Strictures. Ann Surg, Vol. 224, No. 2, pp. 162-167.

[76] Tocchi A.; Mazzoni G.; Liotta G.; Costa G.; Lepre L.; Miccini M.; Masi E.; Lamazza M.A.; & Fiori E. (2000). Management of Benign Biliary Strictures. Arch Surg, Vol. 135, No. 2, pp. 153-157.

[77] Tocchi A.; Mazzoni G.; Lotta G.; Lepre L.; Cassini D.; & Miccini M. (2001). Late Development of Bile Duct Cancer in Patients Who Had Biliary-Enteric Drainage for Benign Disease: A Follow-Up Study of More Than 1,000 Patients. Ann Surg, Vol. 234, No. 2, pp. 210-214 .

[78] Tsalis K.G.; Christoforidis E.C.; Dimitriadis C.A.; Kalfadis S.C.; Botsios D.S.; & Dadoukis J.D. (2003). Management of bile duct injury during and after laparoscopic cholecystectomy. Surd Endosc, Vol. 17, pp. 31-37.

[79] van Gulik T.M. (1986). Langenbuch's cholecystectomy, once a remarkably controversial operation. Neth J Surg, Vol. 38, No. 5, p. 138-141.

[80] Waage A.; & Nilsson M. (2006). Iatrogenic Bile Duct Injury. A Population-Based Study of 152 776 Cholecystectomies in the Swedish Inpatient Registry. Arch Surg, Vol. 141, pp. 1207-1213.

[81] Warren K.W.; & Jefferson M. (1973). Prevention and Repair of Strictures of the Extrahepatic Bile Ducts. Surg Clin North Am, No. 53, Vol. 5, pp. 1169-1190.

[82] Wexler M.J.; & Smith R. (1975). Jejunal mucosal graft: a sutureless technic for repair of high bile duct strictures. Am J Surg, Vol. 129, pp. 204-211.

[83] Wudel L.J.; Wright J.K.; Pinson C.W.; Herline A.; Debelak J.; Seidel S.; Revis K.; & Chapman W. (2001). Bile Duct Injury Following Laparoscopic Cholecystectomy: A Cause for Continued Concern. The Amer Surg, Vol. 67, No. 6, pp. 557-564.

[84] Yeo Ch.J.; Lillemoe K.D.; Ahrendt S.; & Pitt A.P. (2002). Operative Management of Strictures and Benign Obstructive Disorders of the Bile Duct. [In:] Zuidema GD, Yeo ChJ, ed. Shackelford's Surgery of the Alimentary Tract. Vol III. 5th edition. WB Saunders Company, Philadelphia 2002: pp. 247-261.

24

Hepatic Encephalopathy

Om Parkash, Adil Aub and Saeed Hamid
Aga Khan University, Karachi
Pakistan

1. Introduction

The liver is the most important organ for the well-functioning of other organs because of its vital role in nutrition, metabolism and secretion. Any disturbance in normal homeostasis of liver as it happens in acute liver failure (ALF) and chronic liver disease (cirrhosis) will lead to extra hepatic manifestations of liver disease, among them one is encephalopathy. And this encephalopathy caused by liver abnormality is known as Hepatic encephalopathy (HE).(1) HE occurs in 50-70% of patients with chronic liver disease and this is one of the sign of decompensated chronic liver disease. Occurrence of HE associated with poor prognosis with survival of approximately 42% at 1 year.(2)

1.1 Definition

Hepatic encephalopathy(HE) is defined as a reversible and metabolically induced neuropsychiatric complication, most commonly associated with cirrhosis, but may also be a complication of acute or chronic liver disease.(3) The affected patients exhibit alterations in psychomotor functions, personality changes, cognitive impairment and disturbed sleep pattern. Although, precise pathophysiologic mechanisms are not well understood, severe liver damage or the presence of Porto-systemic shunts are thought to be the major mechanisms involved.(4)

According to the classification proposed by the working party in 1998, HE can be graded into 3 types:

1. Type A HE (associated with acute liver failure);
2. Type B HE (observed in patients with Porto-systemic bypass and no intrinsic hepato-cellular disease);
3. Type C HE (associated with cirrhosis or portal-hypertension or Porto-systemic shunt).

    Type C HE can be further divided into three categories:

    i.   Episodic HE (Spontaneous; recurrent; precipitated)
    ii. Persistent HE (Mild; Severe; Treatment dependent)
    iii. Minimal or Overt HE(3)

Overt HE (OHE) is a syndrome of neuropsychiatric abnormalities that can be detected by bedside clinical tests in contrast to minimal HE (MHE) that requires specific psychometric tests for detection.(5) Defining type-C HE into minimal or overt, episodic or persistent and precipitated or spontaneous is clinically relevant since the management of each category is very different. Nowadays MHE has been recognized as the major factor in impairing the health related quality of life (HRQOL) in patients with cirrhosis.(6, 7) And MHE has prognostic significance because it predicts the occurrence of overt HE and is not useful predictor for mortality in cirrhosis.(8)

2. Pathophysiology

The pathophysiology of hepatic encephalopathy is intricate and exact mechanisms leading to HE are not clearly understood. Hepatic encephalopathy pathogenesis has many components which include ammonia, inflammatory cytokines, benzodiazepine like compounds and manganese like substances which impair neuronal function.(9) The role of ammonia has dominated explanations for the pathogenesis of HE but it cannot single handedly explain all the neurological changes seen in HE. Evidence regarding other concurrent factors has emerged over the years and it is thought that these factors either work alone or in synergy to cause astrocytes to swell and fluid to accumulate in brain which causes the symptoms of HE(10). Some factors and conditions also appear to precipitate HE (Box A).

2.1 The ammonia theory

Ammonia is produced predominantly from dietary nitrogenous components, bacterial metabolism of these nitrogenous products in the colon and in small intestine from glutamine by glutaminase enzyme.(11) Eventually this ammonia from gastrointestinal tract enters portal circulation for its final destination of urea cycle in the liver to be converted as urea which will subsequently be excreted by kidneys.(12) Under normal conditions, ammonia is eliminated through urea formation in the liver but in patients with acute liver failure, brain and muscle cells are also involved in the metabolism. Elevated levels of ammonia may cause severe toxicity so it must be removed from the body.(13) Because of liver disease and portosystemic collaterals in cirrhosis, ammonia concentration in blood rises hence crosses the blood brain barrier.(14) In Brain, astrocytes are the only cells capable of metabolizing ammonia and express the enzyme glutamine synthase for the conversion of ammonia into glutamine. So, ammonia detoxification in astrocytes leads to accumulation of glutamine which being an osmolyte, causes movement of water inside the astrocyte and causes cerebral edema i-e 'Trojan horse' hypothesis(14-16). Some of the studies had shown the ammonia induced expression of aquaporin water channel on astrocytes. (17)

This has been seen in autopsies of patients with cirrhosis in which brain tissue had shown swollen astrocytes with enlarged nuclei along with displacement of chromatin to the perimeter of the cell, this condition is known as Alzheimer type II astrocytosis.(18) Acute insult of ammonia leads to calcium dependent glutamate release from astrocytes, which causes increased neuronal activity (as seen in Type A HE). A prolonged exposure to ammonia leads to glutamine induced osmotic stress, which causes compensatory release of myoinositol and taurine from the astrocytes, which may lead to down regulation of glutamate receptors and neuroinhibitory state of HE (as seen in Type C HE). Elevated intracellular ammonia levels also results in altered neurotransmission by agonizing GABA tone.(19)

Hyper ammonia lead to abnormal cerebral blood flow and glucose metabolism and this had been seen in studies of single photon emission tomographic (SPECT) in which redistribution of blood flow form cerebral cortex to subcortical regions had been demonstrated. This abnormality lead to different HE features.(17, 20)

2.2 Inflammation

The partial credit also goes to the inflammation because majority of the cirrhotic patients in the presence of infection develop the HE. This association of markers of inflammatory response in state of systemic inflammatory response (SIRS) and HE, has been demonstrated in different studies.(21, 22) In one of the clinical study, it has been seen that HE or neuropsychological dysfunction improves after the resolution of SIRS.(23) Despite this exact mechanism of inflammation leading to HE is still not known as yet, but possibly it is hypothesized that cytokine mediated changes in blood brain barrier (BBB) permeability, altered glutamate uptake by astrocyte and altered expression of GABA receptors.(23)

TNF released in response to inflammation has been correlated to the symptoms of HE. It causes Astrocytes to release inflammatory cytokines (i-e IL-1, IL-6) which impairs the endothelial Blood-Brain barrier and increases ammonia diffusion into astrocytes. (24)

2.3 Neurosteroids and GABA/Benzodiazepine receptor complex theory

Neurosteroids are mainly produced by myelinating glial cells in response to increased expression of peripheral type benzodiazepine receptor (Trasnslocator proteins), which are activated by ammonia, inflammation and manganese. Neurosteroids increase chloride influx and thereby enhance GABAergic tone, causing symptoms in patients with Type C HE.(25, 26)

GABA mediates its action through GABA-receptor complex (GRC) and acts as an inhibitory neurotransmitter. Increased sensitivity of the trasnslocator proteins also enhances the activation of GABA-GRC complex, hence causing inhibition of neurotransmission.(14, 27) Increased GABAergic tone has been associated with the pathogenesis of HE and this was proved by the reports which had revealed the beneficial effects of benzodiazepine antagonist (Flumazenil).(28) There is an excess of benzodiazepine like compounds in HE that are derived from synthesis by intestinal flora, dietary vegetables and medications.(29, 30) Moreover natural benzodiazepines also accumulate in brain and furthermore cirrhotic patients have the poor capability of clearing the benzodiazepine like compounds.(31) These compounds bind to GABA receptor complex inducing GABA release and neuro-inhibition. A study by Stewart et al group had shown that ammonia itself bind to the GABA receptor complex.(32) It may also potentiate benzodiazepines by up regulating expression of peripheral type benzodiazepine receptor that trigger synthesis of neuro-steroids, which are strong GABA agonists.(33)

Hence GABAergic tone is more likely attributed to elevated levels of benzodiazepines like compounds in patients with cirrhosis.

BCCA and false neurotransmitter theory: Brain neurotransmission is regulated by CNS concentration of amino acids and their precursor. In cirrhotic patients, plasma concentrations of aromatic amino acids (tryptophan, tyrosine, and phenalanine) are elevated and branch chain amino acids (Leucine, isoleucine and valine) concentration are reduced. Aromatic as well as branch chain amino acids share a common transport mechanism into the CNS and as a consequence of increased of aromatic amino acids, neuronal levels may be increased leading to the production of false neurotransmitter subsequently leading to HE.(34)

Serotonin theory: Serotonin, a neurotransmitter which is widely distributed in CNS, has been implicated in the pathogenesis of HE. In cirrhotic patients it has been seen that serotonin metabolism is altered hence leading to serotonergic synaptic deficit. Serotonergic pathway in brain is important for regulation of sleep, locomotion and circadian rhythmicity.(35) Serotonin metabolism is intricately and selectively sensitive to the degree of portosystemic shunting and hyperammonaemia, therefore suggesting a role for serotonin in early neuropsychiatric symptoms of HE.(36)

Zinc theory: Zinc (Zn) element is a component/substrate of urea cycle enzymes. It is assumed that this element is reduced in patients with liver cirrhosis. Zn supplementation increases activities of ornithine transcarbamalyse increasing excretion of ammonia ions. Interestingly till now there is conflicting evidence for this hypothesis of Zn supplementation in He patients.(37, 38)

2.4 Oxidative and nitrosative stress

Exposure of astrocytes to ammonia, inflammatory cytokines, hyponatremia and benzodiazepines leads to enhanced production of RNS & ROS via the Calcium dependent N-methyl-D-aspartate (NMDA) pathway. RNS and ROS cause tyrosine nitration, leading to altered BBB permeability and astrocyte swelling. (39, 40)

2.5 Manganese theory

In normal healthy individuals, Maganese is cleared by liver and excreted into the bile. Manganese is known to stimulate the Translocator proteins located on astrocytes, leading to enhanced neurosteroid synthesis. In cirrhotic patients, it accumulates in the basal ganglia because of decreased excretion of Maganese due to portosystemic shunting and promotes formation of Alzheimer's type 2 astrocytes.(41) Brain magnetic resonance imaging (MRI) in cirrhotic patients has shown changes which are due to accumulation of Maganese in basal ganglia particularly in the palladium, putamen and caudate nucleus.(41)

3. Precipitating factors: (Box A)

The Most of HE episodes are precipitated by an event rather than spontaneous, with infection anywhere in body being the common, though its frequency is decreasing. Hence careful history and examination are necessary to identify the precipitating or contributing factors for HE, most of the time these factors are evident.(42)

Gastrointestinal bleeding commonly precipitates the HE even if it is controlled or stopped bleeding. Sometimes occult chronic gastrointestinal blood loss can also lead to HE, which needs to be evaluated and treated accordingly.(42)

Dehydration is again a very common precipitating factor in cirrhotic patients leading to HE because some of the patients ascites, are diuretics. And aggressive diuresis do induce dehydration leading to metabolic alkalosis and electrolyte imbalances.

• GI Bleeding	• Constipation
• Electrolyte imbalance	• Hypovolemia
• Trauma	• Dehydration
• Infection	• Medications (sedatives, diuretics, psychotropic,)
• Sepsis	• Uremia
• Dietary protein Overload	

Box A. Precipitating Factors for HE

It has also been seen that transjuglar intrahepatic portosystemic shunt (TIPS) in some of the cases can lead to HE. Few other precipitating factors which can sometimes lead to HE, need to be looked into by taking careful history and examination and shown in Box (A)

4. Clinical features

The clinical signs and symptoms of HE may range from mild cognitive impairment to profound coma. These include forgetfulness, alteration in sleep-wake cycle, changes in personality and emotions, hyperreflexia and drowsiness. In more severe cases disorientation, constructional apraxia , asterixis, seizures and eventually coma may develop.(43) It is very important to exclude other causes of altered mental status or encephalopathy (Box B) in suspected patients for appropriate management of HE.

• Subdural Hematoma
• Drug or alcohol intoxication
• Wilson's disease
• Hypoglycemia
• Wernicke's encephalopathy
• CNS Sepsis
• Postictal Confusion

Box B. Differential Diagnosis for HE

Clinically, the most commonly employed criteria used for grading is the West Haven criteria (Table 1) which defines HE semi quantitatively into four grades, based on the presence of specific clinical signs and symptoms and their severity. Further classification of comastose or unconscious patients can be done by using Glasgow Coma Scale which provides a more objective assessment of the conscious state of the patient.(4)

5. Diagnosis

Checking for Elevated Blood ammonia levels is the most commonly used parameter for assessment, but they may also be elevated due to other possible causes (i-e tourniquet use, delayed processing and cooling of sample, disorders related to ammonia and proline metabolism). In acute liver failure, arterial ammonia levels >150 mg/dl may be predictive of brain edema and herniation. However, measurement of arterial ammonia over venous ammonia offers no advantage in Chronic liver disease.(3, 44)

Grade	Intellectual function	Neuromuscular function
0	Normal	Minor abnormalities
1	Personality changes, attention deficits, irritability, depressed state	Tremor and incoordination
2	Changes in sleep-wake cycle, cognitive dysfunction, lethargy, behavioral changes	Asterixis, Speech abnormalities, Ataxic gait
3	Disorientation, unconsciousness, amnesia	Nystagmus, Clonus, Muscular rigidity
4	Stupor and Coma	Unresponsiveness to noxious stimuli, Oculocephalic reflex

Table 1. West Haven classification for grading of HE(1)

Neuropsychometric evaluation usually is done via 'paper and pencil tests' and 'computerized tests'. The routinely used paper and pencil tests include psychometric HE scores (PHES) and The Repeatable Battery for the Assessment of neurological status (RBANS). PHES has been endorsed as a 'gold standard' for diagnosis of MHE and is used to diagnose the cognitive changes that characterize MHE. RBANS in addition to diagnosing the cognitive issues, also scores patient's memory.(45) Some computerized psychometric tests like 'The inhibitory control test' and 'CDR computerized assessment system' are gaining popularity as promising diagnostic tests due to their effectiveness and convenience(46). However, the value of these psychometric tests is limited by methodological problems, training and education, demographic dependence and lack of standardization.(43)

Neurophysiological assessment is done via Electroencephalography (EEG) and the Critical flicker frequency test (CFF). EEG is associated with decreased electrical activity and shows diffuse slowing of alpha waves with eventual development of delta waves.(47) CCF, a light based test, is used for a rapid and reliable quantification of HE. Based on the principle of hepatic retinopathy, it represents the frequency at which discrete light pulses are first perceived by the patient. A CCF of below 39 Hz is diagnostic for MHE and the test results are not dependent on sex, occupation and education level.(48)

Imaging Modalities include different Magnetic resonance techniques(T1-weighted imaging, proton spectroscopy, magnetic transfer ratio, T2- weighted FLAIR sequence and diffusion weighted imaging) to measure cerebral edema, changes in brain activity and concentration of different substances(i-e glutamine, choline). A CT scan can be used to exclude subdural hematoma or other cerebrovascular events that may mimic HE.(48)

6. Treatment

HE treatment has evolved over the last 5 decades and medical science had seen many breakthroughs during this tenure. Treatment can be tailored around multiple key management principles which parallel the pathophysiology of the disease and these principles are:(42)

Management of precipitating factors,

Reduction of ammonia

Modulation intestinal flora

Modulation of neurotransmission

Correction of nutritional deficiencies

Reduction of inflammation/infection

Many treatment options are available for the treatment of HE with the mainstay to eliminate the underlying factors that precipitate HE. It is recommended that all patients should receive the empiric therapy (Box C) for HE, based on the principle of reducing the production and absorption of ammonia. Some strategies that are commonly applied to stop precipitating events are the following:

1. in patients with HE induced by gastrointestinal hemorrhage, stop the bleeding with vasoactive drugs, an endoscopic therapy or an angiographic shunt (TIPS), correct the anemia with a blood transfusion and use a nasogastric tube to facilitate upper gastrointestinal cleansing;
2. Promptly start Antibiotics therapy for infections;
3. Resolve constipation by cathartic and/or bowel enema, electrolyte abnormalities by discontinuing diuretics and correct hypo- or hyperkalemia;
4. Correct deterioration of renal function by stopping diuretics, treating dehydration and discontinuing nephrotoxic drugs
5. if HE is precipitated by the administration of exogenous sedatives, discontinue benzodiazepines and start flumazenil.(49)

- Lactulose (15-30ml orally, twice daily)
- Rifaximin (550mg orally, twice daily)
- Neomycin (500mg orally, four times daily)
- Metronidazole (250mg orally, four times daily)
- Vancomycin (250mg orally, four times daily)
- Sodium Benzoate(5 mg orally, twice daily)
- Flumazenil (1-3 mg IV)

Box C. Empiric Treatment for Hepatic encephalopathy(48)

7. Reduction of ammonia and modulation of neurotransmission

7.1 Nonadsorable disaccharides

Nonadsorable disaccharides (Lacutlose and Lactitol) especially Lactulose are considered the first line therapy for HE despite lack of well-designed randomized controlled trial. They are metabolized by the colonic bacteria and form by products that reduce the colonic PH, hence interfering with mucosal uptake of glutamine and reducing the synthesis and absorption of ammonia. There are other proposed mechanism of lactulose in HE such as lactulose modifies the colonic flora which in turn results in shift of urease containing bacteria with lactobacillus, fourfold increased fecal nitrogen excretion due to increase stool volume and it also helps in reduction of formation potentially toxic short chain fatty acids e.g propionate or butyrate.(50-53)

Lactulose can also be administered orally through a nasogastric tube to unresponsive patients as well as rectally through enemas.

The most common side effects associated with over use include dehydration, electrolyte imbalance and abdominal cramping. Previously it is known to cause no improvement in psychometric test performance and mortality(54). Few years back a study conducted in India had shown significant improvement and health related quality of life and psychometric improvement in patients with HE especially with minimal HE.(7)

The lactulose has got some role in preventing recurrent episodes of HE. It was proved by an open label RCT study from India by Sarin group, which suggested that lactulose is also effective in preventing recurrent episodes of HE.(55)

The recommended dose of lactulose is about 15-30ml given twice a day. Lactitol, an alternative to lactulose is considered equally effective and is used in patients intolerant of lactulose, but it is not available in some countries.(56, 57)

7.2 Antibiotics

Patients intolerant to nonabsorable disaccharides are generally treated with antibiotics, to suppress the bacteria involved in ammonia genesis. There are few antibiotics which have been used for the treatment of HE which had shown limited benefit, which include neomycin, metronidazole, oral vancomycin and very recently Rifaximin.(54)

In fact neomycin was used for treatment of HE for many years based on earlier studies then in early 1990's a double blind randomized controlled trial had no improvement in HE. And also because of its limited systemic absorption which would lead to ototoxicity and nephrotoxicity has lost its use in HE in liver cirrhosis. (58)

Rifaximin, a minimally absorbed oral antibiotic has been approved by FDA for the treatment of chronic HE, on the basis of results of a multicenter, randomized, controlled trials and met analysis.(59) Recently a RCT had shown benefit in prevention of recurrent hepatic encephalopathy over period of 6 months follow up. Subsequently further studies had also shown role of Rifaximin in improving the health related quality of life in patients with HE similarly improvement in Psychometric tests and simulated driving tests.(60-62) The use of this antibiotic is increasing due to few adverse effects and no known drug interactions. The recommended adult daily dose is 1200 mg/day, usually in three divided doses.

Some small studies have also reported the effectiveness of vancomycin and metronidazole, but the data to support their use is not enough.(54)

7.3 Other agents

Acarbose; a hypoglycemic agent and an intestinal a-glucosidase inhibitor which causes decrease in blood ammonia levels and improves mild HE in patients with cirrhosis.(63) It has also been hypothesized that Acarbose promotes the proliferation of intestinal saccharolytic bacterial flora while reducing proteolytic flora that produce mercaptans, benzodiazepine like substances and ammonia as well. This theory was answered in a randomized cross over trial by Gentile S et al group in Italy.(63)

Probiotics and synbiotics modify the gut bacterial flora and reduce ammonia levels. Their use however is still being investigated.(64)

7.4 Agents causing alteration in ammonia metabolism (L-Ornithine L-Aspartate and benzyl benzoate)

Urea cycle plays a key role in ammonia metabolism and its excretion by forming urea in periportal hepatocytes or synthesis of glutamine in perivenous hepatocytes. But in cirrhosis, the activities of carbamyl phosphate synthetase enzyme (Urea synthesis) and of glutamine synthesis (glutamine synthesis) are impaired hence as compensation glutamine increased which in turn lead to increased level of ammonia. Therefore ornithine aspartate and benzoate has been used for reducing the ammonia levels by increasing the metabolism to glutamine and hippurate respectively.

L-ornithine-L-aspartate (LOLA) activates urea cycle and enhances ammonia clearance. LOLA induces an increase of liver and muscle ammonia metabolism, leading to decreased blood levels, and is able to cross the blood-brain barrier, increasing the cerebral ammonia disposal.(65) One or two sachets of LOLA should be administered three times daily.(4)

Other ammonia excretors like sodium benzoate, sodium phenyl acetate and sodium phenyl butyrate are also reported to show improvement but clear efficacy has not been established yet. Sodium phenyl acetate and Ammonal are the only drugs approved by the Food and Drug Administration for the treatment of acute hyperammonemia and associated encephalopathy in patients with urea cycle disorders.(66)

7.5 Agents used in neurotransmission hypothesis

Branch chain amino acids (BCCA): As it has been hypothesized that in liver cirrhosis, there has been reversal of aromatic amino acids (AAA) to BCCA which could lead to encephalopathy in patients with cirrhosis. Encephalopathy is presumably caused by increase in levels of AAA for monoamine neurotransmission which lead to transformed neuronal excitability and causing HE. Hence numbers of studies have been done to evaluate the effects of BCCA on HE. BCCA can be given orally as well as in infusion form.(67, 68)

Agents used for GABA hypothesis pathway: GABA receptor complex is the principal inhibitory network in nervous system and seems to be a contributor to neuronal inhibition in HE. This GABA receptor complex contains barbiturates and benzodiazepine receptor sites, chloride channels and a GABA binding site. In cirrhosis, there is an evidence for increase in benzodiazepine receptor ligands in subjects with HE, therefore effects of benzodiazepine receptor antagonist have been evaluated.(69, 70)

Flumazenil, a $GABA_A$ receptor antagonist also improves the symptoms in patients with grade 3 or 4 HE but its use is limited due to adverse effects(71). It has been seen that response to treatment with flumazenil is rapid onset with few minutes and then with few hours, more than half of these patients deteriorated with 2-3 hours.(72, 73) Because of its short duration effect and variable results of different studies, flumazenil cannot be recommended as routine therapy.

7.6 Other treatment options

7.6.1 Nutritional intervention

In the past, dietary protein restriction was considered an important component of the treatment of HE. Recent evidence however suggests that excessive restriction can raise serum ammonia levels, as a result of reduced muscular ammonia metabolism.(74) It has also been seen that majority of the patients with advanced liver disease had severe protein calorie malnutrition due to multifactorial reasons including the decreased oral intake, catabolic state etc.(75)

A high-protein diet is therefore recommended for improving the symptoms of HE. The European society for Parenteral and Enteral nutrition recommended an energy intake of 35/40 kcal/kg body weight per day and that patients must eat at least 1.2g/kg of protein daily along with Branched-chain amino acids (BCAA's) and vegetable-based protein.(76) Vegetable and dairy based proteins are preferred to animal proteins because of a high calorie-to-nitrogen ratio. Vegetable based proteins increase colonic motility and enhances intestinal nitrogen clearance. They also reduce colonic PH, which prevents ammonia absorption into gut.(77)

Zinc increases the activity of ornithine transcarbamylase (an enzyme in urea cycle) so zinc supplementation is also recommended for HE especially in patients who don't show any response to lactulose or neomycin.(38)

7.6.2 Prognosis once recovered from HE

Patients who recovered from HE can have persistent and cumulative neurologic deficits despite achieving normal mental status after receiving medical therapy. Study for North America had shown that patients with overt HE had persistent deficits in working memory, response inhibition and learning when assessed by psychometric tests. Recurrent episodes are associated with severity of underlying disease.(78, 79)

Conclusion: HE includes variety of neuropsychiatric symptoms and signs among patients with CLD leading to liver failure. Occurrence of HE indicates worse prognosis and should be kept on liver transplant list wherever it is available. Initial treatment includes the identification and correction of precipitating factors such as electrolyte imbalances, GI bleeding, medications, and sepsis. The main treatment modalities include the nonabsorbable disaccharide, principally lactulose and antibiotics like metronidazole or Rifaximin nowadays.

8. References

[1] Nevah MI, Fallon MB. Hepatic encephalopathy, Hepatorenal syndrome, Hepatopulmonary syndrome and Systemic complications of Liver disease. Feldman: Sleisenger and Fordtran's Gastrointestinal and Liver Disease,

Pathophysiology/Diagnosis/Management 9th ed: Saunders, An Imprint of Elsevier 2010. p. 1543-46.

[2] Bustamante J, Rimola A, Ventura PJ, Navasa M, Cirera I, Reggiardo V, et al. Prognostic significance of hepatic encephalopathy in patients with cirrhosis. J Hepatol. 1999 May;30(5):890-5.

[3] Ferenci P, Lockwood A, Mullen K, Tarter R, Weissenborn K, Blei AT. Hepatic encephalopathy--definition, nomenclature, diagnosis, and quantification: final report of the working party at the 11th World Congresses of Gastroenterology, Vienna, 1998. Hepatology. 2002 Mar;35(3):716-21.

[4] Cash WJ, McConville P, McDermott E, McCormick PA, Callender ME, McDougall NI. Current concepts in the assessment and treatment of hepatic encephalopathy. QJM. Jan;103(1):9-16.

[5] Bajaj JS, Wade JB, Sanyal AJ. Spectrum of neurocognitive impairment in cirrhosis: Implications for the assessment of hepatic encephalopathy. Hepatology. 2009 Dec;50(6):2014-21.

[6] Groeneweg M, Quero JC, De Bruijn I, Hartmann IJ, Essink-bot ML, Hop WC, et al. Subclinical hepatic encephalopathy impairs daily functioning. Hepatology. 1998 Jul;28(1):45-9.

[7] Prasad S, Dhiman RK, Duseja A, Chawla YK, Sharma A, Agarwal R. Lactulose improves cognitive functions and health-related quality of life in patients with cirrhosis who have minimal hepatic encephalopathy. Hepatology. 2007 Mar;45(3):549-59.

[8] Romero-Gomez M, Boza F, Garcia-Valdecasas MS, Garcia E, Aguilar-Reina J. Subclinical hepatic encephalopathy predicts the development of overt hepatic encephalopathy. Am J Gastroenterol. 2001 Sep;96(9):2718-23.

[9] Munoz SJ. Hepatic encephalopathy. Med Clin North Am. 2008 Jul;92(4):795-812, viii.

[10] Norenberg MD, Jayakumar AR, Rama Rao KV, Panickar KS. New concepts in the mechanism of ammonia-induced astrocyte swelling. Metab Brain Dis. 2007 Dec;22(3-4):219-34.

[11] Gerber T, Schomerus H. Hepatic encephalopathy in liver cirrhosis: pathogenesis, diagnosis and management. Drugs. 2000 Dec;60(6):1353-70.

[12] Butterworth RF. Complications of cirrhosis III. Hepatic encephalopathy. J Hepatol. 2000;32(1 Suppl):171-80.

[13] Cooper AJ, Plum F. Biochemistry and physiology of brain ammonia. Physiol Rev. 1987 Apr;67(2):440-519.

[14] Sundaram V, Shaikh OS. Hepatic encephalopathy: pathophysiology and emerging therapies. Med Clin North Am. 2009 Jul;93(4):819-36, vii.

[15] Haussinger D, Kircheis G, Fischer R, Schliess F, vom Dahl S. Hepatic encephalopathy in chronic liver disease: a clinical manifestation of astrocyte swelling and low-grade cerebral edema? J Hepatol. 2000 Jun;32(6):1035-8.

[16] Olde Damink SW, Jalan R, Dejong CH. Interorgan ammonia trafficking in liver disease. Metab Brain Dis. 2009 Mar;24(1):169-81.

[17] Rama Rao KV, Norenberg MD. Aquaporin-4 in hepatic encephalopathy. Metab Brain Dis. 2007 Dec;22(3-4):265-75.

[18] Pilbeam CM, Anderson RM, Bhathal PS. The brain in experimental portal-systemic encephalopathy. I. Morphological changes in three animal models. J Pathol. 1983 Aug;140(4):331-45.

[19] Mas A. Hepatic encephalopathy: from pathophysiology to treatment. Digestion. 2006;73 Suppl 1:86-93.

[20] Jalan R, Olde Damink SW, Lui HF, Glabus M, Deutz NE, Hayes PC, et al. Oral amino acid load mimicking hemoglobin results in reduced regional cerebral perfusion and deterioration in memory tests in patients with cirrhosis of the liver. Metab Brain Dis. 2003 Mar;18(1):37-49.

[21] Blei AT. Infection, inflammation and hepatic encephalopathy, synergism redefined. J Hepatol. 2004 Feb;40(2):327-30.

[22] Rolando N, Wade J, Davalos M, Wendon J, Philpott-Howard J, Williams R. The systemic inflammatory response syndrome in acute liver failure. Hepatology. 2000 Oct;32(4 Pt 1):734-9.

[23] Shawcross DL, Davies NA, Williams R, Jalan R. Systemic inflammatory response exacerbates the neuropsychological effects of induced hyperammonemia in cirrhosis. J Hepatol. 2004 Feb;40(2):247-54.

[24] Moldawer LL, Marano MA, Wei H, Fong Y, Silen ML, Kuo G, et al. Cachectin/tumor necrosis factor-alpha alters red blood cell kinetics and induces anemia in vivo. FASEB J. 1989 Mar;3(5):1637-43.

[25] Ahboucha S, Butterworth RF. The neurosteroid system: an emerging therapeutic target for hepatic encephalopathy. Metab Brain Dis. 2007 Dec;22(3-4):291-308.

[26] Baulieu EE. Neurosteroids: a novel function of the brain. Psychoneuroendocrinology. 1998 Nov;23(8):963-87.

[27] Ahboucha S, Butterworth RF. Pathophysiology of hepatic encephalopathy: a new look at GABA from the molecular standpoint. Metab Brain Dis. 2004 Dec;19(3-4):331-43.

[28] Reversal of hepatic coma by benzodiazepine antagonist (Ro 15-1788). Lancet. 1985 Jun 8;1(8441):1324-5.

[29] Lighthouse J, Naito Y, Helmy A, Hotten P, Fuji H, Min CH, et al. Endotoxinemia and benzodiazepine-like substances in compensated cirrhotic patients: a randomized study comparing the effect of rifaximine alone and in association with a symbiotic preparation. Hepatol Res. 2004 Mar;28(3):155-60.

[30] Zeneroli ML, Venturini I, Corsi L, Avallone R, Farina F, Ardizzone G, et al. Benzodiazepine-like compounds in the plasma of patients with fulminant hepatic failure. Scand J Gastroenterol. 1998 Mar;33(3):310-3.

[31] Zeneroli ML, Venturini I, Stefanelli S, Farina F, Miglioli RC, Minelli E, et al. Antibacterial activity of rifaximin reduces the levels of benzodiazepine-like compounds in patients with liver cirrhosis. Pharmacol Res. 1997 Jun;35(6):557-60.

[32] Stewart CA, Reivich M, Lucey MR, Gores GJ. Neuroimaging in hepatic encephalopathy. Clin Gastroenterol Hepatol. 2005 Mar;3(3):197-207.

[33] Ahboucha S, Layrargues GP, Mamer O, Butterworth RF. Increased brain concentrations of a neuroinhibitory steroid in human hepatic encephalopathy. Ann Neurol. 2005 Jul;58(1):169-70.

[34] Fischer JE, Rosen HM, Ebeid AM, James JH, Keane JM, Soeters PB. The effect of normalization of plasma amino acids on hepatic encephalopathy in man. Surgery. 1976 Jul;80(1):77-91.

[35] Lozeva V, Montgomery JA, Tuomisto L, Rocheleau B, Pannunzio M, Huet PM, et al. Increased brain serotonin turnover correlates with the degree of shunting and hyperammonemia in rats following variable portal vein stenosis. J Hepatol. 2004 May;40(5):742-8.

[36] Lozeva-Thomas V. Serotonin brain circuits with a focus on hepatic encephalopathy. Metab Brain Dis. 2004 Dec;19(3-4):413-20.

[37] Yoshida Y, Higashi T, Nouso K, Nakatsukasa H, Nakamura SI, Watanabe A, et al. Effects of zinc deficiency/zinc supplementation on ammonia metabolism in patients with decompensated liver cirrhosis. Acta Med Okayama. 2001 Dec;55(6):349-55.

[38] Marchesini G, Fabbri A, Bianchi G, Brizi M, Zoli M. Zinc supplementation and amino acid-nitrogen metabolism in patients with advanced cirrhosis. Hepatology. 1996 May;23(5):1084-92.

[39] Hermenegildo C, Monfort P, Felipo V. Activation of N-methyl-D-aspartate receptors in rat brain in vivo following acute ammonia intoxication: characterization by in vivo brain microdialysis. Hepatology. 2000 Mar;31(3):709-15.

[40] Schliess F, Gorg B, Haussinger D. Pathogenetic interplay between osmotic and oxidative stress: the hepatic encephalopathy paradigm. Biol Chem. 2006 Oct-Nov;387(10-11):1363-70.

[41] Rose C, Butterworth RF, Zayed J, Normandin L, Todd K, Michalak A, et al. Manganese deposition in basal ganglia structures results from both portal-systemic shunting and liver dysfunction. Gastroenterology. 1999 Sep;117(3):640-4.

[42] Frederick RT. Current concepts in the pathophysiology and management of hepatic encephalopathy. Gastroenterol Hepatol (N Y). 2011 Apr;7(4):222-33.

[43] Haussinger D. [Hepatic encephalopathy: clinical aspects and pathogenesis]. Dtsch Med Wochenschr. 2004 Sep 3;129 Suppl 2:S66-7.

[44] Bernal W, Hall C, Karvellas CJ, Auzinger G, Sizer E, Wendon J. Arterial ammonia and clinical risk factors for encephalopathy and intracranial hypertension in acute liver failure. Hepatology. 2007 Dec;46(6):1844-52.

[45] Weissenborn K, Ennen JC, Schomerus H, Ruckert N, Hecker H. Neuropsychological characterization of hepatic encephalopathy. J Hepatol. 2001 May;34(5):768-73.

[46] Mardini H, Saxby BK, Record CO. Computerized psychometric testing in minimal encephalopathy and modulation by nitrogen challenge and liver transplant. Gastroenterology. 2008 Nov;135(5):1582-90.

[47] Montagnese S, Amodio P, Morgan MY. Methods for diagnosing hepatic encephalopathy in patients with cirrhosis: a multidimensional approach. Metab Brain Dis. 2004 Dec;19(3-4):281-312.

[48] Prakash R, Mullen KD. Mechanisms, diagnosis and management of hepatic encephalopathy. Nat Rev Gastroenterol Hepatol. Sep;7(9):515-25.

[49] Riggio O, Ridola L, Pasquale C. Hepatic encephalopathy therapy: An overview. World J Gastrointest Pharmacol Ther. Apr 6;1(2):54-63.

[50] Ferenci P, Herneth A, Steindl P. Newer approaches to therapy of hepatic encephalopathy. Semin Liver Dis. 1996 Aug;16(3):329-38.

[51] Riggio O, Varriale M, Testore GP, Di Rosa R, Di Rosa E, Merli M, et al. Effect of lactitol and lactulose administration on the fecal flora in cirrhotic patients. J Clin Gastroenterol. 1990 Aug;12(4):433-6.

[52] Mortensen PB. The effect of oral-administered lactulose on colonic nitrogen metabolism and excretion. Hepatology. 1992 Dec;16(6):1350-6.

[53] Mortensen PB, Holtug K, Bonnen H, Clausen MR. The degradation of amino acids, proteins, and blood to short-chain fatty acids in colon is prevented by lactulose. Gastroenterology. 1990 Feb;98(2):353-60.

[54] Bajaj JS. Management options for minimal hepatic encephalopathy. Expert Rev Gastroenterol Hepatol. 2008 Dec;2(6):785-90.

[55] Sharma BC, Sharma P, Agrawal A, Sarin SK. Secondary prophylaxis of hepatic encephalopathy: an open-label randomized controlled trial of lactulose versus placebo. Gastroenterology. 2009 Sep;137(3):885-91, 91 e1.

[56] Blanc P, Daures JP, Rouillon JM, Peray P, Pierrugues R, Larrey D, et al. Lactitol or lactulose in the treatment of chronic hepatic encephalopathy: results of a meta-analysis. Hepatology. 1992 Feb;15(2):222-8.

[57] Camma C, Fiorello F, Tine F, Marchesini G, Fabbri A, Pagliaro L. Lactitol in treatment of chronic hepatic encephalopathy. A meta-analysis. Dig Dis Sci. 1993 May;38(5):916-22.

[58] Strauss E, Tramote R, Silva EP, Caly WR, Honain NZ, Maffei RA, et al. Double-blind randomized clinical trial comparing neomycin and placebo in the treatment of exogenous hepatic encephalopathy. Hepatogastroenterology. 1992 Dec;39(6):542-5.

[59] Jiang Q, Jiang XH, Zheng MH, Jiang LM, Chen YP, Wang L. Rifaximin versus nonabsorbable disaccharides in the management of hepatic encephalopathy: a meta-analysis. Eur J Gastroenterol Hepatol. 2008 Nov;20(11):1064-70.

[60] Bass NM, Mullen KD, Sanyal A, Poordad F, Neff G, Leevy CB, et al. Rifaximin treatment in hepatic encephalopathy. N Engl J Med. 2010 Mar 25;362(12):1071-81.

[61] Sidhu SS, Goyal O, Mishra BP, Sood A, Chhina RS, Soni RK. Rifaximin improves psychometric performance and health-related quality of life in patients with minimal hepatic encephalopathy (the RIME Trial). Am J Gastroenterol. 2011 Feb;106(2):307-16.

[62] Bajaj JS, Heuman DM, Wade JB, Gibson DP, Saeian K, Wegelin JA, et al. Rifaximin improves driving simulator performance in a randomized trial of patients with minimal hepatic encephalopathy. Gastroenterology. 2011 Feb;140(2):478-87 e1.

[63] Gentile S, Guarino G, Romano M, Alagia IA, Fierro M, Annunziata S, et al. A randomized controlled trial of acarbose in hepatic encephalopathy. Clin Gastroenterol Hepatol. 2005 Feb;3(2):184-91.

[64] Liu Q, Duan ZP, Ha DK, Bengmark S, Kurtovic J, Riordan SM. Synbiotic modulation of gut flora: effect on minimal hepatic encephalopathy in patients with cirrhosis. Hepatology. 2004 May;39(5):1441-9.

[65] Poo JL, Gongora J, Sanchez-Avila F, Aguilar-Castillo S, Garcia-Ramos G, Fernandez-Zertuche M, et al. Efficacy of oral L-ornithine-L-aspartate in cirrhotic patients with hyperammonemic hepatic encephalopathy. Results of a randomized, lactulose-controlled study. Ann Hepatol. 2006 Oct-Dec;5(4):281-8.

[66] Jalan R, Wright G, Davies NA, Hodges SJ. L-Ornithine phenylacetate (OP): a novel treatment for hyperammonemia and hepatic encephalopathy. Med Hypotheses. 2007;69(5):1064-9.

[67] Naylor CD, O'Rourke K, Detsky AS, Baker JP. Parenteral nutrition with branched-chain amino acids in hepatic encephalopathy. A meta-analysis. Gastroenterology. 1989 Oct;97(4):1033-42.

[68] Marchesini G, Dioguardi FS, Bianchi GP, Zoli M, Bellati G, Roffi L, et al. Long-term oral branched-chain amino acid treatment in chronic hepatic encephalopathy. A randomized double-blind casein-controlled trial. The Italian Multicenter Study Group. J Hepatol. 1990 Jul;11(1):92-101.

[69] Basile AS, Harrison PM, Hughes RD, Gu ZQ, Pannell L, McKinney A, et al. Relationship between plasma benzodiazepine receptor ligand concentrations and severity of hepatic encephalopathy. Hepatology. 1994 Jan;19(1):112-21.

[70] Basile AS, Hughes RD, Harrison PM, Murata Y, Pannell L, Jones EA, et al. Elevated brain concentrations of 1,4-benzodiazepines in fulminant hepatic failure. N Engl J Med. 1991 Aug 15;325(7):473-8.

[71] Goulenok C, Bernard B, Cadranel JF, Thabut D, Di Martino V, Opolon P, et al. Flumazenil vs. placebo in hepatic encephalopathy in patients with cirrhosis: a meta-analysis. Aliment Pharmacol Ther. 2002 Mar;16(3):361-72.

[72] Barbaro G, Di Lorenzo G, Soldini M, Giancaspro G, Bellomo G, Belloni G, et al. Flumazenil for hepatic encephalopathy grade III and IVa in patients with cirrhosis: an Italian multicenter double-blind, placebo-controlled, cross-over study. Hepatology. 1998 Aug;28(2):374-8.

[73] Gyr K, Meier R, Haussler J, Bouletreau P, Fleig WE, Gatta A, et al. Evaluation of the efficacy and safety of flumazenil in the treatment of portal systemic encephalopathy: a double blind, randomised, placebo controlled multicentre study. Gut. 1996 Aug;39(2):319-24.

[74] Vaquero J, Chung C, Cahill ME, Blei AT. Pathogenesis of hepatic encephalopathy in acute liver failure. Semin Liver Dis. 2003 Aug;23(3):259-69.

[75] Charlton M. Branched-chain amino acid enriched supplements as therapy for liver disease. J Nutr. 2006 Jan;136(1 Suppl):295S-8S.

[76] Plauth M, Cabre E, Riggio O, Assis-Camilo M, Pirlich M, Kondrup J, et al. ESPEN Guidelines on Enteral Nutrition: Liver disease. Clin Nutr. 2006 Apr;25(2):285-94.

[77] Amodio P, Caregaro L, Patteno E, Marcon M, Del Piccolo F, Gatta A. Vegetarian diets in hepatic encephalopathy: facts or fantasies? Dig Liver Dis. 2001 Aug-Sep;33(6):492-500.

[78] Bajaj JS, Schubert CM, Heuman DM, Wade JB, Gibson DP, Topaz A, et al. Persistence of cognitive impairment after resolution of overt hepatic encephalopathy. Gastroenterology. 2010 Jun;138(7):2332-40.

[79] Riggio O, Ridola L, Pasquale C, Nardelli S, Pentassuglio I, Moscucci F, et al. Evidence of persistent cognitive impairment after resolution of overt hepatic encephalopathy. Clin Gastroenterol Hepatol. 2011 Feb;9(2):181-3.

25

Adverse Reactions and Gastrointestinal Tract

A. Lorenzo Hernández[1], E. Ramirez[1]
and Jf. Sánchez Muñoz-Torrero[2]
[1]University Autonoma of Madrid
[2]University of Extremadura
Spain

1. Introduction

Adverse drug reactions are common and there is an increasing interest in recognizing them. There are several studies that try to identify epidemiology, true incidence in hospitalized and not hospitalized patients and the main concerns about their causes and possible solutions. Gastrointestinal tract, mainly haemorrhages and peptic disease are the most common site of adverse drug reactions; that´s the reason why we should recognize this problem and how to manage. Also we try to review the most common drugs affecting gastrointestinal tract. Less common and, usually less severe, liver disease and pancreatitis can be produced by adverse drug reactions. In this chapter we review theses aspects of adverse drug events, particularly, those related to drugs affecting gastrointestinal tract.

2. Definition of adverse drug reactions

An adverse drug event is an unwanted and unintended medical event related to the use of medications. An adverse drug event is considered an adverse drug reaction (ADR) when there is a causal link between the event and use of the drug. An adverse drug reaction is considered serious when the patients outcome is one of the following: death, life-threatening, hospitalization (initial or prolonged), disability –significant, persistent or permanent change, impairment, damage or disruption in the patient's body function/structure or physical activities or quality of life, congenital anomaly or require intervention to prevent permanent impairment or damage [Supplementary information in Appendix 1].

Causality assessment is necessary to determine the likehood that a drug caused a suspected ADR. There are a number of different methods used to judge causation, the first attempts were proposed by Karch and Lasagna (1977), Lecenthal et al. (1979) and Naranjo et a.l (1981). Most of these approaches to assigning causality are based on the following clinical features: temporal relationship between drug exposure and the onset of adverse drug event, characteristic symptoms and laboratory abnormalities and/or histology, and challenge-dechallenge-rechallenge (improvement after stopping the suspected drug and reappearance after starting the agent in question).

ADRs can be considered "on-target" effects, if they are result of exaggerated pharmacology that may be managed by dose reduction or other therapeutic modifications, i.e. hypoglycemia associated with antidiabetic agents. "Off-target" toxicities are frequently more problematic because they may not be predicted from pharmacology and toxicology studies, and they may occur only after prolonged exposure, i.e. hypersensibility reactions associated to antiepileptics. Unexpected ADRs that first appear after marketing authorization of the medication continue trouble clinicians, regulators, and drug sponsors. The most notably cause is the use by large number of patients, providing sufficient statistical power to detect rare events. Other factors include use in special populations, drug inte ractions, renal and hepatic insufficiency, long duration of use and drug withdrawal.

3. Epidemiology of adverse drug reactions

Adverse drug reactions (ADRs) are considered to be among the leading causes of morbidity and mortality. Around 5-25% of hospitals admissions are estimated to be due to ADRs and about 6-15% of hospitalized patients experience serious ADRs (SADRs) causing significant prolongation of hospital stay and projected that adverse drug events are the fourth to sixth leading cause of death in the United States. Most studies are focused on rates of serious and fatal events in hospitalized patients, probably because tracking of ADRs is more established in the inpatients setting. An English study (Kane-Gill, 2010) found an increase in hospitalizations caused by ADR in about 76.8% in ten years. A recent study of administrative health-care data found an annual ADR prevalence rate of 0.5% among ambulatory-care patients; however, the authors acknowledge this is probably an underestimate of true ADR rates. Ambulatory-care patients experiencing an ADR were younger on average than hospitalized patients.

Risk factors of suffering adverse drug events are: women, elderly and polipharmacy mainly. Women were more likely than men to have ADRs in both outpatients and inpatients settings. In the study from Zopf (2008), the OR of women from suffering ADR was 1.562; (95% CI 0.785, 2.013). Other risk factors implicated in adverse drug reactions are elderly, drug-drug interactions, polipharmacy and renal insufficiency. In the study of Sanchez Muñoz (2011), also drug-drug interactions were as important as age and renal insufficiency in producing adverse drug reactions.

Patients affected by adverse dug events are admitted in internal medicine department and geriatrics quite often, but patients hospitalized in Intensive care units and pediatrics also suffer from these problems.

4. Severity of adverse drug reactions – Fatal adverse drug reaction

It has been estimated than fatal ADRs are expected in approximately 0.32% of hospitalized patients, and complications from drug therapy are the most common adverse event in hospitalized patients. If true, then ADRs are the 4th leading cause of death—ahead of pulmonary disease, diabetes, AIDS, pneumonia, accidents, and automobile deaths. However, some studies show greater severity prevalence and fatality rate. In the hospital setting the study from Kaurr, (Kaurr,2011) observed grade severe of adverse reaction in 13.4% patients. In the study from Sánchez Muñoz-Torrero (2010) the reactions were severe in 17% and fatal in 1.6% of hospitalized patients.

These statistics do not include the number of ADRs that occur in ambulatory settings. The exact number of ADRs is not certain and is limited by methodological considerations. However, whatever the true number is, ADRs represent a significant public health problem. In a Sweden study there were reviewed the death reports in one year in relation with adverse drugs reactions. They found 3.1% of deaths associated with fatal adverse drug events, mostly haemorraghes. 89% of patients died at hospital meanwhile only 35% of patients dead at hospital with no relation with drug events.

So most of studies trying to establish epidemiology and cost of adverse drug reactions demonstrate that these events are harmful and we have to make great efforts to diminish the incidence and morbidity.

5. Cost of adverse drug reactions

In western countries, drug-related illnesses account 5% to 10% of inhospital costs, and being associated with a substantial increase in morbidity and mortality. In addition to their impact on human health, ADRs also have significant impact on healthcare costs. These costs are essentially hospital costs, in particular arising from an increase in length of stay caused by an ADR. Although has been estimated that the occurrence of an ADR during hospitalization or leading to hospitalization is responsible in U.S.A. (data from 1997) for a cost of approximately 2800 Euros in an additional length of stay of 2.2 days, several studies have also pointed out that the structure of ADR cost is heterogeneous, a factor which must be taken into account when developing preventive strategies. Although data of costs were not calculated, Sanchez Muñoz-Torrero et al (2010) study found an increase in hospital staying in almost 9 days (18±17 days vs 9.6±5.8, p<0.001), which accounts for more direct and indirect costs of the hospitalization. Also another Spanish (Carrasco Garrido et al, 2010) study found an increase in 19% of hospital costs associated with the appearance of adverse drug events.

6. Potential causes implicated in adverse drug reactions

Older patients are particularly vulnerable to drug-related illness because they are usually on multiple drug regimens, which expose them to the risk of drug interactions (Mallet et al, 2007), and because age is associated with changes in pharmacokinetics and pharmacodinamics (Aronson, 2007).

Onder et al. (2010) developed and validated a risk stratification model (The GerontoNet ADR Risk Score) to identify patients 65 years or older who are at risk for an ADR during hospitalization. They used data from the Italian Group of Pharmacoepidemiology in the Elderly to develop an ADR risk score. The ADR risk score was then validated in a sample of older adults who were admitted to 4 university hospitals in Europe. The number of drugs and history of an ADR were the strongest predictors of ADRs, followed by heart failure, liver disease, presence of 4 or more conditions, and renal failure (Table 1).

Recently Sánchez Muñoz-Torrero et al found that renal function and drug–drug interactions were statistically significant associated with the appearance of ADR. Also duration of hospitalization was associated but it wasn't possible to establish that if duration of hospitalization was the cause or the consequence of ADR. Recently Hamilton et al (2011) reviewed the adverse drug reactions in older people with potentially inappropriate prescriptions.

Variable	OR (95% CI)	Points
≥4 Comorbid conditions	1.31 (1.04-1.64)	1
Heart failure	1.79 (1.39-2.30)	1
Liver disease	1.36 (10.6-1.74)	1
No. of drugs		
≤ 5	1 [Reference]	0
5-7	1.90 (1.35-2.68)	1
≥8	4.07 (2.93-5.65)	4
Previous ADR	2.41 (1.79-3.23)	2
Renal failure	1.21 (0.96-1.51=	1

Abbreviations: ADR, adverse drug reactions; CI, confidence interval; OR, odd ratio.

Table 1. Variables included in the Score (adapted from Onder *et al*)

7. Main drugs implicated in reactions

Drug classes most frequently associated with ADRs in both inpatients and outpatient populations are non steroidal anti-inflamatory drugs (NSAIDs), diuretic, anticoagulants, antiobiotics and antineoplastic agents.

Antibiotic and vaccination reactions are more frequent in the 0 –to-9 year age group.

In adults and elderly people, there a great variety of drugs causing adverse drug reactions. However, it depends the type of hospitalization, the deparment, etc, the type of adverse reactions and drugs implicated are quite different. Pimohamed et al. (2004) found that aspirin was the casual agent in 18% of cases of all admission for ADRs, while other NSAIDs and diuretics were implicates in 12% and 27% respectively. The most common ADRs of NSAIDs were GI bleeding, peptic ulcerations, haemorrhagic cerebrovascular accident, renal impairment, wheezing and rash. Grenouillet-Delacre et al. (2007) found that psychotropic drugs, immunosuppressive drugs, anticoagulants and antibiotics were more than 50% of life-threatening adverse drug reactions at admission to medical intensive care. In Spain, antibiotic and anticoagulants are the drugs more frequently implicated in ADRs appeared during hospitalization but in another epidemiologic study (Carrasco Garrido, 2010) found that main drugs implicated in admission into the hospital were antineoplastics and immunosuppressive therapy. However there are very few studies that show antineoplastics and immunosuppressive therapies as the cause of adverse drug reactions although they are being increasingly used and promote the appearance of infections, medullar aplasia, etc. Also cardiovascular drugs, mainly diuretics and hypotensors drugs account for some common ADRs.

8. Drugs reactions affecting gastrointestinal tract

ADR that cause damage in gastrointestinal tract usually produce GI bleeding/peptic ulcerations, diarrhea (mainly associated to antibiotics), pancreatitis and liver toxicity. About 40% of ADR affect gastrointestinal and liver in hospitalized patients. As said before, gastrointestinal bleeding is the most frequent ADRs causing hospitalization or produced during hospitalization. In this issue, we try to review the ADRs affecting gastrointestinal tract.

8.1 GI bleeding

Mainly non steroidal anti-inflammatory drugs and antiplatelet/anticoagulants are implicated in gastrointestinal bleeding. The most frequent lesion is gastric erosions (about 40.2%), combination of gastric ulcer and gastric erosions (16.1%), gastric ulcer (15.0%), duodenal ulcer (13.8%), normal (13.8%) and duodenal erosions (1.1%). In a recent study 26% of patients admitted because of gastrointestinal bleeding had antiplatelet or anticoagulants as the cause of bleeding. The distribution of lesions was quite similar to the study from Devy, being gastric ulcer the most common lesion involved in the bleeding. Inhibition of cyclooxygenase, leading to inhibition of gastric prostaglandin synthesis, and impaired GI defense mechanisms represent additional mechanisms of drug-induced GI bleeding. In the particular setting of Intensive Care Units (ICUs) the most frequent lesion found in patients is the stress-related mucosal bleeding, in which another causes apart from drugs are implicated. In the study from Wikman-Jorgensen (2011) mortality of upper gastrointestinal bleeding was 3,5%, all in patients with great comorbidity which limited treatment of bleeding.

Drugs most frequently causing bleeding were aspirin in 36%, acenocumarol in 27%, clopidogrel in 18%. Combination of aspirin and clopidogrel are responsible of 6% of upper gastrointestinal bleeding. Aspirin is the drug more frequently implicated but it may chance in the future because of the increasing use of doble antiplatelet treatments and new anticoagulants (Rivaroxaban, Apixaban and Dabigatran). It is possible than in the near future we begin to see hemorrhages with dabigatran because of the recent approval in USA for the use of treatment in atrial fibrillation, including patients with low risk of thromboembolism. The risk of bleeding is bigger with Rivaroxaban as shown in the prophylaxis studies, but the approval for AF is pending.

Also lower gastrointestinal bleeding is increasing because of use of AINES mainly. New techniques for diagnosing lesions in small and large intestine are proving this increase in lower gastrointestinal bleeding. AINES can cause diverticulum perforation, mucosal inflammation, ulceration, causing bleeding in the intestine. Use of aspirin, clopidogrel or anticoagulants and the lower intestinal bleeding is an issue that has to be studied because of its frequency, use and potential harmful in small and large intestine. There´s little information about its presentation and management.

8.2 Diarrhea

Diarrhoea may be defined by frequency or grams of loose grames per day: 3–5 times per day and/or loose stools 200– 300 grams/day (250 mL/day).

It´s estimated that diarrhoea accounts for the 7% of ADRs. There are lot of drugs producing diarrhea as a secondary effect: metformin, some chemotherapies, antibiotics, mainly clavulanic, clindamicin, immunosuppressant... Most of them cause diarrhea only while taking, or only at the beginning of prescription, but some are associated with chronic diarrhoea as metformin. However, the possibility of a drug causing a severe diarrhea is less common except in the case of antibiotics, hipomotility drugs, steroids, proton pump inhibitors because of the possibility of Clostridium difficile diarrhea.

Mechanisms of drugs producing diarrhoea are multiple: osmotic, secretory, motor, exudative, malabsorptive, infectious/inflammatory, and others. Examples of osmotic diarrhoea are enteral nutrition feeding, magnesium salts, etc. Examples of secretory diarrhoea (increase in intestinal ion secretion or diminution in intestinal ion absorption) are digoxin, quinidine, propafenone and theophiline. Examples or rapid intestinal transit are procinetic and macrolids. Exudative diarrhoea (changes in permeability and integrity of intestinal mucosa) are NSAIDs and antineoplastic. Drug-related malabsorption of fats, carbohydrates, and/or bile can also lead to diarrhea. Examples include octreotide (at high doses), highly active antiretroviral therapy, tetracycline, NSAIDs, and antineoplastic agents. Drug-induced infectious/inflammatory diarrhea includes microbial proliferation, pseudomembranous colitis, and histologic colitis. The risk of antibiotic associated diarrhea is higher with broad-spectrum agents (particularly those with antianaerobic activity and activity against Enterobacteriaceae), agents with high luminal concentrations (although oral/enteral administration is not necessarily a risk), longer duration of therapy, and use of multiple antibiotics.

8.3 Constipation and hypomotility

Anticholinergic drugs are responsible of constipation as well as other adverse reactions in patients, particularly elderly patients. Also opioids prescribed for cancer patients, chronic pain, etc are responsible of constipation which can produce paralitic ileum. In the setting of ICU patients hipomotility and constipation appears in 50-80 % of patients, particularly those with mechanically ventilated.

8.3.1 Hypomotility

Hypomotility is produced mainly abnormalities in propulsive motility, disturbances in esophageal and gastric motility, reduction in lower esophageal sphincter pressure. Exogenous cathecolamines can reduce antral contractions and small bowel peristalsis and alter motility patterns. Opioids inhibit neurotransmitters release and altering water and electrolyte absorption.

8.3.2 Constipation

Constipation is produced by changes in neuronal or motor function in the intestine. The most common cause is opioids. They inhibit the release of acetylcholine from the myenteric plexus and promote in the opioid receptors in the intestine a decreased motility and increase in intestinal fluid absorption. Other drugs implicated in constipation are antihistamines, calcium channel blockers, diuretics, tricyclic antidepressants.

8.4 Pancreatitis

Drug induced pancreatitis accounts for 0.1-2% of pancreatitis. Between 1968 and 1993 a total of 525 different drugs from many different substance classes have been reported to the WHO because they were suspected to induce pancreatitis as an unwanted side effect, The three drugs that are responsible of more cases of pancreatitis are mesalazine, azathioprine and simvastatine. Previously recognized patients with more risk of pancreatitis are pediatric and elderly patients, women, advanced HIV disease and inflammatory bowel disease. The interesant review from Balani (2008) showed a table with drugs commonly implicated in pancreatitis: ACE inhibitors, ARA-2, loop diuretics and thiazides, statins, bezafibrate, some antibiotics, pentamidine, azathioprine, mercaptopurine, aminosalicylates, anticonvulsivants and antipsychotics, estrogens, carbimazole, some antineoplastics, codeine, sulindac.

In critically ill patients there's also a review of drugs implicated in pancreatitis (Lat, 2010):

8.4.1 Drugs with a likely association

Drugs with a likely association: Asparaginase, azathioprine, cimetidine, corticosteriopids, corticotrophin, cytarabin, dapsone, didanosine, enalapril, estrogens, furosemide, isonizid, mercaptopurine, mesalamine, methyldope, metronidazole, omeprazol, opiates, pentamidine, pravastatin, salycilates, simvastatin, sulfasalizine, sulfamethoxazole/trimethoprim, sulindac, tetracycline, valproic acid.

8.4.2 Drugs with a potential or questionable association

Drugs with a potential or questionable association: acetaminophen, amiodarone, ampicilin, benzapril, carbamazepine, captopril, ceftriaxone, clarithromycin, cyclosporine, diphenoxylate, cisplatinerythromycin, fluvastatin, gemfibrozil, interferon, ribavirin, ketoprofen, lisinopril, ketoprofen, lisinopril, lovastatin, metformin, naproxen, thiazides, octerotide, penicillin, procainamide, propofol, propoxyphene, ramipril, ranitidine, rifampin.

8.5 Drug-Induced Liver Injury (DILI)

Hepatotoxicity and drug-induced liver injury (DILI) are terms used interchangeably. DILI can be defined as a liver injury induced by a drug or herbal medicines leading to liver test abnormalities or liver dysfunction with reasonable exclusion of other competing etiologies. Most cases of DILI are due to idiosyncratic or unexpected reactions. In contrast to paracetamol-induced hepatotoxicity, which occurs with dose-dependent overdose of the drug. Idiosyncratic drug reactions have been traditionally considered dose independent. However, drugs with well-documented idiosyncratic DILI have been shown to have a dose-dependent component. Idiosyncratic DILI, excluding injury caused by acetaminophen overdose, accounts for 7–15% of the cases of acute liver failure in Europe and the United States and is the most frequent reason for the withdrawal of an approved drug from the market. Estimates of the rate of incidence of DILI leading to hospital referral vary from 2.4 per 100,000 person-years (in a retrospective population-based study of 1.64 million UK subjects) to 13.9 per 100,000 inhabitants (in a prospective analysis in France). Complementary or alternative medicines are used by at least 20% of individuals in Western, Eastern, and African cultures, and reports of DILI have increased. Given its rarity, DILI may not be identified during clinical trials and may come to light only after the culprit drug has obtained market approval and large numbers of patients have been exposed. In addition, in preregistration clinical trials, mild asymptomatic liver injuries, often characterized by asymptomatic elevations in liver enzymes, are commonly seen. However, drugs capable of inducing severe DILI as well as drugs that have a low potential for causing severe injury (e.g., aspirin and heparin) can generate similar patterns of liver injury. It is therefore necessary to develop an approach that can distinguish drugs that are likely to cause severe DILI from drugs that are unlikely to do so.

RUCAM algorithm (Roussel Uclaf Causality Assessment Method) was the first algorithm developed specifically for DILI. After the meeting sponsored by the CIOMS (Paris, 1989), with the support of Russel Uclaf pharmaceutical company, the terminology and diagnosis criteria for causality assessment was proposed. The algorithm was validated using external cases with positive rechallenge (49 cases) and 28 controls (patients with acute liver damage not related to drugs) with available information before occurrence of re-exposure, with results of high sensitivity (86%), specificity (89%), positive predictive value (93%) and negative predictive value (78%) [Algorithm RUCAM are showed in Table 1 and 2 of Appendix 2].

International DILI Expert Working Group of clinicians and scientists reviewed current DILI terminology and diagnostic criteria so as to develop more uniform criteria that could be define and characterize the spectrum of clinician syndromes that constitute DILI. In Appendix 2 of supplementary information you will find threshold criteria for definition of a case as being DILI (Box 1), the pattern of liver injury (Box 2), severity (Box 3), causality assessment (Box 4), and chronicity (Box 5). Consensus was also reached on approaches to characterizing DILI in the setting of chronic liver diseases (Box 6), including autoimmune hepatitis (Box 7).

A very large number of different drugs have been associated with liver injury. There is a clear difference in the documentation or the evidence for hepatotoxicity associated with these drugs. Isoniazid, phenytoin, disulfiram, amoxicillin/clavulanate, halothane and chloromazine are drugs with well characterized hepatotoxicity. More recently antibiotics (amoxicillin/clavunalate, erytromicin, flucloxacillin, trimethoprim-sulpha, nitrofurantoin, isoniazid and rifampicin), analgesics and NSAIDs (diclofenac, dextropropoxyphene, paracetamol, ibuprofen) probably the most common type of drugs associated with DILI. In hospitalized patients, antineoplasic agents seem to commonly lead to DILI and are probably underreported. In a Spanish pharmacovigilance prospective program based on laboratory signals at hospital all patients with liver test abnormalities (x 3 upper limits of normal) were evaluated being antibiotics (19.5%), hormonal contraceptives (14.6%) and anticancer agents (10%) were the most frequent drug-groups associated to liver injury. In out-patients, the single most common drug implicated in ine series was diclofenac. Among patients with acute liver failure resulting from drugs in the US who underwent liver transplantation, paracetamol (acetaminophen) was the most common causative drug, followed by isoniazid, propylthiouracil, phenytoin and valproate.. Herbal and dietary supplements are implicated in approximately 11% of patients who developed acute serious liver disease of unknown cause in Spain.

The expectrum of DILI is varied, acute liver injury with or without jaundice, chronic hepatitis, although rare, liver cirrhosis has been reported to occur with long-standing drug treatment suspected to have caused DILI, and approximately 25-30% of DILI present with symptom of immunoallergic drug reactions. Table 2 showed the most common types of liver injury that have been identified with drugs.

9. Drugs for gastrointestinal diseases and their implication in adverse reactions

Most of adverse reactions with drugs used for treating gastrointestinal diseases are proton pump inhibitors. New antiTNF drugs, steroids and immunosuppressant in general used for

Type	Drugs
Acute liver injury	Isoniazid, disulfiram, paracetamol
Chronic hepatitis	Phenytoin, isoniazid
Autoimmune hepatitis	Minocycline, nitrofurantoin
Granulomatous hepatitis	Carbamazepine, quinidine
Steatohepatitis	Amiodarone, valproate
Cholestatic hepatitis	Flucloxacillin, amoxicillin/clavulanate
Bland cholestasis	Estrogens, nimesulide
Ductopenia	Amoxicillin, Trimethoprim-sulpha
Fibrosis	Methotrexate
Nodular regenerative hyperplasia	Azathioprine, 6-thioguanine

Table 2. Types of DILI (adapted from Björnsson)

inflammatory bowel disease cause also adverse drug reactions but the extended use of IBP makes them responsible of most of the adverse reactions with gastrointestinal drugs: hypergastrinemia, hypomagnesemia, tumors and, recently, enteric infections, pneumonia and osteoporosis (Maffei, 2007). There is a controversy about the probability of some of theses adverse drug reactions with IBPs. In the recent review by Thomson (2010) they failed to found risk of carcinoid tumors, cancer or nosocomial pneumoniae. There still controversy about the risk of osteoporosis with the long term use of IBPs.

10. Strategies to diminish adverse drugs reactions

The main strategies for reducing adverse drug reactions are: drug interaction calculators, renal insufficiency calculators, prescribing programs and collaboration between pharmacists, pharmacologists and clinical physicians.

The world Health Organization defines pharmacovigilance as the science and activities related to the detection, assessment, understanding, and prevention of adverse affects or any other possible drug-related problem. The field has grown significantly in recent years as postapproval safety studies for new medication become increasingly required, encompassing retrospective analysis of heath-care claims databases, meta-analysis, patients registries, and prospective case-control studies.

Recognition, reporting and careful characterization of these troubling, often unexpected ADRs are vital to future prevention of these event because detection of patterns and common features of ADRs can enhance our understanding of new mechanism and risk factors. The expansion of electronic database capabilities in hospital and primare-care setting offers the promise of better safety-based detection and monitoring systems that can detect ADRs earlier and prevent ADRs in the future. Hospital informatics systems linking to electronic medical records and including patient genotype with medication ordering and dispensing will reduce medication errors and inappropriate prescribing while improving detection of ADRs. Also, the review of prescription by pharmacists can achieve a diminution in the appearance of adverse drug reactions.

It´s also important to recognize people specially susceptible to ADRs: elderly, women, polipharmacy, renal insufficiency and presence of drug-drug interactions. In this special population we have to be careful with prescription of new drugs and its dosing.

11. Conclusions

Adverse drug reactions is a very frequent problem that affects specially the gastrointestinal tract, being GI bleeding the most common adverse drug reaction causing hospital admission. Patients predisposed to suffer ADRs are elderly, women, renal insufficiency, polipharmacy and drug-drug interactions. Drugs used for treat gastrointestinal disease are quite sure but can b e implicated in ADRs as IBPs, imunosupre4ssants used for autoimmune hepatitis or inflammatory bowel disease. Recognition of this problem is increasing in frequency and new drugs can be responsible for new ADRs. Collaboration between clinician, pharmacists and pharmacology specialists is needed.

12. Appendix 1

ICH Guideline on E2D post-approval drug safety defined an adverse drug reaction (ADR) and a serious adverse drug reactions (SADR) as follows:

An adverse drug reaction, as established by regional regulations, guidance and practices, is concern noxious and unintended responses to a medicinal product. The phrase "responses to a medicinal product" means that a causal relationship between a medicinal product and an adverse event is at least a reasonable possibility (refer to the ICH E2A guideline). A reaction, in contrast to an event, is characterized by the fact that a causal relationship between the drug and the occurrence is suspected. For regulatory reporting purposes, if an event is spontaneously reported, even if the relationship is unknown or unstated, it meets the definition of an adverse drug reaction".

Serious adverse event / ADR. In accordance with ICH E2A guideline, a serious adverse event or reaction is any untoward medical occurrence that at any dose:

- Results in death
- is life-threatening (NOTE: The term "life-threatening" in the definition of "serious" refers to an event/reaction in which the patient was at risk of death at the time of the event/reaction; it does not refer to an event/reaction which hypothetically might have caused death if it were more severe),
- is a congenital anomaly/birth defect,
- is a medically important event or reaction.

Medical and scientific judgment should be exercised in deciding whether other situations should be considered serious, such as important medical events that might not be immediately life-threatening or result in death or hospitalization but might jeopardize the patient or might require intervention to prevent one of the other outcomes listed in the definition above. Examples of such events are intensive treatment in a emergency room or at home for allergic bronchospasm, blood dyscrasias or convulsions that do not result in hospitalization or development of drug dependency or drug abuse.

13. Appendix 2

Subject Information	
1. Temporal relationship of start of drug to ALT>2x ULN	**Score**
Initial treatment 5–90 days; subsequent treatment course: 1–15 days	2
Initial treatment <5 or >90 days; subsequent treatment course: >15 days	1
From cessation of drug: $\leq$15 days, or $\leq$15 days after subsequent treatment	1
Otherwise	0
2. After drug cessation- difference between peak ALT and upper limits normal	
Decreases >50% within 8 days	3
Decreases >50% within 30 days	2
No information or decrease >50% after >30 days, or inconclusive	0
Decrease <50% after 30 days or recurrent increase	-2
3. Risk factors	
No alcohol use	0
Alcohol use	1
Age $\leq$55 years	0
Age >55 years	1
4. Concomitant drug	
No concomitant drug administered	0
Concomitant drug with suggestive or compatible time of onset	-1
Concomitant known hepatotoxin with suggestive or compatible time of onset	-2
Concomitant drug with positive rechallenge or validated diagnostic test	-3
5. Nondrug causes: Six are primary: recent hepatitis A, B, or C, biliary obstruction, acute alcoholic hepatitis (AST > 2x ALT), recent hypotension Secondary group: Underlying other disease; possible CMV, EBV or HSV infection	
All primary and secondary causes reasonably ruled out:	2
All 6 primary causes ruled out	1
4 or 5 primary causes ruled out	0
< 4 primary causes ruled out (max. negative score for items 4 and 5: –4)	-2
Nondrug cause highly probable	-3
6. Previous information on hepatotoxicity of the drug in question	
Package insert or labelling mention	2
Published case reports but not in label	1
Reaction unknown	0
7. Rechallenge	
Positive (ALT doubles with drug in question alone)	3
Compatible (ALT doubles with same drugs as given before initial reaction) +1	1
Negative (Increase in ALT but <2x ULN, same conditions as when reaction occurred)	-2
Not done, or indeterminate result	0
Total (range of algebraic sum: –8 to +14)	
Score Interpretation: Highly probable >8; Probable 6–8; Possible 3–5; Unlikely 1–2; Excluded <0	

Table 1. RUCAM Hepatocellular Injury Scale

Subject Information	
1. Temporal relationship of start of drug to ALP>2x ULN	Score
Initial treatment 5–90 days; subsequent treatment course: 1–90 days	2
Initial treatment <5 or >90 days; subsequent treatment course: >90 days	1
From cessation of drug: $\leq$30 days, or $\leq$30 days after subsequent treatment	1
Otherwise	0
2. After drug cessation - difference between peak ALP or total bilirubin and ULN	
Decreases $\geq$50% within 180 days	2
Decreases <50% within 180 days	1
Persistence or increase or no information	0
If drug is continued – inconclusive	0
3. Risk factors	
No alcohol use	0
Alcohol use	1
Age $\leq$55 years	0
Age >55 years	1
4. Concomitant drug	
No concomitant drug administered	0
Concomitant drug with suggestive or compatible time of onset	-1
Concomitant known hepatotoxin with suggestive or compatible time of onset	-2
Concomitant drug with positive rechallenge or validated diagnostic test	-3
5. Nondrug causes: Six are primary: recent hepatitis A, B, or C, biliary obstruction, acute alcoholic hepatitis (AST > 2x ALT), recent hypotension Secondary group: Underlying other disease; possible CMV, EBV or HSV infection	
All primary and secondary causes reasonably ruled out:	2
All 6 primary causes ruled out	1
4 or 5 primary causes ruled out	0
< 4 primary causes ruled out (max. negative score for items 4 and 5: –4)	-2
Nondrug cause highly probable	-3
6. Previous information on hepatotoxicity of the drug in question	
Package insert or labelling mention	2
Published case reports but not in label	1
Reaction unknown	0
7. Rechallenge	
Positive (ALT doubles with drug in question alone)	3
Compatible (ALT doubles with same drugs as given before initial reaction) +1	1
Negative (Increase in ALT but <2x ULN, same conditions as when reaction occurred)	-2
Not done, or indeterminate result	0
Total (range of algebraic sum: –8 to +14)	
Score Interpretation: Highly probable >8; Probable 6–8; Possible 3–5; Unlikely 1–2; Excluded <0	

Table 2. RUCAM Cholestatic or Mixed Liver Injury Scale

Any one of the following:
• More than or equal to fivefold elevation above the upper limit of normal (ULN) for alanine aminotransferase (ALT)
• More than or equal to twofold elevation above the ULN for alkaline phosphatase (ALP) (particularly with accompanying elevations in concentrations of 5'-nucleotidase or γ-glutamyl transpeptidase in the absence of known bone pathology
driving the rise in ALP level)
• More than or equal to threefold elevation in ALT concentration and simultaneous elevation of bilirubin concentration exceeding 2× ULN
Level of evidence: 2b (exploratory/retrospective cohort studies)

Box 1. clinical chemistry criteria for drug-induced liver injury (DILI) (adapted from Aithal et al. 2011)

• Pattern of liver injury is based on earliest identified liver chemistry elevations that qualify as DILI (Box 1)
• Pattern of liver injury is defined using R value where R =(ALT/ULN)/(ALP/ULN). This will require estimation of alanine aminotransferase (ALT) (aspartate transaminase is used when ALT is unavailable) and alkaline phosphatase (ALP) from the same serum sample
• ALT activity = patient's ALT/upper limit of normal (ULN); ALP activity = patient's ALP/ULN; R = ALT activity/ALP activity
• Hepatocellular pattern of DILI = R ≥ 5
• Mixed pattern of DILI = R > 2 and < 5
• Cholestatic pattern of DILI = R ≤ 2
• Histological summary should be recorded separately (if liver biopsy has been performed). However, the liver biopsy interpretation will generally not replace the R value for purposes of classification
Level of evidence: 2b (retrospective cohort studies)

Box 2. criteria for classifying the clinical pattern of drug induced liver injury (DILI) (adapted from Aithal et al. 2011)

Category	Severity	Description
1	Mild	Elevated alanine aminotransferase/alkaline phosphatase (ALT/ALP) concentration reaching criteria for DILI* but bilirubin concentration <2× upper limit of normal (ULN)
2	Moderate	Elevated ALT/ALP concentration reaching criteria for DILI* and bilirubin concentration ≥2× ULN, or symptomatic hepatitis
3	Severe	Elevated ALT/ALP concentration reaching criteria for DILI*, bilirubin concentration ≥2× ULN, and one of the following: • International normalized ratio ≥1.5 • Ascites73 and/or encephalopathy, disease duration <26 weeks, and absence of underlying cirrhosis31 • Other organ failure considered to be due to DILI
4	Fatal or transplantation	Death or transplantation due to DILI

Box 3. DILI severity index (adapted from Aithal et al. 2011)

• The Roussel Uclaf Causality Assessment Method (RUCAM) scale should be used for causality assessment (Appendix 2)
• If more than one drug is suspected to be causing DILI, the RUCAM scale should be applied to each drug separately. If such assessments are not practical (e.g., antituberculosis medications), all the drugs involved may be implicated as a single entity.
• If more than one drug is rated "possible" or higher by RUCAM, evaluation should be sought by a specialist to rank the drugs by order of likelihood of causing DILI. This may be done on the basis of the signature pattern of DILI and a review of the literature.
Level of evidence: 1b (validating cohort studies)

Box 4. DILI causality assessment (adapted from Aithal et al. 2011)

• Initial clinical episode met the criteria to qualify as acute DILI (Box 1)
• Initial episode on causality assessment has been considered possible, probable, or highly probable DILI on the basis of Roussel Uclaf Causality Assessment Method scoring criteria (Appendix 2). Persistent DILI is defined as evidence of continued liver injury after withdrawal of the causative agent, beyond 3 months of follow-up for hepatocellular and mixed DILI, and beyond 6 months for cholestatic DILI
• Chronic DILI is defined as evidence of continued liver injury after withdrawal of the causative agent beyond 12 months of follow-up, regardless of the classification of DILI
• There is no new risk factor other than exposure to the suspect drug that would explain the persistence of liver injury, and other causes of chronic liver diseases have been excluded
Level of evidence: 4 (prognostic cohort studies of modest quality)

Box 5. Characteristics of persistent and chronic druginduced liver injury (DILI) (adapted from Aithal et al. 2011)

• Evidence of chronic liver disease is established on the basis of validated methods such as clinical evidence of cirrhosis, histological evidence of chronic liver disease, and imaging in cases of vascular disorder and tumours, as appropriate
• Evidence of drug intake for an appropriate duration preceding the appearance of symptoms, signs, or test results suggestive of chronic liver disease
• Exclusion of other etiologies of chronic disease (outlined in Supplementary Appendix 2, table S3)
Level of evidence: 1b (prospective/validating cohort studies with good follow-up)

Box 6. characteristics of drug-associated chronic liver disease (adapted from Aithal et al. 2011)

• The score is ≥6 points on simplified diagnostic criteria for AIH (scores >6 points with the simplified criteria can be obtained if liver biopsy is performed. Hennes *et al.*()consider a probable diagnostic score to be ≥6)
• Injury resolves on withdrawal of medication that triggered the AIH, with or without immunosuppressive therapy to induce remission
• No relapse within a period of 1 year after withdrawal of all immunosuppressants. This criterion needs further confirmation and cannot be considered pathognomonic because it is quite variable depending on the cohorts analyzed
Level of evidence: 2b (exploratory cohort study)

Box 7. Characteristics of drug-induced autoimmune hepatitis (AIH) (adapted from Aithal et al. 2011)

14. References

Aithal GP, Day CP. Hepatic adverse drug reactions. En: Pharmacovigilance. Chichester: John Wiley & Sons Ltd; p. 429-43 (2006.).

Aithal, G.P., Watkins P.B., Andrade, R.J., Larrey, D., Molokhia, M., Takikawa, H., Hunt, C.M., Wilke, R.A:, Avigan, M., Kaplowitz, N., Bjornsson, E. and Daly, A.K. Case definition and phenotype Standardization in Drug-induced Liver Injury. Clin Pharmacol Ther.89(6): 806-815.

Aronson, J.K. Adverse drug reactions — no farewell to harms. Br J Clin Pharmacol. ;63(2):131-135 (2007).

Balani AR, Grendell JH.Drug Saf. 2008;31(10):823-37.Drug-induced pancreatitis : incidence, management and prevention.

Bates, D.W., Spell, N., Cullen, D.J., Birdick, E., Laird, N., Petersen, L.A., Small, S.D., Boddie, J., Sweitzer, B.J., Leape, L.L. The cost of adverse drug events in hospitalized patients. JAMA. 277(4): 307-311 (2007).

Benichou C, Danan G, Flahault A. Causality assessment of adverse reactions to drugs--II. An original model for validation of drug causality assessment methods: case reports with positive rechallenge. J Clin Epidemiol. 1993 Nov;46(11):1331-1336

Beppu K, Osada T, Shibuya T, Watanabe SPathogenic mechanism of NSAIDs-induced mucosal injury in lower gastrointestinal tract. Nihon Rinsho. 2011 Jun;69(6):1083-7

Björnsson, E., Jerlstad, P., Bergqvist, A. & Olsson, R. Fulminant drug-induced hepatic failure leading to death or liver transplantation in Sweden. Scand. J. Gastroenterol. 40, 1095–1101 (2005).

Björnsson E. Review article: drug-induced liver injury in clinical practice. Aliment Pharmacol ther; 32: 3-12 (2010)

Budnitz, D.S., Pollock, D.A., Weidenbach, K.N., Mendelsohn, A.B., Schoeder, T.J., Annest, J.L. National surveillance of emergency department visits for outpatient adverse drug events. JAMA. 296 (15), 1858-1866 (2006).

Carrasco-Garrido P*, López de Andrés A, Hernández Barrera V, Gil de Miguel A, Jiménez García R. Trends of adverse drug reactions related hospitalizations in Spain (2001-2006). BMC Health Services Research 2010, 10:287. http://www.biomedcentral.com/1472-6963/10/287

Cecile M, Seux V, Pauly V, Tassy S, Reynaud-Levy O, Dalco O, Thirion X, Soubeyrand J, Retornaz F. Adverse drug events in hospitalized elderly patients in a geriatric medicine unit: study of prevalence and risk factors. Rev Med Interne. 2009 May;30(5):393-400.

Cheng, C.M. Hospital systems for detection and prevention of adverse drug events. Clin Pharmacol Ther. 89: 779-781 (2011)

Clark K, Byfieldt N, Dawe M, Currow DC. Treating Constipation in Palliative Care: The Impact of Other Factors Aside From Opioids. Am J Hosp Palliat Care. 2011 May 23.

Classen, D.C., Pestotnik, S.L., Evans, R.S., Loyds, J.F., Burke, J.P. Adverse drug events in hospitalized patients. Excess length of stay, extra cost, and attributable mortality. JAMA. 277 (4),301-6 (1997).

Classen, D.C., Pestonik, S.L., Evans, R.S., Burke, J.P. Computerized surveillance of adverse drug event in hospital patients. Qua.l Saf. Health Care. 14, 221–226 (2005).

Danan G, Benichou C. Causality assessment of adverse reactions to drugs--I. A novel method based on the conclusions of international consensus meetings: application to drug-induced liver injuries. J Clin Epidemiol. 1993 Nov;46(11):1323-1330.

de Abajo, F.j., Montero, D., Madurga, M. & García Rodríguez, L.A. Acute and clinically relevant drug-induced liver injury: a population based case-control study. Br. J. Clin. Pharmacol. 58, 71–80 (2004).

De Valle MB, Av Klinteberg V, Alem N, Olsson R, Björnsson E. Drug-induced liver injury in a Swedish University hospital out-patient hepatology clinic. Aliment Pharmacol Ther 2006; 24: 1187-95

Devi DP, Sushma M, Guido S. Drug-induced upper gastrointestinal disorders requiring hospitalization: a five-year study in a South Indian hospital. Pharmacoepidemiol Drug Saf. 2004 Dec;13(12):859-62

Devlin JW, Mallow-Corbett S, Riker RR. Adverse drug events associated with the use of analgesics, sedatives, and antipsychotics in the intensive care unit. Crit Care Med. 2010 Jun;38(6 Suppl):S231-43.

Fontana RJ, Watkins PB, Bonkowsky HL, Chalasani N, Davern T, Serrano J, Rochon J; DILIN Study Group Drug-induced Liver Injury Network (DILIN) prospective study: rationale, design and condunt. Drug Saf; 32: 55-68 (2009)

Frazier, T.H. & Krueger, K.j. Hepatotoxic herbs: will injury mechanisms guide treatment strategies? Curr. Gastroenterol. Rep. 11, 317–324 (2009).

Gautier, S., Bachelet, H., Bordet, R., Caron, J. The cost of adverse drug reactions. Expert Opinion on Pharmacotherapy. 4(3): 319-326 (2003)

Gurwitz, J.H., Field, T.S., Harold, L.R., Rothschild, J., Debellis, K., Seger, A.C., Cadoret, C., Fish, L.S., Garber, L., Kelleher, M., Bates, D.W. Incidence and preventability of adverse drug events among elder persons in the ambulatory setting. JAMA. 289 (9), 1107 – 1116 (2003).

Grenouillet-Delacre, M., Verdoux, H., Moore, N., Haramburu, F., Miremont-Salamé, G., Etienne, G., Robinson, P., Gruson, D., Hilbert, G., Gabinski, C., Bégaud, B., Molimard, M. Life-threatening adverse drug reactions at admission to medical intensive care: a prospective study in a teaching hospital. Intensive Care Med. Dec;33(12):2150-7 (2007).

Hamilton H, Gallagher P, Ryan C, Byrne S, O'Mahony D. Potentially inappropriate medications defined by STOPP criteria and the risk of adverse drug events in older hospitalized patients.Arch Intern Med. 2011 Jun 13;171(11):1013-9.

Ibanez L, Perez E, Vidal X, Laporte JR. Prospective surveillance of acute serious liver disease unrelated to infectious, obstructive, or metabolic diseases: epidemiological and clinical features, and exposure to drugs. J Hepatol ; 37: 592–600 (2002)

ICH Guideline on E2D Postapproval Safety Data Management: Definitions and Standards for Expedited Reporting. London, 20 November 2003 CPMP/ICH/3945/03.

ICH Guideline on E2A Clinical Safety data Management: definitions and Standards for expedited Reporting E2A. Current Step 4 version, dated 27 October 1994 (CPMP/ICH/377/95)

Johnson, J.A., Bootman, J.L. Drug-related morbidity and mortality; a cost of illness model. Arch. Intern. Med. 155, 1949-56 (1995).

Kane-Gill, S.L., Van Den Bos, J. & Handler, S.M. Adverse drug reactions in hospital and ambulatory are setting identified using a large administrative database. Ann. Pharmacother. 44, 983-993 (2010).

Karch, F.E., Lasagna, L. Toward the operational identification of adverse drug reactions. Clin. Pharmacol. Ther. Mar;21(3):247-254 (1977).

Kaur S, Vinod Kapoor,[1] Rajiv Mahajan,[1] Mohan Lal,[2] and Seema Gupta. Monitoring of incidence, severity, and causality of adverse drug reactions in hospitalized patients with cardiovascular disease. Indian J Pharmacol. 2011 February; 43(1): 22–26.

Kongkaew C, Noyce PR, Ashcroft DM. Hospital admissions associated with adverse drug reactions: a systematic rview of prospectgive observational studies. Ann Pharmacother. 2008 Jul;42(7):1017-25.[1]

Kunac DL, Kennedy J, Austin N, Reith D. Incidence, preventability, and impact of Adverse Drug Events (ADEs) and potential ADEs in hospitalized children in New Zealand: a prospective observational cohort study. Paediatr Drugs. 2009;11(2):153-60.

Kurahara K, Matsumoto T, Iida M.. Characteristics of nonsteroidal anti-inflammatory drugs-induced colopathy Nihon Rinsho. 2011 Jun;69(6):1098-103.

Kutty P, Woods CW, Arlene C. Sena, Stephen R. Benoit, Susanna Naggie,,Joyce Frederick, Sharon Evans, Jeffery Engel, and L. Clifford McDonald. Risk Factors for and Estimated Incidence of Community-associated Clostridium diffi cile Infection, North Carolina, USA1Emerging Infectious Diseases • www.cdc.gov/eid • Vol. 16, No. 2, February 2010

Lancashire RJ, Cheng K, Langman MJ. Discrepancies between population-based data and adverse reaction reports in assessing drugs as causes of acute pancreatitis. Aliment Pharmacol Ther 2003 Apr 1;17(7):887–93.

Lammert C, Einarsson S, Saha C, Niklasson A, Bjornsson E, Chalasani N. Relationship between daily dose of oral medications and idiosyncrativ drug-induced liver injury: sear for signals. Hepatology 2008; 47: 2003-9

Larrey D. Epidemiology and individual susceptibility to adverse drug reactions affecting the liver. Semin Liver Dis; 22: 145–55 (2002).

Lat I, Foster DR, Erstad B. Drug-induced acute liver failure and gastrointestinal complications.Crit Care Med. 2010 Jun;38(6 Suppl):S175-87

Lazarou, J., Pomeranz, B.H., Corey, P.N. Incidence of adverse drug reactions in hospitalized patients: a meta-analysis of prospective studies. JAMA. 279 (15), 1200-5 (1998).

Leape, L.L., Brennan, T.A., Laird, N., Lawthers, A.G., Localio, A.R., Barnes, B.A., Hebert, L., Newhouse, J.P., Weiler, P.C., Hiatt, H. The nature of adverse events in hospitalized patients: results of the Harvard Medical Practice Study II. NEJM. 324 (6), 377-84 (1991).

Leung FW, Rao SS. Approach to fecal incontinence and constipation in older hospitalized patients. Hosp Pract (Minneap). 2011 Feb;39(1):97-104.

Leventhal, J.M., Hutchinson, T.A., Kramer, M.S., Feinstein, A.R. An algorithm for the operational assessment of adverse drug reactions. III. Results of tests among clinicians. JAMA. Nov 2;242(18):1991-1994 (1979).

Maffei M, Desmeules J, Cereda JM, Hadengue A. Side effects of proton pump inhbitors (PPIs). Rev Med Suiss 2007; 5(3): 1934-36, 1938.

Mallet, L, Spinewine, A, Huang, A. The challenge of managing drug interactions in elderly people. Lancet. 370(9582):185-191 (2007).

Mannesse, C.K., Derkx, F.H., de Ridder, M.A., Man in 't Veld, A.J., van der Cammen, T.J. Contribution of adverse drug reactions to hospital admission of older patients. Age Ageing. 29(1):35-39 (2000).

Meier Y, Cavallaro M, Roos M, et al. Incidence of drug-induced liver injury in medical inpatients. Eur J Clin Pharmacol; 61: 135–43 (2005).

Mino-León D, Galván-Plata ME, Doubova SV, Flores-Hernandez S, Reyes-Morales H. A pharmacoepidemiological study of potential drug interactions and their determinant factors in hospitalized patients. Rev Invest Clin. 2011 Mar-Apr;63(2):170-8.

Naranjo, C.A., Busto, U., Sellers, E.M., Sandor, P., Ruiz, I., Roberts, E.A., et al. A method for estimating the probability of adverse drug reactions. Clin. Pharmacol. Ther. Ago;30(2):239-245 (1981).

Nitsche CJ, Jamieson N, Lerch MM, Mayerle JV. Drug induced pancreatitis. Best Practice & Research Clinical Gastroenterology 24 (2010) 143–155

O'Grady, j.G. Acute liver failure. Postgrad. Med. J. 81, 148–154 (2005).

Onder, G., Petrovic, M., Tangíísuram, B., Meinardi, M.C., Markito-Notenboom W.P., Somers, S., Rajkumar, C., Bernabei, R., van der Cammen T.J.M. Development and Validation of a Score to Assess Risk of Adverse Drug Reactions Among In-Hospital Patients 65 years or older. Arch. Intern. Med. 170(13): 1142-1148 (2010).

Ostapowicz, G. et al. Results of a prospective study of acute liver failure at 17 tertiary care centers in the United States. Ann. Intern. Med. 137, 947–954 (2002).

Ouwerkerk J, Boers-Doets COuwerkerk J, Boers-Doets C. Best practices in the management of toxicities related to anti-EGFR agents for metastatic colorectal cancer. Eur J Oncol Nurs. 2010 Sep;14(4):337-49

Pirmohamed M, James S, Meakin S, Green C, Scott AK, Walley TJ, Farrar K, Park BK & Breckenridge AM. Adverse drug reactions as a cause of admission to hospital: prospective analysis of 18 820 patients. BMJ. 329,15-9 (2004).

Ramachandran, R. & Kakar, S. Histological patterns in drug-induced liver disease. J. Clin. Pathol. 62, 481–492 (2009).

Ramirez E, Carcas AJ, Borobia AM, Lei SH, Piñana, E, Fudio S & Frias J A Pharmacovigilance Program From Laboratory Signals for the Detection and Reporting of Serious Adverse Drug Reactions in Hospitalizad Patients. Clin Pharmacol Ther. 87 (1): 74-86.

Russo MW, Galanko jA, Shrestha R, Fried MW & Watkins P. Liver transplantation for acute liver failure from drug induced liver injury in the United States. Liver Transpl. 10, 1018–1023 (2004).

Sánchez Muñoz-Torrero JF, Barquilla P, Velasco R, Fernández Capitán MC, Pacheco N, Vicente L, & all. Adverse drug reactions in internal medicine units and associated risk factors. Eur J Clin Pharmacol (2010) 66:1257–1264

Sgro, C. et al. Incidence of drug-induced hepatic injuries: a French populationbased study. Hepatology 36, 451–455 (2002).

Tai-Yin Wu, Min-Hua Jen, Alex Bottle, Mariam Molokhia, Paul Aylin, Derek Bell, Azeem Majeed. Ten-year trends in hospital admissions for adverse drug reactions in England 1999–2009 J R Soc Med 2010: 103: 239–250. DOI 10.1258/jrsm.2010.100113

Watkins, P.B., Seligman, P.j., Pears, j.S., Avigan, M.I. & Senior, j.R. Using controlled clinical trials to learn more about acute drug-induced liver injury. Hepatology 48, 1680–1689 (2008).

Wawruch M, Macugova A, Kostkova L, Luha J, Dukat A, Murin J, Drobna V, Wilton L, Kuzelova M The use of medications with anticholinergic properties and risk factors for their use in hospitalised elderly patients. Pharmacoepidemiol Drug Saf. 2011 Jun 13. doi: 10.1002/pds.2169.

Wester K, Jönsson A, Spigset O, Druid H, Hägg S. Incidence of fatal adverse drug reactions: a population based study. Br J Clin Pharmacology 2008 / 65:4 / 573–579

White, R.A., Xu, H., Denny, J.C., Roden , D.M., Krauss, R.M., McCarty, C.A., Davis, R.L., Skaar, T., Lamba, J., Savoga, G. The emerging role of electronic medical records in pharmacogenomics. Clin. Pharmmacol. Ther. 89, 379-386 (2011)

Wikman-Jorgensen, López-Calleja E, Safont-Gasó P, Matarranz-del-Amo M, Andrés Navarro R & Merino-Sánchez J. Antiagregation and anticoagulation, relationship with upper gastrointestinal bleeding. Rev Esp Enferm Dig 2011; 103: 360-365.

Zopf Y, Rabe C, Neubert A, Hahn EG, Dormann H. Risk factors associated with adverse drug reactions following hospital admission: a prospective analysis of 907 patients in two German university hospitals. Drug Saf. 2008;31(9):789-98.

26

Selected Algorithms of Computational Intelligence in Gastric Cancer Decision Making

Elisabeth Rakus-Andersson
Blekinge Institute of Technology
Sweden

1. Introduction

Due to the latest research (Engelbrecht, 2007; Rutkowski, 2008) the subject of Computational Intelligence has been divided into five main regions, namely, neural networks, evolutionary algorithms, swarm intelligence, immunological systems and fuzzy systems.

Our attention has been attracted by the possibilities of medical applications provided by immunological computation algorithms. Immunological computation systems are based on immune reactions of the living organisms in order to defend the bodies from pathological substances. Especially, the mechanisms of the T-cell reactions to detect strangers have been converted into artificial numerical algorithms.

Immunological systems have been developed in scientific books and reports appearing during the two last decades (de Castro & Timmis, 2002; Dasgupta & Nino, 2008; Engelbrecht, 2007; Forrest et al., 1997). The basic negative selection algorithm NS was invented by Stefanie Forrest (Forrest et al., 1997) to give rise to some technical applications. We can note such applications of NS as computer virus detection (Antunes & Correia, 2011; Harmer et al., 2002; Zhang & Zhao, 2010), reduction of noise effect (Igawa & Ohashi, 2010), communication of autonomous agents (Ishida, 2004) or identification of time varying systems (Wakizono et al., 2006). Even a trial of connection between a computer and biological systems has been proved by means of immunological computation (Cohen, 2006).

Hybrids made between different fields can provide researchers with richer results; therefore associations between immunological systems and neural networks (Gao et al., 2008) have been developed as well.

In the current chapter we propose another hybrid between the NS algorithm and chosen solutions coming from fuzzy systems (Rakus-Andersson, 2007, 2009, 2010a, 2010b, 2011; Rakus-Andersson & Jain, 2009). This hybrid constitutes the own model of adapting the NS algorithm to the operation decisions "operate" contra "do not operate" in gastric cancer surgery. The choice between two possibilities to treat patients is identified with the partition of a decision region in self and non-self, which is similar to the action of the NS algorithm. The partition is accomplished on the basis of patient data strings/vectors that contain codes of states concerning some essential biological markers. To be able to identify the strings that characterize the "operate" decision we add the own method of computing the patients' characteristics as real values. The evaluation of the patients' characteristics is supported by inserting importance weights assigned to powerful biological indices taking place in the operation decision process. To compute the weights of importance the Saaty algorithm (Saaty, 1978) is adopted.

We introduce the medical task to solve in Section 2. In order to establish the code systems for clinical data the fuzzification of biological markers is discussed in Section 3. In Section 4 we analyze the way of determining the patient characteristics, which should connect the mix of different codes in one value. The adaptation of the NS algorithm to surgery assumptions is made in Section 5. Finally, in Section 6 we test clinical data to prove the action of the model introduced in the paper as an applicable novelty.

2. The description of the medical objective in gastric cancer surgery

Gastric cancer patients are mostly cured by operating on them. Different types of surgery are taken into account. Two of them, namely, the partial resection surgery contra the radical surgery are considered by surgeons when evaluating biological markers in the context of their deviations from normal values (Do-Kyong Kim et al., 2009; de Mello et al., 1983).

Nevertheless, a surgeon often must decide if any operation on a patient is possible. The choice between the status "operate" and "do not operate" will constitute the main problem to solve by engaging different algorithms with their origins in Computational Intelligence. The selection will be made on the basis of three biological markers listed as $X = age$, $Y = CRP\text{-}value$ (C reactive proteins), and $Z = body\ weight$ (Do-Kyong Kim et al., 2009; de Mello et al., 1983). These are considered as the most important indices in gastric cancer surgery decision making.

As a leading method, which should provide us with decisions "operate" against "do not operate", we adapt the NS (Negative Selection) algorithm of immunological computation. To comprehend better some associations between the body immunological system and artificially invented algorithms based on the body protection system let us recall the most essential definitions of immunity.

Immunity refers to the condition, in which the organism can resist diseases. A broader definition of immunity is a reaction to foreign substances (pathogens). The biological immune system (BIS) has the ability to detect foreign substances and to respond them. One of the main capabilities of the immune system is to distinguish own body cells from foreign substances, which is called self/non-self discrimination (Dasgupta & Nino, 2008; Engelbrecht, 2007; Forrest et al., 1997).

This particular ability is assigned to a special kind of lymphocytes called T-cells produced in the bone marrow. The T-cells can differentiate own body cells from pathogenic cells; therefore they play the role of detectors. Both own cells belonging to the self region and foreign pathogen cells forming non-self domain have their special characteristics given in the form of vectors of coded or measured properties.

Let us adapt the meaning of distribution into self and non-self in the medical application sketched as follows. To make a decision concerning an individual patient we assign the immunological region of self to "operate", whereas the non-self field will be identified with "do not operate" (Rakus-Andersson, 2011).

To be able to use the self/non-self discrimination, accomplished by the NS algorithm, we need to create vectors of coded patient data. The own fuzzy technique will be involved to divide reference sets of X, Y and Z into subintervals assisting growth levels of these biological indices. To the subintervals, in turn, the codes are added. We will arrange a code vector assisting the patient's features after examining his/her values of X, Y and Z.

When implementing the NS algorithm we assume that vectors characteristic of self region are available as input data. We do not intend to test too many casual vectors to decide their similarity with self vectors since we want to use the NS algorithm in the effective way. We thus try to generate the strongest population of strings being representatives of the self region.

In order to select this population we provide another own algorithm that converts the code vector to a real value. This value will be recognized as "characteristics of the patient".

3. Fuzzification of *X*, *Y* and *Z* in the creation of code vectors

Before studying the technique of making the self/non-self discrimination to state if the patient can be operated or not we should first be able to compare different strings $v = (x = age, y = CRP, z = body\ weight)$, $x \in X$, $y \in Y$, $z \in Z$, to decide their grades of affinity (coverage). We thus should design sets of codes for each biological parameter.

The markers *age*, *CRP*, and *body weight* are measurable features. Hence, we intend to determine the collections of codes assisting intervals, which correspond to the markers' levels. We want to accomplish a process of fuzzification of the measurable markers in order not to decide lengths of the level intervals intuitively (Rakus-Andersson, 2009, 2010a, 2010b, Rakus-Andersson & Jain, 2009).

A fuzzy set, say, A in the universe X is a collection of elements followed by the membership degrees that are computed by means of the membership function $\mu_A : X \rightarrow [0,1]$. Therefore A is denoted as $A = \{(x, \mu_A(x)), x \in X\}$. A is called normal if at least one element in the set A is assigned to the membership degree equal to 1. The support of A is a non-fuzzy set that consists of elements accompanied by membership degrees greater than 0.

The three quantitative markers X, Y and Z will be then differentiated into levels expressed by lists of terms. The terms from the lists are represented by fuzzy sets (Rakus-Andesson, 2007, 2010b), restricted by the membership functions lying over the domains $[x_{min}, x_{max}]$, $[y_{min}, y_{max}]$ and $[z_{min}, z_{max}]$ respectively.

In conformity with the physician's suggestions we introduce five levels of X, Y and Z as the collections

$$X = "age" = \{ X_1 = "very\ young", X_2 = "young", X_3 = "middle\text{-}aged", X_4 = "old", X_5 = "very\ old"\}$$

$$Y = "CRP\text{-}value" = \{Y_1 = "very\ low", Y_2 = "low", Y_3 = "medium", Y_4 = "high", Y_5 = "very\ high"\}$$

and

$$Z = "body\ weight" = \{Z_1 = "very\ underweighted", Z_2 = "underweighted", Z_3 = "normal", Z_4 = "over\ weighted", Z_5 = "very\ over\ weighted"\}.$$

To accomplish a formal mathematical design of level restrictions let us study the special own technique of their implementations (Rakus-Andersson, 2007, 2010b). In general, we suggest that the linguistic list of terms is converted to a sampling of fuzzy sets $L_1,...,L_m$, where m is an odd positive integer. Each term is represented by the corresponding fuzzy set, whose restriction is supposed to be created as the common formula depending on the lth value, where $l = 1,...,m$. We assume that supports of restrictions $\mu_{L_l}(w)$, $l = 1,...,m$, will cover parts of the reference set $L = [\min(L_1),\max(L_m)]$, $w \in L$. We introduce $E = |L|$ as the length of L.

We divide all expressions L_l in three groups, namely, a family of *"leftmost"* sets $L_1,..., L_{\frac{m-1}{2}}$, the set $L_{\frac{m+1}{2}}$ *"in the middle"* and a collection of *"rightmost"* sets $L_{\frac{m+3}{2}},...,L_m$. To design the membership functions of L_l the s-class function

$$s(w,\alpha,\beta,\gamma) = \begin{cases} 0 & \text{for} \quad w \le \alpha, \\ 2\left(\frac{w-\alpha}{\gamma-\alpha}\right)^2 & \text{for} \quad \alpha \le w \le \beta, \\ 1-2\left(\frac{w-\gamma}{\gamma-\alpha}\right)^2 & \text{for} \quad \beta \le w \le \gamma, \\ 1 & \text{for} \quad w \ge \gamma, \end{cases} \tag{1}$$

will be adopted. The point $(a, 0)$ starts the graph of the s-function, whereas the point $(\gamma, 1)$ terminates this graph. The parameter β is found as the arithmetic mean of a and γ. In $w = \beta$ the s-function reaches the value of 0.5.

When designing parameters of each class function we want to consider the possibility to obtain the equal lengths of these parts of L_l's supports, which assist membership values greater than or equal to 0.5. The parts are regarded as the important representatives of fuzzy sets as they possess the largest index of the relationship to the set. We thus determine the breadth of each L_l to be $\frac{E}{m}$ on the membership level equal to 0.5.

Let us first design the parameters of the membership function *"in the middle"*. The function of $L_{\frac{m+1}{2}}$ is constructed as a π-function

$$\pi(w) = \begin{cases} s(w,\alpha_1,\beta_1,\gamma_1 = \alpha_2) & \text{for} \quad w \le \gamma_1 = \alpha_2, \\ 1 - s(w,\alpha_2 = \gamma_1,\beta_2,\gamma_2) & \text{for} \quad w \ge \gamma_1 = \alpha_2. \end{cases} \tag{2}$$

We suppose that $L_{\frac{m+1}{2}}$ will be a normal fuzzy set in $\gamma_1 = \alpha_2 = \frac{E}{2}$.

In order to guarantee the breadth $\frac{E}{m}$ on the membership level 0.5, function $L_{\frac{m+1}{2}}$ should take $\beta_1 = \frac{E}{2} - \frac{E}{2m} = \frac{E(m-1)}{2m}$ and $\beta_2 = \frac{E}{2} + \frac{E}{2m} = \frac{E(m+1)}{2m}$. Since $L_{\frac{m+1}{2}}$ is expected to preserve the uniform and symmetric shape then $\alpha_1 = \frac{E}{2} - 2\frac{E}{2m} = \frac{E(m-2)}{2m}$ and $\alpha_2 = \frac{E}{2} + 2\frac{E}{2m} = \frac{E(m+2)}{2m}$. We state $L_{\frac{m+1}{2}}$'s formula as

$$\mu_{L_{\frac{m+1}{2}}}(w) = \begin{cases} 0 & \text{for } w \le \frac{E(m-2)}{2m}, \\[2ex] 2\left(\dfrac{w-\frac{E(m-2)}{2m}}{\frac{E}{m}}\right)^2 & \text{for } \frac{E(m-2)}{2m} \le w \le \frac{E(m-1)}{2m}, \\[2ex] 1-2\left(\dfrac{w-\frac{E}{2}}{\frac{E}{m}}\right)^2 & \text{for } \frac{E(m-1)}{2m} \le w \le \frac{E}{2}, \\[2ex] 1-2\left(\dfrac{w-\frac{E}{2}}{\frac{E}{m}}\right)^2 & \text{for } \frac{E}{2} \le w \le \frac{E(m+1)}{2m}, \\[2ex] 2\left(\dfrac{w-\frac{E(m+2)}{2m}}{\frac{E}{m}}\right)^2 & \text{for } \frac{E(m+1)}{2m} \le w \le \frac{E(m+2)}{2m}, \\[2ex] 0 & \text{for } w \ge \frac{E(m+2)}{2m}. \end{cases} \tag{3}$$

For the *"leftmost"* family $L_1,..., L_{\frac{m-1}{2}}$ we make suggestions that the top segments of functions lying on the membership level 1 will have the same lengths. Moreover, the last *"left"* function $L_{\frac{m-1}{2}}$ should have the intersection point with *"in the middle"* function on the membership level 0.5. Each upper segment of L_t, $t = 1,..., \frac{m-1}{2}$, will be thus equal to $\frac{\frac{E}{2}}{\frac{m-1}{2}+1} = \frac{E}{m+1}$. Particularly, $\alpha_{L_{\frac{m-1}{2}}} = \frac{E(m-1)}{2(m+1)}$ after multiplying the length of the distinct upper segment by the number of the last left function. We have already found $\beta_1 = \frac{E(m-1)}{2m}$ of the *"in the middle"* function $L_{\frac{m+1}{2}}$. Due to the previously made assumption the functions $L_{\frac{m-1}{2}}$ and $L_{\frac{m+1}{2}}$ should intersect each other in point $\left(\frac{E(m-1)}{2m}, 0.5\right)$; therefore $\beta_{L_{\frac{m-1}{2}}} = \frac{E(m-1)}{2m}$. The difference between $\alpha_{L_{\frac{m-1}{2}}}$ and $\beta_{L_{\frac{m-1}{2}}}$ is evaluated to be $\frac{E(m-1)}{2m(m+1)}$. To find a uniform slope of $L_{\frac{m-1}{2}}$ we determine $\gamma_{L_{\frac{m-1}{2}}} = \beta_{L_{\frac{m-1}{2}}} + \frac{E(m-1)}{2m(m+1)} = \frac{E(m-1)(m+2)}{2m(m+1)}$.

Since the beginning of $L_{\frac{m-1}{2}}$ is planned to be placed in $(\min(L_1), \ 1)$ then $\mu_{L_{\frac{m-1}{2}}}(w) = 1 - s\left(w, \frac{E(m-1)}{2(m+1)}, \frac{E(m-1)}{2m}, \frac{E(m-1)(m+2)}{2m(m+1)}\right)$. The membership function of $L_{\frac{m-1}{2}}$ is thus expanded as

$$\mu_{L_{\frac{m-1}{2}}}(w) = \begin{cases} 1 & \text{for } w \le \frac{E(m-1)}{2(m+1)}, \\[2ex] 1-2\left(\dfrac{w-\frac{E(m-1)}{2(m+1)}}{\frac{E(m-1)}{m(m+1)}}\right)^2 & \text{for } \frac{E(m-1)}{2(m+1)} \le w \le \frac{E(m-1)}{2m}, \\[2ex] 2\left(\dfrac{w-\frac{E(m-1)(m+2)}{2m(m+1)}}{\frac{E(m-1)}{m(m+1)}}\right)^2 & \text{for } \frac{E(m-1)}{2m} \le w \le \frac{E(m-1)(m+2)}{2m(m+1)}, \\[2ex] 0 & \text{for } w \ge \frac{E(m-1)(m+2)}{2m(m+1)}. \end{cases} \tag{4}$$

All constraints characteristic of the *"leftmost"* family of fuzzy sets will be given after inserting parameter $\delta(t) = \frac{2}{m-1} \cdot t$, $t = 1,\ldots,\frac{m-1}{2}$, in (4) to form it as (Rakus-Andersson, 2007)

$$\mu_{L_t}(w) = \begin{cases} 1 & \text{for} \quad w \leq \frac{E(m-1)}{2(m+1)}\delta(t), \\[2ex] 1 - 2\left(\dfrac{w - \frac{E(m-1)}{2(m+1)}\delta(t)}{\frac{E(m-1)}{m(m+1)}\delta(t)}\right)^2 & \text{for} \quad \frac{E(m-1)}{2(m+1)}\delta(t) \leq w \leq \frac{E(m-1)}{2m}\delta(t), \\[2ex] 2\left(\dfrac{w - \frac{E(m-1)(m+2)}{2m(m+1)}\delta(t)}{\frac{E(m-1)}{m(m+1)}\delta(t)}\right)^2 & \text{for} \quad \frac{E(m-1)}{2m}\delta(t) \leq w \leq \frac{E(m-1)(m+2)}{2m(m+1)}\delta(t), \\[2ex] 0 & \text{for} \quad w \geq \frac{E(m-1)(m+2)}{2m(m+1)}\delta(t). \end{cases} \tag{5}$$

Parameter $\delta(t)$ takes the value of 1 for $t = \frac{m-1}{2}$, which means that $\delta(\frac{m-1}{2})$ in (5) has no influence on the shape of the last left function. However, the introduction of $\delta(t)$ in (5) induces the narrowing effects in the supports of the other left function shapes. To preserve the same lengths of upper segments corresponding to membership 1 and middle segments attached to membership 0.5 we adjust $\delta(t)$, assisting the left function L_t, to be equal to $\frac{1}{\frac{m-1}{2}}$ multiplied by the function number t.

In order to start the implementation of the *"rightmost"* family functions let us note that the first right function $\mu_{L_{\frac{m+3}{2}}}(w)$ should possess $\mu_{L_{\frac{m-1}{2}}}(w)$'s inverted shape. We generate the membership function of $L_{\frac{m+3}{2}}$ by

$$\mu_{L_{\frac{m+3}{2}}}(w) = \begin{cases} 0 & \text{for} \quad w \leq E - \frac{E(m-1)(m+2)}{2m(m+1)}, \\[2ex] 2\left(\dfrac{w - \left(E - \frac{E(m-1)(m+2)}{2m(m+1)}\right)}{\frac{E(m-1)}{m(m+1)}}\right)^2 & \text{for} \quad E - \frac{E(m-1)(m+2)}{2m(m+1)} \leq w \leq E - \frac{E(m-1)}{2m}, \\[2ex] 1 - 2\left(\dfrac{w - \left(E - \frac{E(m-1)}{2(m+1)}\right)}{\frac{E(m-1)}{m(m+1)}}\right)^2 & \text{for} \quad E - \frac{E(m-1)}{2m} \leq w \leq E - \frac{E(m-1)}{2(m+1)}, \\[2ex] 1 & \text{for} \quad w \geq E - \frac{E(m-1)}{2(m+1)}. \end{cases} \tag{6}$$

The function of $L_{\frac{m+3}{2}}$ is symmetrically inverted to the function of $L_{\frac{m-1}{2}}$ over interval $[\min(L_1),$ $\max(L_m)]$.

Hence, the membership function $\mu_{L_{\frac{m-1}{2}}}(w) = 1 - s\left(w, \frac{E(m-1)}{2(m+1)}, \frac{E(m-1)}{2m}, \frac{E(m-1)(m+2)}{2m(m+1)}\right)$ will be changed into $\mu_{L_{\frac{m+3}{2}}}(w) = s\left(w, E - \frac{E(m-1)(m+2)}{2m(m+1)}, E - \frac{E(m-1)}{2m}, E - \frac{E(m-1)}{2(m+1)}\right)$.

To generate the *"rightmost"* family of sets $L_{\frac{m+3}{2}},\ldots,L_m$ we need to create a new parameter $\varepsilon(t) = 1 - \frac{2}{m-1}(t-1)$, $t = 1,\ldots,\frac{m-1}{2}$, which will be inserted in (6). The construction of $\varepsilon(t)$, when comparing to the creation of $\delta(t)$, is authorized by the fact that $t = 1$ should be followed by $\varepsilon(1) = 1$, whereas $t = \frac{m-1}{2}$ is helped by $\varepsilon(\frac{m-1}{2}) = \frac{2}{m-1}$. Formula (7) constitutes a common base for deriving membership functions

$$\mu_{L_{\frac{m+3}{2}+t-1}}(w) =$$

$$\begin{cases} 0 & \text{for} \quad w \le E - \frac{E(m-1)(m+2)}{2m(m+1)}\varepsilon(t), \\[2ex] 2\left(\dfrac{w-\left(E-\frac{E(m-1)(m+2)}{2m(m+1)}\varepsilon(t)\right)}{\frac{E(m-1)}{m(m+1)}\varepsilon(t)}\right)^2 & \text{for} \quad E - \frac{E(m-1)(m+2)}{2m(m+1)}\varepsilon(t) \le w \le E - \frac{E(m-1)}{2m}\varepsilon(t), \\[2ex] 1-2\left(\dfrac{w-\left(E-\frac{E(m-1)}{2(m+1)}\varepsilon(t)\right)}{\frac{E(m-1)}{m(m+1)}\varepsilon(t)}\right)^2 & \text{for} \quad E - \frac{E(m-1)}{2m}\varepsilon(t) \le w \le E - \frac{E(m-1)}{2(m+1)}\varepsilon(t), \\[2ex] 1 & \text{for} \quad w \ge E - \frac{E(m-1)}{2(m+1)}\varepsilon(t). \end{cases} \qquad (7)$$

The functions of fuzzy sets $L_1,...,L_m$ intend to maintain the same distances on the membership level 0.5. This property allows assigning to $L_1,...,L_m$ the relevant parts of their supports possessing the same length. The relevant parts of fuzzy sets consist of the sets' elements that reveal the membership degree values greater than or equal to 0.5. When forming the supports of the same length, in turn, we warrant the partition of $[\min(L_1),\max(L_m)]$ in equal subintervals standing for L_l levels, $l = 1,...,m$. Apart from that, the "*leftmost*" and "*rightmost*" functions also keep the same distances on the membership level 1. This feature provides us with a harmonious arrangement of function shapes.

All steps of the discussed algorithm, which initiates three sets of membership functions corresponding to a list of terms, can be sampled in the block scheme. We need to follow the steps of the scheme together with formulas (3), (5) and (7) to write the excerpt of a computer program. We emphasize that the only data, used in the algorithm, are the length of the reference set and the number of functions. We do not need to specify the sets' borders in the process of the program initialization, as most of programmers do, since the borders are computed automatically by formulas (3), (5) and (7). The steps of the algorithm flow chart are sampled in Fig. 1.

The procedure discussed above has started introduction of membership functions typical of levels of X, Y and Z which, in turn, represent *age*, *CRP* and *body weight*.

For five levels of $X = [0, 100]$, $L = X$, $w = x$, $m = 5$, $E = 100$, the leftmost family is revealed by

$$\mu_{X_t}(x) = \begin{cases} 1 & \text{for} \quad x \le 33.33(0.5t), \\[1.5ex] 1-2\left(\frac{x-33.33(0.5t)}{13.33(0.5t)}\right)^2 & \text{for} \quad 33.33(0.5t) \le x \le 40(0.5t), \\[1.5ex] 2\left(\frac{x-46.66(0.5t)}{13.33(0.5t)}\right)^2 & \text{for} \quad 40(0.5t) \le x \le 46.66(0.5t), \\[1.5ex] 0 & \text{for} \quad x \ge 46.66(0.5t), \end{cases} \qquad (8)$$

for $t = 1, 2$ due to (5).

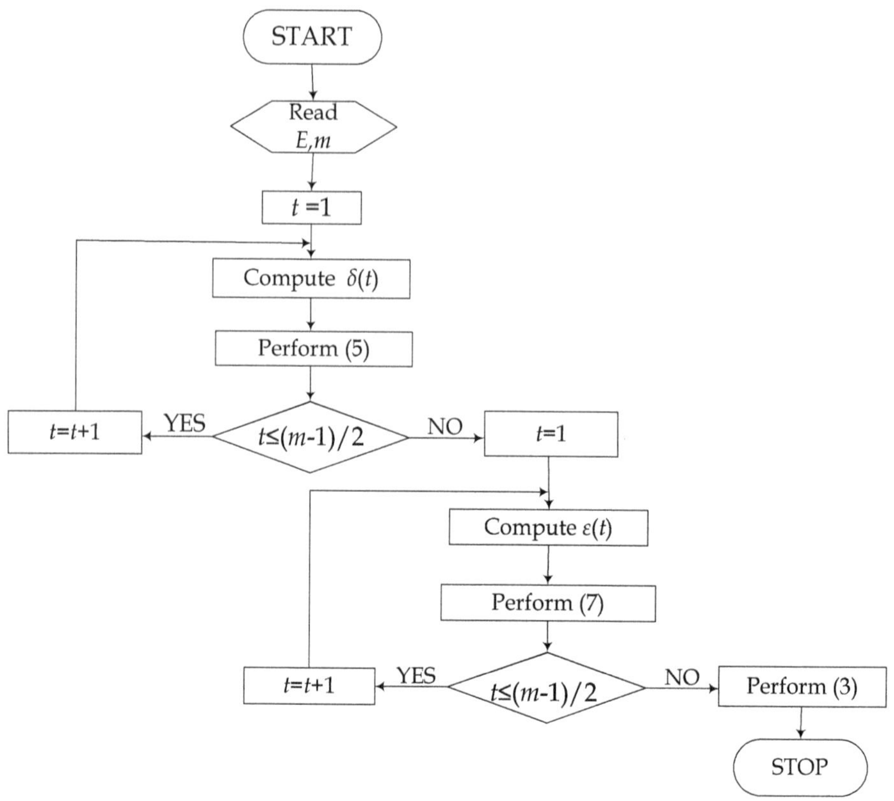

Fig. 1. The flow chart of the $L_1,\ldots,L_m$ implementation

The rightmost family of X-levels, composed with conformity with (7), is stated as

$$\mu_{X_{4+t-1}}(x) = \begin{cases} 0 \text{ for } x \leq 100 - 46.66(1 - 0.5(t-1)), \\[2mm] 2\left(\dfrac{x-(100-46.66(1-0.5(t-1)))}{13.33(1-0.5(t-1))}\right)^2 \\ \text{for } 100 - 46.66(1-0.5(t-1)) \leq x \leq 100 - 40(1-0.5(t-1)), \\[2mm] 1 - 2\left(\dfrac{x-(100-33.33(1-0.5(t-1)))}{13.33(1-0.5(t-1))}\right)^2 \\ \text{for } 100 - 40(1-0.5(t-1)) \leq x \leq 100 - 33.33(1-0.5(t-1)), \\[2mm] 1 \text{ for } x \geq 100 - 33.33(1-0.5(t-1)), \end{cases} \tag{9}$$

for t = 1, 2.

The "*in the middle*" X-level "*middle-aged*" has, in accord with (3), the constraint

$$
\mu_{X_3}(x) = \begin{cases}
0 & \text{for} \quad x \le 30, \\
2\left(\frac{x-30}{20}\right)^2 & \text{for} \quad 30 \le x \le 40, \\
1 - 2\left(\frac{x-50}{20}\right)^2 & \text{for} \quad 40 \le x \le 50, \\
1 - 2\left(\frac{x-50}{20}\right)^2 & \text{for} \quad 50 \le x \le 60, \\
2\left(\frac{x-70}{20}\right)^2 & \text{for} \quad 60 \le x \le 70, \\
0 & \text{for} \quad x \ge 70.
\end{cases}
\tag{10}
$$

All levels of X are sketched in Fig. 2.

The parts of X_1–X_5 supports should be consisted of elements, which have the strongest connections with the X_1–X_5 fuzzy sets. Therefore we only select the elements having the membership degrees greater than or equal to 0.5.

To make the partition of X in subintervals representing levels X_1–X_5 we return to formulas (8), (9) and (10). Due to (8), to find the subinterval of X assisting X_1 when $t = 1$, we concatenate the intervals $x \le 33.33(0.5 \cdot 1)$ and $33.33(0.5 \cdot 1) \le x \le 40(0.5 \cdot 1)$, leading to [0, 20]. We have chosen these intervals, which contain elements of X_1 furnished with membership degrees greater than or equal to 0.5. For $t = 2$, set in two first intervals of (8), we aggregate $x \le 33.33(0.5 \cdot 2)$ and $33.33(0.5 \cdot 2) \le x \le 40(0.5 \cdot 2)$ in [0, 40]. This generates the interval [0, 40]–[0, 20] = [20, 40] typical of X_2. By (10) we find [40, 60] = [40, 50] + [50, 60] as an essential part of X_3. The insertion of $t = 2$ in (9) produces a joint of

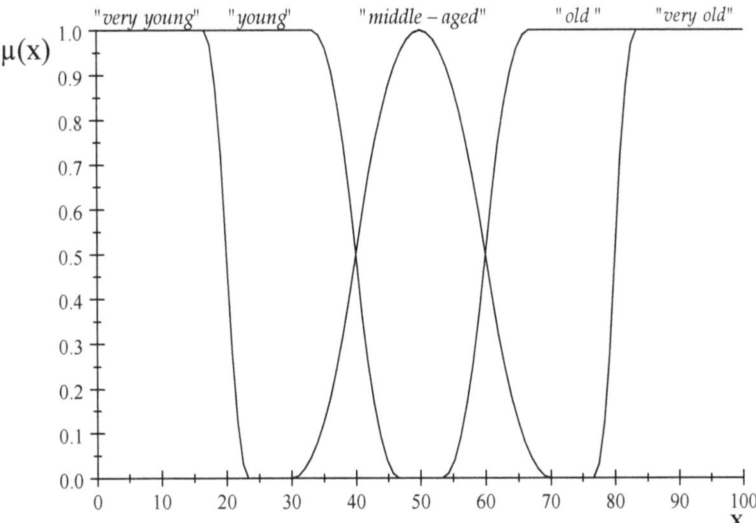

Fig. 2. The fuzzy sets X_1–X_5

$100 - 40(1 - 0.5(2 - 1)) \le x \le 100 - 33.33(1 - 0.5(2 - 1))$ and $x \ge 100 - 33.33(1 - 0.5(2 - 1))$ to be a common interval [80, 100] regarded as the domain of X_5. By setting $t = 1$ in the last intervals of (9) we get the field [60, 100]. It means that X_4 will be given by [60, 80] = [60, 100]–[80, 100]. We are furnished with the same intervals after accomplishing the close analysis of Fig. 2 on the membership level 0.5.

Let us now initiate the associations among the terms of X, characteristic intervals of these terms and assigned to them codes due to the scheme

name of X-level	representative interval	code
X_1	0–20	0
X_2	20–40	1
X_3	40–60	2
X_4	60–80	3
X_5	80–100	4

We emphasize the role of an elegant mathematical design of X's membership functions, which allows making the partition of the X-domain in equal intervals. Definitely, we obtain the same results when dividing the length of X by the number of levels to get a length of one part but the effects computed by means of membership functions only confirm this intuitive calculation. Moreover we can modify the arbitrary lengths of X-subintervals by making changes in the formulas of $\delta(t)$ and $\varepsilon(t)$.

By applying the same technique to $Y = [0, 60]$, $L = Y$, $w = y$, $m = 5$, $E = 60$ we generate the code pattern

name of Y-level	representative interval	code
Y_1	0–12	0
Y_2	12–24	1
Y_3	24–36	2
Y_4	36–48	3
Y_5	48–60	4

Lastly, if $Z = [40, 120]$ for men, $L = Z$, $w = z$, $m = 5$, $E = 80$ then

name of Y-level	representative interval	code
Z_1	40–56	0
Z_2	56–72	1
Z_3	72–88	2
Z_4	88–104	3
Z_5	104–120	4

If we collect clinical data, concerning a patient examined then we will be now capable to create code vectors taking place in the discrimination NS algorithm.

Example 1

An eighty one-year-old man, whose CRP is 17 and weight is 91, will be given by the vector $v = (4, 1, 3)$.

In order to measure the affinity (coverage) of two code vectors v_1 and v_2 of the same length over the same alphabet we are furnished with the r-contiguous bit matching rule, which provides us with a true match(v_1, v_2) if v_1 and v_2 agree in r contiguous locations.

Example 2

For $v_1 = (3, 1, 3)$ and $v_2 = (3, 1, 2)$, when $r = 2$, match(v_1, v_2) is true.

4. The selection of the most representative data vectors for the decision "operate"

We have already mentioned that we need the "operate" types of patient data vectors as the entries of the NS discrimination algorithm. We thus want to prepare typical data strings for the decision "operate" in advance.

Let us first treat the vector $v = (x, y, z)$ as the string of integers $v = (x\ y\ z)$, where x, y and z can take the code values 0, 1, 2, 3, 4. We form the function $f(x\ y\ z) = x + y + z$ to measure the common code value of the data vector. To make the selection of "operate" type vectors even more accurate let us assign the weights of power-importance to the biological indices considered in the operation decision. In the gastric cancer operation decision we first concentrate our attention on the changes of CRP- values, which points out CRP as the most decisive factor. The analysis of CRP is followed by the judgment of age and, finally, we check the values of body weights. Hence, we state the ranking of the symptom importance as $CRP \succ age \succ body\ weight$, provided that $\succ$ means "more important than".

A procedure for obtaining a ratio scale of importance for a group of m elements (in the considered case – biological markers) was developed by Saaty (Saaty, 1978). Assume that we have m objects (symptoms) and we want to construct a scale, rating these objects as to their importance with respect to the decision. We ask a decision-maker to compare the objects in paired comparison. If we compare object j with object k, $j, k = 1,...,m$, then we will assign the values b_{jk} and b_{kj} as follows

1. $b_{kj} = \dfrac{1}{b_{jk}}$.

2. If objective j is more important than objective k then b_{jk} gets assigned a number according to the following scheme:

Intensity of importance expressed by the value of b_{jk}	*Definition*
1	Equal importance of x_j and x_k
3	Weak importance of x_j over x_k
5	Strong importance of x_j over x_k
7	Demonstrated importance of x_j over x_k
9	Absolute importance of x_j over x_k
2, 4, 6, 8	Intermediate values

If object k is more important than object j, we assign the value of b_{kj}.

Having obtained the above judgments an $m \times m$ importance matrix $B = \left(b_{jk}\right)_{j,k=1}^{m}$ is constructed. The importance weights are decided as components of this eigenvector that corresponds to the largest in magnitude eigenvalue of the matrix B.

Example 3

For priorities $Y = CRP \succ X = age \succ Z = body\ weight$ we determine the contents of B as

$$B = \begin{array}{c} \\ X \\ Y \\ Z \end{array} \begin{array}{ccc} X & Y & Z \\ \left[\begin{array}{ccc} 1 & \frac{1}{3} & 3 \\ 3 & 1 & 5 \\ \frac{1}{3} & \frac{1}{5} & 1 \end{array}\right] \end{array}$$

The largest eigenvalue ($\lambda = 3.033$) of B has the associated eigenvector $V = (0.37, 0.92, 0.15)$. V is composed of coordinates that are interpreted as the importance weights w_1, w_2, w_3 sought for X, Y, Z.

Let us rearrange the form of function f by adding the weights of importance to the vector code values. The new pattern of f is designed as $f(x\ y\ z) = w_1x + w_2y + w_3z$. The function value yields the patient's characteristics given by a combination of codes stated for different symptoms.

Example 4

The patient vector $v = (3, 1, 2)$ has the characteristics $f(3\,1\,2) = 0.37 \cdot 3 + 0.92 \cdot 1 + 0.15 \cdot 2 = 2.33$.

Due to the physician's expertise we assume that we can operate patients who are characterized by codes of age equal to 1, 2 and 3, codes of CRP recognized as 0, 1 and 2 and codes of body weight determined as 1, 2 and 3. The minimal patient characteristics to be operated is thus $f(1\,0\,1) = 0.37 \cdot 1 + 0.92 \cdot 0 + 0.15 \cdot 1 = 0.52$, whereas the maximal data characteristics, classifying the patient for the operation is given by $f(3\,2\,3) = 0.37 \cdot 3 + 0.92 \cdot 2 + 0.15 \cdot 3 = 3.4$. We conclude that the patient who is capable to be operated should have the characteristics $f(x\ y\ z)$ included in the interval [0.52, 3.4]. It is worth emphasizing that the decisions are made with respect to the decisive power of biological markers *age*, CRP and *body weight*.

Example 5

We test $v = (4, 2, 4)$. As $f(4\,2\,4) = 0.37 \cdot 4 + 0.92 \cdot 2 + 0.15 \cdot 4 = 3.92$, which lies beyond the boundaries of the "operate" interval, then the patient with data $v = (4, 2, 4)$ should not be operated. For vectors $v_1 = (3, 2, 2)$, $v_2 = (2, 0, 2)$, $v_3 = (3, 1, 3)$, $v_4 = (3, 1, 2)$ the decision will be made as "operate".

The flow chart, sketched in Fig. 3, will show the selection of vectors typical of the decision "operate".

The vectors v_1, v_2, v_3 and v_4 will be included in the experimental population of representative data strings for the positive decision of the operation. We intend to use them in the next part of the chapter, when discussing the action of the NS algorithm adapted to the operation model.

5. The negative selection algorithm

After coding the patient data and selecting the initial data, which are given into account for the decision "operate", we can make a choice between two alternatives concerning the cure

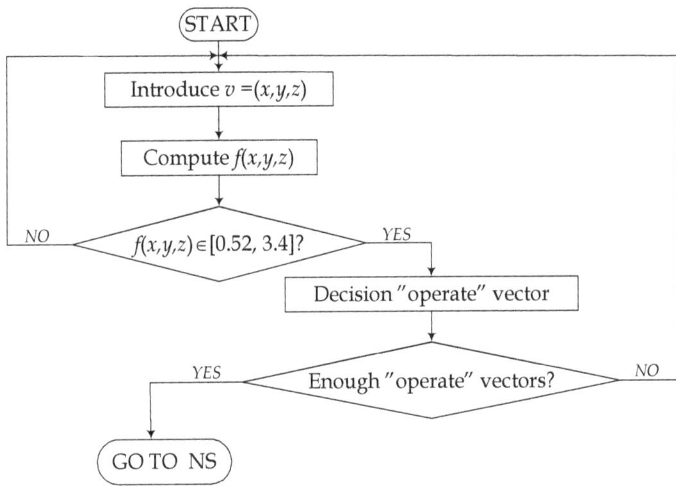

Fig. 3. The flow chart of the selection of "operate" type vectors

of gastric cancer patients. We intend to adapt the technique of an immunological algorithm based on the T cell behaviour. We use the negative selection algorithm NS proposed by Forrest (Forrest et al., 1997).

The goal of NS is to cover the non-self space with a set of detectors. For the sake of the surgery aim, already outlined in Section 2, the algorithm should lead to discrimination of the statements "operate" and "do not operate" provided that vectors characteristic of type "operate" are available. This assumption is motivated by the surgeon's intention to cure the patient from his/her cancer disease by making surgery if the patient's state allows accomplishing it. The patient data reports, which register his/her parameters in the case of operating, are clearly interpretable. However, the physician can have some doubts when he denies an operation for the patient. Therefore we have used the strings confirming the "operate" decision as the more convincing vectors in the entrance of NS.

We distinguish two steps in the surgery NS algorithm prepared on the basis of the general NS (Dasgupta & Nino, 2008; Engelbrecht, 2007; Forrest et al., 1997):

1. Generation of detectors, which should possess the property vectors corresponding to the decision "do not operate" on a patient. These strings are not recognized as obviously as the strings of "operate"; that is why we get some help from the algorithm in generating their patterns.
2. Selection of the surgery settlements "operate" or "do not operate" for any patient data vector due to the matching criterion concerning detectors.

In the first step a set of detectors is generated. To accomplish this task we use as an input a collection of vectors found by the method of preparing "operate" strings, which have been discussed in Section 4. Candidate detectors that match any of the "operate" type vector samples are eliminated whereas unmatched ones are kept. We adopt the *r*-contiguous bit matching rule for the patient data vectors as a measure of "the distance" between the "operate" type and the "do not operate" decision.

In the second step of NS the stored detectors, generated in the first stage, are used to check whether new incoming samples of patient data vectors correspond to the "operate" type or to the "do not operate" type. If an input sample, characterizing a patient, matches any detector then the patient should not be operated. When we cannot find a match between detectors and the incoming patient data vector it will mean that the decision about the surgery should be made. Figure 4 collects all steps of the surgery NS algorithm in the flow chart.

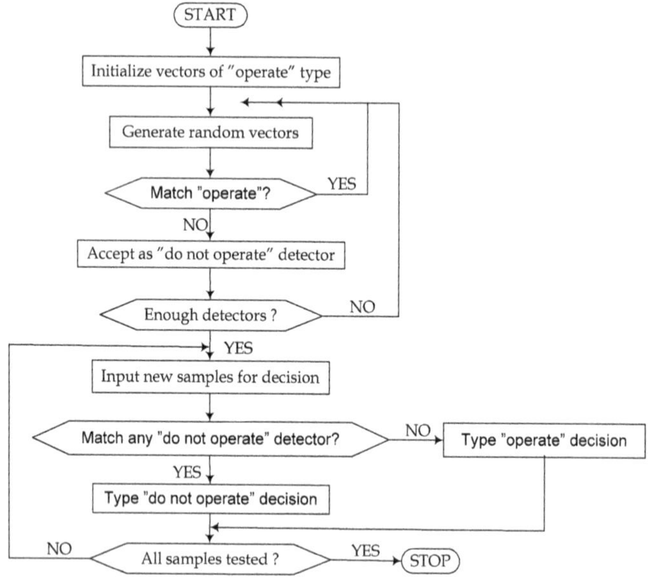

Fig. 4. The flow chart of the surgery NS algorithm

6. The surgery decision based on the NS algorithm

We wish now to follow the steps of the surgery NS algorithm to study its action in practical decision cases concerning the operation decision.

Let us thus go through the following example.

Step 1. *Initialization*

As the input data we introduce the set $V = \{v_1, v_2, v_3, v_4\}$, which consists of four patient data vectors characteristic of the "operate" type. The length of each vector is decided to be three in conformity with previously made suggestions. In Section 4 we have already initialized

$v_1 = (3, 2, 2),$
$v_2 = (2, 0, 2),$

$v_3 = (3, 1, 3)$,
$v_4 = (3, 1, 2)$.

The vectors emerge the clinical data concerning elderly patients whose the *CRP-* values are not very high. The patients' weights are not radically deviated from normal standards either. Hence, they have been operated in conformity with the surgeon's determination.

We now wish to generate the set D of four detectors d_1, d_2, d_3, d_4 that should not match any of $v_j, j = 1,...,4$. At the beginning of the procedure D is an empty set.

To measure the match grade between v_j and candidates to be detectors we state, e.g., $r = 2$ in the r-contiguous bit matching rule.

Step 2. *Introduction of random candidates to act as detectors*

We present $d = (3, 1, 1)$ and check matches between d and each $v_j, j = 1,...,4$, as

match((3, 2, 2), (3, 1, 1)) is false,
match((2, 0, 2), (3, 1, 1)) is false,
match((3, 1, 3), (3, 1, 1)) is true,
match((3, 1, 2), (3, 1, 1)) is true.

Since d matches v_3 and v_4 then it cannot be classified as a detector.

We prove the next candidate $d = (4, 3, 1)$ to make matches between d and each $v_j, j = 1,...,4$, in the form of

match((3, 2, 2), (4, 3, 1)) is false,
match((2, 0, 2), (4, 3, 1)) is false,
match((3, 1, 3), (4, 3, 1)) is false,
match((3, 1, 2), (4, 3, 1)) is false.

All matches are false, which means that $d_1 = d$ is the first detector placed in D. The set of detectors now contains one element $d_1 = (4, 3, 1)$. We repeat the procedure until we determine four detectors in set D. D is finally formed as

$D = \{(4, 3, 1), (2, 3, 4), (4, 4, 1), (3, 4, 0)\}$.

Step 3. *Operation decision making*

In the second phase of the algorithm we test data strings to organize them in either the "operate" type or in the "do not operate" type decisions. If the data vector matches any detector from D then the decision is made as "do not operate" (the non-self region). Otherwise, for all false matches between the data vector and $d_k, k = 1,...,4$, we accept the operation (the self region).

We introduce $v = (3, 2, 3)$. The matches to detectors are determined as

match((4, 3, 1), (3, 2, 3)) is false,
match((2, 3, 4), (3, 2, 3)) is false,
match((4, 4, 1), (3, 2, 3)) is false,
match((3, 4, 0), (3, 2, 3)) is false.

As all matches to detectors are false we conclude the performance of surgery (decision "operate").

Another test vector $v = (3, 4, 1)$ is inserted into the checking system. The match results are shown as

match((4, 3, 1), (3, 4, 1)) is false,
match((2, 3, 4), (3, 4, 1)) is false,
match((4, 4, 1), (3, 4, 1)) is true,
match((3, 4, 0), (3, 4, 1)) is true.

Vector v converges to two detectors, which means the decision to be referred to "do not operate".

By setting $r = 2$ in the contiguous bit matching rule we have preserved a margin of imprecision in decision making, since we do not demand all contiguous vector codes to be equal. This gives a certain chance of operating for the patients whose mix of biological indices cannot be precisely judged. For $r = 3$ the decision will be quite strict.

The method of making medical decisions by means of immunological systems is an applicable novelty. The example has a more didactic and experimental meaning than a real medical investigation. If we really want to use the method for making decisions in the surgery discipline we should, at first, extend the length of data strings by introducing more biological markers. A very dense set of initial vectors from "self" ("operate") ought to be chosen by the algorithm belonging to Section 4. Nevertheless, the proposal of combining fuzzy systems and weighted characteristics of vectors with the NS algorithm to create the hybrid can start a new applied domain in medicine.

7. Conclusion

In the process of creation of a new medical application model we have inserted some elements of fuzzy systems into the negative selection immunological algorithm. This hybrid, attached to two disciplines of Computational Intelligence, has found a practical application in surgery decision making. As self and non-self constitute two regions of the NS partition of objects then we could identify these regions with decisions "operate" against "do not operate" in the case of curing gastric cancer patients. The action of the modified NS could help us to determine the surgery or its lack for individual patients with respect to their clinical data entry vectors.

To make the action of the NS algorithm more efficient we have complemented the method by preparing the population of the most representative vectors standing for the "operate" type. The vectors have been converted to real values giving the common characteristics of a patient. In that characteristics the weights of importance, assigned to biological markers, will play the essential role in the final judgment of the vectors' influence on the decision "operate".

We wish to add that the excerpts from fuzzy systems, involved in NS, come from own research, which has been concentrated on the creation of compact parametric formulas. These formulas concern the generation of a family of membership functions without predetermining their borders in advance.

All parts of the methodology have been prepared in the form of numerical algorithms given by flow charts. This allows composing a common computer program to test large samples of vectors in a real clinical application.

We emphasize that the proposal is a novel contribution in medical applications and should be still tested on larger samples of data. We can expect that, in future investigations, an introduction of the neural artificial perceptron model instead of the NS algorithm will provide us with similar results concerning surgery decisions. As an extension of the model we also wish to adapt the real-value negative selection algorithm in order to insert measured values of biological markers in data vectors instead of codes. This procedure should improve the reliability of a decision. Having results from more models we can select the most efficient one to work on its further development.

8. Acknowledgment

The author thanks the Blekinge Research Board in Sweden for the grant funding the current research. The author is also grateful to Associate Professor Henrik Forssell for supporting these investigations with medical advice and data.

9. References

Antunes, M. & Correia, M.E. (2011). Tunable Immune Detectors for Behavior-Based Network Intrusion Detection, *Artificial Immune Systems: 10th International Conference, ICARIS 2011*, Cambridge, UK, pp. 334–347, LNCS, vol. 6825, Springer, ISBN 978-3-642-22370-9

De Castro, L.N. & Timmis, J. (2002). *Artificial Immune Systems*, Springer, ISBN 978-1-85233-594-6, Berlin Heidelberg

Cohen, I.R. (2006). Immune System Computation and the Immunological Homunculus, LNCS, vol. 4199, pp. 49–52, ISBN 978-3-540-45772-5

Dasgupta, D. & Nino, F. (2008). *Immunological Computation: Theory and Applications*, Auerbach Publishers Inc., ISBN 978-1-420-06545-9, London

Do-Kyong Kim, Sung Yong Oh, Hyuk-Chan Kwon, Suee Lee, Kyung A Kwon, Byung Geun Kim, Seong-Geun Kim, Sung-Hyun Kim, Jin Seok Jang, Min Chan Kim, Kyeong Hee Kim, Jin-Yeong Han & Hyo-Jin Kim (2009). Clinical Significances of Preoperative Serum Interleukin-6 and C-reactive Protein Level in Operable Gastric Cancer, *BMC Cancer* 9, pp. 155–156, ISSN 1471-2407

Engelbrecht, A.P. (2007). *Computational Intelligence*, Wiley & Sons Ltd., ISBN 978-0-470-03561-0, Chichester

Forrest, S., Hofmeyr, A.S. & Somayaji, A. (1997). Computer Immunology, *Communications of the ACM*, vol. 40, nr 10, pp. 88–96, ISSN 1017-4656

Gao, X.Z., Ovaska, S.I., Wang, X. & Chow, M.Y. (2008). A Neural Networks-based Negative Selection Algorithm in Fault Diagnosis, *Neural Computing & Applications*, vol. 17, nr 1, pp. 91–98, ISSN 1433-3058

Harmer, P.K., Williams, P.D., Gunsch, G.H. & Lamont, G.B. (2002). An Artificial Immune System Architecture for Computer Security Applications, *IEEE Transactions on Evolutionary Computation*, vol. 6, nr 3, pp. 252–280, ISSN 1089-778X

Igawa, K. & Ohashi, H. (2009). A Negative Selection Algorithm for Classification and Reduction of the Noise Effect, *Journal of Applied Soft Computing*, vol. 9, nr 1, pp. 431–438, ISSN 1568-4946

Ishida, Y. (2004). *Immunity-Based Systems: A Design Perspective*, Springer, ISBN 3-540-00896-9, Berlin Heidelberg New York de Mello, J., Struthers, L., Turner, R., Cooper, E.H. & Giles, G.R. (1983). Multivariate Analyses as Aids to Diagnosis and Assessment of Prognosis in Gastrointestinal Cancer, *Br. J. Cancer*, nr 48, pp. 341–348, ISSN 0007-0920

Rakus-Andersson, E. (2007). *Fuzzy and Rough Techniques in Medical Diagnosis and Medication*, Springer, ISBN 978-3-540-49707-3, Berlin Heidelberg

Rakus-Andersson, E. & Jain, L. (2009). Computational Intelligence in Medical Decisions Making, *Recent Advances in Decision Making*, Springer, Berlin Heidelberg, pp. 145–159, ISBN 978-3-642-02186-2

Rakus-Andersson, E. (2009). Approximate Reasoning in Surgical Decisions, *Proceedings of the International Fuzzy Systems Association World Congress – IFSA 2009*, Instituto Superior Technico, pp. 225–230, ISBN 978-989-95079-6-8

Rakus-Andersson, E. (2010a). One-dimensional Model of Approximate Reasoning in Surgical Considerations, *Developments in Fuzzy Sets, Intuitionistic Fuzzy Sets, Generalized Nets and Related Topics*, vol. II, System Research Institute of Polish Academy of Sciences, pp. 233–246, ISBN 139788389475305

Rakus-Andersson, E. (2010b). Adjusted s-parametric Functions in the Creation of Symmetric Constraints, *Proceedings of the 10th International Conference on Intelligent Systems Design and Applications - ISDA 2010*, Cairo, Egypt, pp. 451–456, ISBN 978-1-4244-8135-4

Rakus-Andersson, E. (2011). Hybridization of Immunological Computation and Fuzzy Systems in Surgery Decision Making, *Proceedings of the 15th Conference on Knowledge Expert Systems – KES 2011*, Kaiserslauntern, Germany, LNCS/LNAI, vol. 6884, Springer, Berlin Heidelberg, pp. 399–408, ISBN 978-3-642-23865-9

Rutkowski, L. (2008). *Computational Intelligence: Methods and Techniques*, ISBN 978-3-540-76287-4, Springer, Berlin Heidelberg

Saaty, T.L. (1978). Exploring the Interface between Hierarchies, Multiplied Objectives and Fuzzy Sets, *Fuzzy Sets and Systems* 1, pp. 57–58, ISSN 0165-0114

Wakizono, M., Hatanaka, T. & Uosaki, K. (2006). Time Varying System Identification with Immune Based Evolutionary Computation, *Proceedings of SICE-ICASE, 2006*, Busan, Korea, pp. 5608–5613, ISBN 89-950038-4-7

Zhang, Q. & Zhao, H. (2010). The Research of Generation Algorithm of Detectors in a New Negative Selection Algorithm, *Proceedings of the International Conference on Technology Management and Innovation 2010*, paper 78, ISBN 13-978-0-791-85961-2

Printed in the USA
CPSIA information can be obtained
at www.ICGtesting.com
LVHW071546220224
772595LV00006B/60